Tools for Learning

Tools for Learning is an on-line review area that provides a variety of activities designed to help students study for their class. Students will find chapter outlines, review questions (written by the author), flashcards, figure labeling exercises, and links to a variety of tutorials and other useful learning tools to help students master the basic science material.

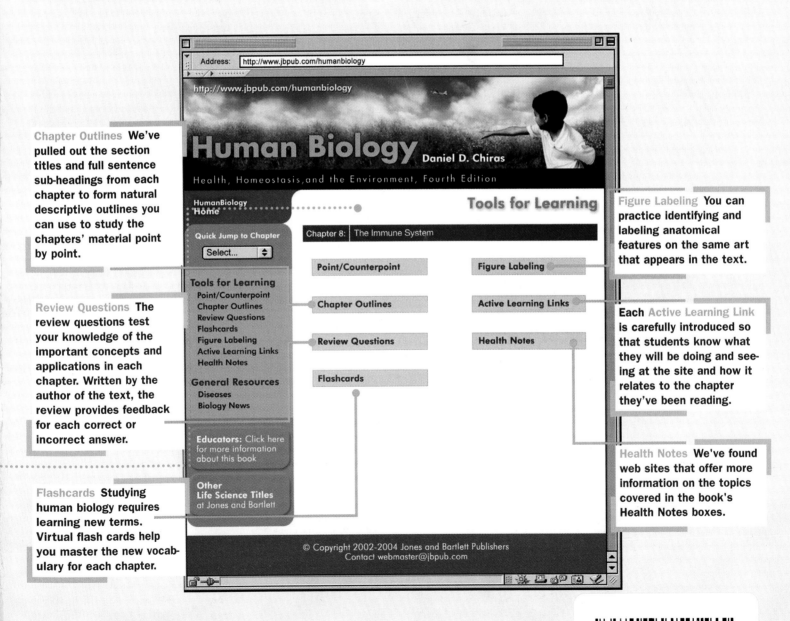

Chapter Outlines We've pulled out the section titles and full sentence sub-headings from each chapter to form natural descriptive outlines you can use to study the chapters' material point by point.

Review Questions The review questions test your knowledge of the important concepts and applications in each chapter. Written by the author of the text, the review provides feedback for each correct or incorrect answer.

Flashcards Studying human biology requires learning new terms. Virtual flash cards help you master the new vocabulary for each chapter.

Figure Labeling You can practice identifying and labeling anatomical features on the same art that appears in the text.

Each Active Learning Link is carefully introduced so that students know what they will be doing and seeing at the site and how it relates to the chapter they've been reading.

Health Notes We've found web sites that offer more information on the topics covered in the book's Health Notes boxes.

To find out more about HumanBiology, please e-mail info@jbpub.com, or call your Jones and Bartlett sales representative at 800-832-0034.

D1372026

Daniel D. Chiras

UNIVERSITY OF DENVER

Human Biology

Health, Homeostasis, and the Environment

FOURTH EDITION

JONES AND BARTLETT PUBLISHERS

Sudbury, Massachusetts

BOSTON   TORONTO   LONDON   SINGAPORE

World Headquarters
Jones and Bartlett Publishers
40 Tall Pine Drive
Sudbury, MA 01776
978-443-5000
info@jbpub.com
www.jbpub.com

Jones and Bartlett Publishers Canada
2406 Nikanna Road
Mississauga, ON L5C 2W6
CANADA

Jones and Bartlett Publishers International
Barb House, Barb Mews
London W6 7PA
UK

JONES AND BARTLETT'S COMMITMENT TO THE ENVIRONMENT

As a book publisher, Jones and Bartlett is committed to reducing its impact on the environment. This and many other Jones and Bartlett titles are printed using recycled post-consumer paper. We purchase our paper from manufacturers committed to sustainable, environmentally sensitive processes. We employ the Internet and office computer network technology in our effort toward sustainable solutions. New communication technology provides opportunities to reduce our use of paper and other resources through online delivery of instructors' materials and educational information—and of course, we recycle in the office.

Production Credits
Chief Executive Officer: Clayton Jones
Chief Operating Officer: Don W. Jones, Jr.
Executive Vice President, Publisher: Robert Holland
V.P., Design and Production: Anne Spencer
V.P., Manufacturing and Inventory Control: Therese Bräuer
Editor in Chief–College: J. Michael Stranz
Senior Developmental Editor: Dean DeChambeau
Associate Editor: Christine Whitney
Senior Production Editor: Lianne Ames
Text Design: Anne Spencer
Editorial Production Service: Kathy Smith
Typesetting: Graphic World
Cover and Frontispiece Design: Kristin Ohlin
Cover Photo: ©Tony Stone/Joe McBride
Printing and Binding: Courier Kendallville
Cover Printing: Courier Kendallville

Library of Congress Cataloging-in-Publication Data
Chiras, Daniel D.
    Human biology : health, homeostasis, and the environment / Daniel D. Chiras.—4th ed.
        p.cm.
    Includes index.
    ISBN 0-7637-1880-7 (pbk.)
     1 Human biology. I. Title

    QP36 .C46 2002
    612—dc21
         2001046289

Printed in the United States of America
05 04 03 02 01   10 9 8 7 6 5 4 3 2 1

 Printed on recycled paper

This book is dedicated to my family: my mother and father, for their love and support; my sons, Skyler and Forrest, for their joyous laughter and bright smiles; and Linda, for her patience, kindness, and unwavering love.

About the Author

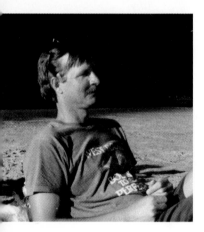

D R. CHIRAS received his Ph.D. in reproductive physiology from the University of Kansas Medical School in 1976. In September 1976, Dr. Chiras joined the Biology Department at the University of Colorado in Denver in a teaching and research position. Since then, he has taught numerous undergraduate and graduate courses, including general biology, cell biology, histology, endocrinology, and reproductive biology. Dr. Chiras also has a strong interest in environmental issues and has taught a variety of courses on the subject.

Currently an adjunct professor at the University of Denver and the University of Colorado at Denver, Dr. Chiras has also been a visiting professor at the University of Washington, where he taught environmental science. Most of his time is spent writing books and articles.

Dr. Chiras is the author of numerous technical publications on ovarian physiology, critical thinking, sustainability, environmental education, natural building, and renewable energy. He has also written numerous articles for newspapers and magazines on environmental issues. Dr. Chiras has written the environmental pollution section for World Book Encyclopedia's annual publication, *Science Year*, since 1993, and has written over 100 articles on human biology and environmental issues for *World Book Encyclopedia, Encyclopedia Americana,* and *Grolier's Multimedia Encyclopedia.*

Dr. Chiras has published five college and high school textbooks, including *Environmental Science: Creating a Sustainable Future* (Jones and Bartlett) and *Natural Resource Conservation: An Ecological Approach* (with John P. Reganold). Dr. Chiras's high school textbook, *Environmental Science: A Framework for Decision Making,* was selected as the official book of the U.S. Academic Decathlon, a nationwide competition involving thousands of American high school students in over 3000 schools.

Dr. Chiras's books for general audiences include *Beyond the Fray: Reshaping America's Environmental Response* and *Lessons from Nature: Learning to Live Sustainably on the Earth,* which outlines ways to apply ecological principles to create a sustainable society. He has also published *Study Skills for Science Students* and *Essential Study Skills* (Brooks Cole). His newest book is *The Natural House: A Complete Guide to Healthy, Energy-Efficient, Environmental Homes* (Chelsea Green). He is currently at work on a book on passive solar heating and cooling that will be published by Chelsea Green in fall 2002.

In addition to writing, teaching, and lecturing, Dr. Chiras plays an active role in the environmental movement. He is founder of the Sustainable Futures Society in Evergreen, Colorado, and currently serves on their board of directors. He is also a member of the Board of Directors of the Advanced Technology Environmental Education Library.

Besides his active scientific and environmental pursuits, Dr. Chiras is an avid bicyclist, organic gardener, river runner, and musician. He and his two sons live in Evergreen, Colorado, in a passive solar home supplied by solar and wind power and constructed from recycled materials, including 800 used automobile tires.

Work in progess.

Finished product.

Brief Contents

Contents

x

Chapter 11 The Nervous System: Integration, Coordination, and Control   239

Chapter 14 The Endocrine System

Part 3   Heredity and Reproduction

Chapter 15 Chromosomes, Cell Division, and Cancer

Chapter 16 **Principles of Human Heredity**

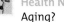
Part 4   Evolution and Ecology

Preface

HUMAN BIOLOGY: HEALTH, HOMEOSTASIS, AND THE ENVIRONMENT, FOURTH EDITION, is written for the introductory human biology course. This book contains a wealth of information on the human body. It presents basic concepts of chemistry that will help you understand the chemistry of living things. It also explores the fascinating world of the cell and examines the structure and function of the tissues and organs that make up our bodies. The book looks at evolution, ecology, and environmental issues, too.

Like other books, this one has a central organizing theme, homeostasis. Homeostasis is a kind of internal balancing act that evolved to help regulate internal conditions vital for our survival. You will explore many fascinating processes that help control levels of chemicals in blood, body temperature, and cell function. You will see how the proper functioning of these mechanisms is essential to maintaining health. You will also see how homeostasis and personal health are dependent on a healthy environment. We'll look at indoor air quality, water pollution, air pollution, and even stress levels in our environment to see how they affect our health.

In writing *Human Biology*, I had several goals in mind. First, this book was written to teach you about the human body. This knowledge, in turn, helps you understand and take care of yourselves and make informed health decisions both now and in the future. Second, this book promotes scientific literacy, that is, an understanding of how scientific information is gathered and the way it influences our lives. Furthermore, it provides background material so that you can understand new scientific discoveries and the way they influence our lives. This will aid you in understanding some of the thorniest political issues of our times. Third, this book promotes critical thinking skills, which will be valuable to you throughout your lives. Fourth, the discussions of the environment assist you in understanding our relationship to the environment, and ways we affect it—sometimes to our own detriment. Fifth, this book helps you begin to learn systems thinking—that is, thinking in terms of whole systems and understanding how the parts interact.

Organization

Human Biology is divided into four parts. Part I outlines basic biological and chemical principles vital to your understanding of the human organism. Part I contains a discussion of science and the scientific method and introduces critical thinking skills that are applied throughout the book. It closes with an overview of the cell, the basic building block of all organisms.

Part II examines the fascinating structure and function of human beings. The chapters in this section describe how the major organ systems operate. Homeostasis is emphasized in these chapters as a unifying principle of biology.

Part III discusses cell division, heredity, and genetic engineering. It also includes a discussion of reproduction and development.

Finally, Part IV focuses on the big picture. It looks at evolution—how we got here—and basic principles of ecology, the study of ecosystems. The final chapter surveys the problems modern society has created in the natural world and offers solutions for redirecting human society onto a sustainable course—one that ensures well-functioning homeostatic mechanisms.

A Bold New Approach to Teaching Chemistry

In the last edition, I took a bold new approach to teaching chemistry to human biology students. Instead of discussing all the chemistry you need to know in one chapter early on in the book, I have introduced just the basics of chemistry in Chapter 2, with a brief overview of the major biological molecules.

Specific information on the important biological molecules—carbohydrates, lipids, proteins, amino acids, and nucleic acids—is provided as you need the information. For example, you learn about proteins and lipids in the section on plasma membranes in Chapter 3, "The Life of the Cell," just before you learn about the structure of the plasma membrane. You then learn a little about carbohydrates in the discussion of energy in that chapter.

More information on carbohydrates, lipids, and proteins is presented in the nutrition chapter. DNA and RNA are presented in detail in the discussion of molecular genetics. We have placed an icon in the table of contents so you and the instructors can see where the basic chemistry has been moved.

This approach has at least two benefits. First, it helps prevent chemistry overload—the deluge of seemingly isolated facts about chemistry that so many students find difficult to grasp and impossible to remember. Second, it offers information on chemistry in context, so that it is easier to learn and retain. It shows the relevancy of chemistry to your understanding of important topics.

New to the Fourth Edition

This text has been thoroughly updated. New examples, new ideas, and new discoveries have been presented in many areas including nutrition, heart health, immunology, cancer, genetics, genetic engineering, and environmental issues.

I've added some new ideas in the critical thinking section that will help you understand how scientific information is often presented in the popular media. You will explore new discoveries in Parkinson's disease and Alzheimer's disease—what causes them and how they could be cured.

There's exciting new information that explains why Americans are experiencing a dramatic rise in allergies, asthma, and sugar diabetes. You'll even learn about the potential benefits of eating chocolate! New treatments for cancer, including efforts that attempt to cut off a tumor's blood supply, are featured in this edition. There's fascinating new information on antibiotic resistance—notably how many potentially harmful bacteria are becoming resistant to antibiotics and even how antibiotics in sewage effluent may be creating resistant strains.

You'll study exciting new developments in treating viral infections and spinal cord injuries. This book will also teach you new discoveries in AIDS research. There's even new research on how we smell and taste.

For diabetics, there's exciting new research on ways to better monitor blood glucose levels without having to prick the skin three times a day. This book also describes new developments, notably, an insulin-containing nasal spray, that could make administering insulin much less painful. In the section on genetic engineering, you will read about genetic techniques such as cloning that scientists are using to help protect endangered species. You will also read about some of the downsides of genetic engineering, for example, the researchers who accidentally produced a potentially lethal mouse virus.

In a continuing effort to provide you with the latest information, many authors of the Point/Counterpoint essays have updated their work. The publisher and I have added or replaced many photographs and drawings with new ones in our quest to improve the value of this book. This edition also features some new health notes, designed to present new and exciting information of great relevance to you now and in the future.

Special Features

Human Biology is a user-friendly book. In this edition, I've tried hard to make sure the material is presented in a friendly style. Complex subjects are simplified somewhat, and numerous analogies are used to make material more meaningful. For the most part, this book concentrates on basic information—key facts and concepts essential to students of human biology. You will find numerous examples sprinkled throughout the book, too. I

have defined many terms, and also added pronunciations of many difficult words. The following features are included to make the your learning experience fun, interesting, and memorable.

Scientific Discoveries That Changed the World

Science is as much a body of facts as it is a process of discovery. To highlight some of the key discoveries in human biology, I've included numerous essays called "Scientific Discoveries That Changed the World." These cover such topics as the discovery of cells, the structure of DNA, the circulation of blood, and the mechanism of gene control. This feature highlights the work of some of the world's most important scientists and illustrates how scientific discoveries have changed our view of the world. They also further your understanding of the scientific method and illustrate the fact that scientific advances usually require the efforts of many scientists, sometimes working in seemingly unrelated areas.

Health Notes

The Health Notes emphasize information that is vital to you both now and in the future. They present practical advice on such topics as proper diet, exercise, stress management, hair loss, heart disease, cancer prevention, and aging. I have updated the Health Notes and added five new ones on the perils of recreational drug use, breast cancer, breast augmentation, the use of maggots to destroy dead tissue in wounds, and the use of leeches to restore blood flow in body parts reattached by microsurgery. Much of this is cutting-edge news. All of it is information you will need throughout your life. You may want to hold on to this book and refer back to it from time to time.

Point/Counterpoints

Many discoveries in biology have had profound impacts on our lives. Today, however, new discoveries often present profound ethical challenges and result in considerable debate. The use of genetic engineering and fetal cell transplantation, for instance, have sparked lively debate. This book presents a number of modern-day controversies in a highly successful feature, the Point/Counterpoints. Some of the Point/Counterpoints debate social and political issues that require a good biological background and others focus on scientific debates.

Each Point/Counterpoint consists of two brief essays written by distinguished writers and thinkers. These essays present opposing views on important issues of our times such as the use of animals for laboratory research, genetic engineering, food irradiation, fetal cell transplantation, cancer testing, and physician-assisted suicide. There are very practical debates as well, such as the Point/Counterpoint on circumcision.

Point/Counterpoints not only help inform you of current issues, they offer a chance to practice critical thinking skills. Additional discussions, questions, and links to web pages supporting differing views on the issues are available at the Jones and Bartlett web site *HumanBiology*. Here's a list of the Point/Counterpoint essays:

Controversy over the Use of Animals in Laboratory Research (Chapter 1)

Controversy over Food Irradiation (Chapter 2)

Fetal Cell Transplantation (Chapter 3)

Tracking People with AIDS (Chapter 8)

Prioritizing Medical Expenditures (Chapter 10)

Are We in a Cancer Epidemic? (Chapter 15)

Are Current Procedures for Determining Carcinogens Valid? (Chapter 17)

Controversy over Herbicide Resistance in Crops Developed Through Genetic Engineering (Chapter 18)

The Medical Debate over Circumcision (Chapter 19)

Physician-Administered Euthanasia (Chapter 20)

Why Worry About Extinction? (Chapter 23)

Critical Thinking Skills

As noted earlier, Chapter 1 presents a number of "rules" for improving critical thinking skills. These guidelines will help you become more discerning thinkers, a skill that could prove useful in this and many other college courses—not to mention the benefit it will have in later life.

Additional emphasis is placed on critical thinking throughout the text. Each chapter, for example, contains a Thinking Critically exercise. At the beginning of the chapter, I outline a problem or present the results of a study and ask you to apply your critical thinking skills. A brief analysis is offered at the end of the chapter.

Some chapters also include an Exercising Your Critical Thinking Skills located at the end of the chapter. These exercises also call on you to apply your critical thinking skills and include case studies, hypothetical scenarios, or summaries of news or scientific reports. Each exercise emphasizes one or two of the critical thinking rules presented in the first chapter. Critical thinking questions are also included after each Point/Counterpoint and in the Test of Concepts questions.

Health, Homeostasis, and the Environment Sections

The health of the Earth's organisms and the environment in which they live are closely connected. To illustrate these connections, most chapters conclude with a Health, Homeostasis, and the Environment section. These features describe the importance of homeostasis and demonstrate some of the ways in which the physical, chemical, social, and psychological environments affect our health by upsetting homeostasis.

In-Text Summaries

To help you learn key concepts, virtually all chapter section heads are written as summary statements. These statements capture key concepts presented in the material that follows. These in-text summaries provide you with a way to review major concepts as you prepare for exams.

End-of-Chapter Summaries

At the end of each chapter is a summary of the material covered in the chapter. You can use the chapter headings to glean key concepts and the End-of-Chapter summaries to review the most important factual information presented in the chapter.

Test of Concepts

Each chapter contains a number of brief essay questions that enable you to assess your understanding of the material. These questions go beyond the regurgitation of facts. The in-text summaries, detailed end-of-chapter summaries, and tests of concepts should provide an excellent study guide.

Art Program

This book contains a remarkable collection of drawings and photographs. In this edition, we've added some new figures and refined many others. These colorful illustrations supplement the text and make the more complex concepts and processes understandable. In this edition, we have added explanatory boxes to some of the art, which describe the key processes illustrated in the figures.

Web Enhancement (www.jbpub.com/humanbiology)

This fourth edition is linked to a extensive web site, *HumanBiology*, developed exclusively for this book by the author and Jones and Bartlett Publishers. The *HumanBiology* web site offers students an unprecedented degree of integration between their text and the online world. For example, the web site introduces students to independent web sites that represent both sides of the topics debated in the text's Point/Counterpoints. *HumanBiology* provides access to the latest biology news and information on the diseases introduced in the book. Each Health Notes topic is linked to sites with more information. This close linkage means the text always remains current. When we provide a link to an independent site, a brief description places the site in context *before* the student connect to it.

To help study for exams, *HumanBiology* also contains Tools for Learning, an online student review area. Students will find complete chapter outlines, review questions with feedback (written by the author), hundreds of flash cards, figure labeling exercises, and links to a variety of interactive tutorials. An illustrated description of *HumanBiology* is provided just inside the front cover of this book.

A Note to Instructors about Using HumanBiology in Their Course

Students use the web in a variety of ways. For example, it can be a source of background material for term papers assigned by an instructor. Students can also use the links we have created to other web sites to further their understanding of human biology—to increase their breadth and depth of knowledge. This information helps them become more knowledgeable citizens, more health conscious, and better informed when it comes to making health-care decisions.

Students can also use the web to find information to help them in class discussions and class debates. Many instructors use the Point/Counterpoints in the book to stimulate debate. Because of space limitations, however, most Point/Counterpoint authors cannot fully develop their arguments. A trip to the web can help students uncover information that will expand their knowledge and assist them in class debates.

Ancillary Materials

Jones and Bartlett Publishers offers an impressive variety of traditional print and interactive multimedia ancillaries to assist instructors and aid students in mastering human biology. Additional information and review copies of any of the following items are available through your Jones and Bartlett Sales Representative.

Instructor's ToolKit CD-ROM

This CD-ROM contains full-color art files of the text's illustrations for computer projection and Microsoft PowerPoint™ Lecture Outline Slides. Also included are the complete text files for the instructor's manual and test bank, an electronic test bank and test-generating

software, and concept maps of key systems. Written by Jay Templin of Montgomery Community College, Pottstown, PA, the instructor's manual contains lecture outlines, learning objectives, key terms, concept questions, and teaching tips—including ideas for using the Point/Counterpoints in class. The test bank contains over 2,000 questions in a variety of formats.

Study Guide

Written by Jim Blahnik of Lorain County Community College, the study guide contains a section on developing good study skills, chapter overviews, chapter outlines, learning objectives, study tips pertinent to each chapter, art labeling exercises, concept map exercises, and practice tests.

Color Transparencies

Qualified adopters may choose either a standard or a customized set of high-quality color transparancies. The standard set contains one hundred of the most frequently used illustrations from the text. Or you can select the illustrations that work best for your lectures and Jones and Barlett will create a custom set of color transparencies.

Acknowledgments

A project of this magnitude is the fruit of a great many people. I wish to thank the thousands of scientists and teachers who have contributed to our understanding of human biology. A special thanks to the extraordinary teachers who have made tremendous contributions to my education, especially the late Weldon Spross, Edward Evans, the late Dr. H. T. Gier, Dr. Gilbert Greenwald, Dr. Howard Matzke, and Dr. Douglas Poorman. Their teaching techniques have made me a better teacher and textbook author, and for that I'm extremely grateful.

I am also deeply indebted to many people for their assistance during the writing of this book. A great debt of gratitude to the folks at Jones and Bartlett. Many thanks to Victoria Jones, ever affable and a joy to work with. Many thanks to those who assisted with the production of the book, including Dean DeChambeau, Lianne Ames, and Kathy Smith. Much appreciation for their calmness throughout, cordiality, attention to detail, and diligence. Additional thanks must be extended to Christine Whitney who coordinated the supplements and to Kathy Smith who researched photos for the new edition. I greatly appreciate the efforts of Jones and Bartlett's many sales representatives who have helped make this book a success. It has been a pleasure and an honor to have worked with such a fine and talented group of people.

Thanks also to the many authors who contributed the Point/Counterpoints in this book. Your work will make this a more exciting journey for students as they begin to appreciate different perspectives of crucial issues.

Throughout this time, my two delightful sons, Skyler and Forrest, have offered considerable support and a counterbalance to the stresses and strains of a project of this magnitude. You're the light of my life, guys. Thanks, too, to my partner, Linda Stuart, for her friendship and inspiration.

Finally, a special thanks to all the reviewers on this and previous editions who offered many useful comments throughout this project. Their insights and attention to detail have been greatly appreciated. Below is a list of those who have reviewed the manuscript.

Reviewers

D. Darryl Adams
  Mankato State University
Donald K. Alford
  Metropolitan State College
David R. Anderson
  Pennsylvania State University—
  Fayette Campus
Felix Baerlocher
  Mount Allison University
Jack Bennett
  Northern Illinois University
Charles E. Booth
  Eastern Connecticut State
  University
J. D. Brammer
  North Dakota State University
Judith Byrnes-Enoch
  Empire State College
Vic Chow
  City College of San Francisco
Ann Christensen
  Pima Community College
Peter Colverson
  Mohawk Valley Community College
Francoise Cossette
  University of Ottowa
John D. Cowlishaw
  Oakland University
Penni Croot
  SUNY Potsdam
Richard Crosby
  Treasure Valley Community College

John Cummings
  Waynesburg College
Jeffrey Dean
  Vanderbilt University
Debby Dempsey
  Northern Kentucky University
Melanie DeVores
  Sam Houston State University
Stephen Freedman
  Loyola University of Chicago
Sheldon R. Gordon
  Oakland University
Martin Hahn
  William Paterson College
John P. Harley
  Eastern Kentucky University
Robert R. Hollenbeck
  Metropolitan State College
Carl Johnson
  Vanderbilt University
Wendel J. Johnson
  University of Wisconsin, Marinette
Florence Juillerat
  Indiana University—Purdue
  University
Ruth Logan
  Santa Monica College
Charles Mays
  DePauw University
David Mork
  St. Cloud State University

Donald J. Nash
  Colorado State University
Emily C. Oaks
  State University of New York—
  Oswego
Lewis Peters
  Northern Michigan University
Richard E. Richards
  University of Colorado at Colorado
  Springs
Lynette Rushton
  South Puget Sound Community
  College
Miriam Schocken
  Empire State College
Richard Shippee
  Vincennes University
Beverly Silver
  James Madison University
Mary Vetter
  University of Regina
David Weisbrot
  William Paterson College
Richard Weisenberg
  Temple University
Terrance O. Weitzel, Jr.
  Jacksonville University
Roberta Williams
  University of Nevada—Las Vegas
Tommy Wynn
  North Carolina State University

Study Skills

College is a demanding time. For many students, term papers, tests, reading assignments, and classes require a new level of commitment to their education. At times, the workload can become overwhelming.

Fortunately, there are many ways to lighten the load and make time spent in college more profitable. This section offers some helpful tips on ways to enhance your study skills. It teaches you how to improve your memory, how to become a better note taker, and how to get the most out of what you read. It also helps you prepare better for tests and become a better test taker.

Mastering these study skills will require some work, mostly to break old, inefficient habits. In the long run, though, the time you spend now learning to become a better learner will pay huge dividends. Over the long haul, improved study skills will save you lots of time and help you improve your knowledge of facts and concepts. That will no doubt lead to better grades and very likely a more fruitful life.

General Study Skills

- Study in a quiet, well-lighted space. Avoid noisy, distracting environments.
- Turn off televisions and radios.
- Work at a desk or table. Don't lie on a couch or bed.
- Establish a specific time each day to study, and stick to your schedule.
- Study when you are most alert. Many students find that they retain more if they study in the evening a few hours before bedtime.
- Take frequent breaks—one every hour or so. Exercise or move around during your study breaks to help you stay alert.
- Reward yourself after a study session with a mental pat on the back or a snack.
- Study each subject every day to avoid cramming for tests. Some courses may require more hours than others, so adjust your schedule accordingly.
- Look up new terms or words whose meaning is unclear to you in the glossaries in your textbooks or in a dictionary.

Improving Your Memory

You can improve your memory by following the PMC method. The PMC method involves three simple learning steps: (1) paying attention, (2) making information memorable, (3) correlating new information with facts you already know.

Step 1 Paying attention means taking an active role in your education—taking your mind out of neutral. Eliminate distractions when you study. Review what you already know and formulate questions about what you are going to learn before a lecture or before you read a chapter in the text. Reviewing and questioning help prime the mind.

Step 2 Making information memorable means finding ways to help you retain information in your memory. Repetition, mnemonics, and rhymes are three helpful tools.

- Repetition can help you remember things. The more you hear or read something, the more likely you are to remember it, especially if you're paying attention. Jot down important ideas and facts while you read or study to help involve all of the senses.
- Mnemonics are useful learning tools to help remember lists of things. I use the mnemonic CARRRP to remember the biological principles of sustainability: conservation, adaptability, recycling, renewable resources, restoration, and population control.
- Rhymes and sayings can also be helpful when trying to remember lists of facts.
- If you're having trouble remembering key terms, look up their roots in the dictionary. This often helps you remember their meaning.
- You can also draw pictures and diagrams of processes to help remember them.

Step 3 Correlating new information with the facts and concepts you already know helps tie facts together, making sense out of the bits and pieces you are learning.

- Instead of filling your mind with disjointed facts and figures, try to see how they relate with what you already know. When studying new concepts, spend some time tying information together to get a view of the big picture.
- After studying your notes or reading your textbook, go back and review the main points. Ask yourself how this new information affects your view of life or critical issues and how you may be able to use it.

Becoming a Better Note Taker

- Spend 5 to 10 minutes before each lecture reviewing the material you learned in the previous lecture. This is extremely important!
- Know the topic of each lecture before you enter the class and spend a few minutes reflecting on facts you already know about the subject that's going to be discussed.

- If possible, read the text before each lecture. If not, at least look over the main headings in the chapter, read the topic sentence of each paragraph, and study the figures. If your chapter has a summary, read it too.
- Develop a shorthand system of your own to facilitate note taking. Symbols such as = (equals), > (greater than), < (less than), w/ (with), and w/o (without) can save lots of time so you don't miss the main points or key facts.
- Develop special abbreviations to cut down on writing time. E might stand for energy, AP might be used for air pollution, and AR could be used to signify acid rain.
- Omit vowels and abbreviate words to decrease writing time (for example: omt vwls & abbrvte wrds to dcrs wrtng tme). This will take some practice.
- Don't take down every word your professor says, but be sure your notes contain the main points, supporting information, and important terms.
- Watch for signals from your professor indicating important material that might show up on the next test (for example, "This is an important point . . .").
- If possible, sit near the front of the class to avoid distractions.
- Review your notes soon after the lecture is over while they're still fresh in your mind. Be sure to leave room in your notes written during class so you can add material you missed. If you have time, recopy your notes after each lecture.
- Compare your notes with those of your classmates to be sure you understood everything and did not miss any important information.
- Attend all lectures.
- Use a tape recorder if you have trouble catching important points.
- If your professor talks too quickly, politely ask him or her to slow down.
- If you are unclear about a point, ask during class. Chances are other students are confused as well. If you are too shy, go up after the lecture and ask, or visit your professor during his or her office hours.

How to Get the Most Out of What You Read

- Before you read a chapter or other assigned readings, preview the material by reading the main headings or chapter outline to see how the material is organized.
- Pause over each heading and ask a question about it.
- Next, read the first sentence of each paragraph. When you have finished, turn back to the beginning of the chapter and read it thoroughly.

- Take notes in the margin or on a separate sheet of paper. Underline or highlight key points.
- Don't skip terms that are confusing to you. Look them up in the glossary or in a dictionary. Make sure you understand each term before you move on.
- Use the study aids in your textbook, including summaries and end-of-chapter questions. Don't just look over the questions and say, "Yeah, I know that." Write out the answer to each question as if you were turning it in for a grade, and save your answers for later study. Look up answers to questions that confuse you. This book has questions that test your understanding of facts and concepts. Critical thinking questions are also included to sharpen your skills.

Preparing for Tests

- Don't fall behind on your reading assignments, and review lecture notes as often as possible.
- If you have the time, you may want to outline your notes and assigned readings. Try to prepare the outline with your book and notes closed. Determine weak areas, then go back to your text or class notes to study these areas.
- Space your study to avoid cramming. One week before your exam, go over all of your notes. Study for two nights, then take a day off that subject. Study again for a couple of days. Take another day off from that subject. Then make one final push before the exam, being sure to study not only the facts and concepts, but also how the facts are related. Unlike cramming, which puts a lot of information into your brain for a short time, spacing will help you retain information for the test and for the rest of your life.
- Be certain you can define all terms and give examples of how they are used.
- You may find it useful to write flash cards to review terms and concepts.
- After you have studied your notes and learned the material, look at the big picture—the importance of the knowledge and how the various parts fit together.
- You may want to form a study group to discuss what you are learning and to test one another.
- Attend review sessions offered by your instructor or by your teaching assistant, but study before the session and go to the session with questions.
- See your professor or class teaching assistant with questions as they arise.
- Take advantage of free or low-cost tutoring offered by your school or, if necessary, hire a private tutor to help you through difficult material. Get help quickly,

though. Don't wait until you are hopelessly lost. Remember that learning is a two-way street. A tutor won't help unless you are putting in the time.

- If you are stuck on a concept, it may be that you have missed an important point in earlier material. Look back over your notes or ask your tutor or professor what facts might be missing and causing you to be confused.
- If you have time, write and take your own tests. Include all types of questions.
- Study tests from previous years, if they are available legally.
- Determine how much of a test will come from lecture notes and how much will come from the textbook.
- Purchase a study guide, if one is available, and use it to review material and test your knowledge.
- Check out your instructor's web site or the author's web site. They often have valuable study aids, such as review questions and practice quizzes.

Taking Tests

- Eat well and get plenty of exercise and sleep before tests.
- Remain calm during the test by breathing deeply.
- Arrive at the exam on time or early.
- If you have questions about the wording of a question, ask your professor.
- Skip questions you can't answer right away, and come back to them at the end of the session if you have time.
- Read each question carefully and be sure you understand its full meaning before answering it.
- For essay questions and definitions, organize your thoughts first on the back of the test before you start writing.

Now take a few moments to go back over the list. Check off those things you already do. Then, mark the new ideas you want to incorporate into your study habits. Make a separate list, if necessary, and post it by your desk or on the wall and keep track of your progress.

Life in the Balance

AN INTRODUCTION TO HUMAN BIOLOGY

Thinking Critically

Your local newspaper reports the results of an experiment a student in one of the local high schools performed to test the effects of a special diet on cholesterol content in chicken eggs. He obtained 20 chickens from two different breeders. Half of the chickens were fed his special diet; the other half were fed a diet of standard chicken feed, which he purchased at the local feed store. The boy found that cholesterol levels in the eggs from the group fed his special diet were lower than the other group. The story created quite a stir in the local media—so much so that the boy's father is trying to acquire funding to market his son's new feed. What problems do you see with this study? ■

Human health is dependent on a healthy lifestyle and a healthy environment.

To begin our exploration of human biology and gain some perspective on our species, we will travel back in time about 3.5 million years to the grasslands of Africa where the first recognizable humanlike organism roamed (**FIGURE 1-1**). Scientists dubbed this creature Australopithecus afarensis (aus-TRAL-owe-PITH-a-CUSS A-far-EN-suss).

Standing only 3 feet tall and walking upright, our earliest ancestors subsisted in large part on a diet of roots, seeds, nuts, and fruits. They supplemented their primarily vegetarian diet with **carrion** (CARE-ee-on), animals that had been killed by predators or that had died from other causes. They may also have captured and killed other animals for meat.

Weak and slow compared to other large animals, our earliest ancestors could have easily ended up as an evolutionary dead-end. Fortunately, though, they possessed several anatomical features that tipped the scales heavily in their favor. Undoubtedly, one of the most important characteristics of all was their brain, a feature that would in time thrust humans to a position of evolutionary dominance.

Although, as one humorist quipped, to an insect a human is just something good to eat, our preeminence in the biological world is indisputable. Today, as testimony to our success, human beings inhabit a world of marvelously complex technology, which even the least tech-

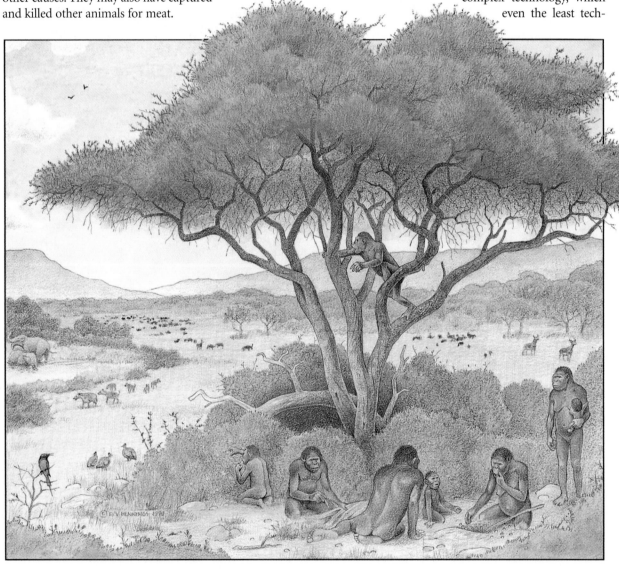

FIGURE 1-1 Australopithecus afarensis   Current scientific evidence suggests that *Australopithecus afarensis* was the first humanlike ape. Its skeletal remains indicate that it walked upright.

(a)

FIGURE 1-2 What Price Progress? Technological development and economic progress are double-edged swords. Although they provide many benefits *(a)* such as the space shuttle and the wonderful discoveries made in space, they do come with extraordinary impacts, *(b)* as in environmental pollution and habitat loss, as evidenced in denuded hillsides cleared to provide wood for human use.

(b)

nologically literate can use thanks to user-friendly interfaces. Rather than collecting nuts and berries from the plants around us, today many people purchase their food from modern grocery stores supplied by highly mechanized farms throughout the world. Many farmers are now using satellites and remote sensing devices, and computerized machinery to produce better crops. Rather than roaming in small bands, the vast majority of the world's people live in cities and towns that offer amenities our ancestors would have never dreamed possible. Instead of being restricted to whimsical gazing into space, we travel there ourselves. And, in recent years, no longer content with what nature provides, our scientists have begun to tinker with the genetic material of the cell to alter plants and animals to increase food production. Some scientists have even begun to manipulate our hereditary material.

From most perspectives, the human experiment has been an overwhelming success (**FIGURE 1-2A**). However, growing evidence shows that our victory has not occurred without a huge price tag. Examples of the cost of our success are many: overpopulation, polluted skies, vanishing forests, and lost species (**FIGURE 1-2B**). Growing evidence, in fact, suggests that human civilization could destroy millions of years of evolutionary history

For better or for worse, humans have become a major player in **evolution** itself, a process of biological change that occurs in distinct groups of organisms, known as **populations.** Evolution results in structural, functional, and behavioral changes in populations. These changes, in turn, result in organisms better equipped to cope with their environment—that is, better able to survive to reproduce.

in a relatively brief time span if we persist along our current path. It is at this point in our evolutionary history that we take up our study of human biology.

Like other texts, the bulk of this book will take you on a journey through the human body. On this journey, you will learn a great deal about yourself—how you got here, how you inherited certain characteristics from your parents, and how your body functions. You will learn the basics of nutrition and how broken bones mend. You will discover how your immune and nervous systems operate. You will explore many common diseases and—perhaps more important—how to prevent them. You will find that many of the diseases afflicting modern humans result from the stressful, polluted, human-engineered environments we've created that reflect a lifestyle that often places convenience and efficiency ahead of healthy patterns of existence. In essence, then, you will be looking at human beings in the modern context.

The information you learn from this book will prove useful to you in many ways. It will also help you understand important political debates over issues such as genetic engineering, pollution, and vaccination. As you proceed through this book, though, be sure to take some time to marvel at the wonders of the human body—the intricate details of the cell, the fascinating structure and function of the body's organs, and the intriguing manner in which the various parts work together.

Health and Homeostasis: Life's Essential Balancing Act

In this book, you will see how human health depends on numerous internal mechanisms that have evolved over many millions of years. These internal processes help to maintain a fairly constant internal condition, a state often referred to as *homeostasis* (home-e-oh-STAY-siss).

Homeostasis Is a State of Relative Constancy

The term **homeostasis** comes from two Greek words, *homeo,* which means "the same," and *stasis,* which means "standing." Literally translated, homeostasis means "staying the same." Thus, many people refer to homeostasis as a state of internal constancy. Unfortunately, this view is not entirely accurate. In reality, homeostasis is not a static state; rather, it is a dynamic (ever-changing) state. Let me explain by using body temperature as an example.

Humans are warm-blooded creatures. We generate body heat internally and maintain body temperature at a fairly constant level—about 98.6 °F. In reality, though, body temperature varies during the day, falling slightly at night when we sleep and rising during the daylight hours. It increases even more when we participate in strenuous physical activity.

Like many other internal conditions, then, body temperature fluctuates within a range. This is what is meant when we say that body temperature is in homeostasis: it is in a dynamic state, but remains more or less the same.

Homeostasis is achieved through a variety of automatic mechanisms that compensate for internal as well as external changes. As Chapter 4 illustrates, homeostatic mechanisms require **sensors,** structures that detect internal and external change—for example, changes in air temperature. Sensors elicit a response that offsets the change, helping to maintain a fairly constant state. On cold days, for example, our bodies often shiver. Shivering is a rhythmic contraction of muscles that generates body heat when the outside temperature drops. It is one of several homeostatic mechanisms in warm-blooded animals triggered by cold.

Homeostatic mechanisms also maintain fairly constant levels of nutrients in the blood, which is essential for normal body function. If nutrient levels fall too low or climb too high, serious problems can arise. For example, glucose (a type of sugar) is essential to the function of all body cells, especially brain cells. If glucose

FIGURE 1-3 Predator Control The fox plays an important role in controlling rodent populations.

levels in the blood fall too low, brain cells are deprived of energy, and a person may go into shock. If levels go too high, other problems arise. Consequently, the blood glucose concentration must be maintained at a fairly constant level. The concentration of blood glucose is regulated by two hormones you will study in Chapter 3.

Homeostatic mechanisms also exist in larger biological systems or ecosystems. An **ecosystem** is a biological system consisting of organisms and their environment. Homeostatic mechanisms help achieve balance in ecosystems, a phenomenon referred to in this book as **environmental homeostasis.**

A highly simplified example illustrates the point. In the grasslands of Kansas, rodent populations generally remain fairly constant from one year to the next. This phenomenon results, in part, from **predators** (animals that hunt and kill other organisms). Predators such as coyotes, foxes, and hawks feed on rodents, and thus help to control rodent populations (**FIGURE 1-3**).

Although predators are a crucial element in maintaining environmental homeostasis in the grasslands of Kansas and virtually all other natural systems, weather, food supplies, and a host of other factors also contribute. In short, it is the net effect of these factors that determines population sizes. The balance can be quite complex. Excess rain may result in a bumper crop of seeds, upon which rodents feed. This, in turn, may lead to a rise in the rodent population. Predator populations may increase in response to the expanding rodent population. Drought in succeeding years, however, may trim rodent populations; their decline results in a decline in predator populations. Homeostatic mechanisms in ecosystems maintain a balance between food supply and populations of organisms.

Some homeostatic mechanisms can also be thought of as ways in which ecosystems recover from changes.

Landslides in the Pacific Northwest, for instance, sometimes occur after heavy rains and can deposit huge quantities of sediment in salmon streams. This, in turn, buries spawning grounds and kills fish. Over time, however, sediment is usually purged by flowing water in streams, which restores gravel beds where fish spawn and allows populations to recover. On the hillside, grasses, shrubs, and trees may take root, stabilizing the slope and preventing future landslides.

Because of these and other similar mechanisms, ecosystems undisturbed by human activity tend to persist for thousands of years—barring natural geological and climactic changes. However, when human disturbances occur frequently or are severe, the changes may overwhelm the recuperative capacity of the environment. In such instances, disruption may lead to destruction. Today, pollution, mining, overgrazing, deforestation, and many other human activities threaten the environment in this manner.

In this book, the term *homeostasis* is used to refer to the balance that occurs at all levels of biological organization—from cells to organisms to entire ecosystems. The abundance of homeostatic mechanisms in nature suggests their evolutionary significance. Maintaining "balance" is essential to the continuation of life. Without it, cells would fall into disarray, organisms would perish and ecosystems would be destroyed!

Human Health and the Health of Ecosystems Are Closely Tied

Scientists have found that the health of the environment and the health of organisms, including human beings, are interdependent. Alterations in the environment—for example, adverse changes in the chemical composition of the air—can have impacts on human health. Polluted air, water, and soils take a toll on humans and other species. According to a recent study by the Environmental Protection Agency, over 76 million Americans (nearly one of every three people) live in cities where the ground-level pollutant ozone poses a threat to health. Ozone is a chemical pollutant derived from automobile exhaust that irritates the eyes and the lungs. Ozone also destroys the tiny air sacs in the lung, resulting in **emphysema,** a disease that kills its victims slowly and painfully (**FIGURE 1-4**).

Ozone is just one of many pollutants in our environment. Dozens of cancer-causing chemicals are also found in our drinking water, food, and air; these chemicals can alter cells in the body, causing some to proliferate uncontrollably. Unthwarted growth forms cancerous tumors that are often fatal. From a strictly human perspective, it should become clear that planet care is the ultimate form of self-care.

Human Health also Depends on a Healthy Psychological and Social Environment. The health of organisms requires more than a clean environment. It requires social and psychological conditions conducive to mental health. Stressful environments can lead to serious ailments in those individuals unfortunate enough to be stuck in them. Health, Homeostasis, and Environment sections at the end of chapters illustrate the connection between our social/psychological environment and our health—a connection, until recently, rarely mentioned in discussions about human health.

(a)

(b)

FIGURE 1-4 Emphysema Pollutants in cigarette smoke and air pollution destroy the tiny air sacs in the lung, which are necessary for the absorption of oxygen into the blood and the release of carbon dioxide. As the air sacs break down, the surface area of the lung decreases, making it harder for victims of this progressive disease to breathe. *(a)* Section through a normal lung; *(b)* section through an emphysemic lung.

Although humans are the central focus of this book, it is important to note that many other species share this world with us. They, too, are profoundly affected by the condition of the environment. In the Pacific Northwest, for example, scientists are finding that chemicals called *nonylphenols* (no-nil-FEE-nalls), which are found in pesticides, plastics, and other products, are making their way into surface waters from sewage treatment plants and, in the case of pesticides, from farmfields. These chemicals alter the hormonal function of young salmon, rendering them unable to get rid of the excess salt that enters their body once they migrate into the ocean, causing them to quickly perish. Scientists are also finding that many drugs that people take are excreted in their urine and end up in sewage effluent and in our waterways. These chemicals could have profound effects on other species. Scientists are particularly concerned about antibiotics. Bacteria in waterways that are exposed to antibiotics could evolve resistance. Humans who ingest these bacteria could become deathly ill. Doctors worry that they won't have antibiotics to treat the resistant strains. Countless other examples could be cited to show the connection between the health of the environment and the health of species.

Health Is a State of Physical and Mental Well-Being

Before we move on, it is important to understand what health is. For many years, human health was defined as the absence of disease (**FIGURE 1-5A**). As long as a person had no obvious symptoms of a disease, that person was considered healthy. Although such a person may have had clogged arteries from a lifetime of eggs-and-bacon breakfasts, it wasn't until symptoms of heart disease—for example, chest pain—became apparent that the patient was considered unhealthy.

In recent years, many health experts have sought to create a much broader and more useful definition of the term *health.* Today, human health considerations take into account two broader categories: physical *and* emotional well-being.

Physical health refers to the state of the body—how well it is working. Physical health can be measured by checking temperature, blood pressure, blood sugar levels, and a host of other variables. Abnormalities in these measurements may be a signal that one's physical health is in jeopardy, even though there are no obvious symptoms of illness. Medical scientists use the term **risk factors** to refer to abnormal conditions such as high blood pressure or high blood cholesterol levels that put a person at risk for disease. The presence of one or more risk factors is a sign of less-than-perfect health. Obviously, the more risk factors there are, the worse one's physical health (**FIGURE 1-5B**).

The new concept of health is very different from the old one because it says that even though a person feels healthy and doesn't exhibit obvious signs of disease, such as a failing heart, the presence of risk factors must be taken into account. As shown in **FIGURE 1-5B**, the absence of risk factors results in the best health. A few risk factors mean health is only good. More risk factors mean health must be considered poor, even though the indi-

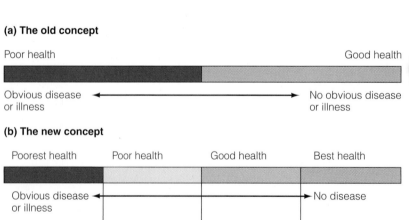

(a) The old concept

Poor health		Good health

Obvious disease or illness ← → No obvious disease or illness

(b) The new concept

Poorest health	Poor health	Good health	Best health

Obvious disease ← → No disease
or illness

Many risk factors	More risk factors	A few risk factors	No risk factors

Poor fitness			Good fitness

Poor mental health			Good mental health

FIGURE 1-5 Old and New Concepts of Health

TABLE 1-1
Healthy Habits
Sleep seven to eight hours per day*
Eat breakfast regularly
Eat a balanced diet
Avoid snacking on junk food (sweets or fatty foods) between meals
Maintain ideal weight
Do not smoke
Avoid alcohol or use it moderately
Exercise regularly
Manage stress in your life
*Not all people need this much sleep. If you're one of them, don't try to force yourself to sleep more than you need.

vidual may not have had a heart attack or some other problem—yet.

Consider the example of high blood pressure. A person with high blood pressure often feels fine, especially early on. In the long run, though, a person with high blood pressure is much more likely to suffer a heart attack than a person with normal blood pressure. Therefore, all other things being equal, a person with high blood pressure is less healthy than one with normal blood pressure.

Scientists also use the term *risk factor* to refer to activities that predispose someone to disease. Smoking and a fatty diet, for example, are risk factors for strokes and heart attacks.

Physical health is also measured by level of physical fitness. If you can't walk up a set of stairs without gasping for air, you're not considered very physically fit. You're more likely to have other problems later in life—for example, heart disease.

Along with physical health goes emotional well-being. Especially relevant today is the ability to cope with the stresses and strains of modern life. Inability to cope may lead to physical ill health, such as high blood pressure, heart disease, and stroke.

In essence, then, mental and physical fitness are measures of our psychological and physical abilities to meet the demands of everyday life. Fit people are able to cope with day-to-day psychological stresses and are able to walk up a flight of stairs without becoming short of breath. (If you can't, it may be time to seek counseling and start an exercise program.)

Maintaining good health is a lifelong job. **TABLE 1-1** lists numerous healthy habits. By incorporating these habits into your lifestyle, you can increase your chances of living a long, healthy life.

Health Is Dependent on Properly Functioning Homeostatic Mechanisms

As pointed out earlier, physical health depends on properly functioning homeostatic mechanisms—that is, regulatory controls in the body that help maintain homeostasis. When these controls function improperly or break down completely, illness results. Persistent stress, for example, can disrupt several of the body's homeostatic mechanisms, leading to disease.

Stress Results in Disease by Disrupting Homeostatic Mechanisms

Stress is prevalent in many of our lives, so let's examine it more carefully. Most people cope with infrequent or short-term stress fairly well. Stress causes little harm when it occurs infrequently. If it is prolonged, however, stress can increase the risk of cardiovascular disease (diseases of the heart and arteries). Persistent stress may also increase the risk of ulcers and weaken the immune system. In addition, it may increase the likelihood of developing mental disorders. Fortunately for us, stress can be alleviated by exercise, relaxation training, massage, acupuncture, and other measures discussed in Health Note 1-1.

This discussion is not meant to imply that all diseases result from homeostatic imbalance. Some are produced by genetic defects; others are caused by bacteria or viruses. But even in these instances, diseases often result from an upset in regulatory mechanisms of the body that disrupt homeostasis. An excellent example is acquired immune deficiency syndrome, or AIDS. AIDS is caused by a virus that attacks certain cells of the immune system. This, in turn, results in a reduction in a key protective mechanism of the body, which is vital to homeostasis. In other diseases, temporary upsets in homeostasis may make us more susceptible to infectious agents. According to a recent study, people under stress are twice as likely to suffer from colds and the flu as those who are not.

Section 1-2

Evolution: The Unity and Diversity of Life

Homeostasis is a central theme of this book because it is so essential to life and is now threatened by modern culture. Another key concept of biology and a subtheme of

Health Note 1-1

Maintaining Balance: Reducing Stress in Your Life

Hard as you try, you can't avoid stress; it's a normal occurrence in everyday life.

Most writings on the subject define **stress** as a mental or physical tension. It's what we feel when we're exposed to stressful situations. Physical danger, for instance, may result in a feeling of stress. Humans have evolved mechanisms that deal very successfully with such danger. But nonlifethreatening situations, like a blind date or a final exam, can also evoke feelings of stress.

Stress can be real or imagined. Either way, it elicits the same response in the body: an increase in heart rate, an increase in blood flow to the muscles and a decrease in blood flow to the digestive system, a rise in blood glucose levels, and a dilation of the pupils. All of these physical changes in the body help prepare us to respond to the stress. Once the stimulus is gone, though, the body returns to normal. That is, it is said to recover. So the first thing we must recognize about stress is that the body doesn't discriminate between stressors—the sources of the stress. The response is always the same.

In pondering the effects of stress on the human body, two considerations are paramount: the duration of the **stressor** (the source of the stress response) and our ability to cope with stress.

In general, the source, be it physical or mental, may be short-lived (acute) or long-term (chronic)—or somewhere in between. Long-term exposure is of greatest concern, for it prevents recovery.

A prolonged period of stress may lead to disease, for during the state of stress, the body's immune system—the system that protects us from bacteria and other microorganisms that lead to disease—is depressed. Thus, prolonged immune-system suppression may make a person more susceptible to infectious disease—bacteria and viruses that cause colds and flu and other diseases. In addition, during a prolonged period of stress, changes occur in the blood vessels that accelerate the accumulation of cholesterol, which clogs the arteries and may eventually result in strokes and heart attacks.

Studies show that severe stress, if prolonged, can cause great physical harm. It may interfere with performance at home, at work, and at school.

Some argue that a little stress may actually help improve a person's performance. Healthy people recognize the stress they're feeling and channel its energies into productive work. This leads us to the second consideration: how people cope with stress. A study of upper-echelon executives in American corporations shows that, despite the daily stresses and strains of the corporate pressure cooker, these people live longer, on average, than people of the same sex in the general population. Why? The answer is that they handle stress well. Some psychologists believe that these people have a sense of being in control, despite the stress of their work. They have clear objectives and meet them with a strong sense of purpose. Ultimately, such people view their jobs as a challenge, not a threat.

Unfortunately, not all people are so lucky. Studies suggest that many people are not in a position of control; they feel expendable and often view themselves as victims. For them, stress is a bad thing and may be associated with many severe and chronic diseases.

To a large degree, then, the effect stress has on us depends on the duration of exposure and our attitudes: what we think about ourselves and our environment. Researchers are finding that stress turns against us when we feel insignificant, powerless, and overwhelmed.

What can be done to deal with stress? One of the most important strategies is preventive. For example, it's important to select an environment and create a lifestyle that is as stress-free as possible. For some people, that means living in the country, rather than a crowded city. For others, it may mean choosing a major in college that suits their personality. The possibilities are limitless.

But this strategy may not be possible. You may have to be in a stressful environment. In this case, it's up to you to take direct action to learn to cope with stress or lessen its impact. Coping with stress requires mental strategies. Lessening its impact requires physical strategies. Let's consider the physical strategies first.

One of the easiest routes is to lessen the impact of stress through exercise. Studies show that a single workout at the gym, a ride on your bicycle, a vigorous hike, or a day of cross-country skiing reduces tension for two to five hours. Even better is a regular exercise program, which reduces the overall stress in your life. An individual who is easily stressed may find that stress levels decline after several weeks of exercise.

Exercise can be supplemented by relaxation training, another physical strategy. As you prepare for a difficult test or get ready for a date that you are nervous about, tension often builds in your muscles. Periodically stopping to release that tension helps you reduce physical stress. For some people, getting up and stretching or taking a walk can reduce the tension. Others find it useful to tighten their muscles forcefully, then let them relax. Massage therapy and acupuncture have also been used to successfully reduce stress. Cassette tapes can teach you relaxation methods. If that's not for you, consider signing up for stress-reduction classes from a trained therapist. The more you practice relaxation, the better you will become at relieving tension.

Stress from within is often blown out of proportion. By dealing with the thoughts that exaggerate your stress, you can eliminate stress before it begins. This is a mental strategy. Start paying attention to the thoughts that provoke anxiety in your life. Are they exaggerated? If so, why? For example, are you nervous before exams? Why? Do you always study adequately? Could you prepare better? Would better preparation reduce your anxiety? Finding the source of your anxiety and taking positive action to alleviate it are helpful ways of reducing stress.

Stress reduction is not always so easy. Test anxiety, for example, may be deeply rooted in feelings of insecurity and inadequacy. Many people struggle with low self-esteem their entire life. A trained psychologist can help you find the roots of your problem and assist you in learning to feel better about yourself. Psychological help is as important as medical help these days. Given the complexity and pace of our society, there is no shame in seeking counseling.

Biofeedback is another form of stress relief. A trained health care worker hooks you up to a machine that monitors heart rate, breathing, muscle tension, or some other physiological indicator of stress (**FIGURE 1**). During a biofeedback session, your trainer will help you relax, and then perhaps discuss a stressful situation. When one of the indicators shows that you are suffering from stress, a signal is given off. Your goal is to consciously reduce the frequency of the signal. For example, if your heart started beating faster when you thought about taking an exam, a clicking sound might be heard. By deep breathing and relaxing, you consciously slow down your heart rate, and the clicking sound slows down, and then disappears. Learning to recognize the symptoms of stress and to counter them is the goal of biofeedback. Eventually, you should be able to do it without the aid of a machine.

You can also reduce tension by managing your time and your workload efficiently. Numerous books on this subject can help you learn to budget your time more effectively. Efficient time management alone can often keep you from feeling stressed. Learning to study more efficiently can also reduce stress. (See the Study Skills section at the beginning of the book.)

If these techniques don't work, you may want to see a doctor. He or she can prescribe medications that relieve tension. Sleep medications and

FIGURE 1 Biofeedback Student in a biofeedback session.

antidepressants are often prescribed, as well. Herbal remedies are also available. Valarien root and Kava Kava are two commonly used herbs by people who suffer from stress.

It is important to challenge yourself in college, but be realistic in what you expect of yourself. If you must work, for example, sign up for a class load that you can handle. Even if you are not working, take a reasonable class load, and be sure to exercise regularly and get plenty of sleep.

Relieving stress in our lives helps us reduce the risk of cardiovascular disease. It helps us relax and enjoy life. Lest we forget, it also makes us more pleasant to be around. All in all, it is best to start learning early in life how to reduce or cope with stress. Lessons learned now will be useful for years to come.

Visit *Human Biology's* Internet site for links to web sites offering more information on this topic.

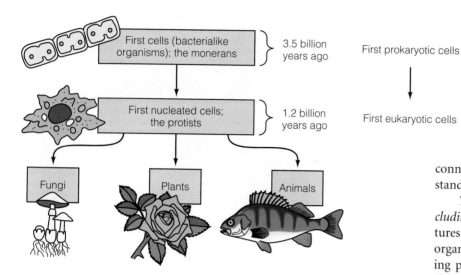

FIGURE 1-6 Evolution of the Prokaryotic and Eukaryotic Cells This diagram illustrates the evolutionary history of life. Organisms fall into one of five major groupings, or kingdoms. The first life-forms were the monerans, which are single-celled prokaryotic organisms. They gave rise to the protistans, single-celled eukaryotic organisms. Eukaryotic protistans, in turn, gave rise to plants, fungi, and animals.

this book is **evolution.** A few words on the subject are essential to your understanding of human biology and the unique evolutionary predicament we're in.

All life-forms alive today exist because of evolution. In fact, every cell and every organ in the human body is a product of millions of years of evolutionary refinement. Even the intricate homeostatic mechanisms described in the previous section evolved over long periods.

FIGURE 1-6 shows the five major groups or **kingdoms** of organisms that exist today. This simple diagram also illustrates evolutionary relationships. The simplest, bacterialike organisms, belonging to a group called the **monerans,** were the first to evolve. They gave rise to a more complex set of organisms, known as the protistans. The **protistans** consist of single-celled organisms such as amoebas and paramecia. During the course of evolution, the protistans gave rise to three additional groups: plants, fungi, and animals, the kingdom to which we humans belong.

This common lineage is responsible for the striking similarities among the Earth's organisms, even in remarkably different organisms. For example, all organisms rely on the same type of genetic material. Similarities also exist on other levels besides the biochemical one. A comparison of certain anatomical features, such as the bones in a person's arm and the wings of birds, reveals an eerie resemblance.

Humans Are Similar to Other Organisms in Many Ways

An analysis of living things turns up seven common features, typically referred to as the characteristics of life. A brief look at these not only shows our evolutionary

connection with other organisms, but helps us understand people better.

The first characteristic of life is that all organisms, including humans, are made of cells. Cells are tiny structures that are the fundamental building block of living organisms. Cells, in turn, consist of molecules, nonliving particles composed of smaller units called **atoms.** Glucose molecules, for instance, contain carbon, hydrogen, and oxygen atoms. Molecules, in turn, combine to form the parts of the cell.

The second characteristic of life is that all organisms grow and maintain their complex organization by taking in molecules and energy from their surroundings. As you will see in subsequent chapters, humans must expend considerable amounts of energy to maintain their complex internal organization. In fact, 70%–80% of the energy that adult humans need is used just to maintain our bodies—to transport molecules in and out of cells, to synthesize proteins, and to perform other basic body functions. The rest is used for activity—walking, running, talking, and so on.

The third characteristic of life is that all living things exhibit a feature called metabolism. **Metabolism** refers to the chemical reactions in organisms. These reactions consist of two types—those in which food substances are built up into living tissue (anabolic reactions) and those in which food is broken down into simpler substances, often releasing energy (catabolic reactions). In human body cells, thousands of reactions occur each second to maintain life.

The fourth characteristic of life is homeostasis. Simply put, all organisms rely on homeostatic mechanisms. In the constantly shifting world of many organisms, maintaining a constant internal environment is a never-ending task.

The fifth characteristic common to all forms of life is irritability. In biological parlance, irritability does not refer to grouchiness, although some of us clearly fit this description. Rather, **irritability** refers to the ability to perceive and respond to stimuli. A young girl demonstrates this vital property when she withdraws her hand from a hot stove or closes her eyes in response to bright light.

(a)

(c)

(b)

FIGURE 1-7 Sexual and Asexual Reproduction *(a)* Sexual reproduction takes place when a sperm unites with an egg. *(b)* Asexual reproduction takes place when an amoeba divides, producing identical offspring. *(c)* Small cellular buds in some organisms like this hydra enlarge to produce genetically identical offspring, which eventually break free from the parent.

The ability to perceive and respond to stimuli allows all organisms to respond to their environment and is, therefore, an important survival tool. Not surprisingly, evolution has resulted in some rather remarkable ways by which organisms detect stimuli. The human eye is one of them.

The sixth characteristic of life is reproduction and growth. All organisms are capable of reproduction and growth. Two types of reproduction are known to exist: sexual and asexual. **Sexual reproduction** (**FIGURE 1-7A**) occurs in organisms that produce offspring by combining sex cells, sperm and eggs. In vertebrates such as birds and mammals, these cells come from male and female individuals.

Asexual reproduction is common in single-celled organisms such as the amoeba (**FIGURE 1-7B**). In these and other single-celled organisms, reproduction generally occurs by simple cell division of a parent cell. When it divides, it forms two identical offspring.

Some multicellular organisms reproduce asexually by budding. **Budding** is a process in which new individuals are produced from small outgrowths called **buds.** Tiny buds enlarge and soon develop into a fully formed organism. **FIGURE 1-7C** shows budding in an aquatic organism known as a hydra. Like cell division in unicellular organisms, budding produces generation after generation of identical offspring.

The seventh characteristic of life is evolution. Evolution is a process that leads to structural, functional, and behavioral changes in species, known as **adaptations.** Favorable adaptations increase an organism's chances of survival and reproduction.

Evolutionary change occurs through the interplay of genetic variation and environment. **Genetic variation** refers to naturally occurring genetic differences in various members of a population. These differences result in variations in structure, function, and behavior of organisms—adaptations. Those adaptations that give members of a population an advantage over others in survival and reproduction tend to persist.

Charles Darwin, the nineteenth century British naturalist who spent much of his life studying evolution, proposed a **theory of natural selection,** which explains the role of the environment in evolution. In essence, he found that the environment acts as a selective agent, weeding out organisms less able to survive.

Darwin described natural selection as a process in which adaptations, if useful, are preserved. As a result, natural selection is a process by which organisms become better adapted to their environment. Because organisms endowed with beneficial variations are more likely to survive and reproduce, they pass on the favorable genetic material to their offspring. Over time, the genetic composition of the species may change. Individuals of a species may become better camouflaged or faster and thus better able to escape being eaten or to capture prey.

The details of evolution are discussed in Chapters 21 and 22. It is important to point out here, however, that individuals do not evolve, only populations do. Put another way, although evolution results from the emergence of adaptations in individuals, it occurs only when there is a shift in the genetic composition of a population. Profound shifts can result in the formation of entirely new species.

Humans Are One Form of Life on Earth and Have Many Unique Characteristics

Sobering as it may seem, humans are just one of evolution's many delightfully interesting products. Nonetheless, humans are also a unique form of life. Several features distinguish us from other species.

One of the key differences between humans and other animals is our ability to acquire and use complex languages. Another distinguishing feature is our culture. Culture has been defined in many ways. Humorist Will Cuppy remarked that culture is anything we do that monkeys don't. **Culture** can be defined as the ideas, values, customs, skills, and arts of a given people in a given time. While other species may have some rudiments of culture, for instance, some communication skills, humans are unique in the biological world because of the complexity and splendor of our cultural achievements (**FIGURE 1-8A**).

Humans differ in other ways as well. One noteworthy difference is our ability to plan for the future. Although a few other animals seem to share this ability, most of what appears to be planning is probably the result of instinct. A bird's nest-building activities, for example, are programmed by its genetic material and are probably not the result of conscious planning. In contrast, building skyscrapers requires an extraordinary amount of forethought.

Another unique characteristic of humans is our unrivaled ability to reshape the environment. The ability of our minds to shape images and the ability of our hands to translate those images into reality have given us a power almost beyond our control. Despite the benefits of our remarkable technologies, attempts to control nature sometimes backfire, creating larger problems. Efforts to control upstream flooding on the Mississippi River, for instance, have led to more frequent floods and more damage downstream, as witnessed by the floods of 1993 (**FIGURE 1-8B**). By building levees along the river, upstream communities prevent water from spilling over their banks, but this protection delivers a larger slug of water to downstream sections.

The marvelous human achievements over the past 200 years have led many to think of our species as the crowning accomplishment of nature. This view, however, can be dangerously misleading. It makes us think

(b)

(a)

FIGURE 1-8 Human Culture: Progress and Setbacks
(a) Architecture is one of our greatest achievements. But in reshaping our environment, we often suffer enormous backlashes. (b) The use of earthen walls, or levees, along the Mississippi River has increased considerably in the past hundred years in an effort to stop flooding. Levees and other measures to control the river have led to more frequent flooding in downstream areas.

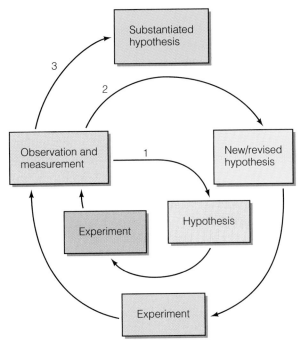

FIGURE 1-9 Scientific Method Scientific study begins with observation and measurement. These activities lead to hypotheses that can be tested by experiments. New and revised hypotheses are derived from experimentation.

of ourselves as separate from nature and immune to its laws, which we are not. It also leads many to believe that nature (the environment) is at our disposal and that we can do with it as we like.

To live on the planet without destroying the natural world around us, disrupting evolution, and ruining the prospects of the human race requires a new way of thinking and acting, one that fosters a cooperative relationship between humans and nature. Barry Commoner, a biologist, put it best when he said that "nothing can survive on the planet unless it is a cooperative part of a larger, global life." It is our challenge to find a way to build such a way of life. Although not the main focus of this book, a few seminal ideas are presented here, especially in the Health, Homeostasis, and the Environment sections and in Chapters 23 and 24.

Section 1-3

Science, Critical Thinking, and Social Responsibility

Over the millenia, human societies have accumulated enormous amounts of information about the world around us. The systematic study of the universe and its many parts today falls into the realm of science.

The term *science* comes from the Latin word *scientia*, which means "to know" or "to discern." Today, **science** is defined as knowledge derived from observation, study, and experimentation. It is also a method of accumulating knowledge. In other words, it involves ways of learning facts as well as an immense body of knowledge.

Many people I talk to seem to view science as a dull and uninteresting endeavor best left in the hands of a select few. In reality, science is an exciting endeavor that often involves enormous creative energy. Because it teaches us about the workings of the world around us, it can be a source of great fascination. As the sometimes zany paleontologist Robert Bakker, a consultant to the company that made the dinosaurs for the movie *Jurassic Park,* once noted, science is "fun for the mind."

Science also has a practical side, as pointed out earlier in this chapter. It provides information that improves our lives in many ways. It helps us understand fascinating and important phenomena such as the weather and the spread of disease. A knowledge of science makes us better voters, better able to discern fact from fiction in a political debate. An understanding of science can help us decide on the safest forms of energy to meet future demands. And an understanding of science, notably human biology, can help us make informed health care decisions.

The Scientific Method Generally Involves Observations, Hypotheses, and Experiments

The methods of science are not as foreign as you might think. In fact, most of us use the scientific method nearly every day of our lives. When your car fails to start, for example, or when your computer acts up, you very likely engage in the type of thinking that scientists use to gather information and test ideas. This process, called the **scientific method,** is summarized in **FIGURE 1-9**. As shown, the scientific method generally begins with observations and measurements. In some cases, these may be part of carefully conducted experiments. Others may occur more haphazardly. A scientist on vacation in the tropics, for instance, may notice a phenomenon that sparks her curiosity and leads to in-depth studies—and a good reason to return to the tropics for a research expedition!

To see how the scientific method works, let us look at a familiar example. Suppose you sat down at a computer, turned on the switch, but nothing happened. You might also have noticed that the lights in the room hadn't come on. These two observations would lead to a **hypothesis** (pronounced high-POTH-eh-siss), a tentative explanation of the phenomenon. From your observations, you might hypothesize that the electricity in your house was cut off.

You would then test your hypothesis by performing an **experiment.** An experiment is a deliberate procedure designed to test some supposition. In this case, all you would need to do would be to traipse into the kitchen and try the light switch. If the lights in the kitchen worked, you would reject your original hypothesis and form a new one. Perhaps, you hypothesize, the circuit breaker to your study had been tripped. To test this idea, you would "perform" another experiment, locating the circuit breaker to see if it was turned off. If the circuit breaker was off, you would conclude that your second hypothesis was valid. To substantiate your conclusion, you would throw the switch, and then test your computer and the room light.

This simple process involving observations and measurements, hypothesis, and experimentation forms the foundation of the scientific method. Although scientific experimentation may be much more complicated than discovering the roots of a computer failure, the process itself is the same.

Theories Are Broad Generalizations Based on Many Experimental Observations

Scientific method leads to the accumulation of scientific facts (really, tested hypotheses). Over time, as our knowledge accumulates, scientists are able to assemble knowledge and gain broader understanding of the way the world works. These broad generalizations are known as **theories.**

Theories are supported by numerous facts that have been established by careful observation, measurement, and experimentation. Unlike hypotheses, theories cannot be tested by single experiments because they encompass many bits of information. Atomic theory, for instance, explains the structure of the atom and fits numerous observations made in different ways over many decades.

A theory commands respect in science because it has stood the test of time. This does not mean that theories are always correct. As history bears out, numerous theories have been modified or discarded as new scientific evidence was gained. Even widely held theories that have persisted for hundreds of years have been overturned. In 140 A.D., for example, the Greek astronomer Ptolemy (TAL-eh-me) proposed a theory that placed Earth at the center of our solar system. This was called the **geocentric theory.** For nearly 1500 years, the geocentric view held sway. Many astronomers vigorously defended this position while ignoring observations that did not fit the theory. In 1580, the astronomer Nicolaus Copernicus dared to expound a new theory—the **heliocentric view,** which places the sun at the center of the solar system. His work stimulated considerable contro-versy, but it eventually prevailed because it better fit the observations.

Because theories may require modifications or rejection, scientists must be willing to analyze new evidence that throws into question their most cherished beliefs. For the most part, though, theories are talked about as if they were fact. Some people even object to calling a theory a "theory" for fear that it sounds tentative.

Another word about theories before we move on. The word *theory* is commonly misused in everyday conversation. A friend, for instance, might say, "My theory about why Jane missed the party is that she didn't want to see her ex-boyfriend." Jane's feelings aside, this is hardly worthy of the status of a theory. What your friend really meant was his "hypothesis," for his explanation was truly a tentative explanation that could be tested by experimentation—in this case, a phone call to Jane.

Science Helps Shape Our Lives and Our Values

Science and the scientific process are essential to modern existence. We wouldn't have the microwave oven or DVD player if it weren't for science. Science can also influence political decisions regarding health care, environmental protection, and a host of other issues.

Many decisions in the public-policy arena, however, are not made solely on the basis of scientific facts. Rather, they are heavily influenced by values—what we view as right or wrong—and economic needs. When human values are framed in the absence of scientific knowledge, however, they can lead to a lopsided way of viewing the world. The political and economic decisions that emerge may be fundamentally flawed.

Although many people do not realize it, science can even influence human values. Environmental values, for instance, are influenced by information gained from the study of ecology. Ecology helps us understand the interconnectedness of living things. It helps uncover relationships that are not obvious to most people, such as the role of bacteria in recycling nutrients. In widening our understanding of the relationships among living organisms and the environment, science helps us understand our dependence on other species and thus helps us act more thoughtfully and compassionately. It widens our ethical and cognitive boundaries, assisting us in living sustainably on the Earth.

Critical Thinking Helps Us Analyze Problems, Issues, and Information More Clearly

Another benefit of your study of science is that it can help you learn to think more critically. **Critical thinking**

TABLE 1-2

Critical Thinking Rules

When analyzing an issue or fact, you may find it useful to employ these rules:

1. Gather complete information.

2. Understand and define all terms.

3. Question the methods by which data and information were derived:
   Were the facts derived from experiments?
   Were the experiments well executed?
   Did the experiment include a control group and an experimental group?
   Did the experiment include a sufficient number of subjects?
   Has the experiment been repeated?

4. Question the conclusions:
   Are the conclusions appropriate?
   Was there enough information on which to base the conclusions?

5. Uncover assumptions and biases:
   Was the experimental design biased?
   Are there underlying assumptions that affect the conclusions?

6. Question the source of the information:
   Is the source reliable?
   Is the source an expert or supposed expert?

7. Don't expect all of the answers or complete information.

8. Examine the big picture.

9. Look for multiple causes and effects.

10. Watch for thought stoppers.

11. Understand your own biases and values.

is not being "critical" or judgmental. Rather, it's a process that allows one to objectively analyze problems, facts, issues, and information. Ultimately, critical thinking permits people to distinguish between beliefs (what we believe to be true) and knowledge (facts that are well supported by research). In other words, critical thinking is a process by which we separate judgment from facts. It is our most ordered kind of thinking. It is not just thinking deeply about a subject, although that is necessary. Critical thinking subjects facts and conclusions to careful analysis, looking for weaknesses in logic and other errors of reasoning. Critical thinking skills, therefore, are essential to analyzing a wide range of problems, issues, and information.

TABLE 1-2 summarizes 11 critical thinking rules that will come in handy as you read the newspaper, watch the news, listen to speeches, and study new subjects in school. Here is a brief description of each rule.

The first rule of critical thinking is: gather complete information. Critical thinking requires facts. Don't sit back and accept everything you read and hear. If you do, you may at times run the risk of learning only what the media or biased special-interest groups want you to think. Question what you learn, and seek other sources of information. Gathering lots of information keeps you from falling into the trap of mistaking ignorance for perspective. By keeping an open mind to alternative views and continually being on the lookout for new facts, you can develop an enlightened viewpoint.

The second rule of critical thinking is: understand and define all terms. Critical thinking requires a clear understanding of all terms. As you study biology, or almost any subject, you will encounter hordes of new terms. Although sometimes tedious, learning new terms is essential. Without a clear understanding of the terminology, you will not be able to master this or any other subject.

Understanding terms and making sure that others define them in discussions also bring clarity to issues and debates. The Greek philosopher Socrates, in fact, destroyed many an argument in his time by insisting on clear, concise definitions of terms. As you analyze any information or issue, always be certain that you understand the terms, and make sure that others define their terms as well.

The third rule of critical thinking is: question the methods by which the facts are derived. In science, many debates over controversial topics hinge on the methods used to discover new information. The first question you should ask is: was the information gained from careful experimentation, or is it an offshoot of casual, unscientific observations?

Proper experimentation in biology usually requires two groups: experimental and control. The **experimental group** is the one that is tested or manipulated in some way. The **control group** is not. Valid conclusions come from such comparisons because, in a properly run experiment, both groups are treated identically except in one way. The difference in treatment is technically known as the *experimental variable*. Consider an example to illustrate this point. In order to test the effect of a new drug on laboratory mice, a good scientist would start with a group of mice of the same age, sex, weight, genetic composition, and so on. These animals would be divided into two groups, the experimental and control groups. Both groups would be treated the same throughout the experiment, receiving the same diet and being housed in the same type of cage at the same temperature. The only difference between the two should be the drug given to the experimental group. Consequently, any observed differences between the groups

Scientific Discoveries that Changed the World 1-1

Debunking the Theory of Spontaneous Generation

**FEATURING THE WORK OF
ARISTOTLE, REDI, AND PASTEUR**

The Greek philosopher and scientist Aristotle, who lived from 384 to 322 B.C., proposed a theory to explain the origin of living things. It was called the **theory of spontaneous generation.** It asserted that living things arose spontaneously from innate matter. Mice, he believed, arose from a pile of hay and rags placed in the corner of a barn. Flies could be produced by first killing a bull, then burying it with its horns protruding from the ground. After several days, one of the horns would be sawed off and flies would emerge. People, it was said, emerged from a worm that developed from the slime in the bottom of a mud puddle.

As absurd as the idea of spontaneous generation sounds to us today, the view remained compelling to many scientists well into the nineteenth century, despite observations that contradicted the theory, such as the phenomenon of childbirth itself.

Debunking the theory of spontaneous generation engaged some of the best scientific minds of the day. Although many scientists were involved in gunning down the theory of spontaneous generation, two promi-

nent scientists, Francesco Redi and Louis Pasteur, played pivotal roles.

Redi, an Italian naturalist and physician, was one of the first scientists to refute spontaneous generation through experimentation. Around 1665, Redi performed a simple but compelling experiment to determine whether ordinary houseflies were spontaneously generated in rotting meat. He began by placing three small pieces of meat in three separate glass containers. The first one was covered with paper. The second was left open, and the third was covered with gauze. Left at room temperature, the meat quickly began to rot and attract flies. Soon, the meat in the open container began to seethe with maggots, larvae hatched from fly eggs. The paper-covered container showed no evidence of maggots, nor did the meat in the gauze-covered container, although maggots did appear in the gauze itself. Redi's conclusion from this experiment was that maggots (which give rise to flies) do not come from the meat itself but from the eggs deposited by flies.

Redi's experiments convinced many people that flies and other organisms did not arise by spontaneous generation, but this did not put the debate to rest. Soon after Redi's

now-famous experiment, in fact, a Dutch linen merchant by the name of Anton Leeuwenhoek discovered bacteria using simple microscopes he had built. This discovery revived arguments for spontaneous generation on the microscopic level. Many scientists asserted that although flies and other organisms did not arise spontaneously, microorganisms probably did—testifying to the allure of ingrained ideas. As evidence, they cited studies showing that microorganisms could arise from boiled extracts of hay or meat. According to die-hard proponents of spontaneous generation, nonliving plant and animal matter was thought to possess a vital, or life-generating, force that could give rise to microorganisms.

The debate over spontaneous generation persisted for the next 200 years even though a number of studies showed that a sterilized medium sealed from the outside air remained free of bacteria, disproving spontaneous generation. But supporters of spontaneous generation claimed that these experiments were flawed. They argued that experimenters had eliminated some vital force needed to give rise to new life.

In 1861, Louis Pasteur published the results of an experiment that

could be attributed to the treatment (the experimental variable).

Besides having an experimental group and a control group, good experimentation requires an adequate number of subjects to ensure that any observed differences are real. Individual variation is natural. As a rule, the smaller the number of animals in each group, the less reliable the data because of variation. In laboratory experiments, at least 10 test animals are required for both control and experimental groups for reliable statis-

tical analysis. Groups larger than 10 are even better. For human health studies, much larger groups are generally used.

As you analyze new findings, first check to see how they were derived. If the results were obtained from experimentation, were the experiments well planned and executed? Did the experiment have a control group? Were the control and experimental groups treated identically except for the experimental variable? Did the experimenters use an adequate number of subjects? Even helped put this debate to rest. He placed sterilized broth in a sterilized swan-necked flask, a flask with a long curved neck (**FIGURE 1**). The design of the flask permitted air to enter, eliminating criticism that he had destroyed any vital forces necessary for spontaneous generation, but it blocked airborne bacteria from entering. (Airborne bacteria probably deposited on the tube leading to the flask and were prevented from entering the broth.) In his experiments, Pasteur clearly showed that bacteria could not arise spontaneously. Only when the broth was open to the air did bacteria emerge.

Besides helping to put an end to the debate about the origin of living organisms, Pasteur's work helped lay the foundation for the modern understanding of infectious disease. Before his simple but convincing experiments, some scientists argued that the diseases we now call infectious were caused by a malfunction in one or more body parts. This malfunction, they claimed, resulted in the production of poisons that caused the illness. The microbes present in the diseased individuals, they went on to say, arose spontaneously as a result of the malfunction and were not the cause of the disease per se.

This brief history points out three important lessons. First, scientific discovery is usually the result of many scientists, each working on different parts of the puzzle. Often, though, one scientist is credited for an important discovery that is, in reality, built on a foundation of scientific research by many others. Second, this brief discussion also shows how discoveries open up new ways of thinking. Third, it illustrates the persistence of ideas that shape the way we think and the resistance people often exhibit to new ideas even in the face of contradictory evidence.

FIGURE 1 Pasteur's Experiment   Pasteur's simple but elegant experiment helped debunk the theory of spontaneous generation. *(a)* These specially designed swan-necked flasks allowed air to enter, but prevented bacteria from entering the broth. *(b)* The broth was boiled to kill microorganisms. *(c)* Microorganisms appeared only if the flasks' necks were removed. *(d)* No microbes grew if the neck remained intact.

if all of these conditions are met, beware. In science, one experiment is rarely adequate to permit you to draw firm conclusions. Careful scrutiny, for example, may show small but significant design flaws: perhaps mice being tested in a drug study were resistant to the drug under examination or were hypersensitive to it. As a rule of thumb, wait for scientific verification of the results. A second researcher may repeat the experiment with similar results. In some cases, a new researcher may find different results.

Nowhere is caution more necessary than when you encounter announcements of scientific breakthroughs on the television news and in magazine and newspaper articles. Ever eager to showcase new scientific studies before they have been verified by others, the media sometimes does a grave disservice to the advancement of scientific knowledge; further study may show that earlier findings were invalid. Unfortunately, the media often fails to publish the results from follow-up studies that contradict previous ones. Scientific journals often

Point/Counterpoint

Controversy over the Use of Animals in Laboratory Research

Animal Research Is Essential to Human Health

Frankie L. Trull

Frankie L. Trull *is president of the Foundation for Biomedical Research, a nonprofit educational organization dedicated to improving the quality of human and animal health by promoting public understanding and support of the ethical use of animals in scientific and medical research.*

Virtually every major medical advance of the last 100 years—from chemotherapy to bypass surgery, from organ transplantation to joint replacement—has depended on research with animals. Animal studies have provided the scientific knowledge that allows health care providers to improve the quality of life for humans and animals by preventing and treating diseases and disorders, and by easing pain and suffering.

Some people question animal research on the ground that data from animals cannot be extrapolated to humans. But physicians and scientists agree that the many similarities that exist provide the best insights into the complex systems of both humans and animals. Knowledge gained from animal research has contributed to a dramatically increased human life span, which has increased from 47 years in 1900 to more than 76.7 years in 1998. Much of this increase can be attributed to improved sanitation and better hygiene; the rest of this increased longevity is a result of health and medical advances made possible in part through animal research.

Research on animals has also led to countless treatments, techniques, and medical technologies. Animal research was indispensable in the development of immunization against many diseases, including polio, mumps, measles, diphtheria, rubella, and hepatitis. One million insulin-dependent diabetics survive today because of the discovery of insulin

and the study of diabetes using dogs, rabbits, rats, and mice. Organ transplantation, considered a dubious proposition just a few decades ago, has become commonplace because of research on mice, rats, rabbits, and dogs.

Animal research has contributed immeasurably to our understanding of tumors, and has led to the discoveries of most cancer treatments and therapies. Virtually all cardiovascular advances, including the heart-lung machine, the cardiac pacemaker, and the coronary bypass, could not have been possible without the use of animals. Other discoveries made possible through animal research include an understanding of DNA; X-rays; radiation therapy; hypertension; artificial hips, joints, and limbs; monoclonal antibodies; surgical dressings; ultrasound; the artificial heart; and the CAT scan.

Animal research will be essential to medical progress in the future as well. With the use of animals, researchers are gaining understanding into the cause of—and treatments for—AIDS, Alzheimer's disease, cystic fibrosis, sudden infant death syndrome, and cancer in the hopes that these problems can be eliminated. Although many nonanimal research models have been developed, no responsible scientist believes that the technology exists today or in the foreseeable future to conduct biological research without using animals.

Despite distortions and exaggerations put forth by those opposed to animal research, occurrences of poor animal care are extremely rare. Researchers care about the welfare of laboratory animals. Like everybody else, scientists don't want to see animals suffer or die. In fact, treating animals humanely is good science. Animals that are in poor health or under stress will provide inaccurate data.

Many people are under the false impression that laboratory animals are not protected by laws and regulations. In fact, many safeguards are in place to guarantee the welfare of animals used in research. A federal law, entitled the Animal Welfare Act, stipulates standards for care and treatment of laboratory animals, and the U.S. Public Health Service (PHS), the country's major source of funding for biomedical research, sets forth requirements with which research institutions must comply in order to qualify for grants for any biomedical research involving *any* kind of animal.

Both the Animal Welfare Act and the PHS animal welfare policy mandate review of all research by an animal care and use committee set up in each institution to ensure that laboratory animals are being used responsibly and cared for humanely. The committee, which must include one veterinarian and one person unaffiliated with the institution, has the power to reject any research proposal and stop projects if it believes proper standards are not being met.

Although animal research opponents portray the medical community as deeply divided over the merits of animal experimentation, the percentage of physicians opposed to animal research remains very small. A 1989 survey by the American Medical Association of a representative sample of all active physicians found that 99% believed animal research had contributed to medical progress, and 97% supported the continued use of animals for basic and clinical research.

The general public, when presented with the facts, has also been supportive of animal research. This support must not be allowed to erode through apathy or misconceptions. Should animal research be lost to the scientific community, the victims would be all people: our families, our neighbors, our fellow humans.

Vivisection: A Medieval Legacy

Elliot M. Katz

Vivisection, an outdated and extremely cruel form of biomedical research, is the purposeful burning, drugging, blinding, infecting, irradiating, poisoning, shocking, addicting, shooting, freezing, and traumatizing of healthy animals. In psychological studies, baby monkeys are separated from their mothers and driven insane; in smoking research, dogs have tobacco smoke forced into their lungs; in addiction studies, chimpanzees, monkeys, and dogs are addicted to cocaine, heroin, and amphetamines, then forced into convulsions and painful withdrawal symptoms; in vision research, kittens and monkeys are blinded; in spinal cord studies, kittens and cats have their spinal cords severed; in military research, cats, dogs, monkeys, goats, pigs, mice, and rats die slow, agonizing deaths after being exposed to deadly radiation, chemical, and biological agents.

Started at a time when the scientific community did not believe animals felt pain, vivisection has left a legacy of animal suffering of unimaginable proportions. Descartes, the father of vivisection, asserted that the cries of a laboratory animal had no more meaning than the metallic squeak of an overwound clock spring. Though the research community considers vivisection a "necessary evil," a growing number of scientists and health professionals see vivisection as simply *evil*.

As a veterinarian, I was taught that vivisection was essential to human health. My eyes were finally opened to the full horrors and futility of vivisection when years later, faculty members and campus veterinarians at the University of California informed me that animals were dying by the thousands from severe neglect and abuse; that vivisectors and campus officials were denying and concealing the abuses; and that experiments were conducted whose only benefit was to the school's finances and researchers' careers. I discovered that animal "care" committees, typically cited as assurance that animals are used responsibly, are in fact "rubber stamp" committees composed mostly of vivisectors who routinely approve each other's projects. Over the years, I have witnessed an ongoing pattern of university officials denying documented charges of misconduct, attempting instead to discredit critics of vivisection, ultimately defending even the most ludicrous and cruel experiments as necessary and humane.

I discovered that assertions by the biomedical community that vivisection is an essential and indispensable part of protecting the public's health are simply untrue. Vivisection can and should be ended. It is scientifically outdated and morally wrong. There is a plethora of modern biomedical technology that can be used to improve society's health without harming animals. The advent of sophisticated scanning technologies, including computerized tomography (CT), positron emission tomography (PET), and magnetic resonance imaging (MRI), has given scientists the ability to examine people and animals noninvasively. This technology has isolated abnormalities in the brains of patients with Alzheimer's disease, epilepsy, and autism, revolutionizing diagnosis and treatment of these diseases. Tissue and cell cultures are being increasingly used to screen cancer and AIDS drugs. Progress with AIDS has come from areas entirely unrelated to animal experimentation. Human skin cell cultures are used to test new products and drugs for toxicity and irritancy.

Why, then, is vivisection so entrenched and defended with an almost religious fervor? Dr. Murry Cohen summed it up when he stated, "Change is difficult for most people, but it is particularly painful for scientific and medical bureaucracies, which fight to maintain the status quo, especially if required change might imply admission of previously held incorrect ideas or flawed axioms." Vivisection continues today because of vested interests, habit, economics, and legal considerations, not for the real advancement of science and public health.

When presented with the facts, members of the public almost unanimously express their desire to see an end to the horrors of vivisection. Thousands of professionals like myself have reevaluated the sense, efficacy, and worth of vivisection and have formed or joined organizations working to end this outdated and cruel form of research. The ending of vivisection will lead to improved public health and restore to medicine and science much needed excellence and compassion for all beings, human and nonhuman alike.

Elliot M. Katz, *DVM (here with companion, Manco) is a graduate of the Cornell University School of Veterinary Medicine. He is president and founder of In Defense of Animals, a national animal rights organization.*

Sharpening Your Critical Thinking Skills

1. Summarize the main points of each author.
2. Do these authors use data or ethical, anecdote (stories or experiences) arguments to make their cases?
3. Do you have a view on this issue? What factors weigh most heavily in making up your mind?

Visit *Human Biology's* Internet site for links to web sites offering more information on this topic.

favor studies that have positive results, too. Researchers who write up a study that shows no effect, may have a difficult time publishing their results. Ultimately, the public—even the scientific community—is left with a false impression of reality.

One further note. Many nutrition studies rely on information gathered by recall. For example, recent studies on the effects of dietary fiber that showed that fiber (in cereals) was not effective in reducing cancer of the colon and rectum, relied on the ability of 80,000 nurses to estimate how much fiber they had eaten on a daily basis since 1980. A similar study of men yielded nearly identical results. Although the results may be valid, a far better research design would be one in which subjects are asked to record what they eat on a daily basis over a long period of time.

The fourth rule of critical thinking is: question the conclusions derived from facts. Surprisingly, even if an experiment is run correctly, there's no guarantee that the conclusions drawn from the results will be correct. How can that be? The answer may lie in bias, ignorance, and error. Bias refers to beliefs that taint the interpretation of results. Ignorance is a lack of full knowledge. This, in turn, may lead a scientist to misinterpret his or her results. Finally, error does occur, in spite of our best efforts.

Two questions should be asked when one analyzes the conclusions of an experiment: (1) Do the facts support the conclusions? and (2) Are there alternative conclusions? An example will illustrate the importance of these questions.

One of the earliest studies on lung cancer showed that people who consumed large quantities of table sugar (sucrose) had a higher incidence of lung cancer than those who ate moderate amounts. The researchers concluded that lung cancer was caused by sugar. Did the facts support this conclusion? A reexamination of the patients showed that the group with lung cancer had a noticeably higher percentage of smokers. It turns out that smokers consume more sugar. Thus, the association between sugar and lung cancer was false. Tobacco smoke was the culprit.

This example illustrates an important principle of biological and medical research: correlation does not necessarily mean causation. In other words, two factors that appear to be related (correlated) may, in fact, not be linked at all.

The fifth rule of critical thinking is: look for assumptions and biases. This rule is related to the previous rule, questioning conclusions, but is so important that it warrants closer examination. Biases and hidden assumptions are to thinking what cyanide is to food, a

poison. Unfortunately, biases and hidden assumptions run rampant in the media.

In many contemporary debates over a wide range of issues, proponents often present information that supports their point of view. This selective inclusion of supportive data and exclusion of contradictory information is often an expression of a hidden agenda. What often happens is that people make up their mind about an issue, then seek out information that supports their point of view. Several of the Scientific Discoveries boxes presented in this book illustrate the pervasive nature of biases and hidden assumptions.

The sixth rule of critical thinking is: question the source of the facts—that is, who is telling them. Closely related to the rule on assumptions and biases, this rule calls on us to learn about the people who performed various research studies or analyses. It calls on us to familiarize ourselves with the people taking various positions. Bias can influence both researchers and analysts. Be especially wary of political operatives. Their penchant for "putting a spin" on things often results in doctored truths. Scientists may also get carried away, making more of their results than they should. Furthermore, many colleges and universities have public relations and media departments that issue press releases when a researcher makes a startling finding. They, too, may "hype up" new findings. Notoriety gained by such publicity is good for the ego and may also enhance a researcher's ability to secure additional research funding. It's also good for the image and funding of the college or university.

Sometimes a study of the biographies of the people delivering the information is as instructive as an examination of their conclusions. An association with a partisan group may be a red flag, warning that bias may have influenced their conclusions. So, beware of "experts" who have a hidden agenda or such a narrow focus that they miss the big picture. So-called experts from industry who swear under oath to the safety of their product may be biased or even deceitful.

Also beware of people who may not know as much as you think they should. Although we think of physicians as experts on human health, most of them received little or no training in nutrition in medical school. Many medical students still graduate without a full understanding of the role of nutrition in preventing disease and promoting good health.

The seventh rule of critical thinking is: do not expect all of the answers. Although this rule may seem contradictory at first, and maybe a little absurd in a section that seeks to sharpen your thinking, remember that hard and fast answers are not always available in science.

As scientists work out the details, we must be patient and therefore comfortable with incomplete knowledge that produces uncertainty. Consider an example.

Many atmospheric scientists believe that the temperature of the Earth is warming as a result of the observed increase in carbon dioxide and other gaseous pollutants produced by modern society. These pollutants trap heat in the atmosphere, much like a blanket or the glass in a greenhouse. Many of these scientists have staked their reputation on global warming and cite an impressive body of information in support of their view. A few scientists disagree, however. They think that too many uncertainties exist to allow a firm conclusion. Thus, global warming may be an issue on which critical thinkers might reserve opinion, although evidence continues to mount in favor of those who claim that global warming truly is occurring.

The eighth rule of critical thinking requires us to examine the big picture. Many examples of this critical thinking rule exist. Health is one of those areas where a "big-picture" view is essential. Many illnesses, for instance, result from lifestyle. Stress, diet, exercise, smoking, and drinking, for instance, all impact our health. An individual suffering from constant colds may need to look at the big picture—his or her lifestyle—to find the cause. While it may be expedient to go to a doctor to get an antibiotic to combat a bacterial infection or a flu shot to prevent getting the flu, if one doesn't take steps to reduce stress and other unhealthy lifestyle factors, persistent illness could plague that person for years. The rule, then, is to be aware of events in their context.

The ninth rule of critical thinking is: look for multiple causes and effects. Be wary of dualistic thinking. The self-proclaimed "thinking man," *Homo sapiens,* exhibits remarkable intelligence. But as intelligent as our species is, we frequently succumb to simplistic thinking when analyzing problems and devising solutions.

In the 1970s, for example, one noted ecologist argued vigorously that the world's environmental problems stemmed from overpopulation—too many people for the available resources. Another equally notable scientist argued that the problems were due to technology and its by-product, pollution.

A more critical analysis of the environmental crisis shows that our problems are the result of many factors. Overpopulation and technology are but two of many. Inadequate laws and education must be factored into the equation. So must various psychological and cultural elements—for instance, our view of nature as something to overcome. Many more could be added to the list.

Critical thinking demands a broader view of cause and effect. Look at a variety of parameters when you assess problems. Avoid simplistic thinking by considering as many contributing factors as you can.

The tenth rule of critical thinking reminds us to watch for thought stoppers. Professor Ann Causey, a colleague of mine, reminds us of the ability of thought stoppers to inhibit critical thinking. Thought stoppers are words or phrases that cause us to temporarily suspend our critical faculties. They elicit an overwhelming emotional response or call upon myths and other half-truths that we've heard so often that we accept them blindly. In the political arena, we call this "putting a spin" on something.

If someone derails your thinking, stop for a moment or two to assess the situation. Have you been derailed by a half-truth, a myth, or an emotional roadblock that will fall apart upon closer scrutiny?

Finally, the eleventh rule of critical thinking is: understand your own biases, hidden assumptions, and areas of ignorance. So far, this discussion on critical thinking has concentrated on ways you can uncover mistakes in reasoning that other people make. But what about your own mistakes? What about your biases, hidden assumptions, and areas of ignorance that affect your ability to think critically? Are you blissfully going through life thinking everyone else has it wrong? Uncomfortable as it may be, it's essential to grapple with your own weaknesses. Only then can you become a truly critical thinker.

As you read this text, you will be presented with examples to help you sharpen your critical thinking skills. The Point/Counterpoints will help you practice these rules.

Summary

Health and Homeostasis: Life's Essential Balancing Act

1. Humans, like all other organisms, have evolved mechanisms that ensure relative internal constancy *(homeostasis)*. These homeostatic mechanisms are vital to survival and reproduction.

2. Homeostatic mechanisms exist at all levels of biological organization, from cells to organisms to ecosystems.

3. The health of all species and ecosystems is dependent on the functioning of homeostatic mechanisms. When these mechanisms break down, illnesses often result.

4. Human *health* has traditionally been defined as the absence of disease, but a broader definition of health is now emerging. Under this definition, good health implies a state of physical and mental well-being.

5. Physical well-being is characterized by an absence of disease or symptoms of disease, a lack of risk factors that lead to disease, and good physical fitness.

6. Mental health is also characterized by a lack of mental illness and a capacity to deal effectively with the normal stresses and strains of life.

7. Human health and the health of the many species that share this planet with us depend on a properly functioning, healthy ecosystem. Thus, alterations of the environment can have severe repercussions for all species, including humans.

Evolution: The Unity and Diversity of Life

8. The *theory of evolution* says that all life evolved from earlier forms. The process of evolution results in improvements in existing species—that is, modifications that make a species better suited to its environment. It may also lead to the formation of new species.

9. Evolution is responsible for the great diversity of life-forms. However, because the Earth's organisms evolved from early cells that arose over 3.5 billion years ago, all organisms, including humans, share many common characteristics. Thus, evolution is responsible for the unity of life as well. Items 10–16 list the common characteristics of all life-forms.

10. All organisms, including humans, are made up of cells.

11. All other organisms grow and maintain their complex organization by taking in chemicals and energy from the surroundings.

12. All living things house many chemical reactions. These reactions are collectively referred to as *metabolism.*

13. All organisms possess homeostatic mechanisms.

14. All organisms exhibit *irritability*—the capacity to perceive and respond to stimuli.

15. All organisms are capable of reproduction and growth.

16. All organisms are the product of evolutionary development and are subject to evolutionary change.

17. Although humans are similar to many other organisms, we also possess many unique abilities. One of the key differences is culture. In addition, not only can we humans plan for the future, but we also possess enormous abilities to reshape the Earth through ingenuity and technology. This, however, does not imply that humans are in any way superior to other forms, nor that we are separate from nature—just that we are unique.

Science, Critical Thinking, and Social Responsibility

18. *Science* is both a systematic method of discovery and a body of information about the world around us.

19. Scientists gather information and test ideas through the *scientific method.* The scientific method begins with observations and measurements, often made during experiments. Observations and measurements often lead to *hypotheses,* explanations of natural phenomena that can be tested in *experiments.* The results of experiments help scientists support or refute their hypotheses.

20. The body of scientific knowledge also contains *theories* or broad generalizations about the way the world works. Theories can change over time as new information becomes available.

21. Scientific discovery can influence ethics. New knowledge about our place in the biosphere, for example, may temper our current notions of human dominance and help people the world over to build a more sustainable relationship with nature.

22. *Critical thinking* is a useful tool in science and is best defined as careful analysis that helps us distinguish knowledge from beliefs or judgments.

23. Critical thinking provides a way to analyze issues and information. It requires that you first define an issue, then study the evidence.

24. Table 1-2 summarizes the critical thinking rules.

www.jbpub.com/humanbiology

Connect to this book's web site: www.jbpub.com/humanbiology
The site features eLearning, an online review area that provides quizzes, chapter outlines, and other tools to help you study for your class. You can also follow useful links for in-depth information, research the differing views in the Point/Counterpoints, or keep up on the latest environmental and health news.

Critical Thinking

Thinking Critically—Analysis

This analysis corresponds to the Thinking Critically scenario that was presented at the beginning of this chapter.

This experiment has several major flaws. First, the boy used chickens from two different farms, so the chickens could have been genetically dissimilar. Differences in genetics could have been responsible for the differences in cholesterol content in the eggs. Second, although differences were found in the cholesterol content of the eggs of the two groups, we don't know if they were statistically significant. Good statistical analysis is necessary to determine whether measured differences are substantial enough to be attributable to the treatment. Another problem is the small sample size. Before I donated any money to this new venture, I'd want to see it performed on a larger group of genetically similar chickens. The fourth problem is that no mention was made of the dif-ferences between the two feeds. A careful analysis is essential to solidify one's confidence.

Clearly, this simple experiment has some flaws, but there's an even larger problem that we haven't addressed yet—notably the underlying supposition that cholesterol in eggs raises blood cholesterol levels. As it turns out, the liver produces lots of cholesterol. It's responsible for most of the cholesterol floating around in our bloodstreams. Furthermore, recent studies have shown that eggs don't contain as much cholesterol as was once thought and that eating foods rich in saturated fat (like bacon) is linked to elevated cholesterol levels in your bloodstream. (You'll learn more about this in Chapter 5 on nutrition.) Because of these findings, the American Heart Association has raised its recommendation for egg consumption from three a week to one a day for healthy people. To control cholesterol, you're better off cutting back on foods that have a high content of saturated fat like hamburgers and bacon.

Test of Concepts

1. How would you define life?
2. In what ways are a rock and a living organism (for example, a bird) similar, and in what ways are they different?
3. Describe the concept of homeostasis. How does it apply to humans? How does it apply to ecosystems? Give examples from your experiences.
4. Using your critical thinking skills debate the statement "planet care is a form of self-care."
5. Using the definition of health and the list of healthy habits in Table 1-1, assess your own health. What areas need improvement?
6. In what ways are humans different from other animals? In what ways are they similar?
7. Describe the scientific method, and give some examples of how you have used it recently in your own life.
8. How do a hypothesis and a theory differ?
9. Can you think of an example in which a single group of animals (including humans) serves as an experimental group and a control group in the same experiment? If you can't, ask one of your campus biologists for some ideas.
10. List and discuss the critical thinking skills presented in this chapter.
    Which skills seem to be most important for the kind of thinking you normally do?
11. A graduate student injects 10 mice with a chemical commonly found in the environment and finds that all of his animals die within a few days. Eager to publish his results, the student comes to you, his adviser. What would you suggest the student do before publishing his results?
12. Given your knowledge of scientific method and critical thinking, make a list of reasons why scientists might disagree on a particular issue or research finding.

CHAPTER

The Chemistry of Life

2

Cholesterol crystal.

Thinking Critically

In 1971, Joseph Chatt and his
colleagues at the University of Sussex in England synthesized two compounds
with the same chemical formula. However, he found that the crystals formed by
one compound were sapphire-green; the crystals formed by the other were
bright green.

Chatt hypothesized that he had created two compounds that have the same
molecular weight and atomic composition but differ in chemical or physical
properties because the atoms are linked in different ways. But, when Chatt
subjected his compounds to X-ray analysis, which helps determine the structure
of molecules, he found that the atoms of his compounds were in the same
relative positions. The only difference appeared to be in the chemical bond
between two atoms (oxygen and molybdenum), which was longer in the bright
green compound than in the sapphire-green one.

Assuming that impurities are rare in single, well-formed crystals, Chatt's
group concluded that the color difference in the two compounds resulted from
differences in the length of a single bond, a phenomenon not previously
reported.

At first, Chatt's findings were discounted, because chemists believe that
molecular bonds have characteristic lengths. Most scientists concluded that his
experiments were flawed. Can you find any reason(s) in the above information
that might have led Chatt to an incorrect conclusion? ■

Surveys of public knowledge often prove to be embarrassing. In a poll of world geography a few years ago, for example, Americans from 18 to 24 years of age only scored tenth among industrial nations in their knowledge of simple geographic facts. Many Americans couldn't locate Egypt or Germany on a world map, and 14% of those polled couldn't locate the United States!

Nowhere is public lack of knowledge more blatant than in the field of chemistry. Considering the importance of chemistry to our lives, it is surprising how little most people know about it. Why is chemistry so important to us?

Chemistry is important, in part, because it has so many useful applications. In recent decades, thousands of new drugs have been developed by scientists. These chemicals have helped humankind combat a wide range of often deadly or debilitating diseases. One of the most notable examples is antibiotics. Not only have these chemicals reduced suffering, they have also greatly reduced mortality, especially among infants.

Advances in chemistry have also led to countless improvements in household products that make our lives safer. House paints are a case in point. At one time, most paints contained lead-based pigments. Because lead is toxic to the nervous system, chips of paint flaking off walls and ceilings pose a health hazard to young children, who routinely put foreign objects in their mouths as they explore their new world. Modern paints lacking lead-based pigments are a definite improvement.

The truth of the matter is that almost everything we touch or look at in our daily lives has been brought to us or improved by chemists. But chemistry is also important in other ways. A little knowledge of chemistry, for example, can help us understand environmental problems such as ozone depletion, urban air pollution, and acid rain. Closer to home, it can help us determine which solvent to use to remove dirt or stains from carpets. On a more personal level, a knowledge of chemistry helps people who want to live long, healthy lives make informed decisions on diet.

But why study chemistry at the beginning of a biology course? The answer is simple. First, cells and organisms are made up of chemicals. These chemicals undergo many reactions that are the basis of life. In order to understand the structure and function of cells and organisms, you must understand some basic principles of chemistry.

This chapter introduces you to several key principles of chemistry, most of which form the foundation for the study of modern biology. We begin with a discussion of atoms and molecules, then look at water, acids, bases, and buffers. This information could prove useful to you throughout your life. The major biological molecules encountered in the study of biology are discussed in subsequent chapters.

Section 2-1

Atoms and Subatomic Particles

The world in which we live is composed of a wide variety of physical matter such as wood, water, plastic, metal, and air. **Matter** is defined as anything that has mass and occupies space. Technically, **mass** is a measure of the amount of matter in an object. Thus, a water balloon has a greater mass than an air-filled balloon, as anyone who has ever been hit by the former will tell you.

Atoms Are the Fundamental Unit of All Matter

Matter is composed of tiny particles called **atoms.** The word *atom* comes from the Greek *atomos,* which means "incapable of division." The ancient Greek philosophers who proposed the existence of atoms believed that all matter consisted of small particles that lacked any internal structure. Over time, though, evidence has shown that atoms consist of smaller particles, called **subatomic particles.** In this chapter, we will examine three of the most important subatomic particles: electrons, protons, and neutrons (**FIGURE 2-1**). **Protons** (PRO-tauns) have the greatest mass of all and are located in the center of the atom, the **nucleus** (**FIGURE 2-1**). Each proton has a positive charge. **Neutrons** (NEW-trauns) are uncharged particles with slightly less mass than protons. Like protons they are also found in the nucleus. Because protons are positively charged and neutrons have no charge, the nucleus of an atom is positively charged.

FIGURE 2-1 The Atom The atom consists of two regions. The central nucleus contains protons and neutrons and makes up 99.9% of the mass. Surrounding the nucleus is the electron cloud, where the electrons spin furiously around the nucleus. (Figure not drawn to scale.)

Surrounding the positively charged nucleus is a region called the **electron cloud.** It contains tiny, negatively charged particles, **electrons** (ee-LECK-trauns), that move rapidly through a large volume of space.

Most of the mass of an atom can be attributed to the protons and neutrons, which are packed into a tiny space. These particles are so heavy that a single cubic centimeter (about $\frac{1}{3}$ teaspoon) would weigh 100 million tons. However, most of the volume of an atom is composed of the electron cloud. Consequently, the late Carl Sagan, one of America's leading astronomers, remarked that atoms are mostly space, or "electron fluff."

Atoms are electrically neutral because they contain the same number of protons and electrons. Thus, the positive charges cancel out the negative ones.

The Elements Are the Purest Form of Matter

Early scientists accounted for the diversity of matter by assuming that there must exist a number of pure substances and that these substances could be combined into an infinite variety of different forms. They called these pure substances *elements*. Today, modern chemists define an **element** as a pure substance (for example, gold or lead) that contains only one type of atom. Put another way, elements are substances that cannot be separated into different substances by ordinary chemical means.

At this writing, 92 naturally occurring elements are known. Another dozen or so can be made in the laboratory. Of the 92 naturally occurring elements, only about 20 are found in organisms. Four elements in this group: carbon, oxygen, hydrogen, and nitrogen (remember: COHN) comprise 98% of the atoms of all living things.

Elements are listed on a chart called the **periodic table of elements** (**TABLE 2-1**; Appendix A). The periodic table is a handy summary of vital statistics on each element. As illustrated in **TABLE 2-1**, most elements are represented on the table by a one- or two-letter symbol. The element hydrogen, for example, is indicated by H. Oxygen is designated by O, and carbon is represented by C.

Above each symbol on the periodic table is its atomic number. The **atomic number** of an element is the number of protons found in the nuclei of the element's atoms. Because all atoms are electrically neutral, the atomic number also equals the number of electrons in the atoms.

As you can see, below the chemical symbol for each element is another number, called the mass number. The **mass number** is the average mass of the atoms of

---

TABLE 2-1

A Simplified Periodic Table

I	II	III	IV	V	VI	VII	VIII
1 ← Atomic number H ← Atomic symbol Hydrogen 1.0 ← Mass number							2 He Helium 4.0
3 Li Lithium 7.0	4 Be Beryllium 9.0	5 B Boron 11.0	6 C Carbon 12.0	7 N Nitrogen 14.0	8 O Oxygen 16.0	9 F Fluorine 19.0	10 Ne Neon 20.2
11 Na Sodium 23.0	12 Mg Magnesium 24.3	13 Al Aluminum 27.0	14 Si Silicon 28.1	15 P Phosphorus 31.0	16 S Sulfur 32.1	17 Cl Chlorine 35.5	18 Ar Argon 40.0
19 K Potassium 39.1	20 Ca Calcium 40.1						

Note that each element is represented by a one- or two-letter symbol. Elements are listed according to their atomic number (the number of protons). Their atomic mass is also shown.

each element. The mass number is approximately equal to the number of protons and neutrons in a given atom. Because electrons have virtually no mass, they contribute very little to the mass of an atom. As shown in **TABLE 2-1**, carbon has an atomic mass of 12.

Isotopes Are Alternative Forms of Atoms, Differing in the Number of Neutrons They Contain

Although I just said that elements are made of identical atoms, I was stretching the truth a little. Fact is, there are very slight differences in some of the atoms of a given element. In fact, most elements are made up of mixtures of two or more variants of the same atom, which are called **isotopes** (EYE-so-topes). Isotopes differ only in the number of neutrons they contain. This doesn't not affect the atom very much. For instance, it does not change its chemical reactivity. Hydrogen, for example, has three slightly different atomic forms. The most common hydrogen atom contains one proton, one electron, and no neutrons. The next most common form has one proton, one electron, and one neutron. The least common hydrogen atom has one proton, one electron, but two neutrons. The three forms, or isotopes, of hydrogen are chemically identical—that is, they react the same.

Additional neutrons don't change the chemical nature of the atom, they just make some atoms of an element slightly heavier than others. It also makes some atoms a bit unstable. To achieve a more stable state, many isotopes release **radiation**—small bursts of energy, or tiny energetic particles—from their nuclei. Radiation carries away energy and mass from an atom's nucleus and helps atoms achieve more stable states. Radioactive isotopes are called **radionuclides** (ray-dee-oh-NEW-klides).

Radiation has provided numerous benefits to humankind. For example, scientists have discovered a wide variety of uses for radiation in medicine and research, including X-rays and radioactive chemicals used in medical tests. One of the most important advancements is the use of radioactive isotopes as markers in experiments (Scientific Discoveries 2-1). Another extremely important application is the use of naturally occurring radioactive isotopes to date rocks and fossils. Information from this technique has helped scientists pinpoint important evolutionary events and has given us important insights into the history of life on Earth.

Despite the many benefits of radiation, its use has not occurred without some risks. For example, radiation exposure damages molecules in body cells and

causes changes (mutations) in the genetic material that can result in birth defects and cancer. Despite these and other problems, radiation is widely used. It is now even being used to sterilize foods, thus eliminating the need to refrigerate foods. The Point/Counterpoint in this chapter examines the pros and cons of this procedure.

The Making of a Molecule

The diversity of matter in the world around us is, as noted above, a result of the presence of a wide range of elements, each with its own unique properties. It also arises from the fact that atoms of various elements can combine to form compounds and molecules. The term **compound** refers to a substance made up of two or more atoms. Each compound has a unique chemical formula that indicates the ratio of atoms found in it. For instance, HCl is the chemical formula of hydrochloric acid. It contains one hydrogen atom and one chlorine atom. The chemical formula of the flammable gas methane is CH_4; it contains one carbon atom for every four hydrogen atoms.

The term **molecule** refers to the smallest particle of a compound that still retains the properties of that compound. Methane gas given off by rotting vegetation, for instance, is a chemical compound consisting of methane molecules. Hydrogen gas is a chemical compound consisting of hydrogen molecules, each one of which contains two hydrogen atoms.

Atoms Bond to Form More Stable Configurations

Atoms in molecules are joined together by chemical bonds. There are two types of bonds that form *between* atoms: ionic and covalent. In both instances, the electrons are responsible for creating the bonds that hold atoms together.

Ionic Bonds Are Electrostatic Attractions Between Two Oppositely Charged Particles

Ionic bonds are formed when two atoms react in such a way that electrons are transferred from one atom to another. This creates two charged particles, or **ions** (EYE-ons). The atom that loses its electron becomes positively charged, and the one that gains an electron is negatively charged. This exchange results in the formation of a weak electrostatic force between the two charged particles. This force holds them together and is referred to as an *ionic bond*. **FIGURE 2-2** shows how an ionic bond forms between a chlorine atom and a sodium atom.

Scientific Discoveries that Changed the World 2-1

The Discovery of Radioactive Chemical Markers

Featuring the Work of Schoenheimer

Biochemist Rudolf Schoenheimer (1898–1941) and his colleagues offered science a chemical tool that would yield important new information and result in significant scientific and medical advances: radioactively labeled molecules—that is, common biological molecules containing one or more radioactive atoms (isotopes).

A radioactive atom incorporated in a biological molecule is akin to a radiotransmitter collar on a grizzly bear. The atom emits tiny bursts of radioactivity, which permit scientists to track molecules on their course

through the body, in much the same way that the collar emits radio signals that allow biologists to electronically track the bear through its forbidding terrain.

Marking common molecules like amino acids with radioactive atoms permits scientists not just to track molecules but to follow what happens to them along the way. Before the emergence of this technique, substances such as fatty acids or amino acids administered to an animal were lost almost immediately, because they were indistinguishable from molecules in the body.

Radioactive markers permit scientists to follow marked molecules as they progress through the body's maze of biochemical reactions. Radioactive markers also permit scientists to determine where chemicals are stored and how they are removed from the body. In fact, many of the physiological processes you will read about in this book were investigated by using radioactively labeled molecules.

Before Schoenheimer's discovery, the inability to track molecules resulted in a huge gap in our knowledge about metabolism and other

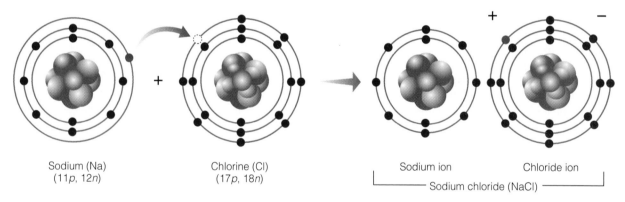

Sodium (Na)   Chlorine (Cl)   Sodium ion   Chloride ion
(11*p*, 12*n*)   (17*p*, 18*n*)
                                            └──── Sodium chloride (NaCl) ────┘

FIGURE 2-2 Ions and Ionic Bonds   Sodium (Na) and chlorine (Cl) atoms differ in their electron affinity. Sodium has a weaker affinity and tends to give up an electron to atoms like chlorine. As a result, sodium becomes a positively charged ion and chlorine a negatively charged ion. The oppositely charged ions attract each other, forming an ionic bond.

Covalent Bonds Are Formed by the Sharing of Electrons Between Atoms

In contrast to ionic bonds, covalent bonds occur when two atoms "share" electrons. This arrangement usually produces a much stronger bond. When atoms are bound by covalent bonds, the electrons they share actually orbit around both atoms. This holds the atoms together. **FIGURE 2-3** illustrates the formation of hydrogen gas, H_2, from two hydrogen atoms.

Consider methane (CH_4), a gas that consists of four hydrogen atoms covalently bonded to one carbon atom.

H atom   H atom H_2 molecule

(a)   (b)

FIGURE 2-3 Covalent Bond   Nonpolar covalent bonds are characterized by a sharing of electrons. *(a)* The shaded regions represent the hydrogen atoms' electron clouds. *(b)* Two atoms bound together by a covalent bond. The electrons orbit around both nuclei, holding them together to create a molecule.

body functions. Futile attempts to "tag" molecules with nonradioactive molecular markers generally failed, because the altered molecules differed so much from their natural substances that they were treated differently by the body.

Through experimentation, Schoenheimer showed that radioactively labeled molecules were so similar to the unlabeled molecule that they reacted identically. This made them ideal markers and opened the door to many additional discoveries.

From Schoenheimer's brilliant experiments, a new picture of life has emerged. He and his colleagues showed that molecules of the body such as DNA, which had previously been considered stable, are actually in a continuous state of flux. Even apparently dormant fat deposits in the body were ever-changing. Additional studies eventually showed that amino acids were rapidly broken down and rebuilt into new ones.

Since their introduction in the 1930s, radioactive markers have also enjoyed great popularity in medicine where they're often used to determine the functional status of various organs. Radioactive iodide ions, for instance, can be administered to a patient to assess the function of the thyroid gland, a hormone-producing gland in the neck.

Radioactively labeled molecules are helping scientists unravel the mysteries of body functions. Labeled glucose molecules, for instance, can be used to determine the relative activity of different parts of the brain, permitting scientists to map brain functions accurately.

These are but a few examples of the tremendous contribution of radioactively labeled molecules to medicine and science.

To understand how this molecule forms, we turn first to the central atom, carbon.

Carbon atoms have six electrons, two in a region or *shell* close to the nucleus and four in an outer shell. Carbon reacts with four hydrogen atoms to form methane. This arrangement results in a full outer shell containing eight electrons.

Many other atoms react similarly, filling the outer shell during covalent bonding. When filled, the outer shell of many atoms contains 8 electrons. Thus, chemists have coined the term **octet rule** (meaning a group of eight) to explain this behavior. You can use it to predict how atoms will react.

Covalent bonding can be represented by using dots and Xs for the outer-shell electrons of an atom. **FIGURE 2-4** uses this technique to show the electron sharing in a molecule of methane. In this example, carbon is represented by the letter C surrounded by four outer-shell electrons, indicated by dots. Each hydrogen atom is represented by H, and the outer-shell electron of each hydrogen atom is indicated by an X. As illustrated, each hydrogen atom shares its electron with the carbon atom, giving the carbon atom four additional electrons and thus creating a full outer shell for carbon. The shell contains 8 electrons.

Another important molecule is water, H_2O. As the formula indicates, a water molecule consists of a single atom of oxygen bonded to two atoms of hydrogen. Oxygen atoms contain eight electrons, two in the inner shell and six in the outer shell. By combining with two hydrogen atoms, oxygen fills its outer shell.

The bonds between carbon and hydrogen in methane and oxygen and hydrogen in water involve the sharing of one pair of electrons—one from each atom. These bonds are referred to as **single covalent bonds.** In chemical nomenclature, they are often indicated by a single line joining two atoms, as in H–H.

Some atoms share two pairs of electrons with another atom, forming **double covalent bonds.** Oxygen, for instance, can share two of its outer-shell electrons with a carbon atom, forming a double covalent bond (C=O), as shown in **FIGURE 2-5** (page 32). Other atoms can share three pairs of electrons, forming triple covalent bonds (**FIGURE 2-5**).

FIGURE 2-4 Covalent Bonding Simplified You can keep track of the electrons being shared in covalent bonds by representing the outer-shell electrons as dots or Xs. See the text for explanation.

Point/Counterpoint

Controversy over Food Irradiation

Food Irradiation: Too Many Questions
Donald B. Louria, MD

Donald B. Louria, MD *teaches at the UMDNJ-New Jersey Medical School, where he is Chairman Emeritus of the Department of Preventive Medicine and Community Health.*

The debate about the safety of irradiating foods raises six issues:

1. The safety issue. Irradiated food does not become radioactive, but the radiation does cause chemical changes in food molecules. The major concerns are genetic damage in those consuming the foods and nutrient loss after irradiation.

A highly controversial, but flawed, study on small numbers of malnourished children in India suggested that consumption of freshly irradiated wheat could produce chromosomal abnormalities. However, a study of a much larger group of healthy adults in China showed no such abnormalities. The proponents of food irradiation have criticized the Indian study and pointed to the larger study they feel showed no chromosome damage. But, that does not answer the concerns. If food irradiation becomes an accepted technique, millions of malnourished people will eat irradiated foods. What is needed is a careful study of possible genetic damage involving adequate numbers of children and adults. I am prepared to believe that consumption of irradiated foods is unlikely to produce significant harm, but such a belief must be supported by proper data.

2. The nutrition issue. Irradiated food loses some of its nutritional value; the extent of loss of vitamin content depends on the type of food and the dose of radiation—the higher the radiation dose, the greater the loss. Irradiation proponents suggest the effects of irradiation on vitamin content are not different from that of conventional food processing (such as heating). But, some evidence suggests that, when irradiated foods are processed (frozen, thawed, heated), there is an accelerated loss of vitamins. Furthermore, some foods that would be irradiated (fruits, vegetables) are eaten raw so the arguments about heating would not apply. Proponents also maintain that the diet in the United States contains redundant vitamins, so some loss through irradiation would not be of concern. Of course, this would not be true for millions of people in other countries, as well as those below the poverty line in the United States and those over age 60 who often have low blood vitamin concentrations.

Arguing that our diet contains adequate vitamins and that destroying the vitamin content of foods by irradiation is of no importance is not likely to be viewed well by many Americans.

3. The necessity for this technology. Proponents say food irradiation will reduce diarrheal illnesses. That is true, but the potential benefits have been exaggerated. There are 200 million diarrheal episodes a year in the United States; of these, only about one-third are food borne and, in most cases, the cause is unknown so food irradiation is not the answer to diarrheal disease in the United States. But, it would reduce substantially diarrheal illnesses due to several bacteria (salmonella, listeria, and E. coli). Proper cooking procedures are just as effective as food irradiation and that, combined with more intensive surveillance of food production and distribution, reduces the need to use irradiation.

4. Helping to solve world hunger. Will irradiating foods prolong their shelf lives and thus, feed the world? Shelf lives will definitely be increased; that is an important benefit for the less-developed world, but the proponents have provided no adequate data on the extent of the benefit. If the trade-off is longer shelf life, but less nutritious foods, that would be unacceptable to many people.

5. The issue of competing technologies. During the next decades, scientists will develop foods that have longer shelf lives and are more nutritious. Advances in biotechnology are likely to give us useful alternatives to food irradiation. Other technologic advances will greatly improve our ability to detect microbial contamination of foods before they are allowed to reach the marketplace.

6. The environmental pollution issue. Food irradiation is a technology that will result in numerous irradiation plants in the United States. The few irradiation plants operating in the United States have, in some cases, contaminated their workers and the environment. Imagine the potential for contamination if there were hundreds of such plants using radioactive materials.

Food irradiation does have potential benefits, but it also raises substantial concerns. Whether we should adopt the technology is obviously a matter for continuing debate. Certainly, the technology should not be adopted until the issue of potential genetic damage has been resolved and there is agreement that the public will always be informed not only that a given food has been irradiated, but also the extent, if any, of nutritional damage.

Food Irradiation: Safe and Sound

George G. Giddings

Irradiated foods are safe and wholesome. The ionizing radiation process applied to foods offers certain proven public health and economic benefits without significant public health risks when carried out according to well-established principles and procedures. Decades of worldwide research and testing by competent, knowledgeable, objective, and responsible scientists have led to this conclusion. This conclusion is also supported by some 30 years of experience in the radiation sterilization of medical devices and other health care products to prevent infections, plus a growing list of industrial and consumer products, including foods and their raw materials, ingredients, and packaging materials. The technology is so pollution-free that the EPA exempts it from environmental impact statements.

There has been organized political opposition to food irradiation by a network of special-interest activists serving various political agendas, notably the antinuclear/anti-irradiation one. This network includes a handful of scientists and medical professionals from other fields who act as "expert witnesses" against food irradiation to serve their hidden agendas. For example, they still point to an old Indian study on irradiated wheat and a few children as suggestive of risk even though it was dismissed in the mid-1970s. Opponents point to minor losses of certain vitamins where in fact irradiation is gentler towards vitamins and other nutrients than

comparable food processes and even cooking. Their campaign is doomed to failure in the face of the unshakable facts, including a growing appreciation for public health and other proven benefits of food irradiation, and its growing worldwide regulatory approval, industrial usage, and public acceptance. The American Medical Association and World Health Organization are among the many professional bodies that have endorsed food irradiation.

Food irradiation is undoubtedly the most versatile physical process yet applied to food substances in terms of the range and variety of objectives it can accomplish. Radiation can

- inhibit the sprouting of foods, such as potatoes and onions, and delay spoilage
- rid fruits, vegetables, and grains of insect pests
- prevent parasites from infecting consumers of fish and meats
- rid foods of microbial pathogens such as the salmonellae
- delay microbial spoilage of a wide variety of animal and plant products by reducing microbe levels
- sterilize packaging materials, eliminating microorganisms that would otherwise contaminate products
- sterilize a wide variety of prepared or cooked foods such as meat, poultry, and fishery products, which have already been used to feed astronauts in space and immune-compromised patients

All of these beneficial effects and more can be, and are, being readily accomplished by the application of

ionizing (gamma, electron, and X-ray) radiation according to well-established principles and procedures. Nevertheless, irradiation must compete with a number of other new technologies. As a result, it is not likely to be applied to all, or even a high percentage, of the national and world food supply. It will therefore be used in cases in which it is clearly the best all-around choice.

George G. Giddings, Ph. D., *has been involved in food irradiation research and development since 1963 and has written and spoken extensively on the subject.*

Sharpening Your Critical Thinking Skills

1. What is food irradiation? Why is it used?
2. List and summarize the key points of each author.
3. Using your critical thinking skills, analyze each author's position. Are you inclined to agree with either one on all issues? Why or why not?
4. In your opinion, what is the best course for the development and implementation of this technology?
5. What facts would you need to know to form a personal conclusion about this issue?

Visit *Human Biology's* Internet site for links to web sites offering more information on this topic.

Structural formula	Lewis dot formula
O ‖ C	xx x O x xx •• • C • Oxygen has six electrons (x) in its outer shell; it shares two of its electrons with carbon. Carbon has four electrons (•) in its outer shell; it shares two of its electrons with oxygen.

(a) Double covalent bond

Structural formula	Lewis dot formula
—C≡C—	x • C x C • x Each carbon atom shares three of its electrons.

(b) Triple covalent bond

FIGURE 2-5 Double and Triple Covalent Bonds *(a)* When atoms share two pairs of electrons, a double covalent bond is formed. Chemists have devised several ways to draw these bonds. In the formula on the left, each line represents a pair of shared electrons. On the right, electrons are indicated by Xs and dots. *(b)* On rare occasions, atoms share three pairs of electrons, creating triple covalent bonds.

Polar Covalent Bonds Occur Any Time There Is an Unequal Sharing of Electrons by Two Atoms

The electrons shared between two atoms in a covalent bond are not always shared equally. Unequal sharing occurs when one of the two atoms has a slightly higher affinity (attraction) for electrons than the other. For example, oxygen and hydrogen join to form a single covalent bond, but oxygen has a slightly higher affinity for electrons than hydrogen. Consequently, the electron of the hydrogen atom tends to spend more time around the oxygen atom than around the hydrogen atom. Because of this, the oxygen atom has a slightly negative charge. The hydrogen atom is visited less frequently by the electron and has a slightly positive charge (**FIGURE 2-6A**).

FIGURE 2-6 Hydrogen Bonding *(a)* Slightly unequal sharing of electrons in the water molecule creates a polar molecule. Electrons tend to spend more time around the oxygen nucleus, making it slightly negative. The hydrogen atoms are, therefore, slightly positive, as indicated by the symbols δ+. *(b)* Because of the polarity, hydrogen atoms of one molecule are attracted to oxygen atoms of another. The attraction is called a hydrogen bond.

The result is a **polar covalent bond.** A polar covalent bond is a covalent bond whose atoms bear a slight charge—either positive or negative.

The presence of polar covalent bonds in molecules makes entire molecules polar. This, in turn, has profound implications to life on Earth, as you will soon see. Consider one of the most important of all polar molecules, water.

As **FIGURE 2-6A** illustrates, water contains two polar covalent bonds and, therefore, has three slightly charged atoms. The slightly charged atoms are often attracted to oppositely charged atoms on *neighboring* molecules (**FIGURE 2-6B**).

Polar molecules are also formed when hydrogen atoms covalently bond to atoms such as nitrogen and fluorine, which, like oxygen, have a slightly higher affinity for electrons than hydrogen.

Hydrogen Bonds Form Between Slightly Charged Atoms Usually on Different Molecules

Covalent bonds occur between atoms of a molecule. They are the bonds that hold the atoms together. But neighboring molecules can also be attracted to one another, thanks to the presence of polar covalent bonds in them. Take water for an example. In a glass of water, positively charged hydrogen atoms of water molecules attract negatively charged oxygen atoms of other water molecules. The electrostatic attractions *between* the positively charged hydro-

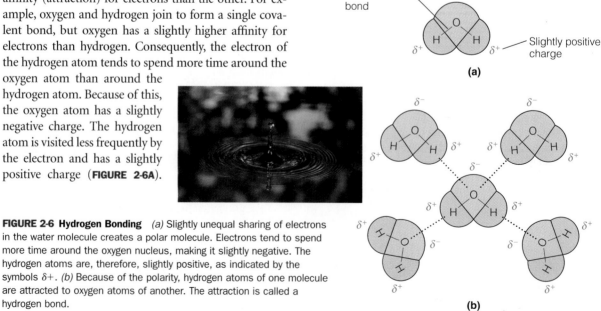

TABLE 2-2	
Comparison of Organic and Inorganic Compounds	
Organic	**Inorganic**
Consists primarily of molecules containing carbon and hydrogen	Usually consists of positively and negatively charged ions
Atoms linked by covalent bonds	Usually consists of atoms joined by ionic bonds
Often consists of large molecules that contain many atoms	Always contains small numbers of atoms

gen atoms of *one* water molecule and the negatively charged oxygen atoms of *another* are called **hydrogen bonds.** This is an electrostatic attraction responsible for many of the unique properties of water and absolutely essential to life on Earth (discussed later). Hydrogen bonds are also found in other biologically important molecules that will be discussed in subsequent chapters.

Chemical Compounds Fall into Two Broad Groups: Organic and Inorganic

Chemists classify compounds as either organic or inorganic. **Organic compounds** contain molecules that are made primarily of carbon atoms. Many organic molecules are quite large. That's because carbon atoms can be joined to one another like the beads of a necklace. These long chains of carbon atoms form the "backbone" of many organic compounds. Attached to the backbone are a number of other atoms, most often hydrogen, oxygen, and nitrogen. In organic molecules, all atoms are covalently linked.

Inorganic compounds are defined primarily by exclusion—

FIGURE 2-7 Perspiration Cools the Body Perspiration is an automatic homeostatic response that helps rid the body of heat.

that is, they are compounds that are *not* organic. Inorganic molecules are generally small molecules. They usually consist of atoms joined by ionic bonds, as opposed to organic compounds, which are always covalently bonded. Sodium chloride and magnesium chloride are examples of inorganic compounds.

As you will see in the study of biology, not all rules apply 100% of the time. In this instance, not all inorganic compounds contain ionic bonds. Water, for example, is an inorganic compound whose atoms are joined by covalent bonds. **TABLE 2-2** summarizes the main features of each type of compound.

Section 2-3

Water, Acids, Bases, and Buffers

Now that you've learned a few basics of chemistry, let's look at water, a biologically important molecule.

Water Is Vital to Life

Scientific historian and naturalist Loren Eiseley once wrote that "if there is magic on the planet, it has to be water." This remarkable substance produces billowy clouds, icicles that hang from the limbs of trees, and elegant waterfalls. Aesthetically pleasing as water is, though, it is also of great practical importance to humans and all other living organisms.

Water is a major component of all cells and organisms. In fact, nearly two-thirds of the human body is water. Thus, if you weigh 100 pounds, nearly 70 pounds of your body weight is water. Water is an important biological **solvent,** a fluid that dissolves other chemical substances. Human blood, for example, contains large amounts of water that dissolve and transport nutrients, hormones, and wastes throughout our bodies.

Water also participates in many chemical reactions in the body—for example, in the breakdown of protein (described later). In addition, water serves as a lubricant. Saliva, which is largely water, lubricates food in the mouth and esophagus, the tube that transports food from our mouths to our stomachs. A watery fluid in the joints called *synovial fluid* enables bones to slide over one another, thus facilitating body motion.

Finally, water helps us regulate body temperature. Perspiration, for example, rids our bodies of heat, for when it evaporates, water draws off heat (**FIGURE 2-7**). People sometimes suffer heatstroke in hot humid climates because the excess water in the atmosphere reduces evaporation. This causes heat to build up, which can cause a person to collapse.

Water Molecules Dissociate into Hydrogen and Hydroxide Ions

Water molecules are fairly stable; nonetheless, some molecules break apart, forming two charged units known as ions as shown in the following reaction:

$$H_2O \rightleftharpoons H^+ + OH^-$$

water   hydrogen ion   hydroxide ion

Because the hydrogen and hydroxide ions formed in this reaction can react with one another to re-form water molecules, this reaction is said to be *reversible*. The double arrow in the reaction formula indicates that it is reversible.

Although water can dissociate, the ratio of water molecules to the ions, H^+ and OH^-, in the human body is about 500 million:1. Nevertheless, even the slightest change in the hydrogen ion concentration can alter cells and organisms, shutting down biochemical pathways and sometimes killing organisms. It is not surprising, then, that the human body contains a number of homeostatic mechanisms to ensure a constant level of these ions.

Acids Are Substances That Add Hydrogen Ions to Solution; Bases Remove Hydrogen Ions

In pure water, the concentrations of H^+ and OH^- ions are equal.[1] A solution containing an equal number of these ions is said to be *chemically neutral*.

Chemical neutrality can be upset by adding or removing H^+ or OH^-. For example, when added to water, hydrochloric acid (HCl) dissociates into hydrogen ions (H^+) and chloride ions (Cl^-). This substance, therefore, increases the hydrogen ion concentration. Scientists call a substance that adds hydrogen ions to a solution an **acid.** Solutions with proportionately more H^+ than OH^- are said to be acidic. **Bases** are substances that remove H^+ from solution. Sodium hydroxide, for example, dissociates when added to aqueous solutions, forming Na^+ and OH^-. The hydroxide ions react with hydrogen ions in the solution, forming water molecules. As sodium hydroxide is added to a solution of pure water, the hydrogen ion concentration declines, and the hydroxide ion concentration increases. A solution with a greater concentration of OH^- than H^+ ions is said to be *basic*.

Acidity is measured on the **pH scale** (**FIGURE 2-8**). As illustrated, the pH scale ranges from 0 to 14. Neutral substances are assigned a pH of 7. Basic substances have a pH greater than 7, and acidic substances have a pH less than 7.

The pH scale is logarithmic (law-gah-RITH-mick). This means that the pH scale mathematically condenses a wide range of numbers onto a fairly small scale. The lesson in all of this is: Don't be fooled by a small change in pH. One pH unit represents a tenfold change in acidity. Accordingly, a solution with a pH of 3 is 10 times more acidic than one with a pH of 4 and 100 times more acidic than one with a pH of 5.

Most biochemical reactions occur at pH values between 6 and 8. Human blood, for example, has a pH of 7.4. So important is this to normal body function that a slight shift in the pH of the blood for even a short period can be fatal. Fortunately, evolution has "provided" us with numerous homeostatic systems that maintain required pHs in the body.

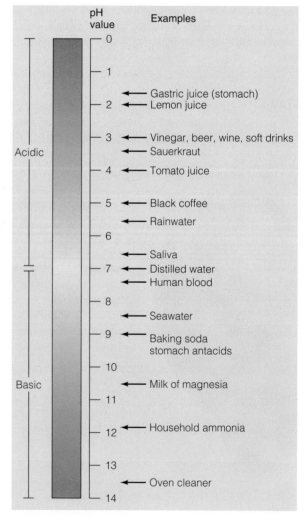

FIGURE 2-8 The pH Scale

---

[1]Concentration is the amount of solute (dissolved substance) in a given amount of solvent (usually water).

Homeostasis Is Ensured in Part by Buffers, Molecules That Help Maintain pH within a Narrow Range

Biological systems operate within a narrow pH range maintained by a relatively simple homeostatic mechanism created by buffers. **Buffers** (BUFF-firs) are chemicals found in organisms and ecosystems, particularly soil and water, that protect against drastic shifts in pH. How do they work?

Buffers can be likened to "hydrogen-ion sponges." They help maintain a constant pH by removing hydrogen ions from solution when levels increase. Buffers give back the hydrogen ions when levels fall.

One of the most prevalent of all buffers is carbonic acid. Found in the blood of animals, carbonic acid is formed from water and carbon dioxide, a waste product of cellular energy production. In blood, carbonic acid dissociates into bicarbonate and hydrogen ions:

$$H_2CO_3 \rightleftharpoons H^+ + HCO_3^-$$

carbonic acid   hydrogen ion   bicarbonate
(weak acid)   (weak base)

In our blood and in lakes and rivers where carbonic acid is also present, this chemical reaction shifts back and forth in response to changing levels of hydrogen ions. Thus, when hydrogen ions are added to water, they combine with bicarbonate ions, driving the reaction to the left. But when the hydrogen-ion concentration falls, the reaction is driven to the right. In either case, the pH of the blood remains constant.

Section 2-4
Overview of Other Biologically Important Molecules

This introduction to chemistry is intended to give you a foundation upon which to add to your chemical literacy. In your study of biology, you will encounter chemistry terms and many chemical compounds. Your studies will reveal four major groups of biological molecules: (1) carbohydrates; (2) lipids; (3) amino acids, peptides, and proteins; and (4) nucleic acids. Rather than describe each one in detail here, I will present a few important facts. These molecules are discussed in more detail in subsequent chapters.

Carbohydrates are organic molecules that range in size from very small molecules such as the blood sugar glucose, which cells use to generate energy, to very large ones such as starch. The large molecules are actually composed of many small molecules. Carbohydrates supply energy to cells. Pastas and cereals are a great source of carbohydrates.

Lipids (LIP-ids) are a rather diverse group of molecules that includes fats and steroids such as cholesterol. Some lipids are a source of energy and others are important structural components of cells. Lipids form a layer of insulation beneath the skin of many animals, including whales and humans. Lipids are found in many foods, especially meat, nuts, fried foods such as french fries, and numerous snack foods such as potato chips.

Most readers have heard the terms *amino acids, proteins, and peptides*. **Proteins** are long molecules (polymers) consisting of many smaller molecules, the **amino acids.** Found in many foods, especially meats and milk products, proteins are important structural elements of cells, as you will see in the next chapter. Many proteins are **enzymes,** special molecules that speed up chemical reactions in the body. **Peptides** are very small proteins—chains of amino acids.

The fourth group of biologically important molecules is the **nucleic** (new-CLAY-ick) **acids.** This structurally complex group includes DNA, the genetic material found in cells. These molecules are long chains of smaller molecules called *nucleotides* (NEW-klee-oh-tides). Another nucleic acid is RNA. Its structure and function are discussed in Chapter 17.

Health, Homeostasis, and the Environment
Tracking a Chemical Killer

Cancer is the ultimate symbol of homeostatic imbalance. That is, it results from a failure of the body's homeostatic system. Cancer occurs when body cells lose control and begin to divide unremittingly, producing tumors. These tumors eventually kill the person unless they're destroyed. Cancer sometimes results from environmental imbalances, excesses of chemical toxins, or some other cancer-causing agents in our environment as the following story reveals.

For 2000 years, the people in Lin Xian, China, 250 miles south of Beijing, have been dying in record numbers from cancer of the esophagus, the muscular tube that transports food to the stomach. So prevalent is the disease that one of every four persons once succumbed to this ruthless killer, whose incidence is higher there than anywhere else in the world.

In 1959, scientists began a systematic study of 70,000 people in the valley around Lin Xian in an attempt to discover origins of the disease and put an end to the scourge. This disease would lead scientists on a lengthy journey of investigation that would show how

FIGURE 2-9 Tracking a Deadly Killer In Lin Xian, China, the link between esophageal cancer and the soil was uncovered by medical researchers.

minute imbalances in the environment can produce internal chemical imbalances that result in cancer.

Scientists first found that esophageal cancer in Lin Xian was the result of a group of chemicals called *nitrosamines* (NYE-trose-ah-MEANS). Nitrosamines, they discovered, were being produced in the stomachs of the residents from two other chemical compounds: nitrites and amines. But where did they come from?

Research showed that residents had abnormally high levels of nitrites, which came from nitrates in the vegetables that residents ate (**FIGURE 2-9**). The amines were present in moldy bread, a delicacy in the region. But why the excess of nitrates in vegetables? And why the higher-than-normal levels of nitrites in people?

Chemical analyses of the soil in which the region's crops were grown showed that the topsoil around Lin Xian was deficient in molybdenum (meh-LIB-deh-num), an element required by plants in minute quantities (**FIGURE 2-9**). This deficiency caused the plants to concentrate nitrates. It also reduced vitamin C production by plants. Nitrates from plants were apparently being converted to nitrites in the stomachs of the residents. Low levels of vitamin C in the plants they ate actually promoted the conversion of nitrates to nitrites. When the residents were given vitamin C tablets, their nitrite levels dropped.

Ultimately, then, a soil deficiency, caused either by intensive agriculture, which depletes the soil, or from a natural deficiency, put the local residents who ate moldy bread rich in amines at high risk for esophageal cancer.

To reduce the risk of esophageal cancer, the villagers now coat wheat and corn seeds with molybde-

num. As a result, nitrite levels in vegetables have dropped 40%, and vitamin C levels have increased 25%. Although it is still too early to tell whether restoring the soil's nutrient balance will put a halt to this deadly killer, scientists are optimistic.

Summary

1. An understanding of chemistry is essential to understanding biology because all cells and organisms are composed of molecules and many life processes are nothing more than chemical reactions.

Atoms and Subatomic Particles
2. The physical world we live in is composed of matter. Matter is anything that has mass and occupies space.
3. All matter is composed of tiny particles called *atoms*.

4. Atoms contain many *subatomic particles,* three of the most important being electrons, protons, and neutrons.
5. Negatively charged particles, *electrons,* are the smallest of these three subatomic particles; they are found in the electron cloud around the dense, central *nucleus.*
6. *Protons* are positively charged particles that are located in the nucleus with *neutrons,* which are noncharged. Neutrons and protons are large and massive compared to electrons.

7. Atoms are electrically neutral because the number of electrons always equals the number of protons.
8. A pure substance such as gold or lead containing only one type of atom is known as an *element.* The elements are listed on the *periodic table* by *atomic number,* which is the number of protons in the nucleus.
9. Most elements are made up of mixtures of two or more *isotopes,* atoms with slightly different atomic masses result-

ing from the presence of additional neutrons.

10. Additional neutrons often make isotopes unstable. To achieve a more stable state, many isotopes release *radiation*—small bursts of energy, or tiny energetic particles—from their nuclei.

11. Radiation has proved to be a useful tool in medicine and science, but it can also damage cells of organisms, leading to birth defects and cancer.

The Making of a Molecule

12. Atoms react with one another to form organic and inorganic compounds. Their reactivity is a result of the interaction of electrons.

13. Two types of bonds are found between atoms, ionic and covalent.

14. In general, atoms tend to react with others to form complete outer shells, creating more stable atomic configurations.

15. During some atomic reactions, electrons are transferred from one atom to another. Transferring an outer-shell electron from one atom to another creates two oppositely charged ions. An electrostatic attraction forms between them and is referred to as an *ionic bond*.

16. *Covalent bonds* form between atoms that share one or more pairs of electrons. This sharing of electrons holds the atoms together.

17. Unequal sharing of electrons results in the formation of a *polar covalent bond*, which is often sufficient to result in the formation of *polar molecules*. Polar molecules are frequently attracted to one another by *hydrogen bonds*, weak electrostatic attractions between the oppositely charged atoms of neighboring molecules.

Water, Acids, Bases, and Buffers

18. *Organic molecules* are compounds made up primarily of carbon and hydrogen. The atoms of these generally large molecules are held together by covalent bonds.

19. *Inorganic molecules* are much smaller molecules whose atoms are often linked by ionic bonds.

20. Water is an important inorganic molecule and a major component of all body cells. It serves as a solvent, which transports many substances in the blood, body tissues, and cells. It also participates in many chemical reactions, serves as a lubricant, and helps regulate body temperature.

21. Although fairly stable, water molecules can dissociate, forming hydrogen and hydroxide ions.

22. In pure water, the concentration of these ions is equal and water has a pH of 7. Adding *acidic substances* increases the concentration of hydrogen ions, causing the pH to fall.

23. Substances that remove hydrogen ions from solution cause the pH to climb and are called *bases*.

24. A solution with a pH less than 7 is acidic; a solution with a pH greater than 7 is basic.

25. Biological systems contain *buffers*, chemical compounds that offset changes in the concentration of hydrogen and hydroxide ions. Buffers are therefore an important component of chemical homeostasis in organisms and the environment.

Overview of Other Biologically Important Molecules

26. Carbohydrates, lipids, amino acids, proteins, and nucleic acids are biologically important molecules. They vary considerably in structure and function. Details of their structure and function are covered in later chapters.

Critical Thinking

Thinking Critically— Analysis

This analysis corresponds to the Thinking Critically scenario that was presented at the beginning of this chapter.

The phrase that may have raised a red flag in your mind while you were reading this exercise is "Assuming that impurities are rare in single, well-formed crystals." Beware of conclusions based on assumptions. They may prove to be wrong.

But this may not be readily apparent at first. In 1985, in fact, chemists at the Ruhr University in Germany reported the synthesis of another pair of isomers like Chatt's, but from tungsten-containing compounds. These isomers were, according to the scientists, also chemically and structurally identical except for the length of one metal-oxygen bond. Several other laboratories also reported

similar findings, creating a great deal of excitement among scientists, for it appeared that a long-held belief of the constancy of bond length was about to topple.

Theoretical chemists began proposing explanations for this exciting phenomenon. In 1988, Nobel Prize-winning chemist Roald Hoffman and his colleagues published one explanation. However, as chemists began to repeat the experiments (a process essential to good science) to learn more about the isomers, enthusiasm began to fade. In one replication of Chatt's experiment, scientists found that impurities in samples resulted in different colored crystals. After the German experiment was repeated, it was shown that those results had also resulted from contamination.

"Bond-stretch isomerism," as it was called, nearly became accepted theory based on the widely accepted, but faulty, assumption that impurities are rare in single, well-formed crystals. Obviously, this was not the case.

Test of Concepts

1. Why is the matter on Earth so varied in its appearance?
2. Describe the structure of an atom, using a diagram to illustrate your answer.
3. Define the following terms: atomic number, mass number, and isotope.
4. How are ionic and covalent bonds different? Describe what holds the atoms together in both cases. In what ways are the bonds similar?
5. Describe how polar covalent bonds form and why they result in the formation of hydrogen bonds.
6. Temperature is a measure of the speed of molecules: the higher the temperature, the higher the speed. With this information and your knowledge of water and hydrogen bonds, why does water have a higher boiling point than a nonpolar liquid like alcohol?
7. Describe the biological significance of water.
8. How does the body regulate H^+ levels in the blood? Describe the process.

www.jbpub.com/humanbiology

Connect to this book's web site: www.jbpub.com/humanbiology
The site features eLearning, an online review area that provides quizzes, chapter outlines, and other tools to help you study for your class. You can also follow useful links for in-depth information, research the differing views in the Point/Counterpoints, or keep up on the latest environmental and health news.

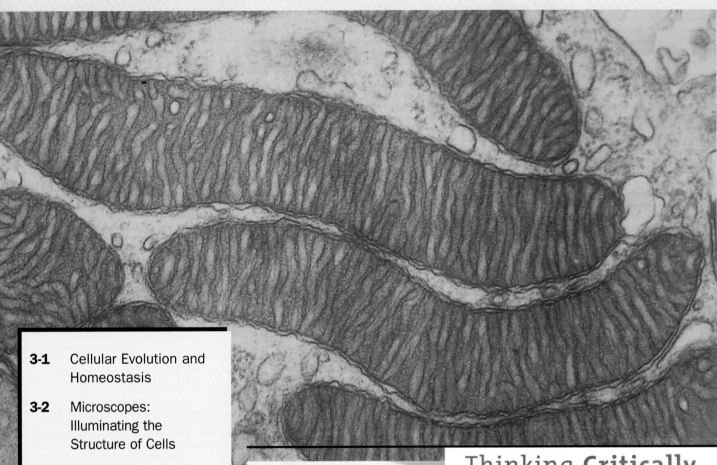

CHAPTER 3

The Life of the Cell

Thinking Critically

Researchers at a major medical college in your area have discovered that cells live longer when cultured (grown) in petri dishes containing a certain vitamin. They suggest that this vitamin might help people live longer. A local newspaper runs with the story, and your friends are thinking of taking the vitamin supplement in hopes of living longer lives. What advice would you give your friends before they embark on this course of action? ■

Mitochondria, energy factories of human cells.

In Sweden, Mexico, and now the United States medical researchers are experimenting with a controversial procedure called *fetal cell transplantation.* By transplanting normal, healthy cells from human embryos into adults, medical scientists hope to be able to cure a number of chronic, debilitating diseases. Scientists believe that fetal cells can replace defective cells in the organs and tissues of adults. This procedure may someday make a significant contribution to medical science, reducing pain and suffering in tens of thousands of people worldwide—people who have little hope of a cure. Already, studies are showing that fetal cell transplantation successfully cures some patients of a debilitating disease known as Parkinson's disease, which currently afflicts actor Michael J. Fox.

Although promising, fetal cell transplantation poses a number of technical challenges. It also poses several significant moral and political dilemmas, which are discussed in the Point/Counterpoint in this chapter.

This chapter focuses on the cell and some key biological molecules. The information presented here forms a foundation on which a good understanding of human biology can be built. This material will also help you understand the details of fetal cell transplantation. Before we examine the structure and function of cells, though, we take a journey back in time to trace the evolution of the cell.

Cellular Evolution and Homeostasis

Two Types of Cells Exist: Prokaryotes and Eukaryotes

All organisms are composed of one or more cells. However, fossil evidence shows that the very first organisms were single-celled. They appeared on Earth approximately 3.5 billion years ago and were the dominant form of life for over 2 billion years.

These first cells and their modern relatives (the bacteria) are known as **prokaryotes** (pro-CARE-ee-oats). Prokaryotes (*pro* = before; *karyon* = nucleus) are single-celled organisms that contain a single circular strand of DNA (**FIGURE 3-1A**).

Prokaryotic organisms formed the Earth's first major group (kingdom) of organisms, the **monerans** (moe-NARE-ens), briefly introduced in Chapter 1. Unlike the more complex cells that make up humans and other multicellular organisms, prokaryotic cells possess few of the internal structures.

Over time, the prokaryotes gave rise to more complex single-celled organisms, the **eukaryotes** (*eu* = true; *karyon* = nucleus; pronounced you-CARE-ee-oats). The cells of these organisms contain DNA within a membrane-bound structure, the **nucleus** (**FIGURE 3-1B**). Eukaryote cells first appeared in the oceans about 1.2 billion years ago. They formed the Earth's second kingdom, the **protistans** (pro-TEES-tans).

(a)

FIGURE 3-1 Prokaryotes and Eukaryotes
(a) Magnified many thousands of times, this bacterium is a typical prokaryote. It contains DNA, but the DNA is not located within a nucleus. (b) Also greatly magnified, this cell is a typical eukaryote. Its DNA is membrane-bound, and it contains numerous cellular organelles.

(b)

The Formation of Complex, Multicellular Organisms Resulted from Evolution

During evolution, single-celled eukaryotic organisms gave rise to three additional groups of organisms, known as **kingdoms.** They were the plants, fungi, and animals.

The evolution of the three new kingdoms was characterized by two major developments: (1) multicellularity, the development of organisms composed of many cells; and (2) cellular specialization, the emergence of cells that perform specific tasks.

Multicellularity and cellular specialization increased the complexity of life on Earth. It made new ways of existence possible. For example, the emergence of cells that contract when stimulated made possible a wide variety of animal species. Cells that could conduct impulses made possible the evolution of sensory systems found today in numerous animal species. Growing complexity also required control mechanisms to ensure that the parts worked in unison. Over time, distinct body systems of multicellular animals, such as the nervous and endocrine systems, evolved and took control over a wide variety of body functions, most of which contribute to the maintenance of homeostasis. As pointed out in Chapter 1, homeostasis is necessary for the proper functioning of the cells and, thus, of the body as a whole.

Despite dramatic evolutionary changes that have led to a diverse array of life-forms, the cell's basic features have endured, reinforcing the principle of evolution that successful patterns tend to persist. This chapter focuses on general cell characteristics. Although this knowledge is applicable to a wide range of organisms, our focus will remain on humans. Before we peer into the internal architecture of the human cell, however, let's take a look at the microscope, an important tool that makes our journey possible.

Microscopes: Illuminating the Structure of Cells

Cells are exceedingly small and, with few exceptions, cannot be seen with the naked eye. Our knowledge of them has depended on the **microscope,** a device consisting of a lens or combination of lenses that enlarges tiny objects. (For a discussion of the discovery of cells, see Scientific Discoveries 3-1.)

Microscopes fit into two broad categories: (1) **light microscopes,** which use ordinary visible light to illuminate the specimen under study; and (2) **electron microscopes,** which use a beam of electrons to create a visual image of the specimen.

Both types of microscopes enlarge minute images and allow us to see details of the cell. However, light microscopes provide less magnification and allow us to see less detail than the electron microscope. Light microscopes magnify objects from 100 to 400 times their original size (**FIGURES 3-2**). Electron microscopes enlarge objects 100,000 times their original size. For a comparison, see **FIGURES 3-2** and **3-3**. One type of electron microscope, known as a *scanning electron microscope,* allows scientists to see a three-dimensional view of cells (**FIGURES 3-3**). Photographs from both light and electron microscopes are used in this book to elucidate the structure of important cells, tissues, and organs.

(a)

(b)

FIGURE 3-2 The Light Microscope *(a)* In the ordinary light microscope, the image is illuminated by light that is cast from a mirror or (in this case) a light bulb located below the object. Two lenses (one in the eyepiece and one just above the object) magnify the object. *(b)* Light micrograph of a section of the lining of the urinary bladder.

Fetal Cell Transplantation

Fetal Tissue Transplants: Auschwitz Revisited

Tom Longua

Tom Longua has been an educator for 39 years and is currently instructor of anatomy and physiology at the Denver Academy of Court Reporting. He has been active in the pro-life movement since 1974 and is a member of the board of directors of Colorado Right to Life.

Persons who advocate medical research using tissue from aborted babies claim it has genuine medical value. But that premise is just plain false. On April 22, 1999, both the *New York Times* and *Washington Post* ran stories about a four-year trial by the National Institute of Neurological Disorder, in which a group of Parkinson patients had fetal cells implanted into their brains, while others had a "sham" operation in which no cells were implanted.

In patients over 60 (those most susceptible to Parkinson's), no difference was observed between the two groups, either on the neurologists' examinations or on the patients' own perception of their condition. Even among younger patients—for whom the treatment allegedly "worked"—there was no difference between the two groups in initiating walking, walking balance, the number of falls, tremors, "freezing" (sudden loss of all movement), and dyskinesia.

But even if the claims were true, should a civilized society allow research on human beings who may be killed, albeit legally, even though they are innocent of any crime?

After World War II, Nazi doctors who experimented on prisoners in concentration camps were tried at Nuremberg for "crimes against humanity." The prosecutor opened his case with this statement:

The defendants in this case are charged with. . . . Atrocities committed in the name of medical science. . . . The wrongs which we seek to condemn and punish have been so calculated, so malignant, and so devastating, that civilization cannot tolerate their being ignored, because it cannot survive their being repeated.

Yet with research involving tissue from elective abortions, we are committing the same "crimes against humanity." Even the claimed justification is the same.

- Nazi doctor August Hirt: "Wouldn't it be ridiculous to send the bodies to the crematory oven without giving them an opportunity to contribute to the progress of society?"
- Lawrence Lawn, a doctor involved in research with tissue from elective abortions: "We are simply using something which is destined for the incinerator to benefit mankind."

Proponents of such research claim that it is acceptable if it is "separated" from abortions that are freely chosen anyway. Again, this argument echoes the Nazi doctors' defense at Nuremberg: "We caused no deaths. They [the victims] were all consigned to death by legal authorities; with . . . professional correctness we tried to salvage some good from their plight."

But "separation" is a myth. As the Auschwitz research depended on the "acceptability" of killing prisoners, fetal tissue research depends on the "acceptability" of killing helpless, innocent human beings in the first place. (Certainly there is nothing wrong with using tissue from ectopic pregnancies or miscarriages; but this debate concerns babies who are purposely killed simply because they are unwanted.) Moreover, new abortion techniques have been contrived specifically for the purpose of securing usable (and salable) tissue. So much for "separation."

But besides the perverseness of the practice itself, such research will have other detrimental effects:

- It will certainly increase the number of abortions. Some medical journals claim that fetal tissue could be used to treat a vast array of diseases. In a 1988 guest editorial in the *Wall Street Journal*, Dr. Emanuel Thorne estimated that the 1.6 million annual abortions in America would not be enough

to keep up with the demand for such tissue. While there have been well-publicized cases of women becoming pregnant to create organ or tissue sources for their parents and other children, it is unlikely that many women would get pregnant to create tissue that might be "useful" for others (although stranger things have happened). But with money to be made, the abortion industry will certainly pressure women who are undecided about having abortions, using the argument that the tissue will serve some "benevolent" purpose. Indeed, retired Aurora abortionist James Parks bragged, "[My patients] say, 'Thank God, some good is going to come out of this.'" (*New York Times*, 11/19/89)

- In a 1991 article on this topic, this writer said, "[This research] will lead to trafficking in human 'spare parts.'" Well, eight years later, Congress launched an investigation into exactly that grisly practice, finding that it was occurring, and that it was extremely lucrative. As the Associated Press reported on October 10, 1999, Congressman Tom Tancredo (R-CO), "displayed a brochure . . . that lists prices for fetal parts, including '$50 for eyes, $150 for lungs and hearts and $999 for an eight-week brain.'"
- Advocacy of fetal tissue research will hinder other—and ethical—research to find cures for some diseases. There are many potential treatments being studied, such as autografts and use of patients' own stem cells, but some researchers have abandoned those possibilities because of the much-touted (albeit dishonestly) fetal tissue approach.

Advocates of fetal tissue research like to depict themselves as "humanitarians." But then, so did the doctors on trial at Nuremberg.

Human Fetal Tissue Should Be Used to Treat Human Disease

Curt R. Freed

Despite its legalization, abortion remains a controversial issue and will continue to stir debate in the future. In the United States, the debate centers on whether a woman has the right to control her reproduction. The future developments of this political debate are uncertain, but recent elections suggest that pro-choice candidates have been victorious when elections are based on the abortion issue.

Currently, over 1 million legal abortions are performed in the United States each year; most abortions are performed in the first trimester. For nearly all women, having an abortion is an anguishing choice filled with regret and ambivalence. Nonetheless, the difficult personal decision to terminate a pregnancy is made. After the abortion, fetal tissue is usually discarded.

As an alternative to throwing this tissue away, research has shown that fetal tissue may be useful for treating patients with disabling diseases. For over 50 years, research in animals has demonstrated that fetal tissue has a unique capacity to replace certain cellular deficiencies and so may be useful for treating some chronic diseases of humans. These diseases include Parkinson's disease, diabetes, and some immune system disorders.

Cadaver fetal tissue offers the promise of helping large numbers of Americans with crippling diseases. Parkinson's disease, for example, affects hundreds of thousands of Americans. By reducing the ability to move, the disease can end careers and turn people into invalids. The disease is caused by the death of a small number of critically important nerve cells that produce a chemical called dopamine. Experiments in animals and early experiments in humans indicate that fetal dopamine cells transplanted into the brains of these patients may restore a patient's capacity to move and may even eliminate the disease. Patients whose minds work perfectly well and whose bodies are otherwise normal may become healthy and productive citizens once again.

Using cadaver tissue to treat humans has been debated for nearly 40 years. As kidney, cornea, and other organ transplants were developed in the 1950s, many objected to recovering organs from cadavers. In the intervening decades, opinion has changed so that the practice of recovering these organs from cadavers has gone from a provocative and controversial practice to an accepted policy endorsed by most states. In fact, in most states, a check-off box on the back of driver's licenses is used to give permission for organ donation in the event of the death of the driver. Because abortions are induced, some argue that fetal tissue should be regarded differently from other cadaver tissue. Given the facts that abortion is legal and that fetal tissue is ordinarily discarded, there should be no moral dilemma in using fetal tissue for therapeutic purposes. As with the use of all human tissue for transplant, specific informed consent by the woman donating the tissue must be obtained.

Some have proposed that using fetal tissue for therapeutic purposes will increase the number of abortions. This is preposterous. It strains the imagination to think that a woman would get pregnant and have an abortion simply on the chance that the aborted fetal tissue might be used to treat a patient unknown to her. An unwanted pregnancy is an intimate and deeply personal crisis; it is inconceivable that the pregnancy would be seen primarily as a philanthropic opportunity.

Politics and medicine have frequently mixed in the past and will continue to do so in the future. As a physician, I think it is important to try to improve the health of patients with serious diseases. Legally acquired fetal cadaver tissue that would otherwise be discarded should be used to treat humans with disabling diseases.

Curt R. Freed, M.D., is a professor of medicine and pharmacology at the University of Colorado School of Medicine in Denver. He has written some 70 articles on medical topics as well as numerous abstracts, chapters, and reviews.

Sharpening Your Critical Thinking Skills

1. Summarize the positions of each author.
2. Using your critical thinking skills, analyze the view of each author. Is each stand well substantiated? Do the author's biases play a role in each argument?
3. Do you see this debate as scientific or ethical? Explain your answer.
4. Each position is based on at least one key argument. Can you pinpoint them?
5. Which viewpoint do you agree with? Why? What factors (biases) affect your decision?

Visit *Human Biology's* Internet site for links to web sites offering more information on this topic.

Scientific Discoveries that Changed the World 3-1

The Discovery of Cells

Featuring the Work of Hooke, Leeuwenhoek, Brown, Schleiden, Schwann, and Virchow

FIGURE 1 Thin Slice of Cork   Hooke discovered tiny, boxlike compartments that reminded him of a honeycomb. He called them cellulae, meaning "little rooms."

One of the fundamental principles of biology is known as the **cell theory.** The cell theory consists of three parts: (1) all organisms consist of one or more cells, (2) the cell is the basic unit of structure of all organisms, and (3) all cells arise from preexisting cells. Although this may seem rather elementary, it was not so obvious to early scientists, who labored with relatively crude instruments and without the benefit of many facts we now take for granted.

One of those scientific pioneers who opened our eyes to the world of cells was Robert Hooke, a seventeenth-century British mathematician, inventor, and scientist. Equipped with a relatively crude microscope, Hooke observed just about everything he

could lay his hands on—which he described in his book *Micrographia,* published in 1665.

One especially useful description was that made on a thin slice of cork (**FIGURE 1**). Peering through his microscope, Hooke beheld a network of tiny, boxlike compartments that reminded him of a honeycomb. He called these compartments cellulae, meaning "little rooms." Today, we know them as cells.

Hooke did not really see cells but, rather, cell walls, the structures that surround the plasma membranes of plant cells. The cytoplasm and cellular organelles had disappeared.

Hooke's work was complemented a few years later by Antony van Leeuwenhoek, a Dutch shopkeeper who spent much of his free time de-

FIGURE 3-3 The Electron Microscope
(a) Scanning electron microscope.
(b) Scanning electron micrograph of the lining of the urinary bladder.

(a)

(b)

Section 3-3

An Overview of Cell Structure

In humans, most cells exhibit a high degree of structural and functional specialization. Very few look alike. But we won't worry about the differences. Instead, we'll focus on generalities as we examine a fictional entity, the typical animal cell. This structure, shown in **FIGURE 3-4**, is a potpourri of structures found in the various body cells. Don't look for it under the microscope, because it only exists on the pages of biology textbooks. You may want to refer to **TABLE 3-1** as you study the following material and as you review this material later.

The Cell Consists of Two Main Compartments

Human cells are the product of millions of years of evolution. As illustrated in **FIGURE 3-4**, human cells—like those of other eukaryotes—consist of two basic compartments, the nuclear and the cytoplasmic. The nuclear compartment, or **nucleus,** is the control center of the cell because it contains the genetic information that regulates the structure and function of the cell. As shown signing simple microscopes. Like Hooke, Leeuwenhoek examined just about everything he could find and wrote extensively on his observations. Wayne Becker, a cell biologist at the University of Wisconsin writes, "His detailed reports attest to both the high quality of his lenses and his keen powers of observation." Becker continues: "They also reveal an active imagination, since at one point he reported seeing a 'homunculus' (little man) in the nucleus of a human sperm cell."

Leeuwenhoek discovered bacteria and protozoans (single-celled eukaryotic organisms). Although his microscopes were superior to any others around at that time, they were still crude by modern standards. This fact and the tendency of the scien-

tific community back then to focus only on the observation and description of life-forms stalled progress in our understanding of cells for some time. In fact, more than a century passed before cell biology moved significantly forward.

Aided by improved lenses, the eighteenth-century English botanist Robert Brown noted that every plant cell he studied contained a centrally placed structure, now called a nucleus. A German colleague, Matthias Schleiden, concluded that all plant tissues consisted of cells. One year later, Theodor Schwann, a German scientist, arrived at a similar conclusion regarding animal cells. This discovery laid to rest an earlier hypothesis that plants and animals were structurally different.

Based on earlier research and his own work, Schwann proposed the first two parts of the cell theory—that all organisms consist of one or more cells and that the cell is the basic unit of structure for all organisms. Less than 20 years after the discovery of cell division, the German physiologist Rudolf Virchow added the third tenet of the cell theory, that all cells arise from preexisting cells.

Like other discoveries, the cell theory is the work of many people over many years. Although only a few people are named as having made possible this important discovery, the credit really belongs to an entire line of scientists who, through careful observation and experimentation, have changed our view of the world.

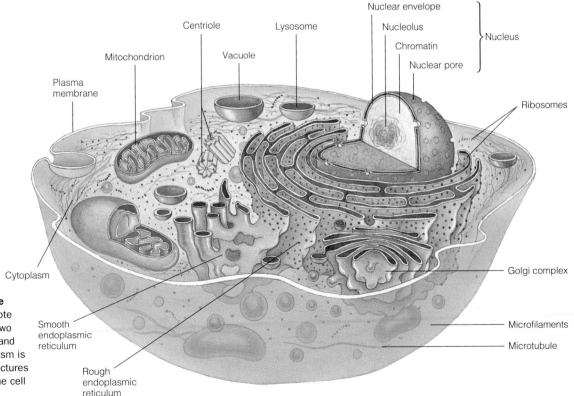

FIGURE 3-4 Structure of the General Eukaryotic Cell Note that the cell is divided into two compartments, the nuclear and the cytoplasmic. The cytoplasm is packed with a variety of structures called organelles in which the cell carries out many functions.

TABLE 3-1

Overview of Cell Organelles

Organelle	Structure	Function
Nucleus	Round or oval body; surrounded by nuclear envelope	Contains the genetic information necessary for control of cell structure and function; DNA contains hereditary information.
Nucleolus	Round or oval body in the nucleus consisting of DNA and RNA	Produces ribosomal RNA
Endoplasmic reticulum	Network of membranous tubules in the cytoplasm of the cell. Smooth endoplasmic reticulum contains no ribosomes. Rough endoplasmic reticulum is studded with ribosomes.	Smooth endoplasmic reticulum (SER) is involved in the production of phospholipids and has many different functions in different cells; round endoplasmic reticulum (RER) is the site of the synthesis of lysosomal enzymes and proteins for extracellular use.
Ribosomes	Small particles found in the cytoplasm; made of RNA and protein	Aid in the production of proteins on the RER and polysomes
Polysome	Molecule of mRNA bound to ribosomes	Site of protein synthesis
Golgi complex	Series of flattened sacs usually located near the nucleus	Sorts, chemically modifies, and packages proteins produced on the RER
Secretory vesicles	Membrane-bound vesicles containing proteins produced by the RER and repackaged by the Golgi complex; contain protein hormones or enzymes	Store protein hormones or enzymes in the cytoplasm awaiting a signal for release
Food vacuole	Membrane-bound vesicle containing material engulfed by the cell	Stores ingested material and combines with lysosome
Lysosome	Round, membrane-bound structure containing digestive enzymes	Combines with food vacuoles and digests materials engulfed by cells
Mitochondria	Round, oval, or elongated structures with a double membrane. The inner membrane is thrown into folds.	Complete the breakdown of glucose, producing NADH and ATP
Cytoskeleton	Network of microtubules and microfilaments in the cell	Gives the cell internal support, helps transport molecules and some organelles inside the cell, and binds to enzymes of metabolic pathways
Cilia	Small projections of the cell membrane containing microtubules; found on a limited number of cells	Propel materials along the surface of certain cells
Flagella	Large projections of the cell membrane containing microtubules; found in humans only on sperm cells	Provide motive force for sperm cells
Centrioles	Small cylindrical bodies composed of microtubules arranged in nine sets of triplets; found in animal cells, not plants.	Help organize spindle apparatus necessary for cell division

in **FIGURE 3-4**, the nucleus is surrounded by a double membrane, the nuclear envelope.

The cytoplasmic compartment lies between the nucleus and the **plasma membrane,** the outermost structure of the cell. It contains a substance known as cytoplasm. **Cytoplasm** is a semifluid material that consists of numerous molecules, including water, protein, ions, nutrients, vitamins, dissolved gases, and waste products.

(a)

FIGURE 3-5 The Cytoskeleton *(a)* Photomicrograph of the cytoskeleton of a human fibroblast (connective tissue cell). The microtubules are yellow, and the microfilaments are red. *(b)* Artist's rendition of the cytoskeleton, showing its two major components: microtubules (tubes made of the protein tubulin) and smaller microfilaments (solid fibers made of actin and myosin proteins).

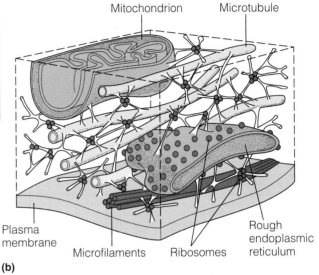

Mitochondrion   Microtubule

Plasma membrane

Microfilaments   Ribosomes   Rough endoplasmic reticulum

(b)

It forms a nutrient pool from which the cell draws chemicals it needs for metabolism. It is also a dumping ground for wastes.

As shown in **FIGURE 3-4**, the cell contains numerous structures called organelles. **Organelles** ("little organs") carry out specific functions (**TABLE 3-1**). Many organelles are bounded by membranes and form subcompartments within the cytoplasm.

Compartmentalization is essential to the smooth functioning of complex cells because it permits cells to segregate many of their functions. This increases the efficiency of cells and helps complex organisms perform many functions simultaneously. In a way, a cell is much like a modern factory with different departments in different parts of the building, each performing specific functions, but all working together toward one end.

The cytoplasm of the cell also contains organelles that are not membrane-bound. These organelles perform many important functions, too (outlined shortly).

Giving shape to the cell is a network of protein tubules and filaments found in the cytoplasm and known as the **cytoskeleton** (**FIGURE 3-5**). Besides giving support, the cytoskeleton helps organize the cell's activities, greatly increasing cellular efficiency. The cytoskeleton facilitates this vital function by binding with enzymes. **Enzymes** are proteins that increase the rate of chemical reactions in cells. As you will see later in the chapter, many chemical reactions in cells of the body occur in series, with one reaction giving rise to a substance that's used in the next. A series of linked reactions is called a **metabolic pathway** and is the cellular equivalent of an assembly line in a factory. The enzymes of the metabolic pathway are the cell's equivalent to assembly line workers.

Molecules enter one end of a metabolic pathway and are modified along their course by enzymes (**FIGURE 3-6**). Eventually, a finished product comes off the line. Because enzymes are arranged along the cytoskeleton in proper order, the product of one reaction is conveniently situated for the next reaction. Without the cytoskeleton, chaos might erupt as in a factory that haphazardly assembles its products.

FIGURE 3-6 Metabolic Pathway Reactions in the cell occur as parts of larger pathways where the product of one reaction becomes the reactant of another, as in this biochemical pathway. This illustrates the early steps in glycolysis, the breakdown of glucose in the cytoplasm of eukaryotic cells. Note that each reaction has its own enzyme (labeled in red). Also note that the names of these, and all other enzymes, end in *-ase*.

Glucose

Hexokinase   ATP / ADP

Glucose 6-phosphate

Phosphoglucose isomerase

Fructose 6-phosphate

Phosphofructokinase   ATP / ADP

Fructose 1,6-bisphosphate

The Structure and Function of the Plasma Membrane

The **plasma membrane**, the outermost part of a cell, is a thin layer of lipids and proteins. The plasma membrane controls what goes in and out of the cell thereby controlling the cell's internal chemical environment—a function essential to cellular homeostasis and survival (**TABLE 3-2**).

TABLE 3-2

Overview of Plasma Membrane Functions

Ensures the cell's structural integrity

Regulates the flow of molecules and ions into and out of the cell

Maintains the chemical composition of cytoplasm and extracellular fluid

Participates in cellular communication

Forms a cellular identification system

The Lipids of the Plasma Membrane Form a Double Layer in Which Many of the Proteins Float Freely

The plasma membrane and all of the other internal membranes of the cell consist of lipids, proteins, and a small amount of carbohydrate (**FIGURE 3-7**). **Lipids** or fats are a chemically diverse group of biochemicals that form waxes, grease, and oils. All are insoluble in water. Lipids serve a variety of functions. Some provide energy. Others serve as insulation and energy storage. Still others play a structural role. Three different lipids are discussed in this book. The first, which is found in the membranes of cells, is the **phospholipid** (FOSS-foh-lip-id). Shown in **FIGURE 3-8**, phospholipids form lollypop-shaped molecules with a polar (charged) head and a nonpolar (uncharged) tail. Most of the lipid molecules in the plasma membrane are phospholipids.

Experimental studies strongly suggest that the phospholipid molecules of the plasma membrane are arranged in a double layer. **FIGURE 3-7** shows the most widely accepted model (theory) of the plasma membrane's structure, the **fluid mosaic model.** As shown, the polar heads of the outer layer of phospholipid mol-

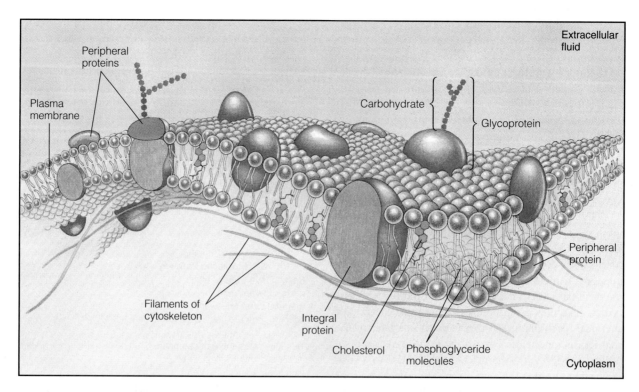

FIGURE 3-7 Fluid Mosaic Model of the Plasma Membrane of Animal Cells   The fluid mosaic model is the most widely accepted theory of the plasma membrane. Phospholipids are the chief lipid component. They are arranged in a bilayer. Integral proteins float like icebergs in a sea of lipids.

FIGURE 3-8 Phospholipids *(a)* Each phospholipid consists of a glycerol backbone, two fatty acids, a phosphate, and a variable group generally designated by the letter R. In this case, the R group is choline, which is polar. *(b)* Because of the R group, the molecule has a polar head. The nonpolar tail region is formed by the two fatty acid chains.

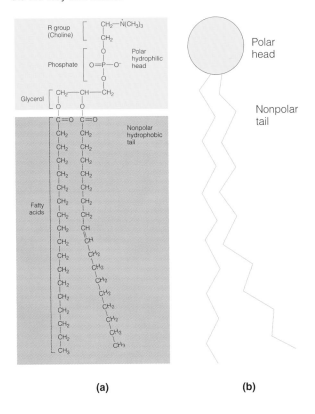

(a)   (b)

FIGURE 3-9 Structure of Amino Acids *(a)* The amino acid is a small organic molecule with four groups, one of which is variable and is designated by the letter R. *(b)* Some representative R groups.

ecules face the watery extracellular fluid, and the polar heads of the inner layer of molecules are directed inward toward the watery cytoplasm.

Interspersed in the lipid bilayer of human cells are large protein molecules known as integral proteins. **Proteins** are large molecular weight compounds made of many smaller molecules, known as amino acids. **Amino acids** contain a central carbon atom, attached to which are an amino group (NH_2) and a carboxylic acid group (COOH)—from which they derive their name (**FIGURE 3-9**). As shown in the figure, the central carbon atom also bonds to a hydrogen and a variable group (denoted by the letter R). To date, approximately 250 amino acids have been discovered in plants and animals or synthesized in the laboratory. However, only 20 of them are found in natural proteins. From this seemingly limited pool of amino acids, cells build thousands of different proteins.

Proteins serve many different functions. One important class of proteins, the **enzymes,** accelerates chemi-

cal reactions in the body. Without enzymes, few reactions would occur. Other proteins play a structural role. **Keratin** (CARE-ah-tin), for example, is a protein in human hair and nails. **Collagen** (coll-AH-gin), the most abundant protein in the human body, forms fibers that are found in ligaments, tendons, and bones.

Proteins are synthesized in the body one amino acid at a time, but a large protein containing hundreds of amino acids is assembled in under a minute. **FIGURE 3-10** shows how amino acids bind. The bond between two amino acids is called a **peptide bond.** As a protein is synthesized, the chain of amino acids begins to twist and bend (**FIGURE 3-11**). Further along in the process, the amino acid structure forms a three-dimensional structure. It is often globular in nature. The integral proteins of the plasma membrane are globular structures that float freely like giant icebergs in their sea of lipid. As illustrated, some of them completely penetrate the plasma membrane; others penetrate only partway. Several integral proteins may join to form pores

FIGURE 3-10 Formation of the Peptide Bond The carboxyl and amino groups react in such a way that a covalent bond is formed between the carbon of the carboxyl group of one amino acid and the nitrogen of the amino group of another. This bond is called a peptide bond.

Primary structure

The primary structure is the sequence of amino acids. It determines to a large extent the complex shape a protein assumes.

Peptide bonds

Amino acids

Secondary structure

The secondary structure results from a bending or coiling of the primary structure. Three general types are found.

Hydrogen bonds

Pleated sheet

Alpha helix

Random coil

Tertiary structure

The tertiary structure results when the secondary structure of a protein is compacted to form the three-dimensional shape on which its function is dependent.

Quaternary structure

The quaternary structure results when two or more globular proteins unite to form a "superprotein."

FIGURE 3-11 Protein Structure

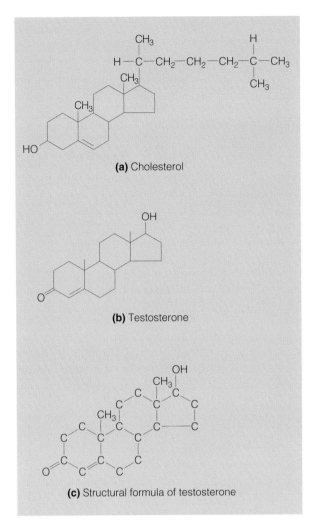

(a) Cholesterol

(b) Testosterone

(c) Structural formula of testosterone

FIGURE 3-12 Steroids Steroids, such as *(a)* cholesterol and *(b)* testosterone, consist of four rings joined together. Parts *(a)* and *(b)* are a shorthand way of drawing *(c)* the structural formula.

steroid. Its chemical formula is shown in **FIGURE 3-12**. Cholesterol and other steroids consist of four ring structures that are joined together. Cholesterol molecules are found in the plasma membranes of cells, wedged in between the phospholipid molecules (**FIGURE 3-8**). Their importance is not well understood. They appear to make the membrane more elastic.

The Plasma Membrane Serves Many Functions and Is Essential to Cellular Homeostasis

The plasma membrane is a vital component of homeostasis. The plasma membrane regulates the flow of molecules and ions into and out of the cell. This helps maintain the precise chemical concentrations inside and outside the cell—both essential for optimal cellular function. (For a review of plasma membrane functions, see **TABLE 3-2** on page 48.)

Because the plasma membrane regulates the molecular traffic, it is said to be **selectively permeable.** Put another way, the plasma membrane selects or controls what enters and leaves the cell. As you will learn in later chapters, the plasma membrane also plays a vital role in cellular communication. Communication is defined very broadly here to include the transmission or receipt of any kind of message. Some hormones in the tissue fluid surrounding cells, for example, attach to specific integral proteins (membrane receptors) in the plasma membranes of cells. Like the ringing of a doorbell, this sends a message to the cell's interior that triggers important changes in the cell's structure and function. Consequently, hormones are said to "communicate" with the cell through its membrane.

The plasma membrane is also part of an elaborate cellular identification system. The cells in each of us have a unique protein "cellular fingerprint."[1] Because the protein composition of the plasma membrane of the cells of each individual is unique, a person's immune system can recognize its own cells and determine when foreign cells—such as bacteria—have invaded. The immune system also identifies cancer cells. Cancer cells proliferate wildly. Their cellular fingerprint also becomes altered, making them unrecognizable or foreign. Once the immune system has identified microbial invaders or tumor cells, the body mounts an attack, often successfully eliminating them. Without this marvelous ability to recognize foreign invaders or altered cells, we

that permit the movement of molecules into and out of the cell. Others may attach to the underlying cytoskeleton, anchoring the plasma membrane in place.

Another group of proteins, the **peripheral proteins,** is found in the plasma membrane. On the cytoplasmic side of the membrane, peripheral proteins often attach to the exposed surfaces of integral proteins. They may also bind to the cytoskeleton.

Plasma membranes contain small but significant amounts of carbohydrate. Most carbohydrates are oligosaccharides (short chains of much simpler sugars). Shown in **FIGURE 3-7**, these segments attach to integral proteins that protrude into the extracellular fluid of cells. A protein combined with a carbohydrate is a **glycoprotein.** The glycoproteins of the plasma membrane are vital to cell function.

Another type of lipid is also found in the plasma membrane. This lipid is cholesterol. Cholesterol is a

---

[1]These proteins are called glycoproteins because they contain smaller carbohydrate molecules.

would very likely perish in rapid order from infections or tumors.

As noted in Chapter 1, human actions often disrupt homeostasis. Perhaps one of the most blatant examples is an organ transplant. During this procedure, surgeons remove damaged organs and replace them with healthy organs from donors. Kidneys, hearts, and skin are the most commonly transplanted organs and tissues. However, unless the tissue or organ comes from an identical twin, who's genetically identical to the recipient, the immune system of the recipient recognizes the cells of a transplanted organ as foreign and attempts to destroy them. To prevent rejection, physicians prescribe drugs that suppress the immune system. Unfortunately, this treatment makes a patient vulnerable to bacterial and viral infections, although newer drugs have less effect on the immune system.

In a sense, then, a change in the body's delicate balance (caused by a transplant) results in a grave imbalance that must be counterbalanced by drugs. As evidence of the seriousness of this tinkering, many early heart transplants failed as patients died from massive infections. Not to be deterred, scientists have developed new drugs that suppress the immune system and prevent the rejection of transplanted tissues and organs without completely eliminating the body's protection from bacteria and viruses. In such instances, the body maintains some ability to control its internal environment and to keep itself free of bacteria and other infectious agents.

Fetal cell transplantation, discussed at the opening of this chapter, represents another means of trying to dupe the immune system. Fetal cells have no protein fingerprint and can therefore be transplanted without triggering an immune reaction.[2]

Molecules Move Through the Plasma Membrane in Five Ways

Cells are bathed in a liquid that fills the tiny spaces between them. This is called **interstitial fluid** (in-ter-STICH-al). This liquid and the cytoplasm of cells contain a great deal of water and a variety of chemical substances that are dissolved or suspended in them. Some of these substances pass through the membrane with ease; others must be transported across the membrane with the aid of special molecules. All told, five basic mechanisms exist for moving molecules and ions across plasma membranes (**TABLE 3-3**).

The Movement of Molecules from High to Low Concentrations Either Directly Through the Membrane Lipid or Through Pores Is Called Simple Diffusion. Lipid-soluble substances pass directly through the membrane via diffusion. Why? Because the plasma membrane is principally made of lipid, and chemical compounds readily dissolve in chemically similar solvents. Steroid hormones, oxygen, and carbon dioxide are all lipid-soluble and therefore pass directly through the lipid bilayer of the plasma membrane with ease (**FIGURE 3-13A**).

---

[2]The immunologic immaturity of fetal cells is probably an evolutionary adaptation that protects fetuses from attack by the mother's immune system.

TABLE 3-3

Overview of Plasma Membrane Transport

Process	Description
Simple diffusion	Flow of ions and molecules from high concentrations to low. Water-soluble ions and molecules probably pass through pores; water-insoluble molecules pass directly through the lipid layer.
Facilitated diffusion	Flow of ions and molecules from high concentrations to low concentrations with the aid of protein carrier molecules in the membrane.
Active transport	Transport of molecules from regions of low concentration to regions of high concentration with the aid of transport proteins in the cell membrane and ATP.
Endocytosis	Active incorporation of liquid and solid materials outside the cell by the plasma membrane. Materials are engulfed by the cell and become surrounded in a membrane.
Exocytosis	Release of materials packaged in secretory vesicles.
Osmosis	Diffusion of water molecules from regions of high water (low solute) concentration to regions of low water (high solute) concentrations.

Diffusion refers to any movement of molecules or ions down a concentration gradient—that is, from high to low concentration. As you will soon see, two types of diffusion exist, simple and facilitated. Movement of lipid-soluble chemicals through the membrane without assistance, as described above, is **simple diffusion.**

Water-soluble materials cannot pass through the lipid bilayer of the plasma membrane and must travel via other routes. Scientists believe that water and many other small water-soluble molecules and ions pass through pores in the plasma membrane and that these pores are formed by integral proteins (**FIGURE 3-13B**).

Movement through membrane pores is another form of simple diffusion. Interestingly, no one has ever even seen a pore in electron micrographs of cell membranes, and their existence is based entirely on physiological research. Nonetheless, researchers believe that some protein pores remain open all the time, thus permitting small molecules and ions to cross the plasma membrane.

Water-Soluble Molecules Can Also Diffuse Through Membranes with the Assistance of Protein Carrier Molecules. **Carrier proteins** are molecules that transport small water-soluble molecules and ions across the membrane in ways not yet completely understood. Carrier proteins "shuttle" molecules across membranes from regions of high concentration to regions of low concentration. This process is called **facilitated diffusion** to distinguish it from simple diffusion through pores or through the lipid bilayer (**FIGURE 3-14A**).

Molecules Are Also Actively Transported Across the Membrane. Another transport mechanism found in plasma membranes is known as active transport. **Active transport** is the movement of molecules across membranes with the aid of protein carrier molecules in the plasma membrane and with energy supplied by a special molecule called ATP (**FIGURE 3-14B**). **ATP** or **adenosine triphosphate** (ah-DEN-oh-seen try-FOSS-fate) is a molecule with an important job. ATP consists of three smaller molecules, shown in **FIGURE 3-15**: a nitrogen-

containing organic base, adenine; a five-carbon sugar, ribose; and three phosphate groups.

ATP is often likened to a form of energy currency. When the cell needs energy, say to move molecules across its membrane, ATP splits off a phosphate, forming ADP (adenosine diphosphate). The breaking of the phosphate bond yields energy that the cell can use directly. The reaction is:

$$ATP \longrightarrow ADP + P_i + Energy$$

Reactions in the body that give off energy often turn the energy over to ADP. That way, new ATP can be formed.

$$ADP + P_i + Energy \longrightarrow ATP$$

(a) Simple diffusion

(b) Diffusion through protein pores

FIGURE 3-13 Membrane Transport *(a)* Lipid-soluble substances pass through the membrane directly via simple diffusion. *(b)* Water-soluble molecules can diffuse passively through pores formed by protein molecules.

FIGURE 3-14 Membrane Transport *(a)* Water-soluble molecules can also diffuse through membranes with the assistance of proteins in facilitated diffusion. *(b)* Other proteins use energy from ATP to move against concentration gradients in a process called active transport.

(a) Facilitated diffusion

(b) Active transport

FIGURE 3-15 Molecular Structure of the Nucleotide ATP
ATP is often called the energy currency of the cell.

ATP serves as a kind of an energy shuttle, picking up energy from reactions that release it and shuttling it to reactions that require it. The energy is stored in the covalent bond between ADP and the last phosphate.

During active transport, molecules and ions are transported from regions of low concentration to regions of high concentration—movement "up," or against, the concentration gradient. Active transport occurs in cells that must concentrate chemical substances to function properly and, like the various forms of diffusion, it is essential for maintaining homeostasis. For example, cells in the thyroid glands in the neck require large quantities of the iodide ion (I^-) to manufacture the hormone thyroxine (thigh-ROX-in). But since levels of I^- in the bloodstream are fairly low, thyroid cells must actively transport iodide ions into the cytoplasm, where the iodide concentration is many times higher.

Ultimately, if thyroid cells had to rely on diffusion, they would probably not be able to produce enough hormone to meet the body's needs. Cells also use active transport to move materials out of their cytoplasm against concentration gradients.

Large Molecules and Cells Are Ingested by Endocytosis. Endocytosis (en-doe-sigh-TOE-siss; literally, "into the cell") is illustrated in **FIGURE 3-16A**. This process requires ATP and consists of two related activities: phagocytosis (fag-oh-sigh-toe-siss) and pinocytosis. **Phagocytosis** ("cell eating") occurs when cells engulf larger particles, such as bacteria and viruses. In humans, phagocytosis is limited to relatively few types of cells—those involved in protecting the body against foreign invaders. **Pinocytosis** (cell drinking) occurs when cells engulf extracellular fluids and dissolved materials. Most, if not all, cells are capable of pinocytosis.

Cells Also Regurgitate Materials, Releasing Large Molecules, Such as Hormones. This process is called **exocytosis** ("out of the cell") and is essentially the reverse of endocytosis (**FIGURE 3-16B**). For example, in the cells of the pituitary gland, which is located under the brain, protein hormones are packaged internally into tiny membrane-bound vesicles. These vesicles migrate to the plasma membranes and fuse with them. At the point of fusion, the membranes break down, and the protein hormone is released into the extracellular fluid. This process is exocytosis.

The Diffusion of Water Across the Plasma Membrane Is Known as Osmosis

Like any other small molecule, water moves from one side of a plasma membrane to the other by diffusion. The diffusion of water across a selectively permeable membrane, however, is given a special name, **osmosis**

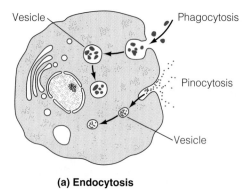

(a) Endocytosis

FIGURE 3-16 Membrane Transport *(a)* Cells can engulf large particles, cell fragments, and even entire cells via endocytosis. *(b)* Exocytosis, the reverse process, rids the cell of large particles.

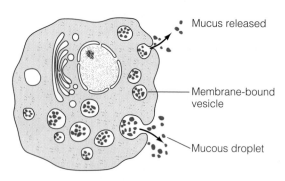

(b) Exocytosis

(oss-MOE-siss; this word comes from a Greek word meaning "to push"). To understand osmosis, consider a simplified example in **FIGURE 3-17**.

In this example, we begin with a large bag made of a special plastic that's selectively permeable. We fill the bag with water and table sugar (sucrose) and then submerge it in a large beaker of distilled water (**FIGURE 3-17**). The bag permits the water (but not the sucrose) to move in and out. Soon after immersion in the distilled water, water molecules will begin to diffuse down the concentration gradient, and the bag will begin to swell. This swelling results from the inward movement of water molecules shown by the arrows in **FIGURE 3-17B**. In this system, water moves from a region of high water concentration (distilled water) to a region of low water concentration (inside the bag).

The concentration difference across the membrane "drives" the water across a selectively permeable membrane. Therefore, whenever two fluids with different concentrations of solute (dissolved substance) are separated by a selectively permeable membrane, water will flow from one to the other, moving down the concentration gradient; the driving force is called **osmotic pressure.** The greater the difference in water concentration, the greater the osmotic pressure, and the more quickly the water moves.[3]

In humans and other multicellular organisms, osmosis helps regulate the concentration of fluid surrounding the cell (also called **extracellular fluid**), keeping it at the same concentration as that of the cells' cytoplasm. In such cases, the extracellular fluid is said to be **isotonic** (having the same strength).

If the fluid surrounding a cell is not isotonic, serious problems can be expected. For example, if blood cells are immersed in a solution that is more concentrated than their cytoplasm, water will move out of the cells, and the cells will shrink. A solution with a solute concentration higher than the cell's cytoplasm is said to be **hypertonic** (having a greater strength). A solution with a solute concentration lower than the cell's cytoplasm is said to be **hypotonic** (having a lesser strength). If red blood cells are placed in such a solution, water will rush in, causing the cells to swell and burst.

Combined with blood pressure and other forces, osmotic pressure plays an important role in the filtering

of blood in the kidney—a function essential to homeostasis (Chapter 10).

Section 3-5

Cellular Compartmentalization: Organelles

We next turn our attention to the **organelles**—structures that carry out many of the key functions of the cell. We begin with the nucleus.

The Nucleus Houses the DNA and Is the Cell's Command Center

As noted earlier, the nucleus is one of the cell's two major compartments. It is also one of the cell's most conspicuous and most important organelles (**FIGURE 3-18**). It is often likened to a cellular command center. The nucleus of the cell consists of (1) the nuclear envelope, (2) the chromatin, (3) the nucleoplasm, and (4) the nucleolus.

The **nuclear envelope** is a double membrane that isolates the nuclear material from the cytoplasm. Minute channels in the envelope, the **nuclear pores**, allow materials to pass into and out of the nucleus (**FIGURE 3-18B**).

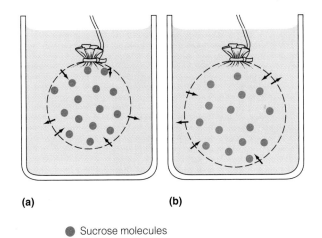

(a)　　　　　**(b)**

● Sucrose molecules

FIGURE 3-17 Osmosis Osmosis is the diffusion of water molecules from a region of higher water concentration (or low solute concentration) to one of lower water concentration (or high solute concentration) across a selectively permeable membrane. *(a)* To demonstrate the process, immerse a bag of sugar water in a solution of pure water. *(b)* Water diffuses into the bag (toward the lower concentration), causing it to swell.

---

[3]Water concentration is measured by the number of water molecules per milliliter. Pure water has a higher water concentration than salt water; that is, there are more water molecules per unit volume in pure water than in salt water.

The bulk of the nucleus contains long, threadlike fibers of DNA and protein, called **chromosomes** (CHROME-ah-zomes). The DNA-protein fibers, known as **chromatin** (CHROME-eh-tin), appear as fine granules in transmission electron micrographs of nuclei (**FIGURE 3-18A**). The DNA in the nucleus is the genetic material. It houses all of the information a cell needs for proper development and functioning—hence the description of the nucleus as a central command center. Just before cell division, the chromosomes coil to form short, compact bodies, highly visible in the light microscopic preparations (**FIGURE 3-19B**). This compaction greatly facilitates the cell division by making it much easier to divide the nuclear contents. A detailed discussion of DNA can be found in Chapter 17.

Proteins, water, and other small molecules and ions are also found in the nucleus, forming a semifluid material known as the **nucleoplasm** (new-KLEE-oh-plazem)—the nuclear equivalent of cytoplasm.

Nucleoli ("little nuclei"; singular, nucleolus) are temporary structures found in the nuclei of cells between cell divisions (**FIGURE 3-4**). They appear as small, clear, oval structures in light micrographs and as dense bodies in transmission electron micrographs. Nucleoli are regions of the DNA actively engaged in the production of RNA, specifically **ribosomal RNA** (also known as **rRNA**; pronounced RYE-bow-zomal). Ribosomal RNA gets its name from the fact that it combines with

certain proteins to form ribosomes. **Ribosomes** are nonmembranous organelles that appear as small, dark granules in electron micrographs and consist of two subunits. Produced in the nucleus, the subunits enter the cytoplasm through the nuclear pores. In the cytoplasm, they combine to play an important part in protein synthesis, described in Chapter 17. A detailed discussion of RNA is also presented in that chapter.

The Mitochondrion Is the Site of Cellular Energy Production in Animal Cells

No factory would operate without a source of energy and a place where that energy is generated. In most industrial nations, a factory's energy comes from power plants fueled by coal or oil or nuclear fuels. Like the factory, the cell also requires energy and a special structure to generate it. This structure is the mitochondrion (MY-toe-CON-dree-on).

The **mitochondrion,** shown in **FIGURE 3-20**, is an organelle that liberates energy from organic molecules, usually sugars and fats. Unlike power plants that generate electricity, mitochondria (plural) crank out ATP. Cells use ATP for many purposes: to synthesize chemical substances, to transport molecules across membranes, to divide, to contract, and to move about.

Although mitochondria vary considerably in form and number from cell to cell depending on the cell's energy requirement, they "share" several common characteristics. All mitochondria, for instance, are membrane-bound. In addition to the outer membrane, which holds the structure intact, all mitochondria contain an inner membrane, which is thrown into folds or **cristae** (CHRIS-tee) (**FIGURE 3-20B**). This membrane therefore divides the mitochondrion into two distinct compart-

Mitochondrion

Cytoplasm

Nuclear pore

Nuclear envelope

Nucleoplasm

Chromatin

(a)

Nuclear pores

(b)

FIGURE 3-18 The Nucleus   *(a)* The nucleus houses the genetic information that controls the structure and function of the cell. The nuclear envelope, made of lipids and proteins like the plasma membrane, actually consists of two membranes, separated by a space. Pores in the membrane allow the movement of molecules into the nucleus, providing raw

materials for the synthesis of DNA and RNA. They also allow RNA molecules to travel into the cytoplasm, where they participate in the production of protein. Chromatin may be densely packed or loosely arranged in the nucleus. *(b)* Colorized scanning electron micrograph of the nuclear membrane, showing numerous pores.

(a)

FIGURE 3-19 **Chromosomes** *(a)* The threadlike chromosomes, made of chromatin fibers consisting of protein and DNA, must condense before the nucleus can divide. *(b)* Condensed chromosomes. Can you think of any advantages to this strategy?

ments, the inner compartment and the outer compartment, each with its own function. They also increase the surface area on which chemical reactions take place.

Mitochondria play a key role in the liberation of energy in the body. During the breakdown of glucose, the principal source of energy, about one-third to two-thirds of the energy released during the chemical reactions is captured by the cell to produce ATP. The rest of the energy once housed in glucose molecules is given off as heat. This "waste" product creates body heat. It, in turn, is necessary for maintaining normal enzymatic function in warm-blooded animals like you and me. Without it, many processes would cease, as would we.

(b)

Three Organelles Are Involved in Manufacturing Protein and Other Cellular Products

Many cells are miniature factories synthesizing a variety of molecules vital for growth, reproduction, and day-to-day maintenance. Many of these molecules are used within the

cell; others, such as hormones, are released from the cell into the bloodstream where they travel to distant cells, eliciting specific responses. This section examines three organelles principally involved in cellular synthesis: the endoplasmic reticulum, ribosomes, and the Golgi complex.

Cytoplasm

Matrix

(b)

Outer membrane   Intermembrane compartment

Inner membrane

Cristae

Proteins of electron transport system

(a)

FIGURE 3-20 **The Mitochondrion** *(a)* Like the nucleus, the mitochondrion is delimited by a double membrane. The inner membrane, however, is infolded, forming cristae. *(b)* Electron micrograph of a mitochondrion. The infolding creates two distinct compartments: an inner compartment filled with a material called matrix, and an outer compartment lying between the two membranes. Compartmentalization is essential for ATP synthesis because it isolates functions. Membranes that form compartments also increase the surface area on which reactions occur.

Endoplasmic Reticulum. Coursing throughout the cytoplasm of many cells is a branched network of membranous channels, the **endoplasmic reticulum** (END-oh-PLAZ-mick rah-TICK-u-lum; meaning intracellular network) (**FIGURE 3-21A**). These membranous channels are derived chiefly from the nuclear envelope and may be coated with ribosomes (**FIGURE 3-21B**). Ribosome-studded endoplasmic reticulum is referred to as the **rough endoplasmic reticulum (RER).** The RER produces a variety of proteins. In the pancreas, it produces digestive enzymes. In certain endocrine glands, it produces protein hormones. In certain blood cells, it produces lysosomal enzymes (described shortly). And in all cells it produces plasma membrane proteins.

The proteins produced by the RER are made on the outside surface of the structure but are quickly transferred into its interior, possibly to protect them from damage. The interior of the RER is yet another specialized compartment. Not only does it protect the proteins, it contains 30–40 enzymes that convert some proteins into glycoproteins. Proteins and glycoproteins are then transferred to yet another organelle, the Golgi complex, for final packaging.

Cells also contain endoplasmic reticulum lacking ribosomes (**FIGURE 3-21C**). Known as the **smooth endoplasmic reticulum (SER),** this organelle specializes in the production of phospholipids, which are needed to replenish the plasma membrane. The SER performs a variety of functions in different cells. In the human liver, for instance, it detoxifies certain drugs, such as barbiturates, one type of sedative. In the stomach of humans and other mammals, the SER of certain cells produces hydrochloric acid, necessary for protein digestion. In the adrenal glands, the SER produces steroid hormones.

Ribosomes. As noted earlier, ribosomes are tiny particles made of protein and ribosomal RNA (rRNA). In the cytoplasm, ribosomes attach to strands of RNA molecules known as **messenger RNA (mRNA).** Messenger RNA molecules are produced in the nucleus of the cell and, as you shall see in Chapter 17, contain all of the information required to synthesize protein.

In the cytoplasm, several ribosomes attach to a single strand of mRNA, forming a structure known as a **polyribosome** or **polysome.** Together, **mRNA** and its attached ribosomes begin to produce protein. If it is a protein destined for inclusion in lysosomes or the plasma membrane or if it is intended for extracellular use (hormones and digestive enzymes), the polysome attaches to the RER, and the protein is transferred into the cisterna. If it is a protein for intracellular use, like those of the cytoskeleton or cytoplasmic enzymes, the polysome remains free within the cytoplasm.

The Golgi Complex. Proteins and glycoproteins manufactured by the RER are transported internally to the

FIGURE 3-21 The Endoplasmic Reticulum *(a)* Created by a network of membranes in the cytoplasm, the endoplasmic reticulum is often studded with small particles, the ribosomes, forming rough endoplasmic reticulum. This is the site of the synthesis of protein for lysosomes and extracellular use (digestive enzymes and hormones). *(b)* Electron micrographs of RER and *(c)* SER.

(a)

(b)

FIGURE 3-22 Protein Synthesis and Secretion *(a)* Protein packed in lysosomes and secretory granules (for later export) is synthesized on the RER and then transferred in tiny transport vesicles to the Golgi complex. Protein is sometimes chemically modified in the cisternae of both the

RER and the Golgi complex. The Golgi complex separates protein by destination and repackages it into secretory granules, which remain in the cytoplasm until secreted by exocytosis. *(b)* Transmission electron micrograph of the Golgi complex.

ends of sacs, the terminal ends (**FIGURE 3-22A**). As these products build up inside the RER, the ends bulge and eventually pinch off, forming tiny membrane-bound **transfer vesicles** (VESS-sick-kuls). The vesicles protect the proteins and glycoproteins as they are transported to the final packaging unit, the Golgi complex.

The **Golgi complex** (GOL-gee) consists of a series of membranous sacs (**FIGURE 3-22B**). It performs three functions. First, it sorts the molecules it receives. The Golgi complex separates lysosomal enzymes from hormones and plasma membrane proteins, ensuring that products end up in the right place. Second, like the RER, the Golgi complex chemically modifies many proteins, often adding carbohydrates or other small molecules. Finally, the Golgi complex packages proteins into lysosomes or secretory vesicles (or secretory granules) (**FIGURE 3-22A**).

Secretory vesicles are membranous organelles that reside in the cytoplasm. They act as temporary storage sites for hormones and digestive enzymes that will eventually be "shipped" to distant sites. When the signal for release comes, secretory vesicles migrate to the plasma membrane and fuse with it. The fused membranes soon dissolve, releasing the contents of the secretory vesicle into the extracellular space. This is an example of exocytosis.

Lysosomes Are Membrane-Bound Organelles That Contain Digestive Enzymes

Lysosomes (LIE-so-ZOMES; literally, digestive bodies) have been likened to tiny time bombs inside cells that, fortunately, rarely go off (**FIGURE 3-23**). Containing numerous digestive enzymes produced by the RER and packaged by the Golgi complex, these organelles—when functioning properly—break down materials that are phagocytized by cells. A better description of the lysosome might be to liken it to a wrecking crew that's kept under lock and key until the cell takes in something it needs to break apart.

As illustrated in the top of **FIGURE 3-23**, material engulfed by the cell (endocytosis) is enclosed in a membrane derived from the plasma membrane. The resultant structure is called a **food vacuole.** Lysosomes attach to food vacuoles and release their enzymes into them. The enzymes then break down the molecules inside the food vacuole into smaller molecules. These, in turn, diffuse into the cytoplasm, where they are often used by the cell. The undigested material left behind is expelled from the cell by exocytosis.

Besides providing the cell with nutrients, lysosomes are cellular custodians that destroy aged or defective cellular organelles, such as mitochondria. Lysosomes may

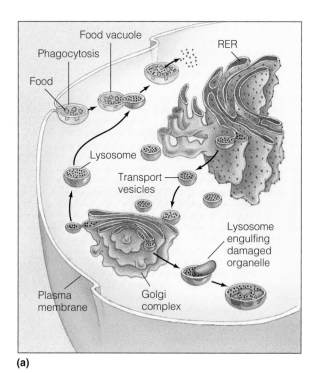

(a)

also digest protein and other molecules that have become defective. This process helps cells maintain their structure and function. How cells recognize defective molecules and organelles remains a mystery.

Lysosomes also rid the body of injured or aged cells. In these cells, lysosomes break open, releasing their enzymes and destroying the cell from the inside out.

Interestingly, lysosomal enzymes are released from damaged cells and, because of this, are the basis of a useful diagnostic tool. During a heart attack, for example, heart muscle cells that die release very specific enzymes into the blood, which can be measured to confirm a physician's diagnosis. Several other diseases can also be detected by blood enzyme levels.

Lysosomes play an important role in embryonic development. In humans, for example, the fingers of an early embryo are webbed (**FIGURE 3-24**). The cells of the webbing, however, are genetically programmed to self-destruct. At a certain point in development, the lysosomes of these cells release their enzymes, which destroy the cells and eliminate the webbing.

Most cells in the human body contain only a few lysosomes; these are used primarily to recycle outdated organelles or perhaps to put an end to the cell when its useful lifetime is over. However, certain cells contain hundreds of lysosomes. An example is the neutrophil (NEW-trowe-PHIL). Neutrophils are one type of blood cell that scavenges the blood and body tissues looking for bacteria and viruses, which they then phagocytize and digest internally with the aid of lysosomes. Thus, neutrophils play an important role in homeostasis by eliminating infectious agents.

Mitochondria   Lysosomes

(b)

FIGURE 3-23 Lysosomes   *(a)* The digestive enzymes of the lysosome are produced on the RER and transported to the Golgi complex for repackaging. Lysosomes produced by the Golgi complex fuse with food vacuoles; this allows their enzymes to mix with the contents of the food vacuole. The enzymes digest the contents, which diffuse through the membrane into the cytoplasm, where they are used. The membrane surrounding the lysosome helps protect the cell from digestive enzymes. *(b)* Electron micrograph of lysosomes within a macrophage. The dark-staining bodies are the lysosomes, filled with digestive enzymes that are used by these cells to break down ingested material.

FIGURE 3-24 The Human Embryonic Hand   The webs between the fingers present during the fetal stage are normally destroyed by lysosomes during development.

FIGURE 3-25 The Sperm Cell The sperm cell is a marvel of architecture, uniquely "designed" to streamline the cell for its long journey to fertilize the ovum. The nuclear material is compacted into the sperm head. The flagellum helps propel the sperm through the female reproductive tract.

(a)

FIGURE 3-26 Flagella *(a)* A sperm flagellum, showing the 9 + 2 arrangement and additional fibers thought to provide support and strength to the vigorously beating tail. *(b)* A basal body is found at the base of each cilium and flagellum. It consists of nine sets of triplets that give rise to the microtubule doublets of the cilium.

Triplet of microtubules

(b)

Flagella Are Organelles That Permit Cellular Motility

Most cells in the human body are part of tissues and organs and remain in the same place throughout their life. One exception is the mammalian sperm cell, which must move out of the body to perform its specialized task: fertilization.

The human sperm cell moves with the aid of a flagellum (fla-GEL-um; plural, flagella; Latin for "whip"). As shown in **FIGURE 3-25**, a flagellum is a long, whiplike extension of the plasma membrane. It contains numerous small tubules, the microtubules, which are shown in **FIGURE 3-26A**. Microtubules produce the motive force. As illustrated, the nine pairs of microtubules of the flagellum are arranged around a central pair. Biologists typically refer to this as the "9 + 2" arrangement. The flagella in sperm have additional fibers outside the central 9 + 2 array, which provide extra strength.

At the base of each flagellum is an anchoring structure, the **basal body** (BAZ-il) (**FIGURE 3-26B**). The basal body gives rise to the flagellum during development and contains nine sets of microtubules (with three microtubules each) but no central pair.

Movement Across the Surface of Cells Is Provided by Cilia

Several fixed cells in the body, such as those lining the trachea (TRAY-key-ah) or wind pipe, contain an or-

ganelle called the cilium (SILL-ee-um). **Cilia** (plural, pronounced SILL-ee-ah) are small extensions of the cell membrane (**FIGURE 3-27**). Like flagella, they have a central core of microtubules in a 9 + 2 arrangement.

Hundreds, even thousands, of cilia can be found on a single cell. In humans, for instance, thousands of cilia protrude from cells lining the trachea (**FIGURE 3-27**). These cilia beat toward the mouth and transport mucus (MEW-kuss) that is produced by other cells to the oral cavity (mouth), where it can be either swallowed or expectorated (spit out). Since the mucus traps dust particles in the air we breathe, the cilia are part of an automatic cleansing mechanism, vital for protecting the lungs and maintaining our health.

At the base of each cilium is a basal body, identical to those found in flagella. The basal body gives rise to the cilium during development and anchors the organelle in place.

Cilia and flagella are structurally similar, but flagella are much longer than cilia and far less numerous. Normal human sperm cells, for example, have one flagellum each, whereas each of the ciliated cells lining the respiratory system and parts of the female reproductive system

FIGURE 3-27 **Cilia** Cilia on cells lining the trachea of the human respiratory tract.

Power stroke   Return stroke

(a) Cilium

Continuous propulsion
(b) Flagellum

FIGURE 3-28 **Beating of Cilia and Flagella** *(a)* Cilia beat with a stiff power stroke—something like a rowing motion. During the return stroke, the cilium is flexible. *(b)* The flagellum beats like a whip, over and over, propelling the sperm cell forward.

(notably the Fallopian tubes) contains thousands of cilia. Flagella and cilia also beat differently. Cilia perform a stiff rowing motion with a flexible return stroke, whereas flagella beat more like whips, undulating in a continuous motion (**FIGURE 3-28**).

Because cilia and flagella often beat continuously, they require a more or less constant supply of energy, provided by ATP. As noted earlier, most ATP is produced by mitochondria, which are located nearby.

Some Cells Move by Amoeboid Motion

Another type of movement is called **amoeboid motion** (ah-ME-boyd). During amoeboid movement, the cell sends out many small cytoplasmic projections, or **pseudopodia** (SUE-dough-POW-dee-ah; "false feet"). Pseudopodia attach to solid surface's "in front" of the cell (**FIGURE 3-29**). Cytoplasm flows into the pseudopodia, moving the cell forward.

In humans, most cells are stationary and don't engage in ameboid motion. There are some cells, however, that move about in the body. One of them is the neutrophil, described earlier. It is a type of white blood cell that is transported in the blood. These cells, however, can escape through the walls of thin-walled blood vessels in body tissues called capillaries. Inside the tissues,

the neutrophils move about by ameboid motion, gobbling up bacteria and damaged cells.

Section 3-6
Energy and Metabolism

Cells get the energy they need primarily from two sources: the breakdown of glucose, a type of carbohydrate, and the breakdown of triglycerides, a type of fat. Under certain circumstances, they can even capture energy from pro-

Pseudopodia

Direction of movement

FIGURE 3-29 **Amoeboid Movement** Some cells in the human body move by amoeboid movement. Studies of the amoeba (shown here) show that cells that move by amoeboid movement send out minute extensions called pseudopodia (false feet), which attach to solid surfaces. Cytoplasm then flows into the pseudopodia, moving the cell forward.

teins (Chapter 5). In this section, we'll look briefly at how cells in humans acquire energy from glucose, a type of sugar. Before we examine this process, however, a few words about glucose and other carbohydrates are in order.

As noted in Chapter 2, carbohydrates are a general class of biological molecules. **Carbohydrates** are organic compounds that range in size from simple sugars such as glucose to very large molecules such as starch. Starch and

other complex carbohydrates, as they are called, contain many molecules of glucose bonded to one another by covalent bonds (Chapter 2). The molecular structures of two simple carbohydrates—ribose, a five-carbon sugar, and glucose, a six-carbon sugar—are shown in **FIGURE 3-30**. These are also known as **monosaccharides.**

Simple sugars such as glucose and fructose (another six-carbon sugar that is found in fruits) can unite by covalent bonds to form **sucrose,** commonly known as table sugar (**FIGURE 3-31**). Sucrose is a **disaccharide,** because it consists of two monosaccharides. As noted earlier, monosaccharides can unite in long, branching chains (**FIGURE 3-32**). These are known as **polysaccharides,** and include such important molecules as starch, glycogen, and cellulose. These molecules will be discussed in more detail elsewhere in the book. For now, let us return to fascinating ways in which cells derive energy from glucose.

Glucose molecules, like other organic molecules, contain energy—a fact that you could demonstrate by holding a spoonful of sugar over a candle. This energy is stored in the covalent bonds that hold the atoms of the molecule in place. Cells can tap into this energy by breaking glucose molecules apart in an orderly series of chemical reactions. This series begins in the cytoplasm and is completed in the mitochondrion. The complete breakdown of glucose is referred to as **cellular respiration**. Cells don't breathe like we do, but they do require oxygen and give off carbon dioxide; hence the name **cellular respiration**.

During cellular respiration, glucose, which contains six carbon atoms, is broken down into six molecules of carbon dioxide and six molecules of water. The overall reaction is

$$\text{glucose} + \text{oxygen} \rightarrow \text{carbon dioxide} + \text{water} + \text{energy}$$

$$C_6H_{12}O_6 + 6\,O_2 \rightarrow 6\,CO_2 + 6\,H_2O + 38\,\text{ATP}$$

FIGURE 3-30 Two Monosaccharides

FIGURE 3-31 Disaccharides   Simple sugars such as glucose and fructose can combine to form the disaccharide known as sucrose.

FIGURE 3-32 Polysaccharides Simple sugars can also combine to form polysaccharides such as glycogen, which is a storage form of glucose in animals and is found in muscle and liver.

Portion of polysaccharide molecule (glycogen)

Glycogen (segment of larger molecule)

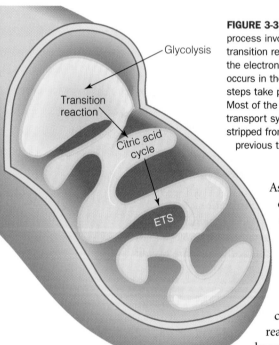

Glycolysis

Transition reaction

Citric acid cycle

ETS

FIGURE 3-33 Cellular Respiration This process involves four steps: glycolysis, the transition reaction, the citric acid cycle, and the electron transport system. Glycolysis occurs in the cytoplasm; the remaining steps take place in the mitochondrion. Most of the ATP is produced in the electron transport system (ETS) from the energy stripped from electrons given off by the previous three stages.

As shown, the complete breakdown of glucose requires oxygen. Without oxygen, glucose can be only partially broken down, and only a fraction of its energy can be captured.

The breakdown of glucose releases lots of energy. A reaction that gives off energy is known as an **exergonic reaction.**

Cells can capture sizable portions of this energy and use it to synthesize ATP from inorganic phosphate (P_i) and ADP. The formation of ATP results in the storage of energy. ATP synthesis is an **endergonic reaction** (energy-requiring). Exergonic and endergonic reactions are often coupled—linked so that energy from one is transferred to the other. The complete breakdown of glucose generates enough energy to produce 38 molecules of ATP from ADP and inorganic phosphate.

The Chemical Breakdown of Glucose Occurs in Four Steps

Cellular respiration is not as simple as the reaction you've just studied may imply. In our cells, the complete breakdown of glucose requires many chemical reactions that occur during four distinct, yet interconnected processes: (1) glycolysis, (2) the transition reaction, (3) the citric acid cycle, and (4) the electron transport system (**FIGURE 3-33**). During respiration each glucose molecule is broken apart to produce 6 carbon dioxide molecules and energy. The energy is captured by the cell

TABLE 3-4

Overview of Cellular Energy Production

Reaction	Location	Description and Products
Glycolysis	Cytoplasm	Breaks glucose into two three-carbon compounds, pyruvate; nets two ATP and two NADH molecules
Transition reaction	Mitochondrion	Removes one carbon dioxide from each pyruvate, producing two acetyl CoA molecules; produces two NADH molecules
Citric acid cycle	Inner compartment of mitochondrion	Completes the breakdown of acetyl cycle CoA; produces two ATPs per glucose; produces numerous NADH and FADH molecules
Electron transport	Inner membrane of mitochondrion	Accepts electrons from NADH and FADH, generated by previous system reactions; produces 34 ATPs

to produce ATP, the only form of energy cells can use. **TABLE 3-4** summarizes the stages of cellular respiration and lists their products. The following paragraphs provide a more detailed summary of cellular respiration for students required to have a more in-depth understanding of this process.

Glycolysis Is the Breakdown of Glucose into Two Pyruvate Molecules. The first phase of cellular respiration in cells is known as glycolysis. **Glycolysis** (gly-COLL-eh-siss) is a metabolic pathway located in the cytoplasm of cells. As **FIGURE 3-34** shows, during glycolysis, glucose is split in half, forming two three-carbon molecules of pyruvic acid, or pyruvate. The energy released during this process nets the cell a modest two molecules of ATP. It also yields two molecules of NADH (nicotine adenine dinucleotide). NADH is a substance (technically a coenzyme) that picks up hydrogens and electrons given off by the reactions. Its importance will be clear shortly.

The Transition Reaction Is an Intermediate Step in Which One Carbon Atom Is Cleaved Off Each Pyruvate. Pyruvate generated in glycolysis diffuses from the cytoplasm into the inner compartment of the mitochondrion and reacts there with a large molecule

FIGURE 3-35 Overview of the Transition Reaction and the Citric Acid Cycle *(a)* The transition reaction cleaves off one carbon dioxide and binds the remaining two-carbon compound temporarily to a large molecule called Coenzyme A. The result is a molecule called acetyl-CoA. It then enters the citric acid cycle. *(b)* Occurring in the matrix of the mitochondrion, the citric acid cycle liberates two carbon dioxides and produces one ATP per pyruvate molecule. Its main products, however, are NADH and FADH$_2$, bearing high-energy electrons that are transferred to the electron transport system.

called Coenzyme A (CoA) as shown in **FIGURE 3-35**. During this **transition reaction,** one carbon atom is cleaved off each pyruvate molecule, forming a two-carbon compound (acetyl group) that binds to Coenzyme A (**FIGURE 3-35**). The product of this reaction is **acetyl CoA** (ah-SEAT-ill). The transition reaction also yields two NADH molecules.

The Citric Acid Cycle Completes the Breakdown of Glucose. Acetyl CoA enters the third stage of cellular respiration, a cyclic metabolic pathway also located inside the inner compartment of the mitochondrion. This elaborate pathway is called the **Krebs cycle,** after the scientist who worked out many of its details, or the **citric acid cycle,** after the very first product formed in the reaction sequence.

During the cycle, the two-carbon compound produced in the transition reaction binds to a four-carbon compound known as **oxaloacetate** (ox-AL-oh-ass-eh-tate). The result is a six-carbon product, citric acid. Citric acid proceeds through a series of chemical reactions, each catalyzed by its own enzyme. Along the way, the molecule is modified many times. During the complex molecular rearrangements, two molecules of carbon dioxide are removed from the six-carbon chain, and oxaloacetate is regenerated at the end, thus ensuring the continuation of the cycle.

As shown in **FIGURE 3-35**, one of the chemical reactions of the citric acid cycle yields an ATP molecule. Because two molecules of pyruvate enter the citric acid cycle for each glucose molecule broken down by

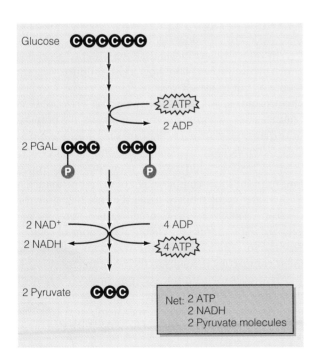

FIGURE 3-34 Overview of Glycolysis During this process, glucose is broken down into two molecules of PGAL, which are converted to pyruvate. The cell nets two ATP and two NADH molecules.

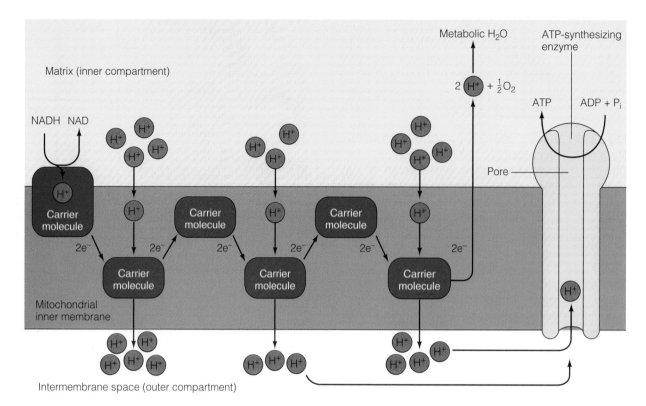

FIGURE 3-36 The Electron Transport System and Chemiosmosis Located on the inner surface of the mitochondrial inner membrane, the electron transport system produces ATP via chemiosmosis, described in the text.

glycolysis, the citric acid cycle nets the cell two ATP molecules. Several other reactions release electrons, which are funneled into the fourth, and final, part of cellular respiration, the electron transport system.

Electrons Given Off During the Citric Acid Cycle and Glycolysis Enter the Electron Transport System. The electrons liberated during certain reactions of the citric acid cycle are passed to one of the two electron acceptors in the mitochondrial matrix: **nicotinamide adenine dinucleotide (NAD)** and **flavine adenine dinucleotide (FAD)**. These molecules, in turn, transfer the electrons to a series of protein carrier molecules embedded on the inner surface of the inner membrane of the mitochondrion (**FIGURE 3-36**). The carrier proteins constitute the **electron transport system (ETS)**.

The electron transport system accepts electrons from FADH and NADH. These electrons are then passed from one protein to another and are eventually given over to oxygen molecules inside the matrix. Dur-

ing their rapid journey along this chain, the electrons lose energy, much like a hot potato passed along by a line of people. The energy lost along the way is used to make ATP. But how does the cell make ATP?

In 1961, British biochemist Peter Mitchell proposed a mechanism to explain how cells produce ATP in their electron transport systems. This hypothesis, called **chemiosmosis,** won Mitchell the Nobel Prize in 1978 (**FIGURE 3-36**). According to this hypothesis, the proteins of the electron transport chain are dual-purpose molecules. That is, they transport electrons, and they also serve as hydrogen-ion pumps, transporting hydrogen ions from the inner compartment of the mitochondrion to the outer compartment using the energy lost by the electrons (**FIGURE 3-36**). As noted earlier, these hydrogens are released from the chemical reactions of cellular respiration. The export of the hydrogen ions to the outer compartment results in their buildup.

Hydrogen ions do not stay put, however. Many of them flow back into the inner compartment through pores in the inner mitochondrial membrane. It is this flow of hydrogen ions, Mitchell hypothesized, that powers ATP synthesis. How?

Just as electrons flowing in a wire provide energy to run motors or to power light bulbs, the flowing hydrogen ions are thought to drive the process of ATP synthesis.

All told, the electron transport system produces 34 ATP molecules per glucose molecule. Because 2 ATPs are generated by glycolysis and 2 are produced in the citric acid cycle, the total output for cellular respiration is 38 ATP molecules per glucose molecule.

As shown in **FIGURE 3-36**, the "de-energized" electrons from the electron transport system eventually combine with hydrogen ions and oxygen to produce water.

Enzymes Are Essential to Virtually All Chemical Reactions Occurring in the Cell

Before moving on, it is important to note that each of the chemical reactions of cellular respiration is regulated by an enzyme. Described earlier, enzymes are protein molecules that greatly accelerate chemical reactions. So important are they that a missing enzyme in a metabolic pathway will very likely shut the pathway down—in much the same way that a missing worker on an assembly line interrupts production.

Each enzyme is a large, globular protein with a small region known as the active site (**FIGURE 3-37A**). The **active site** is an indentation, or pocket, where the chemical reaction occurs. Its shape corresponds to that of the **substrate(s),** the molecule(s) undergoing reaction. Substrates fit into the active site in much the same way that a hand fits into a glove. Because each enzyme has its own uniquely shaped active site capable of binding to one or at most a few chemical substrates, enzymes are said to be specific. This feature allows the cells to regulate chemical reactions very precisely.

Interestingly, although enzymes play an active role in the metabolism of cells, they are unchanged by the reaction. As a result, they can be recycled—used over and over again.

Enzymes can also be controlled by the cells themselves, which provides additional control over cellular metabolism. The most common regulators of enzyme activity are the end products of chemical reactions. When produced in excess, the end products often bind to specific control regions on enzymes. The control regions are called **allosteric sites** (al-oh-STAIR-ick). Allosteric sites are the molecular equivalent of switches. When an end product binds to one, it turns the enzyme off, shutting down the entire metabolic pathway (**FIGURE 3-37B**). In some metabolic pathways, end products may bind directly to the active site of an enzyme. This binding also blocks substrates from entering the site, thereby inhibiting the enzyme and shutting down the metabolic pathway (**FIGURE 3-37C**).

Cellular respiration can be controlled by the buildup of chemicals such as citrate and ATP, both of

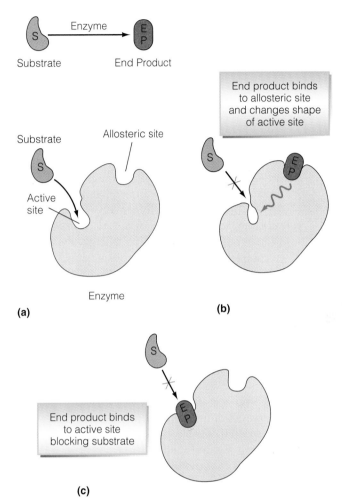

FIGURE 3-37 Enzyme Structure and Function *(a)* Two-dimensional drawing of an enzyme. The active site conforms to the shape of the reacting molecule(s). *(b)* The allosteric site is a molecular switch that regulates enzyme activity. In some metabolic pathways, the end products bind to the allosteric site. This may turn the active site on or off, depending on the enzyme. *(c)* In others, the end products of a reaction bind to the active site itself, blocking it entirely.

which shut down a specific enzyme in the glycolytic pathway.

Fermentation: Tired Muscles, Cheese, and Wine

What do tired muscles, cheese, and wine have in common? The answer is that they're all products of a process called fermentation. Fermentation occurs in human cells when oxygen levels run low. It also occurs in certain microorganisms. Basically, **fermentation** is a chemical reaction in which pyruvic acid produced from glycolysis is converted to one of several other end products (**FIGURE 3-38**). These reactions are important, in part, because they produce energy. Let's look briefly at this process in body cells.

During strenuous exercise, oxygen consumption in muscle cells may exceed replenishment. When this occurs, oxygen levels inside the cells fall. The cells are said to be anaerobic. With oxygen no longer available to accept electrons, the electron transport system (ETS) shuts down. When the ETS falters, so does the citric acid cycle. Fortunately, glycolysis still continues. But in the absence of oxygen, the end product of glycolysis, pyruvate, is converted to lactic acid as shown in **FIGURE 3-38A**.

Thus, rather than shutting energy production down completely, muscle cells continue to generate energy via glycolysis and fermentation. Unfortunately, fermentation is exceedingly inefficient, netting the cell only 2 ATPs for each glucose molecule, compared with 38 during the complete breakdown.

In humans, heavy exercise, such as weight lifting and running, depletes muscle oxygen, making cells become anaerobic, which results in the buildup of lactic acid in muscle cells. This causes muscle fatigue and soreness you feel after you've exercised heavily. Lactic acid, however, diffuses out of the muscle within hours and is carried by the blood to the liver, where it is converted first to pyruvate and then to glucose in a series of chemical reactions that is essentially the reverse of glycolysis. Some of the glucose is used to synthesize glycogen, and the rest is released into the blood, where it is redistributed to body cells and used to generate energy.

Fermentation is also the chief source of energy for many bacteria and other single-celled organisms. Those that live in oxygen-free environments—for example, deep in muddy sediments of lakes and rivers—meet their energy needs by fermentation. Other microorganisms temporarily deprived of oxygen can also satisfy their energy needs through fermentation.

The most common type of fermentation is lactic acid fermentation, discussed above. Many popular foods, such as cheese and yogurt, are produced by lactic acid fermentation. Most cheeses, for instance, are produced from milk and selected lactic acid bacteria. To make cheese, lactic acid bacteria are added to milk. These bacteria break down milk sugar (lactose), releasing glucose molecules in the process. Glucose molecules are then broken down in the glycolytic and fermentation pathways in the bacteria, and lactic acid is produced. Enzymes that digest proteins, known as proteolytic enzymes, are then added to cause the liquid to curdle. The thin watery part (whey) is drawn off, leav-

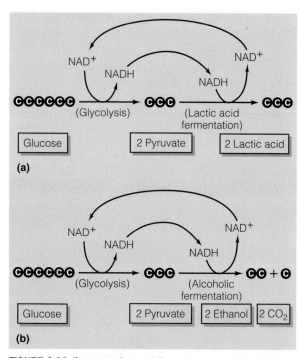

FIGURE 3-38 Fermentation *(a)* Pyruvate, or pyruvic acid, from glycolysis is converted into lactic acid in muscle cells when oxygen levels fall. *(b)* Fermentation can produce a variety of products in bacteria and yeast cells. In certain microorganisms, pyruvate is converted into ethanol and carbon dioxide.

ing behind the unripened cheese (for example, cottage cheese). Additional bacteria and fungi may be added to break down milk fat and protein, yielding specific ripened cheeses, such as blue cheese.

Other microorganisms undergo **alcoholic fermentation,** which, as the name implies, produces ethanol and carbon dioxide from pyruvate (**FIGURE 3-38B**). Alcoholic fermentation is the basis of the production of beer, wine, and hard liquor. Alcoholic fermentation is also the basis of bread making. Yeast cells are added to bread dough. These microorganisms are anaerobic and produce carbon dioxide and ethyl alcohol. The carbon dioxide forms bubbles in the dough, causing it to rise, and the alcohol is driven off during baking, producing the pleasant smell of baking bread.

Health, Homeostasis, and the Environment
Parkinson's and Pollution?

The stability of the internal environment is continuously threatened by disruptive forces, many of them of our own making. Chemical pollution is one of the many forces that can throw our cells and therefore our bodies out of balance. The following paragraphs describe a frightening example of this phenomenon.

In 1983, several relatively young men and women were admitted to a California hospital in a catatonic stupor. Dr. J. W. Langston, the neurologist who treated them, was baffled by their condition. His patients represented a novel medical puzzle unlike any he had ever seen. The patients lay immobile day after day. They could neither talk, nor feed themselves, nor move their limbs. It was as if they had been frozen.

Langston began an intensive study of the patients, all drug addicts. He found that each of them had taken a synthetic, heroinlike drug that had been contaminated with a paralyzing chemical known as MPTP. Made in the basement of one of California's small-time drug pushers, the drug was the latest in a long list of "designer" drugs then on the market. Sloppy chemistry resulted in the contamination.

MPTP attacks nerve cells in a part of the brain called the substantia nigra (sub-STAN-she-ah NIGH-gra). Degeneration of the brain cells in this region has long been thought to cause **Parkinson's disease,** a disorder that usually afflicts older individuals. Parkinson's disease is characterized by tremors, or involuntary rhythmic shaking, of the hands or head. If the disease worsens, patients have difficulty talking and writing. Walking becomes awkward and clumsy. In later stages, memory and thinking can be severely impaired.

Interestingly, individuals exposed to even minute amounts of MPTP develop symptoms similar to those seen in Parkinson's patients. In fact, a Swiss chemist who had worked briefly with the chemical was hospitalized because his body muscles, like those of the addicts whom Langston had encountered, "froze up" on him. Puzzled physicians put him in a mental hospital, assuming that he was suffering from a psychological disorder called catatonic schizophrenia.

MPTP is similar to several common industrial chemicals and pesticides. Some scientists speculated that MPTP-like chemicals in the air, water, and soil might be the underlying cause of the nerve cell damage in Parkinson's disease. However, several studies have failed to show a link between Parkinson's disease and industrial pollution. At a 1985 meeting at the National Institutes of Health, researchers agreed: Parkinson's disease had not been shown to be caused by environmental contamination.

No sooner had the researchers arrived home than a Canadian scientist announced the results of a study in Quebec showing a remarkable correlation between the use of MPTP-like pesticides (for example, paraquat) and the incidence of Parkinson's disease. He argued,

however, that pesticides were probably not the only chemical villain. Many neurotoxins discharged from nearby chemical factories could have been present in the area.

In support of the hypothesis that Parkinson's disease is linked to industrial pollution and pesticide use, researchers note that Parkinson's disease was unheard of before the Industrial Revolution. As industrialization and environmental pollution spread, the incidence of the disease rose. It reached a plateau in the early 1900s. Although no increase has been seen since 1940, some researchers warn that an increase in the use of MPTP-like pesticides and an increase in industrial pollution could substantially raise the incidence of the disease in years to come.

That's not good news, because Parkinson's is a crippling disease. Caused by a lack of a chemical substance in the brain called dopamine, Parkinson's disease can be treated with a drug known as levodopa. But its benefits diminish over years of use. And some patients suffer severe side effects, including severe nausea and vomiting. Several other drugs are also used.

Recent studies show that fetal cell transplants into the affected brain area may eliminate the symptoms of the disease. A year after receiving a fetal cell transplant, 13 of 19 people showed elevated levels of dopamine production. Surgeons can also ablate (destroy) a small region of the brain that appears to be hyperactive in Parkinson's patients. This improves a patient's score on standardized movement tests, although several patients had serious side effects including facial paralysis. Electrodes can also be implanted in the brain to stop uncontrollable movements. Patients are equipped with tiny electronic stimulators, much like pacemakers, that can be switched on or off as needed.

The cause of Parkinson's disease is still unknown. Other factors may also cause the disease. Some researchers think that amalgam fillings in teeth may be play a role in the onset of the disease. Chemicals used in wood stains may be responsible. Very likely, there are many causes.

If the connection between MPTP and other harmful chemicals in our environment proves to be valid, Parkinson's disease could be a case study showing how the function of certain nerve cells may be affected by chemical pollution and how the delicate balance that keeps muscles in check is lost because of a chemical imbalance in the environment. Not only does this illustrate the connection between human health, homeostasis, and environmental conditions, it underscores the importance of a clean environment to a healthy future.

Summary

1. The fundamental unit of all living organisms is the *cell*. All organisms are composed of one or more cells.

2. Two types of cells are found: prokaryotic and eukaryotic. *Prokaryotic cells* lack nuclei and are found in single-celled organisms such as bacteria. *Eukaryotic cells* are structurally more complex cells with membrane-bound nuclei. Some single-celled organisms and all multicellular organisms are eukaryotic.

Cellular Evolution and Homeostasis

3. During cellular evolution, prokaryotic organisms emerged first, about 3.5 billion years ago.

4. Eukaryotes evolved about 2.0 billion years later. The first eukaryotic cells were single-celled organisms.

5. As evolution proceeded, organisms became multicellular and began to acquire specialized cells. Over time, eukaryotes gave rise to three additional kingdoms: plants, fungi, and animals.

6. The increasing complexity of organisms was paralleled by the development of complex systems that ensure homeostasis.

Microscopes: Illuminating the Structure of Cells

7. The *microscope* is one of many scientific instruments used to study cells. Microscopes enlarge objects and allow us to see detail.

8. Microscopes fall into two broad categories: (1) *light microscopes,* which use ordinary visible light to illuminate the specimen; and (2) *electron microscopes,* which use beams of electrons to visualize an image.

An Overview of Cell Structure

9. Cells of the human body differ widely, but all consist of two major compartments, the nuclear and the cytoplasmic.

10. The nuclear compartment, or *nucleus,* contains the genetic information that regulates the structure and function of all eukaryotic cells.

11. The cytoplasmic compartment contains *cytoplasm,* which, in turn, contains numerous *cellular organelles,* structures that perform specific functions.

12. The cytoplasmic compartment is home to the *cytoskeleton,* a network of tubules and filaments that gives cells their three-dimensional shape and also binds to enzymes in metabolic pathways, increasing cellular efficiency.

The Structure and Function of the Plasma Membrane

13. The outermost boundary of the cell, the *plasma membrane,* consists of lipids, proteins, and small amounts of carbohydrate.

14. The plasma membrane ensures the structural integrity of the cell, regulates the flow of materials into and out of the cell, and participates in cellular communication and cellular identification.

15. *Lipids* are a diverse group of organic chemicals characterized by their lack of water solubility. The biologically important lipids serve many functions. Two main lipids were discussed in this chapter: (a) phospholipids and (b) steroids.

16. *Amino acids* are small organic molecules that join by *peptide bonds,* forming a variety of *peptides* (containing fewer than 20 amino acids) and *proteins* (containing more than 20 amino acids).

17. Thousands of different types of proteins are found in human cells; each type is structurally and functionally unique. Their uniqueness results from the sequence of amino acids in a protein.

18. Because it is mostly lipid, the membrane is a natural barrier to water-soluble molecules. Lipid-soluble materials pass through with ease.

19. Water-soluble molecules and ions are believed to pass through pores in the membrane by *diffusion,* the flow of a substance from an area of higher concentration to an area of lower concentration.

20. *Carrier proteins* may also transport water-soluble molecules across the membrane down the concentration gradient. This process is called *facilitated diffusion.*

21. Some molecules are actively transported across the membrane. *Active transport* mechanisms use energy to pump materials into or out of the cell and require a special class of membrane proteins, the transport molecules. Active transport permits cells to transport substances from regions of low concentration to regions of high concentration.

22. Cells engulf liquids and their dissolved materials in a process called *pinocytosis.* Cells may also engulf large molecules and cells by *phagocytosis.* Pinocytosis and phagocytosis are collectively referred to as *endocytosis.*

23. During endocytosis, the plasma membrane indents and surrounds the material to be ingested. The material engulfed by the cell is incorporated in a membranous vesicle, which is taken into the cell.

24. Water is believed to move through tiny pores in plasma membranes. The diffusion of water molecules through a selectively permeable membrane from a region of higher water concentration to a region of lower water concentration is called *osmosis.*

Cellular Compartmentalization: Organelles

25. The *nucleus* is one of the most conspicuous cellular organelles. It houses the DNA, which contains the genetic information that determines the structure and function of the cell.

26. The nucleus is bounded by a double membrane, the *nuclear envelope,* which contains numerous pores that allow many materials (but not the DNA) to pass freely between the nucleus and the cytoplasm.

27. Energy in the cell is produced principally by the breakdown of glucose. Glucose breakdown takes place, in part, in the cytoplasm but mostly in the *mitochondrion.* Energy liberated from glucose molecules is captured by ATP molecules.

28. All mitochondria have two membranes, an outer one and an inner one. The inner membrane is thrown into folds called *cristae.*

29. Cellular energy production captures 30–60% of the energy contained in glucose; the rest is liberated as heat.

30. The *endoplasmic reticulum* is a network of membranous channels in the cytoplasm of the cell and is the main location of cellular protein synthesis.

31. Endoplasmic reticulum may be smooth or rough. *Smooth endoplasmic reticulum* has no ribosomes. *Rough endoplasmic reticulum* contains many ribosomes on its outer surface.

32. Smooth endoplasmic reticulum produces phospholipids (needed to make more plasma membrane), and it has many additional functions in different cells. The rough endoplasmic reticulum is involved in synthesizing protein for extracellular use (for example, hormones) and in the production of enzymes that are contained in *lysosomes*.

33. Proteins produced on the surface of the RER enter the cavity, where they may be chemically modified. Proteins are transferred from the RER to the Golgi complex, where they are sorted, chemically modified, and repackaged into *secretory vesicles* or lysosomes.

34. Secretory vesicles accumulate in the cytoplasm and are released when needed. Lysosomes remain in the cell, where they bind to food vacuoles (material phagocytized or pinocytized by the cell) or destroy malfunctioning cellular organelles.

35. Most cells in the body are fixed. Still other cells can move about in tissues via amoeboid movement.

36. The human sperm cell utilizes another kind of motive force, the *flagellum*, a long, whiplike structure.

37. Some cells contain numerous smaller extensions, called *cilia*, which propel fluids and materials along their surfaces.

38. Both cilia and flagella contain nine pairs of microtubules arranged in a circle around a central pair.

Energy and Metabolism

39. Cells acquire energy from glucose, a carbohydrate.

40. Carbohydrates are a group of organic compounds that consist of simple sugars (monosaccharides) such as glucose, disaccharides such as sucrose, and long chains (polymers) of monosaccharides.

41. The complete breakdown of glucose is called *cellular respiration* and consists of four interdependent parts: glycolysis, the transition reaction, the citric acid cycle, and the electron transport system.

42. Glycolysis is a series of reactions occurring in the cytoplasm of cells. During glycolysis, glucose is split in two. Each molecule of glucose yields two molecules of pyruvic acid, or pyruvate.

43. Glycolysis nets the cell two molecules of ATP and two NADH molecules containing high-energy electrons.

44. Pyruvate produced during glycolysis next diffuses into the mitochondrion and undergoes the transition reaction. This step produces acetyl CoA and two NADH molecules.

45. Acetyl CoA enters the citric acid cycle, which produces two ATPs and numerous molecules of NADH and $FADH_2$. These electron carriers accept high-energy electrons from various reactions in the citric acid cycle and move them to the electron transport system.

46. The electron transport system consists of a series of protein molecules embedded in the inner surface of the inner membrane of the mitochondrion. Electrons from NADH and $FADH_2$ are passed down the chain and are eventually given to oxygen. During this process, numerous molecules of ATP are produced via *chemiosmosis*.

Fermentation:
Tired Muscles, Cheese, and Wine

47. Without oxygen, the electron transport system shuts down, as does the citric acid cycle. At this point, cells must rely on glycolysis and fermentation to generate energy.

48. Fermentation is a chemical reaction in which pyruvate is converted into lactic acid or some other product, such as ethyl alcohol.

49. Lactic acid fermentation is also an important source of food for humans, including cheeses and yogurts, which are made from milk and selected bacteria.

50. Alcoholic fermentation produces ethanol from pyruvate and occurs in certain microorganisms.

51. Wines, beer, and hard liquor are all produced by combining plant by-products (grains or fruits) with microorganisms that are alcoholic fermenters.

Health, Homeostasis, and the Environment:
Parkinson's and Pollution?

52. MPTP is a chemical contaminant in a synthetic, heroinlike drug. MPTP attacks certain cells in the brain, the same cells, in fact, long thought to be associated with *Parkinson's disease,* a disorder that generally afflicts older individuals and that is characterized by involuntary rhythmic shaking of the hands or head.

53. Individuals exposed to even minute amounts of MPTP develop symptoms similar to those seen in Parkinson's patients.

54. MPTP is similar to several common industrial chemicals and pesticides. Some scientists now speculate that MPTP-like chemicals in the air, water, and soil may be the underlying cause of Parkinson's disease.

55. This example illustrates the connection between homeostasis, human health, and environmental quality. It shows how alterations in the level of cellular function can have dramatic effects on the whole body and, if the link between Parkinson's and industrial chemicals proves valid, underscores the importance of protecting human health by protecting the quality of our environment.

Critical Thinking

Thinking Critically—Analysis

This analysis corresponds to the Thinking Critically scenario that was presented at the beginning of this chapter.

First, you might note that one study is never enough to test the validity of a hypothesis. Further work is needed before you can be certain that the results are valid. Some questions to ask are: Did the vitamin increase the lifespan of all cells or just certain types of cells? Were there any other factors responsible for increased lifespan? Was the test done on cells from an infant, a toddler, a youngster, a teenager, or an adult?

Second, you might also suggest that studies on animals would be needed to test this hypothesis. Tissue cultures are very artificial environments. An organism is much more complicated than some of its cells in tissue culture. Many hormones and other substances are present that might alter the effect of the vitamin.

Finally, you might want your friends to consider the potential toxic effects of the vitamins they are thinking about taking. Would vitamin supplements cause more harm than good?

Test of Concepts

1. Describe the concepts of cellular and organismic homeostasis. How are they related? How does environmental homeostasis or environmental quality affect them?
2. Cellular compartmentalization allows for greater efficiency. Why? Give an example to support your argument.
3. Draw a diagram of the plasma membrane, and describe the five routes by which molecules pass through the membrane.
4. In what ways does the plasma membrane participate in cellular communication? How is this function important for the maintenance of homeostasis?
5. Define the terms *osmosis, isotonic, hypotonic,* and *hypertonic.* In what way(s) is osmosis similar to diffusion, and in what way(s) is it different?
6. Describe the organelles involved in the synthesis, storage, and release of protein for extracellular use, starting with the basic instructions needed to make the protein.
7. In what ways are cilia and flagella similar, and in what ways are they different?
8. What is the main energy currency of the cell? Where is it formed? Where does it get its energy?
9. Describe the four phases of cellular energy production.

www.jbpub.com/humanbiology

Connect to this book's web site: www.jbpub.com/humanbiology
The site features eLearning, an online review area that provides quizzes, chapter outlines, and other tools to help you study for your class. You can also follow useful links for in-depth information, research the differing views in the Point/Counterpoints, or keep up on the latest environmental and health news.

Principles of Structure and Function

Thinking Critically

Health care costs are skyrocketing, and many critics are arguing that our health care dollars are being misused. In particular, they argue that expensive procedures, such as organ transplants for indigent people costing taxpayers $150,000 or more each, are draining dollars that could be invested in preventive medicine, such as prenatal care. Analyze this view using your critical thinking skills. ■

Human red blood cell trapped in a fibrin network of a blood clot.

Jenny Hawn has cystic fibrosis, a deadly disease that afflicts the respiratory system and pancreas. One of the main problems with the disease is the production of excess mucus by the cells lining the respiratory tract. This mucus traps bacteria and viruses and can result in frequent lung infections.

Jenny's disease is genetic. Until recently, there's been little hope of curing this young teen or any of the thousands of other children with this disease, which claims most of its victims before they reach the age of 20. Today, however, there may be some hope. Geneticists are experimenting with novel ways to repair the genetic defects in the cells lining Jenny's respiratory tract, the cells that are responsible for excessive mucus production.

To correct the genetic defect, researchers are experimenting with certain cold viruses that infect the cells lining the respiratory tract. Normally, these cells inject their DNA into the lining cells, causing cold symptoms. But researchers cut out the viral genes that cause colds, and splice in new genes that could lead to normal mucus production. By inserting the normal genes into these viruses and exposing a cystic fibrosis patient to the virus, scientists hope to transport good genes into defective cells, creating a lasting cure for a deadly disease.

This research, still in its early stages, is just one many forms of "body work" scientists are now performing. Other researchers are working at a level slightly higher—that is, at the level of tissues and organs (defined shortly). Some scientists are developing genetically engineered pigs whose cells contain human genes. Their hope is that the that pig-human organs could someday be transplanted into people to replace failed livers or kidneys. In fact, they speculate, an organ could be specially made with a person's own genes to prevent tissue rejection. It would be available in a fraction of the time it now takes to find a genetically compatible organ from a suitable donor.

Health Note 4-1 describes other remarkable medical procedures used to repair or rebuild tissues and organs. This chapter presents some basic information about body structure and function, information you will need to understand the human body and many of the exciting research projects you hear about or read about in the news. This chapter also revisits homeostasis, elaborating on what you've already learned and setting the stage for your study of human organ systems, the subject of the next ten chapters.

From Cells to Organ Systems

To begin our study of the structure and function of the human body, we will look at the beginning of life—that is, fertilization. During the process, the sperm and ovum combine to form a zygote (ZIE-goat). The zygote's genetic material (DNA) contains all of the information needed to develop a fully functional adult and to control complex life functions, such as growth, reproduction, and homeostasis.

Cells Unite to Form Tissues, and Tissues Combine to Form Organs

During embryonic development, the zygote divides many times, first producing a ball of cells called a **morula** (MORE-you-lah) (**FIGURE 4-1**). The cells continue to divide and soon a cavity begins to form. This structure is now called a blastocyst. Soon the cells start to undergo a process called **differentiation**. During this phase of development, the embryonic cells become structurally and functionally specialized. Cellular differentiation is akin to the kind of development students undergo as they proceed through an educational system. They start out in kindergarten pretty much interested in the same things: naps, finger painting, and playing in the mud. But as they proceed through primary and secondary school and college, they branch off. Some become physics majors. Others take up medicine. Others pursue the arts. Cells do pretty much the same thing. They start off pretty general, then gradually specialize.

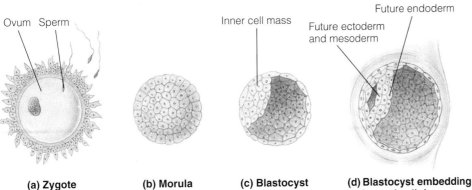

(a) **Zygote**   (b) **Morula**   (c) **Blastocyst**   (d) **Blastocyst embedding in uterine lining**

Ovum Sperm   Inner cell mass   Future ectoderm and mesoderm   Future endoderm

FIGURE 4-1 Early Embryonic Development in Humans *(a)* The fertilized ovum divides mitotically, eventually forming a solid ball of cells, the morula *(b),* which later becomes a hollow blastocyst, shown here in cross section *(c).* The inner cell mass, also shown here in cross section, becomes the embryo, differentiating into *(d)* ectoderm, endoderm, and mesoderm in later stages of development.

The first sign of differentiation occurs in the early embryo with the emergence of three distinct cell types: ectoderm, mesoderm, and endoderm (**FIGURE 4-1D**). These cells can be told apart chiefly by their location in the early embryo. **Ectoderm,** for instance, lies on the outside of the embryo. **Mesoderm** lies in the middle. **Endoderm** is the innermost layer. During embryonic development in humans, ectodermal, mesodermal, and endodermal cells give rise to a variety of highly differentiated cell types, each of which carries out very specific functions. Ectoderm, for instance, gives rise to the skin, eyes, and nervous system. Mesodermal cells give rise to muscle, bone, and cartilage. Endoderm forms the lining of the digestive tract and several digestive glands.

The specialized cells produced from the three embryonic cell layers are often bound together by extracellular fibers and other extracellular materials, forming **tissues** (from the Latin "to weave"). Extracellular materials may be liquid (as in blood), semisolid (as in cartilage), or solid (as in bone). During embryonic development, various tissues combine to form **organs,** discrete structures in the body that carry out specific functions. Organs, like their counterparts in cells, the organelles, provide for a division of labor.

Cells Combine to Form Four Primary Tissues

Four major tissue types are found in humans: (1) epithelial, (2) connective, (3) muscle, and (4) nervous.

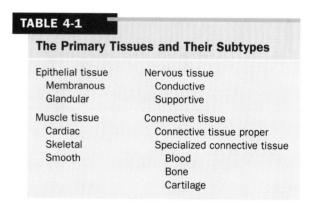

TABLE 4-1	
The Primary Tissues and Their Subtypes	
Epithelial tissue	Nervous tissue
Membranous	Conductive
Glandular	Supportive
Muscle tissue	Connective tissue
Cardiac	Connective tissue proper
Skeletal	Specialized connective tissue
Smooth	Blood
	Bone
	Cartilage

These are called **primary tissues. TABLE 4-1** lists the primary tissues. As you can see, each primary tissue consists of two or three subtypes. Muscle tissue, for instance, comes in three varieties: cardiac, skeletal, and smooth. Cardiac muscle cells are found exclusively in the heart. Skeletal muscle cells are located chiefly in body muscles. Smooth muscle cells are found in the walls of the stomach, intestinal tract, and blood vessels. (More on these later.)

The primary tissues exist in all organs but in varying amounts. The lining of the stomach, for example, consists of a single layer of epithelial (ep-eh-THEEL-ee-ill) cells forming the surface epithelium (**FIGURE 4-2B**). It's a protective coating. Just beneath the epithelial lining is a layer of connective tissue. It

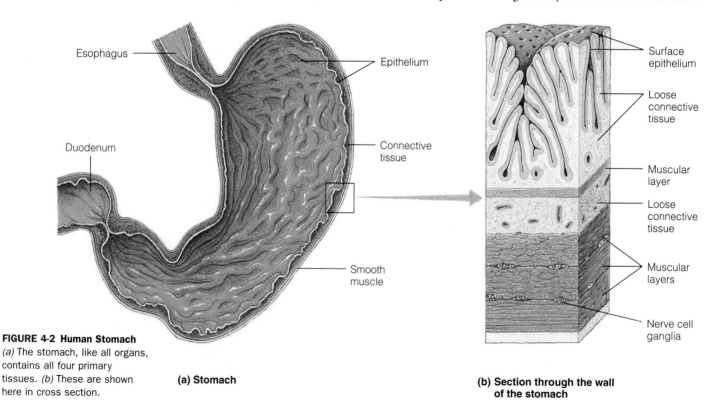

FIGURE 4-2 Human Stomach
(a) The stomach, like all organs, contains all four primary tissues. (b) These are shown here in cross section.

(a) Stomach

(b) Section through the wall of the stomach

(a) Simple epithelia

(b) Stratified epithelia

FIGURE 4-3 Membranous Epithelia *(a)* Single-celled (simple) epithelia *(b)* and stratified epithelia exist in different parts of the body.

holds things together. Beneath that is a thick sheet of smooth muscle cells, which forms the bulk of the stomach wall. Smooth muscle cells are also found in blood vessels supplying the tissues of the stomach. Nerves enter with the blood vessels and control the flow of blood.

Epithelium Forms the Lining or External Covering of Organs and Also Forms Glands

Epithelial tissue exists in two basic forms: glandular and membranous. The **membranous epithelia** consist of sheets of cells tightly packed together, forming the external coverings or linings of organs. Membranous epithelia come in a variety of forms, each specialized to protect underlying tissues. To simplify matters, histolo-

gists (scientists who study the microscopic structure of organisms) divide membranous epithelia into two broad categories: **simple epithelia,** consisting of a single layer of cells, and **stratified epithelia,** consisting of many layers of cells (**FIGURE 4-3**).

The **glandular epithelia,** the second major type of epithelium, consists of clumps of cells that form many of the glands of the body. Epithelial glands arise during embryonic development from tiny "ingrowths" of membranous epithelia, as illustrated in **FIGURE 4-4**. Some glands remain connected to the epithelium by hollow ducts and are called **exocrine glands** (EX-oh-crin; glands of external secretion); products of the exocrine glands flow through ducts into some other body part (**FIGURE 4-4A**). In humans, sweat glands in the skin are exocrine glands. They produce a clear, watery fluid that is released onto the surface of the skin by small ducts. This fluid evaporates from the skin, and cools the body. Salivary glands are another exocrine gland. Located around the oral cavity, the salivary glands produce saliva, a fluid that is released into the mouth via small ducts.

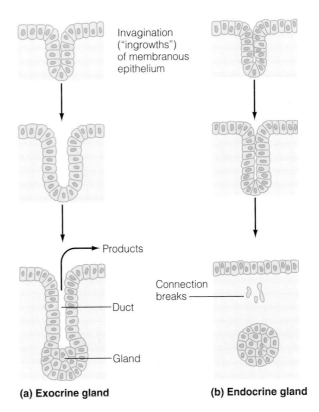

(a) Exocrine gland   **(b) Endocrine gland**

FIGURE 4-4 Formation of Endocrine and Exocrine Glands *(a)* Exocrine glands arise from invaginations of membranous epithelia that retain their connection. *(b)* Endocrine glands lose this connection and thus secrete their products into the bloodstream.

Some glandular epithelial cells break off completely from their embryonic source, as shown in **FIGURE 4-4B**, to form **endocrine glands** (EN-doh-crin; glands of internal secretion). The endocrine glands produce hormones that are released into the bloodstream, where they travel to other parts of the body (Chapter 14).

Epithelial Tissues Illustrate a Basic Biological Principle: That Structure Closely Correlates with Function. One of the basic rules of architecture is that form (the structure of a building) often follows function—in other words, architectural design reflects underlying function. Animals exhibit a similar relationship. This rule is "obeyed" all the way down to the cellular level, so it is not surprising to find a remarkable de-

gree of correlation between structure and function in tissues as well.

The membranous epithelia provide many examples of this relationship. A good example is the outer layer of the human skin, the **epidermis** (ep-eh-DERM-iss), which, among other things, protects us from excessive water loss. Shown in **FIGURE 4-5A**, the epidermis consists of numerous cell layers, known as a **stratified squamous epithelium** (SQUAW-mus). The cells of this epithelium flatten toward the surface and are tightly joined by special connections. The outermost cells become isolated from the blood supply and die, forming a dry protective layer. Together, the thickness of the epidermis, the adhesion of one cell to another, and the dry protective layer of dead cells im-

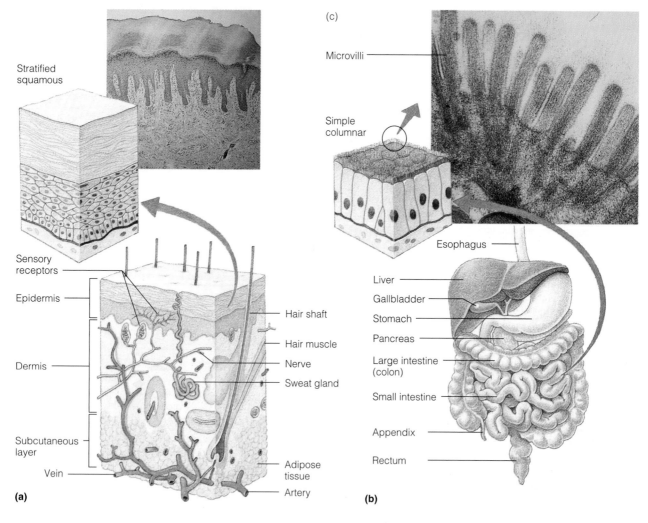

FIGURE 4-5 Comparison of Two Epithelia with Markedly Different Functions *(a)* A cross section of the skin showing the stratified squamous epithelium of the epidermis (above), which protects underlying skin from sunlight and desiccation.

(b) The simple columnar epithelium of the lining of the small intestine, which is specialized for absorption. *(c)* The plasma membranes of the cells lining the intestine are thrown into folds (microvilli) that greatly increase the surface area for absorption.

(a) Loose connective tissue

(b) Dense connective tissue

(c) Cartilage

(d) Adipose tissue

(e) Bone

(f) Blood

FIGURE 4-6 Connective Tissue Connective tissue consists of many diverse subtypes.

Connective Tissue Binds the Cells and Organs of the Body Together

As the name implies, **connective tissue** is the body's glue. Connective tissue binds cells and other tissues together and is present in all organs in varying amounts.

The body contains several types of connective tissue, each with specific functions (**FIGURE 4-6**). Despite the differences, all connective tissues consist of two basic components: cells and varying amounts of extracellular material. Two types of connective tissue will be discussed here: connective tissue proper and the specialized connective tissues—bone, cartilage, and blood.

Connective Tissue Proper Consists of Two Subtypes, Determined by the Relative Proportion of Fibers and Cells. Connective tissue proper is an important structural component of humans and consists of two types: dense connective tissue and loose connective tissue. As the name implies, **dense connective tissue (DCT)** consists primarily of densely packed fibers produced by cells interspersed between them. DCT is found in ligaments and tendons (**FIGURE 4-7A**). **Ligaments** join bones to bones at joints and provide support for joints. I use the mnemonic *LBJ*, which stands for one of our presidents, Lyndon Baines Johnson, if you're a history student, or *l*igaments connect *b*ones to bones at *j*oints if you're a biology student. **Tendons** join muscle to bone and aid in body movement.

DCT is also found at other sites. For instance, the layer of the skin underlying the epidermis, known as the **dermis,** is composed of dense connective tissue, although the fibers are less regularly arranged than those in ligaments and tendons.

If connective tissue were likened to packing materials in a factory, dense connective tissue would be akin to strapping tape that's wrapped around packages—it holds things together. **Loose connective tissue (LCT)** would be more like the styrofoam peanuts or excelsior

pede water loss. They also present a formidable barrier to microorganisms.

Another example of the relationship between structure and function is the epithelium of the small intestine. As shown in **FIGURE 4-5B**, the lining of the small intestine consists of a single layer of columnar cells, uniquely suited to absorb food molecules. These cells are also structurally modified in ways that further enhance food absorption. As shown in **FIGURE 4-5C**, the surfaces of these cells have numerous tiny protrusions known as **microvilli** (MY-crow-VILL-eye), which markedly increase the surface area of the cell available for absorption. The larger the surface area, the more efficient the absorption of food.

(a)

(b)

FIGURE 4-7 Light Micrographs of Connective Tissue
(a) Dense connective tissue.
(b) Loose connective tissue.

used to fill the spaces between products jammed in a box. In other words, it's the body's packing material, but it also holds structures together.

As shown in **FIGURE 4-7B**, LCT contains cells in a loose network of collagen and elastic fibers. Both of these fibers are made of protein. Loose connective tissue forms around blood vessels in the body and in skeletal muscles, where it binds the muscle cells together. It also lies beneath epithelial linings of the intestines and trachea, filling the space and anchoring them to underlying structures.

The chief difference between dense and loose connective tissues lies in the ratio of cells to extracellular fibers. As you can see in **FIGURE 4-7**, dense connective tissue has far more fibers than loose connective tissue.

The extracellular fibers found in dense and loose connective tissue are produced by a connective tissue cell known as the **fibroblast** (FIE-bro-blast). In addition to producing the fibers that hold many tissues together, fibroblasts repair damage created by cuts or tears in body tissues. When the skin is cut, for example, fibroblasts in the dermis migrate into the injured area, where they begin producing large quantities of collagen. The collagen fibers fill the wound, closing it off, creating a temporary patch. The epidermis soon begins to grow over the damaged area, repairing the damage and restoring the integrity of the skin. When the cut is small, the epidermis covers the damaged area completely, leaving no scar, but in larger wounds, the epidermal cells are often unable to grow over the entire wound, leaving some of the underlying collagen exposed and producing a visible scar.

Besides helping to hold the body together, loose connective tissue gives refuge to several cell types that protect us against bacterial and viral infections. One of the most important of the protective cells is the **macrophage** (MACK-row-FAYGE; "big eater"). Containing numerous lysosomes for digesting foreign material, macrophages engulf microorganisms that penetrate the skin and underlying loose connective tissues as a result of injury. This prevents bacteria from spreading to other parts of the body and producing a systemic infection—one that affects the entire organism. Macrophages also play a role in immune protection, which will be discussed in Chapter 8.

Some LCT contains large, conspicuous **fat cells.** The fat cell is one of the most distinctive of all body cells. It contains huge fat globules that occupy virtually the entire cell, pressing the cytoplasm and the nucleus to the periphery. Fat cells occur singly or in groups of varying size. Large numbers of fat cells in a given region form a modified type of LCT known as **adipose tissue** (AD-eh-poze), or, less glamorously, fat. Adipose tissue is an important storage depot for lipids, particularly triglycerides, which are used as an energy source under certain conditions. Fatty deposits also provide insulation for humans and many other mammals and some birds, especially those that live in aquatic environments where heat loss can be substantial.

For humans, fatty deposits often become unsightly. To rid the body of these deposits, individuals can engage in exercise programs and can reduce their intake of food. The combination of the two can prove quite effective. Some individuals opt for a surgical measure called **liposuction** (LIE-poh-suck-shun) (**FIGURE 4-8**). In this procedure, a small incision is made in the skin through which surgeons insert a device to aspirate fat deposits under the skin in various locations, such as the thighs, buttocks, and abdomen. The fat cells extracted from one region can even be transferred to other regions, such as the breast, to resculpt the human body. Liposuction is a relatively safe technique but, like most surgery, not free from risk.

The Specialized Connective Tissues Are Modified to Perform Specific Functions Essential to Homeostasis

The body contains three types of specialized connective tissue: cartilage, bone, and blood.

Cartilage. Cartilage consists of cells embedded in an abundant and rather impervious extracellular material, the matrix (**FIGURE 4-9**). Surrounding virtually all types of cartilage is a layer of dense, irregularly packed connective tissue, the **perichondrium** (PEAR-eh-CON-dree-um; "around the cartilage"). This layer contains the blood vessels that supply nutrients to cartilage cells through diffusion. No blood vessels penetrate the cartilage itself. Because cartilage cells are nourished by diffusion from perichondral capillaries, damaged cartilage heals very slowly. For this reason, joint injuries that involve the cartilage often take years to repair or may not heal at all.

FIGURE 4-8 Liposuction During liposuction surgery, the physician aspirates fat from deposits lying beneath the skin, helping to reduce unsightly accumulations.

FIGURE 4-9 **Light Micrographs of Cartilage** *(a)* Hyaline. *(b)* Elastic. *(c)* Fibrocartilage. *(d)* Intervertebral disk showing location and *(e)* arrangement of fibrocartilage in a protective ring around the soft, spongy part of the disk that absorbs shock.

Three types of cartilage are found in humans: hyaline, elastic, and fibrocartilage. Each serves a special purpose. The most prevalent type is **hyaline cartilage** (HIGH-ah-lynn) (**FIGURE 4-9A**). Hyaline cartilage contains numerous collagen fibers, which appear white to the naked eye. Found on the ends of many bones, hyaline cartilage greatly reduces friction, so bones can move over one another with ease. Hyaline cartilage also makes up the bulk of the nose and is found in the larynx (voice box) and the rings of the trachea, which you can feel below the adam's apple. The ends of the ribs that join to the sternum (breastbone) are composed of hyaline cartilage. In embryonic development, the first skeleton is made of hyaline cartilage. It is later converted to bone.

Elastic cartilage is similar to hyaline cartilage but contains many wavy elastic fibers, which give it much greater flexibility (**FIGURE 4-9B**). Elastic cartilage is found in regions where support and flexibility are required—for example, in the external ears and eustachian tubes (ewe-STAY-shun), the cartilaginous ducts that help equalize pressure in the inner ear (Chapter 12).

Fibrocartilage is the rarest of all cartilage. Like hyaline cartilage, it consists of an extracellular matrix containing numerous bundles of collagen fibers. As shown in **FIGURE 4-9C**, however, fibrocartilage contains far fewer cells than either hyaline or elastic cartilage.

Fibrocartilage is found in the outer layer of **intervertebral disks** (in-ter-VER-tah-braul), the shock-absorbing tissue between the vertebrae (bones) of the spine (**FIGURE 4-9D**). An intervertebral disk consists of a soft, cushiony central region that absorbs shock. Fibrocartilage forms a ring around the central portion of the disk, holding it in place (**FIGURE 4-9E**).

Over time the fibrocartilage ring weakens and may tear, permitting the central part of the disk to bulge outward (or herniate). In so doing, it often presses against nerves that supply various parts of the body. This condition is referred to as a **slipped** or **herniated disk** and usually occurs in the neck or lower back, resulting in a significant amount of pain in the neck, back, or one or both legs, depending on the location of the damaged disk. Pain is generated when the disk presses against nearby nerves.

Surgeons can correct the problem by removing the herniated portion of the disk with a scalpel. Physical therapy, however, is often successful too and is often the first approach. Lasers are also being used to remove herniated disks. In some cases, the entire disk is removed and the vertebrae are then fused. You can reduce your chances of "slipping" a disk in the first place by watching your weight, keeping in shape, sitting upright (not slouching) in a chair, and lifting heavy objects carefully (**FIGURE 4-10**).

Bone. **Bone** is another form of specialized connective tissue. Contrary to what many might think, bone is dynamic, living tissue. Besides providing internal support and protection to internal organs such as the brain, heart, and lungs, bone plays an important role in maintaining optimal blood calcium levels and is, therefore, a homeostatic organ. Calcium is required for many body functions such as muscle

FIGURE 4-10 **Protecting Your Back** When lifting heavy objects, bend your legs and grasp the object, as the man in the top illustration is doing. With your back straight, stand up and lift with your legs.

(a)

(b)

(c)

(d)

FIGURE 4-11 Bone *(a)* Compact and spongy bone, shown in a section of the humerus. *(b)* Light micrograph of compact bone. *(c)* Photomicrograph of spongy bone, showing osteoblasts and osteoclasts. *(d)* Osteoclast digesting surface of bony spicule.

contraction, normal nerve functioning, and blood clotting.

Like all connective tissues, bone consists of cells embedded in an abundant extracellular matrix (**FIGURE 4-11B**). Bone matrix consists primarily of collagen fibers, which give bone its strength and resiliency, interspersed with numerous needlelike salt crystals containing calcium, phosphate, and hydroxide ions, which give bone its hardness. Calcium in bone can be dissolved by weak acids, leaving behind a collagen replica. It can be turned into a thick paste called **de-**

mineralized bone matter (DBM). DBM is rather remarkable stuff, and it is being used to repair severe bone damage.

Two types of bone tissue are found in the body: compact bone and spongy bone (**FIGURE 4-11A**). **Compact bone** is, as its name implies, dense and hard. As illustrated in **FIGURE 4-11B**, the cells in compact bone (**osteocytes**) are located in concentric rings of calcified matrix. These surround a central canal through which the blood vessels and nerves pass. Each osteocyte has numerous processes that course through tiny canals in the bony matrix, known as **canaliculi** (CAN-al-ICK-u-LIE; literally "little canals"). The canaliculi provide a route for nutrients and wastes to flow to and from the osteocytes and the central canal.

Inside most bones of the body is a tissue known as spongy bone. **Spongy bone** consists of an irregular network of calcified collagen spicules (SPICK-yuls). As shown in **FIGURE 4-11C**, on the surface of the spicules are numerous **osteoblasts** (OSS-tee-oh-BLASTS), bone cells that produce collagen, which later becomes calcified. Once these cells are surrounded by calcified matrix, they are referred to as osteocytes.

Between the spicules are numerous cavities. In most of the bones of an adult, these cavities are filled with fat cells and form the **yellow marrow.** In other bones, the cavities are filled with blood cells and cells that give rise to new blood cells, thus forming **red marrow.**

On the surfaces of many bony spicules of spongy bone are large, multinucleated cells called **osteoclasts** (OSS-tee-oh-KLASTS; "bone breakers") (**FIGURE 4-11D**). These cells are part of a homeostatic system that ensures proper blood calcium levels. When calcium levels in the blood fall, osteoclasts are activated by the parathyroid hormone produced by the thyroid gland. Once activated, the osteoclasts digest small portions of the spongy bone. This, in turn, releases calcium into the bloodstream to restore proper levels.

Spongy bone is "remodeled" when bones are subjected to new stresses. For example, the leg bones of a desk-bound executive from Atlanta who goes on a skiing vacation in Jackson Hole, Wyoming, are remodeled as her legs are subjected to the rigors of skiing. This adjustment accommodates the new stresses and strains. During this process, osteoclasts tear down some of the spongy bone, while osteoblasts rebuild new bone in other areas to meet the new stresses. By the end of a two-week ski trip, the executive's bones have been considerably refashioned and are much stronger than when she left home. When she is back at her desk, though, her bones revert to their previous, weaker state.

Blood. Blood is also a specialized form of connective tissue and consists of two components: (1) the formed elements and (2) a large amount of extracellular material, a fluid called *plasma.* The **formed elements** of blood consist of the red and white blood cells and the platelets. They are responsible for 45% of the blood volume. Plasma makes up the remaining 55%. **Red blood cells,** or **erythrocytes,** transport oxygen and small amounts of carbon dioxide to and from the lungs and body tissues. **White blood cells,** or **leukocytes,** are involved in fighting infections. **Platelets** are fragments of large cells (**megakaryocytes**) located in the red bone marrow, the principal site of blood cell formation. Platelets play a key role in blood clotting.

Muscle Tissue Consists of Specialized Cells that Contract when Stimulated

Muscle is found in virtually every organ in the body. Muscle gets its name from the Latin word for "mouse" (mus). Early observers likened the contracting muscle of the biceps to a mouse moving under a carpet.

Muscle is an excitable tissue. When stimulated, it contracts, producing mechanical force. Muscle cells working in large numbers can create enormous forces. Muscles of the jaw, for instance, create a pressure of 200 pounds per square inch, forceful enough to snap off a finger. (Don't try this at home.) Muscle also moves body parts, propels food along the digestive tract, and expels the fetus from the uterus during birth. Heart muscle contracts and pumps blood through the 50,000 miles of blood vessels in the human body. Acting in smaller numbers, muscle cells are responsible for intricate movements, such as those required to play the piano or move the eyes.

As mentioned earlier, three types of muscle are found in humans: skeletal, cardiac, and smooth. The cells in each type of muscle contain two contractile protein filaments, actin and myosin. These very same fibers were first encountered in your study of the microfilamentous network lying beneath the plasma membrane of cells. As you may recall, this layer of fibers is responsible for cytokinesis, the division of the cytoplasm. When stimulated, actin and myosin filaments of muscle cells slide over one another, shortening and causing contraction.

Skeletal Muscle. The majority of the body's muscle is called **skeletal muscle**—so named because it is frequently attached to the skeleton. When skeletal muscle contracts, it causes body parts (arms and legs, for instance) to move. Most skeletal muscle in the body is under voluntary, or conscious, control. In other words, signals from the brain cause the muscle to contract. A notable exception is the skeletal muscle of the upper esophagus, which contracts automatically during swallowing.

Skeletal muscle cells are long cylinders formed during embryonic development by the fusion of many embryonic muscle cells. Because of this, skeletal muscle cells are usually referred to as muscle fibers. Each muscle fiber contains many nuclei (**FIGURE 4-12A**). Because of the dense array of contractile fibers in the cytoplasm of the muscle fiber, the nuclei become pressed against the plasma membrane. As you might suspect, this highly specialized cell cannot divide, and damaged muscle cells cannot be replaced.

Skeletal muscle fibers appear banded, or striated, when viewed under the light microscope (**FIGURE 4-12A**). The striations result from the unique arrangement of actin and myosin filaments inside muscle cells, a topic discussed in Chapter 13.

Cardiac Muscle. Like skeletal muscle, **cardiac muscle** is striated (**FIGURE 4-12B**). Unlike skeletal muscle, cardiac muscle is involuntary; that is, it contracts without conscious control. Found only in the walls of the heart, cardiac muscle cells contain a single nucleus. They also branch and interconnect freely, and individual cells are tightly connected to one another. This adaptation helps maintain the structural integrity of the heart, an organ subject to incredible strain as it pumps blood through the body day and night. The points of connection also provide pathways for electrical impulses to travel from cell to cell, allowing the heart muscle to contract uniformly when stimulated.

Smooth Muscle. **Smooth muscle,** so named because it lacks visible striations, is involuntary. Actin and myosin filaments are present in smooth muscle cells, but are not organized like those found in other types (**FIGURE 4-12C**). Smooth muscle cells may occur singly or in small groups. Small rings of smooth muscle cells, for example, surround tiny blood vessels. When these cells contract, they reduce or shut off the supply of blood to tissues. Smooth muscle cells are most often arranged in sheets in the walls of organs, such as the stomach, uterus, and intestines (**FIGURE 4-2**). Smooth muscle cells in the wall of the stomach churn the food, mixing the stomach contents, and force tiny spurts of liquified food into the small intestine. Smooth muscle contractions also propel the food along the intestinal tract.

Nervous Tissue Contains Specialized Cells Characterized by Irritability and Conductivity

Last but not least of the primary tissues is nervous tissue, which consists of two types of cells: conducting cells and supportive cells. Many of the conducting cells, or **neurons,** are modified to respond to specific stimuli, such as pain or temperature. Stimulation results in bioelectric impulses, which the neuron transmits from one region of the body to another. As noted previously, the ability to respond to stimuli is a characteristic of all living things and is called *irritability*. The ability to transmit an impulse is called *conductivity*. The properties of irritability and conductivity in neurons allow us to be aware of our environment and to respond to internal and external stimuli. The evolution and refinement of the nervous system have been vitally important to our present success.

Nuclei   Muscle fiber

(a)

(b)

(c)

FIGURE 4-12 Light Micrograph of the Three Types of Muscle *(a)* Skeletal. *(b)* Cardiac. *(c)* Smooth.

The supportive cells of the nervous system are a kind of nervous system connective tissue. These cells are incapable of conducting impulses, but they transport nutrients from blood vessels to neurons and also guard against toxins by creating a barrier to many potentially harmful substances. As you will see in Chapter 11, the supportive cells also increase the rate of conduction in neurons with which they are associated. Together, the neurons and their supporting cells form the brain, spinal cord, and nerves of the nervous system, described in more detail in Chapters 11 and 12.

Neurons Share Many Characteristics. At least three distinct types of neurons are found in the body. Despite obvious anatomical differences, they share several common features. We will study these similarities by looking at one of the most common nerve cells, the multipolar neuron, shown in **FIGURE 4-13**. The **multipolar neuron** contains a prominent cell body to which are attached several short, highly branched processes, known as **dendrites** (DEN-drites). (It is the presence of these processes that give this neuron its name, multipolar.) The dendrites receive impulses from receptors or other neurons and trans-

FIGURE 4-13 Multipolar Neurons Attached to the cell body of the multipolar neuron are many highly branched dendrites, which deliver impulses to the cell body. Multipolar neurons have one long, unbranching fiber called the axon, which transmits impulses away from the cell body.

Compartmentalization also occurs at the organismic level in organs.

Organs are discrete structures that have evolved to perform specific functions, such as digestion, enzyme production, and hormone synthesis. Most organs, however, do not function alone. Instead, they are part of a group of cooperative organs, called an **organ system.** The brain, spinal cord, and nerves are all organs that belong to an organ system known as the nervous system.

As you will see in upcoming chapters, components of an organ system are sometimes physically connected—as in the digestive system (**FIGURE 4-14A**). In other cases, they are dispersed throughout the body—as in the endocrine system (**FIGURE 4-14B**). Some organs belong to

mit them to the cell body. Also attached to the cell body of the multipolar neuron is a large, fairly thick process, the **axon** (AXE-on), which transports bioelectric impulses away from the nerve cell body.

Like muscle cells, nerve cells are highly differentiated and cannot divide. When a nerve cell is destroyed, it degenerates and cannot be replaced by cell division. A cut nerve axon, however, may partially regenerate. A new axon may grow from the damaged end, reestablishing previous connections and restoring some sensation or control over muscles. New research may someday provide ways to stimulate regeneration of nerve cells artificially, thus helping physicians to more fully restore nerve function to victims of accidents.

Tissues Combine to Form Organs; Organs Often Function in Groups Called Organ Systems

The cell contains organelles ("little organs") that carry out many of its functions in isolation from the biochemically active cytoplasm. As pointed out in Chapter 3, compartmentalization such as this is an evolutionary adaptation, the importance of which is underscored by its ubiquity.

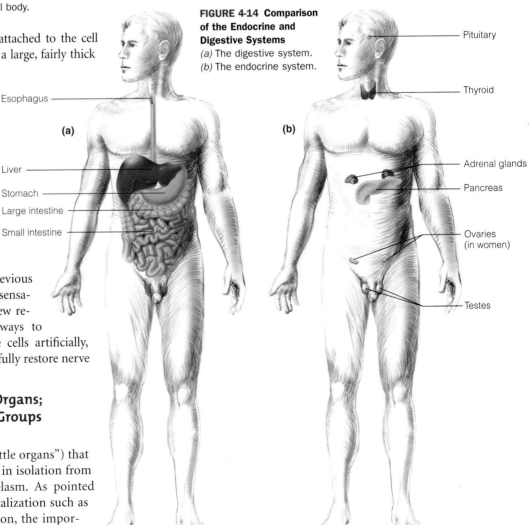

FIGURE 4-14 Comparison of the Endocrine and Digestive Systems (a) The digestive system. (b) The endocrine system.

Esophagus

Liver
Stomach
Large intestine
Small intestine

(a)

(b)

Pituitary

Thyroid

Adrenal glands
Pancreas

Ovaries (in women)

Testes

FIGURE 4-15 Role of the Body Systems in Maintaining Homeostasis

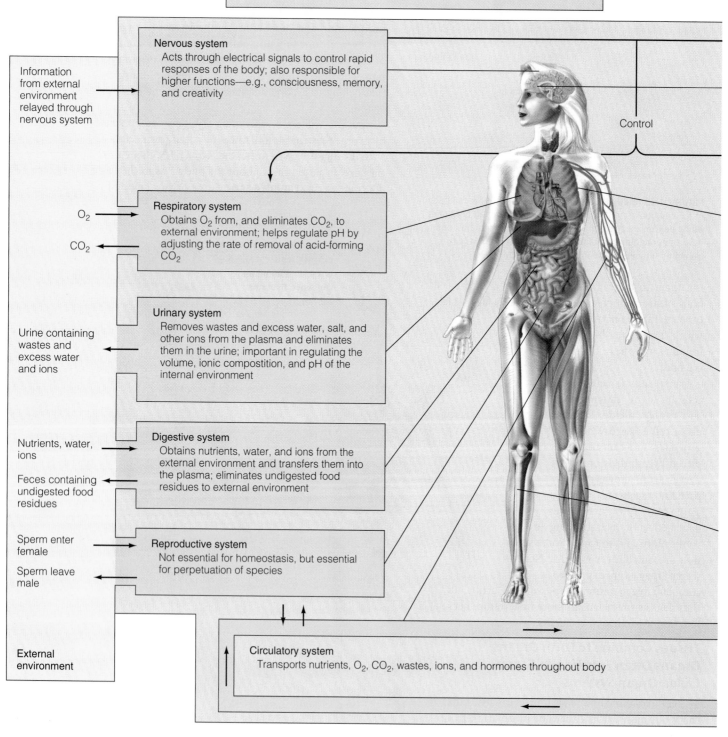

BODY SYSTEMS
Made up of cells organized by specialization to maintain homeostasis

Nervous system
Acts through electrical signals to control rapid responses of the body; also responsible for higher functions—e.g., consciousness, memory, and creativity

Information from external environment relayed through nervous system

Control

O_2

CO_2

Respiratory system
Obtains O_2 from, and eliminates CO_2, to external environment; helps regulate pH by adjusting the rate of removal of acid-forming CO_2

Urinary system
Removes wastes and excess water, salt, and other ions from the plasma and eliminates them in the urine; important in regulating the volume, ionic compostition, and pH of the internal environment

Urine containing wastes and excess water and ions

Nutrients, water, ions

Digestive system
Obtains nutrients, water, and ions from the external environment and transfers them into the plasma; eliminates undigested food residues to external environment

Feces containing undigested food residues

Sperm enter female

Sperm leave male

Reproductive system
Not essential for homeostasis, but essential for perpetuation of species

External environment

Circulatory system
Transports nutrients, O_2, CO_2, wastes, ions, and hormones throughout body

more than one system. For example, the pancreas produces digestive enzymes that are secreted into the small intestine, where they break down food materials. The pancreas is therefore part of the digestive system. The pancreas also contains cells that produce two hormones (insulin and glucagon) that help control blood glucose levels. Thus, the pancreas also belongs to the endocrine system.

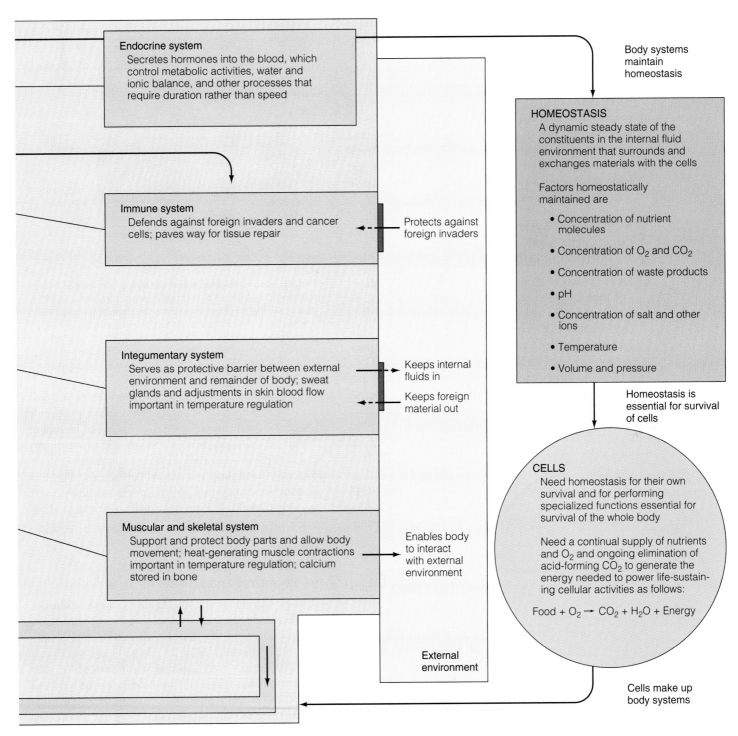

Endocrine system
Secretes hormones into the blood, which control metabolic activities, water and ionic balance, and other processes that require duration rather than speed

Immune system
Defends against foreign invaders and cancer cells; paves way for tissue repair

Integumentary system
Serves as protective barrier between external environment and remainder of body; sweat glands and adjustments in skin blood flow important in temperature regulation

Muscular and skeletal system
Support and protect body parts and allow body movement; heat-generating muscle contractions important in temperature regulation; calcium stored in bone

Protects against foreign invaders

Keeps internal fluids in

Keeps foreign material out

Enables body to interact with external environment

External environment

Body systems maintain homeostasis

HOMEOSTASIS
A dynamic steady state of the constituents in the internal fluid environment that surrounds and exchanges materials with the cells

Factors homeostatically maintained are

- Concentration of nutrient molecules
- Concentration of O_2 and CO_2
- Concentration of waste products
- pH
- Concentration of salt and other ions
- Temperature
- Volume and pressure

Homeostasis is essential for survival of cells

CELLS
Need homeostasis for their own survival and for performing specialized functions essential for survival of the whole body

Need a continual supply of nutrients and O_2 and ongoing elimination of acid-forming CO_2 to generate the energy needed to power life-sustaining cellular activities as follows:

$$Food + O_2 \rightarrow CO_2 + H_2O + Energy$$

Cells make up body systems

The following 10 chapters describe the major organ systems and the functions they perform, paying special attention to their role in homeostasis. **FIGURE 4-15** summarizes the functions of each organ system and lists the role each plays in the overall economy of the human organism. You may want to take a moment to read the descriptions in the light blue boxes before proceeding.

Principles of Homeostasis

The body's many systems perform specific functions that help us move about in our environment and perform work or play. Many systems also contribute to homeostasis. Homeostasis, of course, is essential for the survival of cells, which make up body systems.

Defined in Chapter 1 as a state of relative internal constancy, homeostasis occurs on a variety of levels—in cells, tissues, organs, organ systems, organisms, and even the environment. Homeostatic systems at all levels of biological organization have several common features essential for you to understand before you begin your study of the organ systems.

Homeostatic Systems Maintain Constancy Chiefly through Negative Feedback Mechanisms

Feedback mechanisms control various body processes. The most common type is called **negative feedback.** To understand how negative feedback systems work, let's consider a familiar example, the heating system in a typical house, as it contains many of the features that are present in biological feedback mechanisms (**FIGURE 4-16A**).

In the winter, the heating system (the furnace and thermostat) of a house maintains a constant internal temperature, even though the outside temperature fluctuates sharply. Heat lost through ceilings, walls, windows, and tiny cracks is replaced by heat generated from the combustion of natural gas or oil in the furnace (**FIGURE 4-16A**).

The furnace is controlled by a thermostat, which detects changes in room temperature. When indoor temperature falls below the desired setting, the thermostat sends a signal to the furnace, turning it on. Heat from the furnace is then distributed through the house, raising the room temperature. When the room temperature reaches the desired setting, the thermostat shuts the furnace off. Like all negative feedback mechanisms, the product of the system (heat) "feeds back" on the process, shutting it down.

A graph of a hypothetical house temperature is shown in **FIGURE 4-16B** and illustrates another important principle of homeostasis: Homeostatic systems do not maintain absolute constancy. Rather, they maintain conditions (such as body temperature) within a given range.

All homeostatic mechanisms in humans operate in a similar fashion, maintaining conditions within a narrow range around an operating point. The operating

FIGURE 4-16 Homeostasis and the House *(a)* Heat is maintained in a house by a furnace, which compensates for heat loss. The thermostat monitors the internal temperature and switches the furnace on and off in response to temperature changes. *(b)* A hypothetical temperature graph showing temperature fluctuation around the operating point.

point is akin to the setting on a thermostat. As you will see in later chapters, our bodies maintain fairly constant levels of a great many chemical components, including hormones, nutrients, wastes, and ions. We also maintain physical parameters such as body temperature, blood pressure, blood flow, and others. Fortunately, all of this is done subconsciously and quite automatically. We'd never get anything done if we had to attend to all of these functions ourselves!

All Homeostatic Feedback Mechanisms Require a Sensor (or Receptor) and an Effector

Biological homeostatic mechanisms contain **sensors** that detect change and **effectors** that correct conditions. In your home, the thermostat is the sensor, and the furnace is the effector.

The human body contains many sensors. In your body, for instance, specially modified nerve cell endings in the skin detect temperature changes in the environment. These sensors not only detect changes in the ambient (outside) temperature, but also send signals to the brain, alerting it to such changes. The brain then sends signals to the body to rectify matters—usually to reduce heat loss and increase heat output. The options for generating more heat are many. In other words, the body contains several different types of effectors—in the same way that heat can be generated and conserved in a house many ways (closing curtains, starting a fire in the woodstove, or cranking up the furnace).

One of the main sources of heat in the human body is the breakdown (catabolism) of glucose and other molecules. Chapter 3 noted that the cells of the body break down glucose to make ATP. During this process, heat is given off. Each cell, then, is a tiny furnace whose heat radiates outward and is distributed throughout the body by the blood. Unlike the furnace in your home, the cellular "furnaces" cannot be turned up very quickly. They respond much more slowly than a furnace and are part of a delayed response to low temperature. As winter progresses, metabolism increases, and the body produces more heat.

In order to respond to sudden changes in outside temperature, the body must rely on more rapid mechanisms. If you walked outdoors on a cold winter night dressed only in a light sweater and blue jeans, for example, receptors in your skin would sense the cold and send signals to the brain. The brain, in turn, would send signals to blood vessels in the skin, causing them to constrict, reducing the flow of blood in the skin. The restriction of blood flow through the skin reduces heat loss. If it is cold enough outside, the brain may also send signals to the muscles, causing them to undergo rhythmic contractions, known as shivering. Shivering burns additional glucose, releasing extra heat. (It's like adding additional logs to a fire. The more fuel burned, the more heat you get.) Many voluntary actions may also be "ordered" by the brain to reduce heat loss or generate more heat. For example, you might put on a hat or turn around and go back inside. In humans, conscious acts are often crucial components of homeostasis.

Homeostasis Is Maintained by Balancing Inputs and Outputs

The diagram in **FIGURE 4-17** illustrates the many ways the body regulates the level of various chemicals. Although it may look a bit complicated, it's pretty logical and easily understood if you take a look at one part at a time. Let's start with the input side first—that is, how chemicals enter our bodies.

As illustrated, ions (for example, calcium) and other chemical substances (for example, glucose) are ingested in food or water. Other essential chemicals such as oxygen enter our bodies in the air we breathe. Still other substances (such as certain amino acids) are actually produced in the body. Input from these sources tends to increase internal concentrations.

Now look at the output side. As illustrated, excretion and metabolism tend to lower concentrations. **Excretion** is the loss of materials through a number of specialized body systems. Carbon dioxide, for example, is excreted by the lungs, as is water. Water is also excreted by the kidneys. Metabolism (chemical reactions occurring in the body cells) also removes certain substances from the body. Blood glucose levels, for instance, are decreased by cellular catabolism.

Internal concentrations are kept in balance in large part by input and output. However, internal storage depots (regions where chemicals are stored) also participate in homeostatic balance. For example, glucose molecules in the blood can be stored in the liver. Thus, blood glucose levels are also determined by input and output in storage depots.

The relative importance of the various homeostatic pathways depends on the substance in question. Water, for example, enters the body primarily via the food and liquids we consume. Water is removed by the kidneys, lungs, and skin. For iron, the rate of absorption by the small intestine is a key determinant of blood levels. When iron levels decrease—say, because of a decrease in iron intake—the body reestablishes the balance by increasing the rate of absorption in the small intestine.

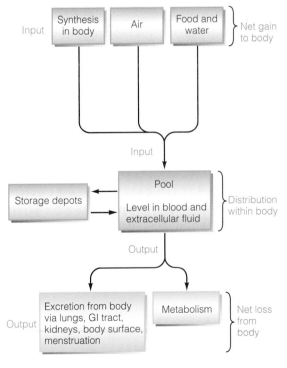

FIGURE 4-17 Generalized View of a Homeostatic System
Inputs and outputs are balanced to maintain more or less constant levels of chemical and physical parameters.

Homeostasis Can Be Upset by Changes in the Input, Output, or Storage

Homeostasis can be thrown out of balance by changes in input, output, and storage. Consider output first. On a hot day, water escapes our bodies very rapidly through perspiration, an adaptation that helps cool us down. Although perspiration is beneficial, it can be quite damaging if water loss is severe. Severe water loss leads to dehydration, which may upset homeostasis—so much so, in fact, that death may occur.

Severe diarrhea—a drastic increase in water output—also results in a dangerous depletion of body fluids. It can be so severe that it too can result in death. In fact, dehydration resulting from severe diarrhea kills millions of children each year in the less developed nations.

Just as changes in the output of a substance drastically alter homeostasis, so do changes in input. For example, going without water for a prolonged period (approximately 3 days) can kill a human being. Excess input can also prove dangerous. Excess salt intake, for example, can result in hypertension (high blood pressure) in some people. Whatever the cause, imbalances in homeostasis can have dramatic impacts on human health.

Homeostatic Control Requires the Action of Nerves, Hormones, and Various Chemicals that Operate over Short Distances

Most homeostatic mechanisms are **reflexes**—that is, automatic physiological responses triggered by various stimuli. Reflexes occur without conscious control. Two types of reflexes exist: nervous system and hormonal.

The Nervous System Reflex. Homeostatic systems controlled by the nervous system are fairly straightforward. As shown in **FIGURE 4-18**, heat from a candle is detected by sensors, or receptors, in the skin. These receptors send nerve impulses to the brain or spinal cord via sensory nerves. The brain and spinal cord, in turn, direct an appropriate response to counterbalance the change. In this example, the spinal cord sends a signal to pull the hand away from the flame.

At any one time, the brain and spinal cord receive thousands of signals from receptors in the body. These signals alert the nervous system to a variety of internal and external conditions. The brain and spinal cord then send out special responses, after integrating (making sense of) the various inputs they have received. The brain and spinal cord control the activity of many effectors, generally muscles and glands.

Hormonal Control. Hormones are chemical substances produced by the endocrine glands. Released into the blood, hormones travel to distant sites, where they

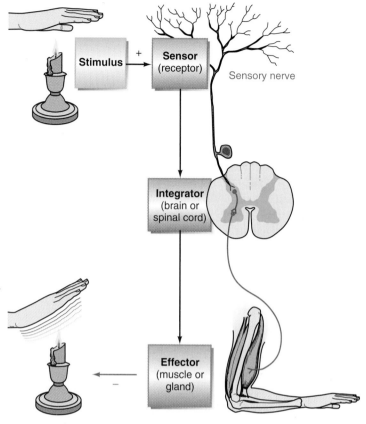

FIGURE 4-18 Nervous System Reflex Reflexes involve some kind of stimulus, a sensor, an integrator, and an effector. The sensor detects a change and sends a signal to the integrator, the brain or spinal cord, which then elicits a response in the effector organs. Negative feedback from the effector eliminates the stimulus.

effect some sort of change. But hormones don't just pour out of endocrine glands in a constant stream. They are released only under certain circumstances and then usually as part of a chemical reflex essential for maintaining homeostasis. Consider an example.

The **parathyroid glands** (pair-ah-THIGH-roid) are four tiny nubbins of tissue embedded in the thyroid gland in the neck. They produce a hormone known as **parathyroid hormone,** or **PTH.** PTH is released from the cells of the parathyroid glands when calcium levels in the blood fall below a certain concentration. PTH then travels in the blood to the bone, where it stimulates osteoclasts, bone-destroying cells described earlier. These cells cause the release of calcium, which raises the calcium level of the blood, returning concentrations to normal.

In this reflex, the cells of the parathyroid gland are the sensors, which detect the drop in blood calcium. The bone is the effector, which produces the desired response (**FIGURE 4-19**). There's no intermediate command center such as the brain.

Some endocrine reflexes do operate through the nervous system, making the lines of cause and effect a bit more difficult to follow. A good example is the thyroid gland, which produces a hormone called **thyroxine** (thigh-ROX-in) (**FIGURE 4-20**). Thyroxine increases the metabolic rate of cells and thus increases heat production in the same way that putting more logs on a fire increases its output of heat.

Thyroxine levels must be kept within a normal range and are monitored by cells in the brain (the receptors). When thyroxine levels fall, these brain cells release a chemical substance TSH-RH (thyroid-stimulating hormone-releasing factor) that travels from its site of production in the brain to another site, the pituitary gland, located just beneath the brain. The pituitary responds by releasing yet another hormone, thyroid-stimulating hormone, TSH. It travels in the blood to the thyroid gland. There, TSH steps up the production of thyroxine, correcting the deficiency.

This reflex has one sensor (cells in the brain), which detects levels of thyroxine, but four effectors: the cells of the hypothalamus that release TSH-RH, the cells of the pituitary that release TSH, the cells of the thyroid that release thyroxine, and body cells that respond to thyroxine by increasing their rate of metabolism.

Local Chemical Control. Nervous and endocrine feedback mechanisms generally occur over considerable distances. In the nervous system, for example, nerves carry impulses from the brain and spinal cord to distant parts of the body, often several feet away. In the endocrine system, the bloodstream carries the messages from endocrine glands to distant effectors. But not all systems require messages that are transported over long distances. In some cases, chemical control is exerted through the extracellular fluid only a cell or two away.

Chemicals that elicit local effects are called **paracrines** (PEAR-ah-crins). Produced by individual cells, paracrines diffuse to neighboring cells. Epidermal growth factor (EGF) produced by skin cells is one example. EGF stimulates cell division when skin cells are damaged or lost, providing a degree of local control over cell growth.

One of the best-known paracrines is a group of chemical substances known as prostaglandins (PROSS-tah-GLAND-ins). **Prostaglandins** comprise a rather large group of molecules with diverse functions.

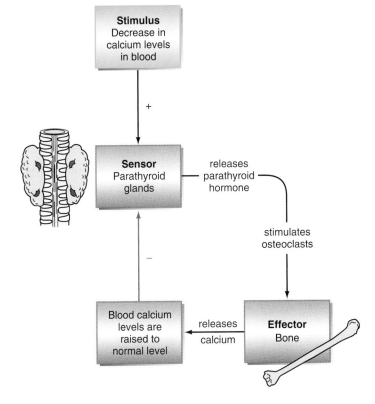

FIGURE 4-19 Endocrine Reflex Not Involving the Nervous System   This reflex operates through the bloodstream. A decrease in calcium in the blood stimulates a series of reactions that restores normal blood calcium levels. A plus sign indicates that the stimulus increases parathyroid gland activity; a minus sign indicates the opposite effect.

FIGURE 4-20 Neuroendocrine Reflex   This reflex involves both the endocrine and nervous systems. Sensors are located in the brain.

Health Note 4-1

The Truth About Herbal Remedies

A male patient is treated by his physician for a painful infection of the prostate gland, one of the sex accessory glands that produces a large portion of the semen. She prescribes an antibiotic and advises the patient to take an herbal remedy, saw palmetto, to help prevent prostatic enlargement, a common problem in older men. A female patient suffering from restlessness and minor problems with sleep is advised by a friend to try some valerian root, another type of herbal remedy. A patient suffering from depression, who wants a "natural" remedy, is advised by her physician to try St. John's Wort.

Herbal remedies are derived from roots, bark, seeds, fruit, flowers, leaves, and branches of plants. In China, some herbal remedies even contain animal parts. An estimated 3000 different medicinal herbs are currently used throughout the world.

Herbal remedies are sold in the United States and in other countries by herbalists, and may be mixed on site. More commonly, people get their herbs in pill, capsule, or liquid form from health food stores, grocery stores, and even large discount stores such as Wal-Mart. In recent years, more and more people have turned to alternative remedies for many conditions they can self-diagnose and treat—and even some that should be attended to by physicians.

Although herbs are the latest craze in the United States, the Chinese and other Asian peoples have been using them for thousands of years. In China, the history of herbal remedies goes back 5000 years. Unbeknownst to many doctors, certain herbs were used routinely in the United States and other developed nations before the advent of modern medicines. Echinacea (ek-eh-NAH-shah), for instance, was widely used to treat colds in the United States prior to the introduction of sulfa drugs (the first generation of synthetic antibiotics). In Germany, herbal remedies are considered prescription medicines and are covered by health insurance.

Herbal treatments not only have a long history of use, but their source, the plants, have been the source of a surprisingly large proportion of the many prescription and over-the-counter drugs in use today. That is, many so-called "modern medicines" contain active ingredients originally extracted from plants. Aspirin, for instance, is derived from the inner bark of willow trees. Wild chimpanzees have been observed chewing willow bark to combat tooth aches. But are herbal treatments effective?

There is no blanket answer to this question. While research shows that many claims about the effectiveness of numerous common herbal preparations appear to be unfounded, not all are. Echinacea, for instance, does appear to enhance the immune system function, and it can be used as a preventative and for treatment of colds and flus. Bilberry, dried blueberries, helps maintain eyesight and improves night vision. It was even used in World War II by the Royal Air Force on night bombing missions. Valerian root is an effective, nonaddicting sleep aid and mild relaxant. Saw palmetto appears to be effective in reducing enlargement of the prostate. Ginger is effective in the treatment of nausea and morning sickness, although it should not be used for an extended time during pregnancy. Garlic lowers serum cholesterol and may have antibacterial properties, a fact discovered by Louis Pasteur. Feverfew seems to help prevent migraine headaches. St. John's Wort is an antidepressant. Hawthorn fights hypertension. The

---

Some stimulate blood clotting; others stimulate smooth muscle contraction.

An interesting evolutionary adaptation akin to paracrines are the **autocrines,** molecules produced by a cell that affect the function of that cell. Autocrines are part of the simplest chemical reflexes in the body. Some prostaglandins function as autocrines. Like hormones, paracrines and autocrines are involved in maintaining homeostasis.

Human Health Depends on Homeostasis, Which, in Turn, Requires a Healthy Environment

This book emphasizes a theme that is important to all of us—notably, that human health is dependent on homeostasis. Homeostasis, in turn, requires a healthy, clean environment. The health of the environment, of course, is also dependent in part on properly functioning homeostatic systems in nature that maintain conditions conducive to life.

The relationship between homeostasis and health is shown in **FIGURE 4-21.** Take a moment to study this diagram. Notice that the body systems (right side of diagram) maintain overall homeostasis, which is essential for proper cell function. Cells make up body systems. They also contain homeostatic mechanisms that are vital to their own function as well as to the overall economy of the organism. Notice too that environmental factors, such as pollution, affect the function of body systems and cells in ways that can upset list goes on. For those interested in finding out more, check out the web sites and books on the subject listed below.

The main advantage of herbs, say some proponents, is that they have no side effects and contain no chemicals; they are also purportedly safe and effective. Unfortunately, this claim is far from true. Herbal remedies contain naturally produced chemicals, and some can have very serious side effects. A number of herbs, for instance, damage the liver, including comfrey—an herb that reportedly promotes bone healing. When taken for long periods, however, its active chemical ingredient is toxic to the liver.

David Kroll, a pharmacologist from the University of Colorado Health Sciences Center, notes further problems. First and foremost, U.S. labeling information is inadequate. Herbs are sold as dietary supplements, and as such, no claims about their use are available. Individuals must often rely on advice from sales clerks. Very little is known about the long-term effects of the wide variety of herbal remedies or their potential interactions with conventional medicines, although our knowledge base is expanding rapidly.

And others warn that without federal regulations that require strict standards for drug content in various herbal remedies, a patient can't know for sure the exact dose he or she is receiving. Some studies have shown that some herbal remedies have none of the active ingredient or smaller than required amounts. In Europe, however, stricter laws require much better controls on product content. In the United States, there's a web site where you can check out various herbal remedies to see if they contain the proper amount of active ingredient to be effective.

Another bit of advice from Dr. Kroll. When given a choice between an over-the-counter remedy and an herbal one, he favors the over-the-counter treatment because of the standardization issue. He also notes that treatment with herbal remedies, as OTC preparations, may delay the diagnosis of more serious conditions. The rule: See a doctor first to be certain that you have what you think you have. And buy products from reputable companies.

Herbal remedies will invariably increase in popularity, and many measures should be taken to make them safer and more effective. Guidelines similar to those in Germany, for instance, could result in more consumer confidence in the quality and content of the product. Canada requires some testing before an herbal preparation can be sold. Although it is not as rigorous as the testing required for pharmaceuticals in the United States, it does help ensure the effectiveness of the remedy. Canada has also established standards for the purity and content of herbal remedies.

The important lesson in all of this is *buyer beware*. Study an herb thoroughly before you take it, or better yet, see a qualified physician who practices both traditional and herbal medicine. More rigorous training of those who dispense herbs might also help raise consumer confidence. In China, herbalists graduate from a five-year program of study. Also needed is more research by herbal "manufacturers" similar to that required of drug companies—to fine tune our knowledge about these increasingly popular forms of treatment.

Visit *Human Biology's* Internet site for links to web sites offering more information on this topic.

FIGURE 4-21 Health, Homeostasis, and the Environment   Human health is dependent on maintaining homeostasis. Homeostasis, however, is affected by the condition of our environment. Stress, pollution, noise, and other environmental factors upset the function of cells and body systems, thus upsetting homeostasis and human health. As a result, human health is dependent on a healthy environment.

Diet and Lifestyle

Environment
(pollution, stress, noise)

create

**Human
Activities**

Diet, Lifestyle, and Environmental conditions affect the function of body cells.

Cells

Homeostasis is essential for cell function.

Cells make up body.

Organ Systems

create

Homeostasis

the internal balance, thus altering human mental and physical health.

Just as human health is affected by the condition of the environment, so too is the health of many other species. For a discussion of herbal remedies that help restore health, see Health Note 4-1.

Section 4-3

Biological Rhythms

The previous discussion may have given you the impression that homeostasis establishes an unwavering condition of stability that remains more or less the same, day after day, year after year. In truth, many physiological processes undergo rhythmic change.

Not All Physiological Processes Remain Constant over Time, But Those That Fluctuate Do So in Predictable Ways

Body temperature varies during a 24-hour period by as much as 0.5°C. Blood pressure may change by as much as 20%, and the number of white blood cells, which fight infection, can vary by 50% during the day. Alertness also varies considerably. About 1:00 P.M. each day, for instance, most people go through a slump. For most of us, activity and alertness peak early in the evening, making this an excellent time to study. Daily cycles, such as these, are called **circadian rhythms** (sir-KADE-ee-an; "about a day"). Circadian rhythms are natural body rhythms linked to the 24-hour day-night cycle.

Many hormones follow daily rhythmic cycles. The male sex hormone testosterone, for example, follows a 24-hour cycle. The highest levels occur in the night, particularly during dream sleep also known as REM sleep.

Dream sleep occurs primarily in the early morning hours—the later the hour, the longer the periods of dream sleep (**FIGURE 4-22**).

Not all cycles occur over 24 hours, however. Some can be much longer. The menstrual cycle, for instance, is a recurring series of events in the reproductive functions of women that lasts, on average, 28 days. During the menstrual cycle, levels of the female sex hormone estrogen undergo dramatic shifts. Estrogen concentrations in the blood are low at the beginning of each cycle and peak on day 14, when ovulation normally occurs. Throughout the remaining 14 days, estrogen levels are rather high. Then they drop off again when a new cycle begins. Estrogen levels follow this cycle month after month in women of reproductive age.

The important point here is that the body is not static. Although many chemical substances are held within a fairly narrow range by homeostatic mechanisms, others fluctuate widely in normal and quite essential cycles. Over the long run, these changes are quite predictable. They also occur within prescribed physiological limits; they do not run out of control. They are part of the body's dynamic balance, just as yearly weather changes are part of the dynamic balance of the planet's climate.

In Humans, Internal Biological Rhythms Are Controlled by the Brain

Just how the body controls its many internal rhythms remains a mystery. Research suggests that the brain controls many biological cycles. One region in particular, the **suprachiasmatic nucleus** (SUE-pra-ki-as-MAT-tick), is thought to play a major role in coordinating several key rhythms.

The suprachiasmatic nucleus (SCN) is a clump of nerve cells in the base of the brain in a region called the hypothalamus. It may regulate other control centers. As a result, the suprachiasmatic nucleus is often referred to as the "master clock." Like a clock, the SCN ticks off the minutes, faithfully imposing its control on the body,

FIGURE 4-22 Stages of Sleep   Numbers indicate the stages of sleep: the higher the number, the deeper the sleep. Note that around midnight sleep is deepest. As morning approaches, a person's sleep is lighter, and REM sleep, or dream sleep, occurs in longer increments.

turning body functions on and off like an automatic timer that controls lights in a home when the occupants are gone. Even in complete, prolonged darkness, the clock ticks on, directing many circadian rhythms.

In humans, research suggests, the master clock operates on a 25-hour cycle. That is, if isolated in a dark room, many of us would fall into a 25-hour sleep-wake cycle. But as with most other biological phenomena, there is considerable variability. Some individuals, for example, operate on 28-hour sleep-wake cycles. Other individuals' cycles are shorter than 24 hours. Sleep researchers believe that in the real world, the more common 25-hour clock is modulated by the 24-hour day-night cycle. In other words, the environment alters the clock and maintains many biological rhythms on a 24-hour cycle.

Ultimate control of the SCN is thought to reside in a gland in the brain known as the **pineal gland** (PIE-knee-al). It secretes a hormone thought to keep the suprachiasmatic nucleus in sync with the 24-hour day-night cycle.

The study of biological rhythms is a fascinating field that has yielded some important information and insights. One practical application is a better understanding of jet lag, that drowsy, uncomfortable feeling people get from the disruption of sleeping patterns caused by long-distance airplane travel. Studies suggest that jet lag occurs when the body's biological clock is thrown out of synchrony with the day-night cycle of a traveler's new surroundings. A businesswoman who travels from Los Angeles to New York, for instance, may be wide awake at 10:00 P.M. New York time because her body is still on Los Angeles time—3 hours earlier. When the alarm goes off at 6:00 A.M., our weary traveler crawls out of bed exhausted, because as far as her body is concerned, it is 3:00 A.M. Los Angeles time.

To avoid the discomfort associated with travel, sleep researchers suggest that you abide by your internal clock, following "home time" when in a new time zone, or, barring that, try to reset your biological clock before you get there. You can do this by going to bed an hour or two earlier when you are traveling from west to east. Do just the opposite for east-to-west travel.

Insomnia is another disruption of sleeping patterns. For more on this topic, see Health Note 4-2.

Research on body rhythms has also shown that people respond to drugs differently at different times of the day and night. By administering drugs at the body's most receptive times, physicians may be able to reduce the doses, lowering toxic side effects and fighting diseases more effectively.

Health, Homeostasis, and the Environment

Tinkering with Our Biological Clocks

Human health is dependent on a healthy environment. Unhealthy environments disrupt homeostasis, leading to health problems of varying magnitudes.

As I've pointed out previously in this book, the health of our environment depends on more than clean air and water. It requires a healthy social and psychological atmosphere with manageable levels of stress. As this section points out, though, many adults are thrown into fairly unhealthy workplaces, a situation caused in part by our society's obsession with economic growth and convenience. Let me elaborate further.

Modern life with its stress, noise, pollution, hectic pace, and weird work schedules can deal a blow to our internal biological rhythms. Dr. Richard Restak, a neurologist and author, notes that the "usual rhythms of wakefulness and sleep . . . seem to exert a stabilizing effect on our physical and psychological health." The greatest disrupter of our natural circadian rhythms, he says, is the variable work schedule, surprisingly common in the United States and other industrialized countries. Today, one out of every four working men and one out of every six working women is on a variable work schedule, shifting frequently between day and night work. In many industries, workers are at the job day and night to make optimal use of equipment and buildings. As a result, more restaurants and stores are open 24 hours a day, and more health care workers must be on duty at night to care for accident victims.

What business owners have forgotten is that for millions of years, humans have slept during the night and been awake during the day. Make a person work at night when he or she normally sleeps, say sleep experts, and you can expect more accidents and lower productivity. Consider an example.

At 4:00 o'clock in the morning in the control room of the Three Mile Island nuclear reactor in Pennsylvania, three operators failed to notice lights indicating that a valve in the system had remained open. When the morning-shift operators entered the control room, they quickly discovered the problem, but it was too late. Pipes in the system had burst, sending radioactive steam and water into the air and into two buildings. John Gofman and Arthur Tamplin, two radiation health experts, estimate that the radiation released from the accident, the worst nuclear accident in U.S. history, will result in at least 300 and possibly as many as 900 additional fatal cases of cancer in the residents living near

Health Note 4-2

Wide Awake at 3 A.M.: Causes and Cures of Insomnia

It's Thursday evening. The final exam in your human biology course is tomorrow. Forty percent of your grade depends on your performance. You've studied hard, but it's well past midnight and you can't get to sleep. It's happened before and you know your ability to think during the test, which is scheduled to start at 8 A.M., will be impaired. That puts more pressure on you, making it more difficult to sleep.

This frustrating problem, which affects almost everyone at some time in life, is just one of several sleep disorders that physicians call *insomnia* (in-SOM-knee-ah). Another common complaint of insomniacs is waking up in the middle of the night and not being able to fall asleep again for several hours, if at all. In other instances, individuals find that they wake up too early; still others complain of sleeping through the night, but waking up feeling unrefreshed. In summary, then, insomnia is best defined as a condition of inadequate or poor quality sleep. It's a problem that

affects a great many people. In a recent study in Canada, for example, two of every five people surveyed said they had trouble sleeping at least once a week. Insomnia affects both men and women, but is more common in women and the elderly.

Insomnia may be transient (short term), intermittent (on and off), or chronic (persistent). Short-term and intermittent insomnia are generally of less concern than chronic insomnia, which can last for years. Chronic insomniacs complain of tiredness, a lack of energy, difficulty concentrating, and irritability. Insomnia can make people more susceptible to common illnesses, such as colds.

What causes insomnia? Perhaps the most common cause of insomnia is a change in one's daily routine. For example, travel, starting a new job or a new semester, going into a hospital, sleeping in a strange environment, moving into a new home, and anxiety over job interviews or tests are some possible

causes. But these are generally short-lived stimuli that rob us of our sleep. Chronic insomnia is often related to more serious problems. Certain diseases that cause pain and nausea, for example, may affect sleep. Chronic anxiety, for example, caused by a project at work that may take five months to complete, with many deadlines along the way, can keep one from falling asleep.

Another very common cause of chronic insomnia is depression. Depression usually manifests itself in the wide-awake-at-3 A.M.-syndrome. A person who is depressed may fall asleep without trouble, but may wake up every evening at 2 or 3 A.M. and may stay awake for a few hours or through the entire night. Depression, which is discussed at length in Health Note 11-1, comes in a variety of shapes and sizes, too—and can last for many years. Common symptoms include persistent sadness and anxiety, feelings of emptiness, worthlessness, and pessimism. Loss of pleasure in activities that one

the troubled reactor, although other experts (especially in the nuclear industry) contest these projections, saying that the accident will not have a noticeable effect. Whatever the outcome of this debate, one thing is certain: The 1979 accident at Three Mile Island will cost several billion dollars to clean up.

Late in April 1986, another nuclear power plant ran amok. This crisis, in the former Soviet Union, was far more severe. In the wee hours of the morning, two engineers were testing the reactor. They deactivated key safety systems in violation of standard operational protocol. Steam built up inside the reactor and blew the roof off the containment building. Workers battled for days to cover the molten radioactive core, which spewed radiation into the sky that spread worldwide.

Although no one will ever know for sure, the Chernobyl disaster, like the accident at Three Mile Island,

may have been the result of workers operating at a time unsuitable for clear thinking. One has to wonder how many plane crashes, auto accidents, and acts of medical malpractice could be traced to judgment errors resulting from our insistence on working against the natural body rhythms.

Making matters worse, many companies that maintain shifts round the clock spread the burden evenly among employees. One week, workers are on the day shift; the next week, they are switched to the "graveyard shift" (midnight to 8:00 A.M.). The next week, they are put on the night shift (4:00 P.M. to midnight). Many workers subject to such disruptive changes report that they often feel run down and have trouble staying awake on the job. Their work performance suffers. When employees who have been on the graveyard shift arrive home, they are physically ex-once enjoyed and a loss of appetite or overeating are also common.

What can be done to treat chronic insomnia? If you have a medical problem, treatment of that problem can be helpful. If you are feeling anxious all of the time, stress-relieving techniques, including psychotherapy, all of which are described in Health Note 1-1, can be helpful. Depression can be treated by psychotherapy, which helps eliminate sources of the problem. Antidepressant drugs are often prescribed for insomniacs, too. Antidepressants such as Prozac, Paxil, Luvox, and Remeron help restore normal brain chemistry by raising levels of serotonin. It may take a few weeks, however, for brain chemistry to begin to improve and for depression to begin to subside. Besides these important steps, experts recommend the following do's and don't's for dealing with insomnia.

- Go to bed and get up at the same time each day.
- Maintain a comfortable temperature in your bedroom—too hot or too cold can make it difficult to sleep.
- Sleep in a quiet, darkened room.
- Exercise regularly during the week—it helps to relieve stress.
- Don't exercise or engage in mentally stimulating activities just before going to bed.
- Exercise early in the afternoon.
- Engage in quiet tasks such as reading or listening to music in the hour or two before going to sleep.
- Try a light bedtime snack with protein just before going to bed.
- Avoid caffeine, which is found in coffees, teas, and caffeinated sodas.
- Don't use alcohol to stimulate sleep.
- Don't fight to go sleep; if you can't fall asleep within a half an hour, get out of bed, engage in some relaxing activity, and then go to bed when you feel tired.

If you need a nap, take one early in the day, before 3 pm. Sleeping pills can be used to treat insomnia, but they are mainly used to treat short-term insomnia that results from occasional stressors. Sleeping pills such as Ambien are usually not taken for more than two weeks because they can actually worsen one's insomnia. Ironically, several common prescription drugs used to treat insomnia-causing depression—including Prozac and Paxil—actually cause sleeplessness in about one-third of the patients taking them. Sleeping pills, both over-the-counter remedies and prescription medicines, can cause a host of side effects, including confusion, heart problems, and decreased sexual desire.

Visit *Human Biology's* Internet site for links to web sites offering more information on this topic.

hausted but cannot sleep because they are trying to sleep at a time when their body is trying to wake them up. What is more, weekly changes in schedule never permit workers' internal clocks to adjust. Studies show that most people require from 4 to 14 days to adjust to a new schedule.

Not surprisingly, workers on alternating shifts suffer more ulcers, insomnia, irritability, depression, and tension than workers on unchanging shifts. Many suffer from impaired judgment on the job and, in some circumstances, they may pose a threat to society.

Thanks to studies of biological rhythms, researchers are finding ways to reset the body's clock. These efforts could lessen the problems shift workers face and improve the performance of those on the graveyard shift. For instance, one simple measure is to place all shift workers on 3-week cycles instead of weekly cycles. This gives their biological clocks time to adjust. And instead of shifting workers from daytime to a graveyard shift, transfer them forward, rather than backward (for example, from a daytime to an evening shift and from an evening shift to the graveyard shift). Studies suggest that moving forward is far easier for workers than shifting backward.

For reasons not well understood, special treatment with bright lights helps reset the biological clock. Patients who suffer from insomnia because their biological clocks are out of phase can receive daily doses of bright light, which somehow reset their internal clocks. Similar treatments are being tested for shift workers. They are a small price to pay for a healthy work force and a safer society.

Summary

From Cells to Organ Systems

1. The basic structural unit of all organisms is the cell. In humans, cells and extracellular material form *tissues*, and tissues, in turn, combine to form *organs*.

2. Four *primary tissues* are found in the bodies of most multicellular animals such as humans: epithelial tissue, connective tissue, muscle tissue, and nervous tissue. Each primary tissue serves a unique function.

3. Organs contain all four primary tissues in varying proportions.

4. *Epithelial tissues* consist of two types: *membranous epithelia,* which form the coverings or linings of organs, and *glandular epithelia,* which form exocrine and endocrine glands.

5. *Connective tissues* bind other tissues together, provide protection, and support body structures. All connective tissues consist of two basic components: cells and extracellular fibers.

6. Two types of connective tissue are found in the body: *connective tissue proper* (dense and loose connective tissue) and *specialized connective tissue* (bone, cartilage, and blood).

7. *Cartilage* consists of specialized cells embedded in a matrix of extracellular fibers and other extracellular material.

8. *Bone* is a dynamic tissue that provides internal support, protects organs such as the brain, and helps regulate blood calcium levels.

9. Bone consists of bone cells (*osteocytes*) and a calcified cartilage matrix. Two types of bone tissue exist: spongy and compact.

10. The *osteoclast,* one type of bone cell, plays a major role in reshaping bone to meet the changing demands of the body and in releasing calcium to help maintain blood calcium levels.

11. *Blood* is another form of specialized connective tissue. It consists of numerous blood cells and *platelets* and an extracellular fluid, called *plasma*.

12. *Muscle* is an excitable tissue that contracts when stimulated. Three types of muscle tissue are found in the human body: skeletal, cardiac, and smooth muscle.

13. *Skeletal muscle* is under voluntary control, for the most part, and forms the muscles that attach to bones. *Cardiac muscle* is located in the heart and is involuntary. *Smooth muscle* is involuntary and forms sheets of varying thickness in the walls of organs and blood vessels.

14. *Nervous tissue* is the fourth primary tissue. It consists of two types of cells: conducting and nonconducting (supportive). The conducting cells, called *neurons,* transmit impulses from one region of the body to another. The *nonconducting cells* are a type of nervous system connective tissue.

15. Tissues combine to form organs in which specialized functions are carried out. Most organs are part of an organ system, a group of organs that cooperate to carry out some complex function.

Principles of Homeostasis

16. The nervous and endocrine systems coordinate the functions of organ systems, helping the body maintain homeostasis, or internal constancy. Homeostasis also occurs on the cellular level.

17. All homeostatic systems maintain constancy by balancing inputs and outputs as well as movement to and from storage depots. Homeostatic systems do not maintain absolute constancy and can be upset by alterations in input or output or by changes in movements in or out of storage depots. Imbalances can seriously affect an individual's health.

18. Homeostatic mechanisms are *reflexes,* occurring without conscious control. They operate by *negative feedback.*

19. Homeostatic reflexes occur at all levels of biological organization and involve two main mechanisms: nervous and hormonal.

20. Nervous and endocrine mechanisms generally occur over considerable distances. In some cases, control is exerted locally through the extracellular fluid.

Biological Rhythms

21. Many physiological processes undergo definite rhythmic changes. These natural rhythms may take place over a 24-hour period or over much longer or shorter periods.

22. The brain controls many biological cycles. A clump of nerve cells (the *suprachiasmatic nucleus*) located in the hypothalamus is thought to play a major role in coordinating several key functions and control centers. It is therefore often referred to as the "master clock."

Health, Homeostasis, and the Environment: Tinkering with Our Biological Clocks

23. The hectic pace of modern life, the shifting work schedules that many people follow, and the stressful environments in which we live can upset internal rhythms, with disastrous consequences.

24. The greatest disrupter of our natural circadian rhythms is the variable work schedule, which is surprisingly common among industrialized nations.

25. Workers on alternating shifts suffer from a higher incidence of ulcers, insomnia, irritability, depression, and tension than workers on regular shifts. Making matters worse, tired, irritable workers whose judgment is impaired by fatigue pose a threat not only to themselves, but also to society.

26. Researchers are finding ways to reset the biological clock, which could lessen the problems shift workers face and thereby increase work performance, particularly of those on the graveyard shift.

Critical Thinking

Thinking Critically— Analysis

This Analysis corresponds to the Thinking Critically scenario that was presented at the beginning of this chapter.

With a little digging—a step vital to critical thinking— you will find that prenatal care consists of visits to doctors for checkups and advice on nutrition and other matters pertinent to pregnant women. Prenatal care is crucial to the development of a healthy fetus. If problems arise, they can be dealt with immediately, not when it's too late and too costly. You will also find that the cost of one organ transplant could supply medical care for 1000 pregnant women, assistance that itself could prevent ailments that necessitate costly transplant procedures.

Given this information, should Americans spend more on prevention and less on dramatic life-saving measures, such as organ transplants? Why?

After you have given your opinion on this matter, put yourself in the position of a parent whose child needs a kidney transplant to survive. How does this perspective affect your position? What lessons can be learned from this?

Test of Concepts

1. Define the following terms: tissues, extracellular material, organs, and organ systems.
2. List the four primary tissues and their subtypes.
3. Describe the similarities and differences in the embryonic origin of endocrine and exocrine glands. Explain why the two secrete differently.
4. Discuss some biological examples showing how structure reflects function.
5. Describe the two types of connective tissue and how they function.
6. Why do cartilage injuries repair so slowly or not at all? Bone is repaired much more easily than cartilage. Why is this true?
7. In what way is bone part of a homeostatic system?
8. Describe the chief differences among cardiac, skeletal, and smooth muscle.
9. What is an organ system? List some examples.
10. Define homeostasis, and describe the major principles of homeostasis presented in this chapter. Use an example to illustrate your points.
11. Homeostatic mechanisms are largely reflexes, involving chemical or nervous impulses. Describe each type of reflex, giving an example. You may find it helpful to include drawings of the systems.
12. Are biological rhythms an exception to the principle of homeostasis?
13. Describe the biological clock, and explain how it is synchronized with the 24-hour day-night cycle.
14. How does shift work upset the biological clock? How can these problems be mitigated?
15. The Health, Homeostasis, and the Environment section makes the point that human health and welfare is threatened by an environment of economic greed that compels people to work when they should be sleeping. Do you agree with this? Why or why not?

www.jbpub.com/humanbiology

Connect to this book's web site: www.jbpub.com/humanbiology
The site features eLearning, an online review area that provides quizzes, chapter outlines, and other tools to help you study for your class. You can also follow useful links for in-depth information, research the differing views in the Point/Counterpoints, or keep up on the latest environmental and health news.

CHAPTER 5

Nutrition and Digestion

Thinking Critically

Kidney stones begin as tiny crystals. These crystals, which are made of calcium and other ions, grow layer by layer and can eventually obstruct the flow of urine, causing considerable pain and discomfort. Because stones are made primarily of calcium, physicians often recommend a dietary solution to patients who have already had a stone: reducing their intake of calcium by cutting back on milk and milk products, such as cheese and yogurt. Sounds logical doesn't it?

Unfortunately, a new study of 45,000 men suggests that a low-calcium diet may actually increase the risk of developing kidney stones. This study showed that men who ate a diet rich in calcium actually had a 34% lower risk of developing kidney stones than men who ate a low-calcium diet. The researchers were perplexed by the results. Their study seemed counterintuitive.

Kidney specialist Gary Curhan offers a hypothesis to explain the results. He believes that a chemical called *oxalate*, which is present in many foods, may be the reason for the results. Oxalate binds to calcium and forms insoluble crystals that make up most kidney stones. Curhan believes that oxalate in the diets of people who ingest normal amounts of calcium binds to the calcium in their intestines. This prevents blood oxalate levels from rising and retards the formation of stones. Low-calcium diets permit an excess of oxalate to enter the body; this oxalate binds to calcium in the kidney and causes stones. How would you test this hypothesis? What lessons can be gleaned here?

Electron micrograph of the villi of the small intestine.

It must be a law of human nature. ask almost any couple, and they will tell you: She lies shivering under the covers on a cold winter night while he bakes. Out on a hike in winter, he stays warm in a light jacket while she bundles up in stocking cap, down coat, and gloves. What causes this difference between many men and women?

Part of the answer may lie in iron—not pumping iron, but dietary iron. Quite simply, many American women do not consume enough iron to offset losses that occur during menstruation, the monthly discharge of blood and tissue from the lining of the uterus. Iron deficiencies in women may reduce internal heat production.[1]

John Beard, a researcher at Pennsylvania State University, published a study that supports this conclusion. Beard compared two groups of women, one with low levels of iron in the blood and another with normal levels. Beard found that body temperature dropped more quickly in iron-deficient women exposed to cold than in those with normal iron levels. He also found that iron-deficient women generated 13% less body heat.

Adding credence to the hypothesis that iron deficiency reduces body heat and makes women colder, Beard gave the iron-deficient women iron supplements for 12 weeks, after which they responded normally to cold. These findings illustrate how important proper nutrition is to normal physiological function, especially homeostasis.[2] You'll see additional examples as we explore nutrition and digestion. What you learn here will help you in many ways. It will help you understand what a healthy diet is and will enable you to evaluate the merits (or lack thereof) of many fad diets..

---

[1]Differences in body temperature between men and women may also result from other factors, such as body mass and surface area. Low blood pressure or poor circulation would also make the extremities feel cold.

[2]Because iron can be toxic if ingested in excess, people considering supplementing their diets with iron tablets should consult a physician.

A Primer On Nutrition

Some people eat to live, but many others seem to live to eat. No matter what your orientation, food probably occupies a central part of your life. If you're like many others, you may often plan your daytime activities around meals. In addition, you spend a good part of your life shopping for, preparing, and eating meals. Depending on your income, 10%–20% of the money you earn goes to buy food. Thus, 1.5–3 hours of each workday goes to providing money for food. (The rest goes to paying income tax!)

If you live to be 65, you will consume over 70,000 meals. Because foods affect your body in many ways, what you eat will determine how you feel in your later years. That's how important nutrition is to your health. Despite the increased emphasis on nutrition today, studies suggest that most Americans pay little attention to their diet. To perform and feel our very best, though, we must eat a balanced diet to acquire the energy and nutrients needed by our cells, tissues, and organs.

A **balanced diet** is attained by eating a variety of foods. In 1992, the U.S. Department of Agriculture released a helpful tool called a **food pyramid**, to help Americans eat better. It places foods in six major groups and prescribes allotments from each group necessary for proper nutrition (**FIGURE 5-1**). Take a few moments to study the pyramid and compare it to your diet. If you would like to assess your eating habits, you can take the test in **TABLE 5-1**. As you can see from **FIGURE 5-1**, a healthy diet consists of plenty of breads, cereals, rice, and pasta. It also includes plenty of fruits and vegetables. Meat and milk products are required, but in lesser

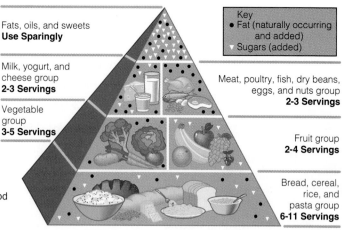

FIGURE 5-1 Food Guide Pyramid Replacing the four food groups, the food pyramid divides food into six groups. Recommended daily intake is shown for each group.

TABLE 5-1

How Healthy Is Your Diet?

This quiz enables you to assess your eating habits. The more points you get, the better your nutritional health is likely to be.

PART I
1. I usually limit my meat, fish, poultry, or egg servings to once or twice a day. — Yes/No
2. I eat red meats (beef, ham, lamb, or pork) not more than about three times a week. — Yes/No
3. I remove fat or ask that fat be trimmed from meat before cooking. — Yes/No
4. I eat no more than one egg per day, including those cooked with other foods. — Yes/No
5. I sometimes have meatless days and eat such protein-rich foods as legumes and nuts. — Yes/No
6. I usually broil, boil, bake, or roast meat, fish or poultry; I usually don't fry it. — Yes/No

Total "YES" answers: _____

PART II
7. I have two or more cups of milk or the equivalent in milk products every day. — Yes/No
8. I drink low-fat or nonfat milk (2% or less butterfat) rather than whole milk. — Yes/No
9. I eat ice cream or ice milk only twice a week or less. — Yes/No
10. I seldom have more than about 3 tsp of margarine or butter per day. — Yes/No

Total "YES" answers: _____

PART III
11. I usually have one serving ($\frac{1}{2}$ c) of citrus fruit or juice (oranges, grapefruit, etc.) each day. — Yes/No
12. I have at least one serving of dark green or deep orange vegetables each day. — Yes/No
13. I eat fresh fruits and vegetables when I can get them. — Yes/No
14. I cook vegetables without fat (if I use margarine, it's measured and added after cooking). — Yes/No
15. I eat fresh fruit for dessert more often than pastries. — Yes/No

Total "YES" answers: _____

PART IV
16. I generally eat whole-grain breads. — Yes/No
17. Most of the cereals I use are whole-grain and good sources of fiber. — Yes/No
18. The cereals I use have little or no sugar added. — Yes/No
19. I use brown rice in preference to white rice. — Yes/No
20. I generally have at least four servings of bread or cereal grain products each day. — Yes/No

Total "YES" answers: _____

PART V
21. I am usually within 5 to 10 lbs of the weight considered appropriate for my height. — Yes/No
22. I drink no more than $1\frac{1}{2}$ oz of alcohol (one to two drinks) per day. — Yes/No
23. I do not add salt to food after preparation and prefer foods salted lightly or not salted at all. — Yes/No
24. I try to avoid foods high in refined sugar and use sugar sparingly. — Yes/No
25. I always eat a breakfast of at least cereal and milk, egg and toast, or other protein-carbohydrate combination with fruit or fruit juice. — Yes/No

Total "YES" answers: _____

For each "yes" answer, give yourself 1 point. How are your points distributed among the various areas of nutrition?

		Excellent	Good	Fair	Poor	Your score
Part I	Meat and meat alternate choices	5–6	4	3	0–2	_____
Part II	Dairy choices	4	3	2	0–1	_____
Part III	Fruit and vegetable choices	5	4	3	0–2	_____
Part IV	Grain choices	5	4	3	0–2	_____
Part V	Weight control, other choices	5	4	3	0–2	_____

How is your overall nutrition score? **Total points earned:** _____

(24–25 is excellent; 19–23 is good; 14–18 is fair; 13 or lower is poor.)

SOURCE: Adapted with permission from Roger Sargent, *Have a Good Life Series*, Greenville, S.C.: Liberty Life.

TABLE 5-2

Macronutrients and Micronutrients

Nutrients	Foods Containing Them
Macronutrients	
Water	All drinks and many foods
Amino acids and proteins	Milk and milk products such as cheese; soy products such as tofu and soy milk; meat, and eggs
Lipids	Milk and milk products, meats, eggs, nuts, oils, and seeds
Carbohydrates	Breads, pastas, cereals, sweets
Micronutrients	
Vitamins	Many vegetables, meats, and fruits
Minerals	Many vegetables, meats, fruits, nuts, and seeds

amounts. Fat is to be minimized. Most people in the more developed countries go wrong by eating too few fruits and vegetables and too much of the upper end of the pyramid: meats, milk products, and fats.

The nutrients we need to survive and prosper physically and mentally can be divided into two broad categories: macronutrients and micronutrients. **TABLE 5-2** lists the basic nutrients and includes some of the foods and beverages that provide them. The following section describes the macronutrients and micronutrients more fully and explains why they are important to the proper functioning of the human body and the maintenance of health.

Macronutrients Are Required in Relatively Large Quantities and Include Four Substances: Water, Carbohydrates, Lipids, and Proteins

Water. Water is one of the most important of all the substances we ingest. Without it, a person can survive only about 3 days. Despite its importance, water rarely shows up on nutrition charts. In part, that is because it is supplied in so many different ways. For example, water constitutes the bulk of the liquids we drink and is present in virtually all of the solid foods we eat; water is even produced internally during cellular metabolism (Chapter 3).

Maintaining the proper level of water in the body is important for several reasons. First, water participates in many chemical reactions in the body. For example, the

Monomers

H₂O

H   HO

FIGURE 5-2 Hydrolysis Hydrolysis is a reaction in which water is added across a covalent bond, causing the bond to split.

breakdown of several large chemicals like starch require water. The breakdown of a chemical using water is called **hydrolysis** (high-DROL-ah-siss). A simplified version is shown in **FIGURE 5-2**. In these reactions, enzymes add water across covalent bonds, causing them to break apart.

Because of water's importance in metabolism, a decrease in its level can impair metabolism, including energy production. According to some studies, athletic performance may drop significantly when the body's water level falls even slightly.

Maintaining an adequate water volume also helps to stabilize body temperature. A decline in the amount of water in your body decreases your blood volume and your extracellular fluid. These declines cause your body temperature to rise, because the heat normally produced by body cells is being absorbed by a smaller volume of water. A rise in body temperature can impair cellular function and can, if high enough, lead to death. This is one reason physicians tell you to drink plenty of water when you are suffering from a fever.

Maintaining proper water levels also helps individuals maintain normal concentrations of nutrients and toxic waste products in the blood and extracellular fluid. If you don't drink enough liquid, your urine will become more concentrated; the rise in the concentration of chemicals in the blood and urine increases your chance of developing a kidney stone, a deposit of calcium, and other materials that can block the flow of urine, causing extensive damage to this organ.

Maintaining proper water levels is so important that animals have evolved a variety of homeostatic mechanisms to carry out this function. Several of these, which are present in humans, are featured in Chapter 10.

Carbohydrates Serve Many Functions in Humans; One of the Most Important Is as a Source of Energy. Carbohydrates are a group of organic compounds that includes such well-known examples as table sugar (sucrose), blood sugar (glucose), and starch. Carbohydrates consist primarily of carbon, oxygen, and hydrogen. Carbohydrates belong to three broad groups: monosaccharides, disaccharides, and polysaccharides.

Monosaccharides are the smallest carbohydrates. They are often simple sugars. These water-soluble molecules contain three to seven carbons, and many of them form ring structures when dissolved in water. One of the most common and most important monosaccharides is **glucose** (GLUE-kose), a six-carbon sugar introduced in Chapter 3. Glucose is made by plants during photosynthesis.

Disaccharides (dye-SACK-are-ides) are carbohydrates that consist of two monosaccharides covalently bonded to each other. The disaccharide sucrose, for instance, consists of two monosaccharides, glucose and fructose.

In animals and plants, many monosaccharides react to form much larger molecules known as polymers. A **polymer** is a general term used to describe any molecule consisting of numerous smaller molecules. Proteins, for instance, are polymers of amino acids. Starch is a polymer containing numerous glucose molecules.

Carbohydrate polymers are called **polysaccharides.** The most common building block of polysaccharides is glucose. Plants synthesize two important polysaccharides from glucose: (1) **starch** and (2) **cellulose** (CELL-you-lose).

Starch molecules produced in the leaves of plants are stored in plant roots (as in potatoes) or seeds (as in wheat and rice) and are an important nutrient for plant-eating animals. In the digestive tract of humans and other animals, starch is broken down into glucose molecules. Glucose enters the bloodstream and is distributed to body cells, where they are broken down to release energy. Glucose can also be stored in cells of the liver and skeletal muscle.

In liver and muscle cells of animals, glucose combines to form yet another polysaccharide, **glycogen** (GLYE-co-gen), which contains thousands of glucose molecules. Glycogen is often called "animal starch" because it serves a similar purpose and has a structure similar to starch found in plants.

Glycogen is an important player in the homeostatic mechanism that ensures constant blood sugar (glucose) levels. When blood glucose levels fall in the periods between meals, the liver breaks down its stored supplies of glycogen. The glucose molecules produced in this process are released into the bloodstream, maintaining serum glucose concentrations needed to keep us alive and well.

The release of glucose from the liver is stimulated by a hormone called **glucagon**. When blood glucose levels fall, glucagon secretion (release) is stimulated. Produced by certain cells in the pancreas, glucagon enters the bloodstream, circulates to the liver, where it stimulates the breakdown of glycogen.

Although muscle cells also store glucose in the form of glycogen, they do not participate in maintaining normal blood sugar levels. This glycogen is used only by muscle cells in times of need.

Animals derive the glucose they need primarily from plant starch. A few animals such as cattle, sheep, and other grazers are able to acquire glucose from cellulose in the plants they consume.

Cellulose molecules are polysaccharides found only in plants. The covalent bonds that join the glucose molecules are slightly different than those in starch. Because of this, cellulose cannot be digested by most animals; they lack the enzymes needed to break the covalent bonds joining its glucose subunits. (**Enzymes** are protein molecules that speed up the rate of many chemical reactions in cells.) Consequently, cellulose passes through the digestive system of most animals relatively unchanged.

Even though it is not digested, cellulose is important to normal body function. In the human diet, for example, nondigestible cellulose is a principal form of **dietary fiber.** For reasons explained shortly, cellulose facilitates the passage of feces through the large intestine and also reduces the incidence of colon cancer.

Some species, such as cows, can digest cellulose, and are therefore able to get the glucose they need to make energy. These species, however, do not digest cellulose on their own. In other words, they don't produce the enzymes needed to cleave the odd covalent bonds in cellulose; they get them from bacteria and other single-celled organisms that live within their stomachs. These organisms secrete celluose-digesting enzymes into the stomach of a cow (and other similar species). They absorb some of the glucose for their own use, but the rest goes to their host. It's not a bad arrangement. In exchange for a generous supply of food, these organisms enable cows and other species to feed on grasses and other plant matter.

Humans need a continuous supply of energy, even the most ardent couch potatoes! Cells, for instance, require energy to carry out the thousands of functions required to grow, to divide, and to transport molecules across their membranes. Surprisingly, 70%–80% of the total energy required by sedentary humans (individuals who get little exercise) goes to perform basic functions—metabolism, food digestion, absorption, and so on. The remaining energy is used to power body movements such as walking, talking, and turning on the television via the remote control. For more active people, these percentages shift considerably. A bicycle commuter, for example, uses proportionately more energy for vigorous muscular activity than an office worker who rides a bus or drives a car to work.

At rest, the body relies on nearly equal amounts of carbohydrate (mostly glucose) and fat (triglycerides) to supply basic body needs. As you may recall from Chapter 3, glucose is broken down (catabolized) during cellular respiration.

The most common source of glucose is the polysaccharide starch. Starch is present in grains and their by-products (pasta and bread). It is also provided by many vegetables. Starch contributes on average about 22% of the total energy requirements of most Americans (**TABLE 5-3**).

TABLE 5-3

Energy Sources in the Average American Diet

Source	Percentage	Ideal Percentage
Fat	42	20–30
Sucrose	24	} 50
Starch	22	
Protein	12	10

In the digestive system of humans, starch is broken down into glucose molecules, which are absorbed into the bloodstream and distributed to body cells. The cells break down some glucose immediately to produce energy. Most of the rest is converted into glycogen in muscles and the liver and stored for later use (**FIGURE 5-3**). This ability to store glucose is vital to our survival. Without it, we'd need to eat constantly.

Between meals and during exercise, the liver breaks down stored glycogen to form glucose, which is released into the bloodstream. As noted earlier, glycogen in muscle is catabolized to provide energy for muscular contraction, but is not released into the bloodstream.

Another important carbohydrate, not involved in energy production, is fiber. **Dietary fiber** is nondigestible polysaccharide (such as cellulose) that is found in fruits, vegetables, and grains. As noted earlier, humans cannot digest cellulose because the body lacks the enzymes needed to break the covalent bonds joining the monosaccharide units (glucose) in the molecule. Consequently, fiber passes through the intestine largely unaffected by stomach acidity or digestive enzymes. So why is it so important to us?

Let me explain. Dietary fiber exists in two basic forms: water-soluble and water-insoluble. **Water-soluble fibers** are gummy polysaccharides in fruits, vegetables, and some grains—including apples, bananas, carrots, barley, and oats. Several studies suggest that water-soluble fiber helps lower blood cholesterol by acting as a sponge that absorbs dietary cholesterol inside the digestive tract. This prevents cholesterol from being absorbed into the bloodstream.

In contrast, **water-insoluble fibers** are rigid cellulose molecules in foods such as celery, cereals, wheat products, and brown rice. Some foods, such as green beans and green peas, contain a mixture of both types.

Water-insoluble fiber such as that in whole wheat bread increases the water content of the **feces** (FEE-seas), the semisolid waste produced by the large intestine. This makes the feces softer and facilitates their transport through the large intestine. Increasing the water content also reduces constipation. To understand why whole wheat bread is good for you, you must understand a little bit about the composition of a grain of wheat and the making of flour.

FIGURE 5-4 shows that wheat grain consists of three parts: (1) the **bran**, or shell, which contains most of the fiber; (2) the

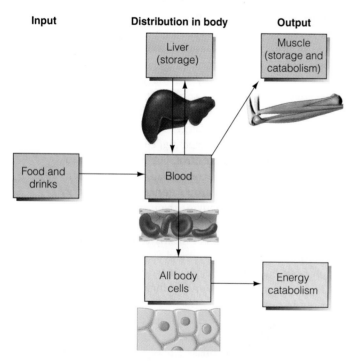

FIGURE 5-3 Glucose Balance   Glucose levels in the blood result from a balance of input and output.

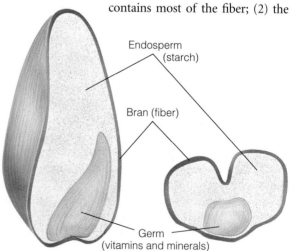

FIGURE 5-4 The Wheat Seed   Parts of a wheat grain and the nutrients and minerals they supply.

endosperm, the starchy portion that provides nutrients for the growing plant; and (3) the **germ**, the vitamin- and mineral-rich portion that becomes a new plant. When the wheat grain is ground, it produces whole-wheat flour, a brown powder containing the entire wheat grain. In contrast, white flour is produced from grain whose bran and germ have been removed. Removing the bran eliminates most, if not all, of the water-insoluble fiber (cellulose). Removing the germ eliminates most of the vitamins and minerals. White flour, therefore, consists mostly of starch. Ironically, some bread makers now fortify their bread with minerals and vitamins—the very same ones they remove to make the bread!

The benefits of water-insoluble fiber were first reported in 1971 by a British missionary surgeon, Denis Burkitt. He noted that rural Africans had a much lower incidence of cancer of the colon and rectum than those of us in the West. In fact, colorectal cancer was practically nonexistent in African men and women. Burkitt hypothesized that the difference could be explained by Ugandans' high-fiber diet. The mechanism, quickly offered by the scientific community, was that fiber caused the moister fecal matter to be moved more rapidly through the large intestine. Additional studies seemed to support Burkitt's hypothesis.

Even though the evidence was still circumstantial, the American Cancer Society began to recommend fiber in 1984 as a means of reducing colorectal cancer. Cereal boxes began to carry these claims. More rigorous clinical studies in the 1980s and early 1990s showed that the protective effect of water-insoluble fiber from cereals was weaker than earlier work had predicted. In 2000, researchers who studied the diets of 88,000 female nurses for nearly 20 years, reported that those who consumed approximately 30 grams of dietary fiber a day had the same risk as those who consumed only 13 grams per day. A similar study in men also yielded negative results. Two additional clinical studies offered the same results for cereal fiber.

Unfortunately, the news media reported that dietary fiber was ineffective in reducing colorectal cancer. The studies focused on cereal fiber. Many nutritionists and researchers believe that a diet of whole fruits and vegetables as well as whole grains does protect us from colorectal cancer. Fiber in cereals apparently does not.

Lipids Are Fat-Soluble Molecules That Serve as a Source of Energy and Are Also Important Structural Components of Cells.

Lipids are a structurally diverse group of organic molecules that are insoluble in water and soluble in nonpolar solvents such as ethyl alcohol. Lipids are the waxy, greasy, or oily compounds found in plants and animals. Fats and oils in animals are energy-rich molecules that serve as an important storage depot. Still other lipids are structural components of cells. Two biologically important lipids will be discussed in this chapter: triglycerides and steroids. (Phospholipids were discussed in Chapter 3.)

Triglycerides. Triglycerides are known to most of us as fats and oils. Cooking oil, for example, is a triglyceride, as is the fat in a steak or the butter on a piece of bread.

Triglycerides are composed of four subunits, each an organic molecule: one molecule of glycerol and three fatty acid molecules (**FIGURE 5-5**). Glycerol is a three-carbon compound; fatty acids are long molecules containing many carbons and hydrogens and a COOH, or **carboxyl group** (car-BOX-ul), on one end.

Triglycerides contain many covalent bonds, each of which stores a small amount of energy. When cells break down (catabolize) triglycerides, these bonds are broken and energy is released. Energy liberated during the breakdown of triglycerides is used to drive a variety of cellular processes. Gram for gram, triglycerides yield more than twice as much energy as carbohydrates.

In humans and many other mammals, triglycerides are stored in fat cells under the skin and in other locations (**FIGURE 5-6**). In adult humans, triglycerides provide about half of the cellular energy consumed at rest, with carbohydrates providing most of the rest. During moderate (aerobic) exercise, triglycerides provide a larger proportion of the body's energy demand, explaining why aerobic exercise like jogging and bicycling helps people lose weight.

Fatty deposits around certain organs also cushion them from damage. Horseback riders, motorcyclists, and runners, for instance, can engage in their sports for hours at a time without damaging their internal organs in part because of nature's natural cushions.

With a few exceptions, fats (from most animals) are solid at room temperature, and oils (from plants and fish) are liquid. The reason for this difference lies in their chemical structures. In fats, the carbon atoms of the fatty acids are joined by single covalent bonds (**FIGURE 5-5**). The remaining bond sites on the carbon atoms are taken up by hydrogens. Thus, the fatty acids are said to be *saturated* with hydrogens. When the carbon backbone of a fatty acid consists solely of single covalent bonds, the structure zigzags but still remains fairly linear (**FIGURE 5-7A**). This allows the triglyceride molecules of a fat to pack together, forming a solid at room temperature.

In contrast, the fatty acids in oils contain a number of double covalent bonds and these molecules are said

FIGURE 5-5 Triglycerides
The triglycerides are the fats and oils. Triglycerides consist of glycerol and three fatty acids, covalently bonded as shown.

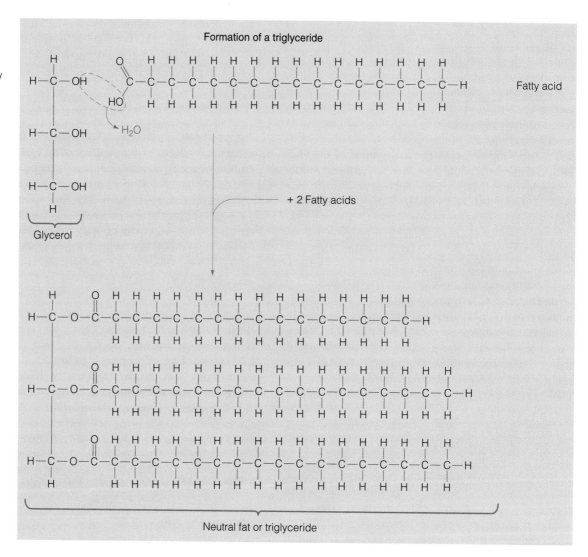

Formation of a triglyceride

Fatty acid

+ 2 Fatty acids

Glycerol

Neutral fat or triglyceride

Fat cells

(a)   (b)

FIGURE 5-6 Fat Cells   *(a)* A light micrograph of fat tissue. The clear areas are regions where the fat has dissolved during tissue preparation. Notice that the cytoplasm is reduced to a narrow region just beneath the plasma membrane. *(b)* A scanning electron micrograph of fat cells.

(a) Saturated fatty acids   **(b)** Unsaturated fatty acids

Distortion resulting from double bonds

FIGURE 5-7 The Difference a Few Double Bonds Can Make
(a) Saturated fatty acids are principally derived from animal fats. The side chains are relatively straight and allow the molecules to pack tightly together, which explains why fats are solid at room temperature. *(b)* Double bonds in unsaturated fatty acids in oils cause the fatty acid chains to bend and thus prohibit tight packing. Oils, derived chiefly from plants, are therefore liquid at room temperature.

to be unsaturated (**FIGURE 5-7B**). Double covalent bonds cause a bend in the fatty acid molecules that is believed to prevent tight packing. This somewhat "looser" arrangement of triglyceride molecules produces a liquid at room temperature.

When numerous double bonds exist in a fatty acid molecule, the molecule is said to be *polyunsaturated.* Studies show that polyunsaturated fats reduce one's risk of developing **atherosclerosis** (AH-ther-oh-skler-OH-siss), a disease that results from a buildup of cholesterol deposits, or **atherosclerotic plaque,** on the walls of arteries (**FIGURE 5-8**). Plaque restricts blood flow to the heart and brain, causing heart attacks and strokes.

For reasons not well understood, saturated fatty acids increase cholesterol production by the liver, so diets rich in saturated fat (animal fats) tend to increase the chances of developing atherosclerosis. Steak, hamburgers, cheese, chicken with its skin on, bacon, whole milk, and many common snack foods contain lots of saturated fat. In fact, fat is often added as a flavoring.

Atherosclerosis is also more common in sedentary people and smokers. Some individuals are genetically predisposed to develop atherosclerosis. Their livers simply produce abnormally high levels of cholesterol.

What is shocking, is that the arteries of many children, teenagers, and young adults are starting to show a surprising amount of plaque. In a recent study of heart

Wall of artery

(a) Normal artery

Wall of artery   Plaque

(b) Atherosclerotic artery

FIGURE 5-8 Atherosclerosis These cross sections of *(a)* a normal artery and *(b)* a diseased artery show how atherosclerotic plaque can obstruct blood flow.

Health Note 5-1

Lowering Your Cholesterol

Let there be no doubt about it: Diseases of the heart and arteries are leading causes of death in the United States.

Atherosclerosis, the accumulation of plaque on artery walls, and the problems it creates are responsible for nearly two of every five deaths in the United States each year. Thanks to improvements in medical care and diet, the death rate from atherosclerosis has been falling steadily in recent years, but it is still a major concern. New research, in fact, shows that atherosclerotic plaque is present even in children as explained in the text.

Researchers believe that atherosclerotic plaques begin to form after minor injuries to the lining of blood vessels. High blood pressure, they think, may damage the lining, causing cholesterol in the blood to seep through the lining. Certain cells, known as macrophages, in the region begin to absorb the cholesterol, becoming **foam cells**, so named because they appear foamy under the microscope. The blood vessel responds by producing cells that grow over the fatty deposit. This thickens the wall of the artery, reducing blood flow. Additional cholesterol is then deposited in the thickened wall, forming a larger and larger obstruction.

Cholesterol deposits impair the flow of blood in the heart and other organs, cutting off oxygen to vital tissues. Blood clots may form in the restricted sections of arteries, further reducing blood flow. When the oxygen supply to the heart is disrupted, cardiac muscle cells can die, resulting in heart attacks and death. Blood clots originating in other parts of the body may also lodge in diseased vessels, obstructing blood flow. Oxygen deprivation can weaken the heart, impairing its ability to pump blood. When the oxygen supply to the heart is restricted, the result is a type of heart attack known as a **myocardial infarction** (my-oh-CAR-dee-ill in-FARK-shun). Victims of a myocardial infarction feel pain in the center of the chest and down the left arm. If the oxygen-deprived area is extensive, the heart may cease functioning altogether.

Atherosclerotic plaque also impairs the flow of blood to the brain. Blood clots catch in the restricted areas and block the flow of blood to vital regions of the brain. Victims may lose the ability to speak or to move limbs. If the damage is severe enough, they may die. Thanks to advances in medical treatment, however, many victims can be saved. And over time, they can recover lost functions as other parts of the brain take over for the damaged regions.

Atherosclerosis and cardiovascular disease have been associated with nearly 40 factors. Several of these risk factors, such as old age and sex (being male), cannot be changed. Other factors are controllable. These include high blood pressure, high blood cholesterol, stress, smoking, inactivity, and excessive food intake. Of all the risk factors, three emerge as the primary contributors to cardiovascular disease: elevated blood cholesterol, smoking, and high blood pressure.

Consider cholesterol. Cholesterol is essential to normal body function. It is part of the plasma membrane and is needed to synthesize certain hormones. Interestingly, in most people, the majority of the cholesterol in the blood is produced by the liver. The liver synthesizes and releases about 700 milligrams of cholesterol per day. Only about 225 milligrams of cholesterol are derived from the food

transplants carried out by the Cleveland Clinic Foundation, researchers found that hearts from healthy, young donors showed signs of heart disease. Eighteen of 77 hearts from donors who died before their thirtieth birthday displayed early signs of heart disease, notably the build up of atherosclerotic plaque in the heart arteries. Five of 32 hearts from teenage donors in this group showed plaque build-up. Some researchers are concerned that the high fat diets of many young children in the affluent industrial nations and the lack of exercise could dramatically increase heart disease in the years to come.

Lowering the level of saturated fat in the diet can be accomplished by switching from whole milk to low-fat milk, reducing the consumption of red meat, trimming fat from chicken and other meats, cutting down on cheese, and cooking with unsaturated vegetable oil instead of animal fat (lard). Watch out for snack foods too. Manufacturers list the total fat and saturated fat content of all packaged foods. Check out the label very carefully. (For more on cholesterol, see Health Note 5-1.)

Vegetable oil can be converted to a solid (margarine) by chemically adding hydrogens to it. This process decreases the number of double bonds and tends to straighten the fatty acid chains, resulting in a solid. Even as such, polyunsaturated margarines, advertised for their health benefits, still contain a large number of double bonds.

we eat each day. Interestingly, the concentration of cholesterol in the blood tends to stay fairly constant. If dietary input falls, the liver increases its output. If the amount of cholesterol in the diet rises, the liver reduces its production. So what's all the fuss about cholesterol in a person's diet?

Even though the liver regulates cholesterol levels, it cannot work fast enough. That is, it may simply be unable to absorb, use, and dispose of cholesterol quickly enough. Consequently, excess cholesterol circulates in the blood after a meal and is deposited in the arteries.

Cholesterol is carried in the bloodstream bound to protein. These complexes of protein and lipid fall into two groups: high-density lipoproteins (HDLs) and low-density lipoproteins (LDLs). HDLs and LDLs function very differently. LDLs, for example, transport cholesterol from the liver to body tissues. In contrast, HDLs are scavengers, picking up excess cholesterol and transporting it to the liver, where it is removed from the blood and excreted in the bile. Research shows that the ratio of HDL to LDL is an accurate predictor of cardiovascular disease. The higher the ratio, the lower the risk of cardiovascular disease.

A high cholesterol level (or hypercholesterolemia) tends to run in families. Thus, if a parent died of a heart attack or suffers from this genetic disease, his or her offspring are more likely to have high cholesterol levels.

To reduce your chances of atherosclerosis, the American Heart Association recommends (1) limiting dietary fat to less than 30% of the total caloric intake; (2) limiting dietary cholesterol to 300 milligrams per day; and (3) acquiring 50% or more of one's calories from carbohydrates, especially polysaccharides (notably, starches found in potatoes, rice, vegetables and other foods). Reductions in saturated fats (animal fats) can also help lower cholesterol levels. You can cut back on saturated fat by reducing your consumption of red meat and trimming the fat off all meats before cooking. You can also increase your consumption of fruits, vegetables, and grains, letting these low-fat foods displace some of the fatty foods you might otherwise have eaten.

Blood cholesterol levels can also be lowered with drugs and exercise. Research spanning several decades shows that a lower cholesterol level translates into a decline in cardiovascular disease.

High cholesterol is also surprisingly common in children, leading many health experts to believe that steps should be taken to prevent problems later in life. In children under the age of 2, however, diets should not be restricted. A diet that is too restrictive may actually impair physical growth and development. What all children need is a well-balanced diet, low in fats, especially animal fat, with sufficient calories from other sources. Such a diet could encourage the eating habits necessary for good health throughout adult life.

Visit *Human Biology's* Internet site for links to web sites offering more information on this topic.

Steroids. Steroids are also present in the plasma membrane. As a group, the **steroids** (STEER-oids) are structurally quite different from the triglycerides and phospholipids. As shown in **FIGURE 3-12** (page 51), steroids consist of three six-carbon rings and one five-carbon ring all joined in one large structure resembling chicken wire. One of the best-known steroids is cholesterol (**FIGURE 3-12A**). **Cholesterol** is a component of the plasma membrane in animal cells (but not in plants). In humans, it is a raw material needed to synthesize other steroids, such as vitamin D, bile salts, and the sex hormones estrogen and testosterone. As noted earlier, cholesterol is also a major component of atherosclerotic plaque. In humans, cholesterol comes primarily from the liver. A lesser amount comes from the diet.

Most Americans consume lipids in excess of what is required. On average, fats provide about 42% of the dietary caloric intake (**TABLE 5-3**). To lower the risk of heart attack, fat intake should only be about 30%, perhaps even lower, and animal fat should be eaten in small quantities. You don't need to eliminate fat. In fact, really low fat diets can be unhealthy. Some patients develop fatty acid deficiencies. Eat fat, but consume it in moderation and limit saturated fats.

Amino Acids and Protein. **Amino acids** and **proteins** are important nutrients. Their structure is discussed in Chapter 3. In healthy, well-nourished individuals, dietary protein is used to supply amino acids. They

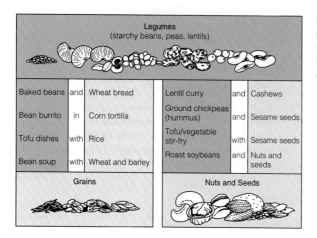

Legumes (starchy beans, peas, lentils)					
Baked beans	and	Wheat bread	Lentil curry	and	Cashews
Bean burrito	in	Corn tortilla	Ground chickpeas (hummus)	and	Sesame seeds
Tofu dishes	with	Rice	Tofu/vegetable stir-fry	with	Sesame seeds
Bean soup	with	Wheat and barley	Roast soybeans	and	Nuts and seeds
Grains			Nuts and Seeds		

FIGURE 5-9 Complementary Protein Sources By combining protein sources, a vegetarian who consumes no animal by-products can be assured of getting all of the amino acids needed. Legumes can be combined with foods made from grains or nuts and other seeds.

are needed to synthesize enzymes, hormones, and structural proteins such as collagen. Dietary proteins, however, cannot be absorbed by the small intestine; they must first be broken down into amino acids by hydrolytic enzymes in the digestive tract.

Proteins in the human body contain 20 different amino acids—all of which can be provided from the diet. The body, however, is capable of synthesizing 12 of the amino acids it needs from nitrogen and smaller molecules derived from carbohydrates and fats. Thus, if they are not present in the diet, they can be made. Two of the twelve are considered **semiessential amino acids.** They are produced in sufficient quantities in adults, but not in growing children. The remaining eight amino acids cannot be synthesized by body cells under any circumstances—that is, they *must* be provided by the diet. These amino acids are called **essential amino acids**. A deficiency of even one of the essential amino acids can cause severe physiological problems. As a result, nutritionists recommend a diet containing many different protein sources so individuals receive all of the amino acids they need.

Proteins are divided into two major groups by nutritionists: complete and incomplete. **Complete proteins** contain ample amounts of all of the essential amino acids. Complete proteins are found in milk, eggs, meat, fish, poultry, cheese, and soy products including soy milk and tofu. **Incomplete proteins** lack one or more essential amino acids and include those found in many plant products: nuts, seeds, grains, most legumes

(peas and beans), and vegetables. Vegetarians who avoid all animal products, including milk and eggs, must acquire the essential amino acids they need by combining incomplete protein sources. Legumes such as beans can be combined with grains or nuts and seeds, as shown in **FIGURE 5-9**. A meal consisting of a legume, for example, baked beans, combined with wheat bread provides all of the amino acids your body needs. A bean burrito and a corn tortilla will do the same.

Although many people think of proteins as a source of energy, proteins are only used for this purpose when dietary intake of carbohydrates and fats is severely restricted or when protein intake far exceeds demand.

Protein deficiencies occur in millions of children throughout the world. The arms and legs of these children are often thin and wiry because their muscle cells break down protein in an effort to provide energy (**FIGURE 5-10**). According to the United Nations, one of every six people in the world, a total of one billion people, suffer from protein malnutrition.

On the other end of the spectrum are the overfed populations of the world. The average American, for example, consumes twice the daily requirement of protein. Amino acids derived from the surplus dietary protein are broken down in the body to produce energy and fat.

FIGURE 5-10 A Protein-Deficient Child This child suffers from severe protein deficiency (kwashiorkor; kwash-ee-or-core). His arms and legs are emaciated because muscle protein has been broken down to supply energy. His belly is slightly swollen because of a buildup of fluid in the abdomen.

Overnutrition is Now Reaching Epidemic Proportions in the More Developed Countries of the World.

Residents of many countries, Americans included, ingest numerous nutrients, besides proteins, in excess. Excess food intake, called **overnutrition**, now rivals **undernutrition**, a lack of food. In the United States, 55% of all American adults are overweight. The percent of the population classified as obese (severely overweight) has climbed from 15% to 23% since 1970. Even children are afflicted, with one of every five now classified as overweight or obese. But the United States is not alone in this regard. Fifty percent of the adults in Russia, the United Kingdom, and Germany are overweight. Even in less developed nations, overnutrition is becoming more commonplace among the wealthier classes. While many struggle to get enough to eat, the wealthy eat too much. The effects of overeating are many: heart attacks, stroke, and late-onset diabetes.

With this overview of the macronutrients, we now turn to the micronutrients.

Micronutrients Are Substances Needed in Small Quantities and Include Two Broad Groups: Vitamins and Minerals

Vitamins. **Vitamins** are a diverse group of organic compounds present in very small amounts in many of the foods we eat. These molecules are absorbed by the lining of the digestive tract without being broken down.

The 13 known vitamins play an important role in many metabolic reactions. Because vitamins are recycled many times during metabolic reactions, they are needed only in very small amounts. In fact, 1 gram of vitamin B-12, about 1 teaspoon, would supply over 300,000 people for a day.

Most vitamins are not synthesized in the cells of the body or, if they can be made, are not produced in sufficient amounts to satisfy cellular demands, making dietary intake essential. Vitamin D, for instance, is manufactured by the skin when exposed to sunlight. However, most Americans spend so much time indoors that dietary input is essential to good health. **TABLE 5-4** lists the vitamins and their functions.

Because vitamins are needed in almost all cells of the body, a dietary deficiency in just one vitamin can cause wide-ranging effects. Vitamins also interact with other nutrients. Vitamin C, for example, increases the absorption of iron in the small intestine. Large doses of vitamin C, however, decrease copper utilization by the cells. Consequently, maintaining good health requires ingesting the proper balance of vitamins and other nutrients. Imbalances can result in upsets in homeostasis.

Vitamins fall into two broad categories: water-soluble and fat-soluble. **Water-soluble vitamins** include vitamin C and eight different forms of vitamin B. Water-soluble vitamins are transported in the blood plasma. Because they are water-soluble, they are readily eliminated by the kidneys and are not stored in the body in any appreciable amount.

Water-soluble vitamins generally work in conjunction with enzymes, promoting the cellular reactions that supply energy or synthesize cellular materials. Contrary to common myth, the vitamins themselves do not provide energy.

Many proponents of vitamin use believe that megadoses of water-soluble vitamins are harmless because these vitamins are excreted in the urine and do not accumulate in the body. New research, however, shows that this is not entirely true. Some water-soluble vitamins, such as vitamin B-6, when ingested in excess, can be toxic. (See **TABLE 5-4** for some examples.)

The **fat-soluble vitamins** are vitamins A, D, E, and K. They perform many different functions. Vitamin A, for example, is converted to light-sensitive pigments in receptor cells of the retina, the light-sensitive layer of the eye. These pigments play an important role in vision. Another member of the vitamin A group removes harmful chemicals (oxidants) from the body.

Unlike water-soluble vitamins, the fat-soluble vitamins are stored in body fat and accumulate in the fat reserves. The accumulation of fat-soluble vitamins can have many adverse effects (**TABLE 5-4**). An excess of vitamin D, for example, can cause weight loss, nausea, irritability, kidney stones, weakness, and other symptoms. Large doses of vitamin D taken during pregnancy can cause birth defects.

Vitamin excess is encountered largely in the more affluent developed countries and usually occurs only in people taking vitamin supplements. Each year, in fact, approximately 4000 Americans are treated for vitamin supplement poisoning. To avoid problems from excess vitamins, nutritionists recommend eating a balanced diet that provides all of the vitamins the body needs, rather than taking vitamin pills. Megadoses, they say, should be avoided.

Vitamin deficiencies, like dietary excesses, can lead to serious problems. A deficiency of vitamin D, for example, can produce **rickets** (RICK-its), a disease that results in bone deformities. Vitamin K deficiencies can result in severe bleeding on injury and internal hemorrhaging. Vitamin C deficiency can result in delayed wound healing and reduced immunity, making people more susceptible to infectious disease.

One of the most common dietary illnesses is caused by a deficiency of vitamin A. This deficiency afflicts over

TABLE 5-4

Important Information on Vitamins

Vitamin	Major Dietary Sources	Major Functions	Signs of Severe, Prolonged Deficiency	Signs of Extreme Excess
Fat-soluble				
A	Fat-containing and fortified dairy products; liver; provitamin carotene in orange and deep green fruits and vegetables	Vitamin A is a component of rhodopsin; carotenoids can serve as antioxidants; retinoic acid affects gene expression; still under intense study	Night blindness; keratinization of epithelial tissues including the cornea of the eye (xerophthalmia) causing permanent blindness; dry, scaling skin; increased susceptibility to infection	*Preformed vitamin A:* damage to liver, bone; headache, irritability, vomiting, hair loss, blurred vision *13-cis retinoic acid:* some fetal defects *Carotenoids:* yellowed skin
D	Fortified and full-fat dairy products, egg yolk (diet often not as important as sunlight exposure)	Promotes absorption and use of calcium and phosphorus	Rickets (bone deformities) in children; osteomalacia (bone softening) in adults	Calcium deposition in tissues leading to cerebral, CV, and kidney damage
E	Vegetable oils and their products; nuts, seeds	Antioxidant to prevent cell membrane damage; still under intense study	Possible anemia and neurologic effects	Generally nontoxic, but at least one type of intravenous infusion led to some fatalities in premature infants; may worsen clotting defect in vitamin K deficiency
K	Green vegetables; tea	Aids in formation of certain proteins, especially those for blood clotting	Defective blood coagulation causing severe bleeding or injury	Liver damage and anemia from high doses of the synthetic form menadione
Water-soluble				
Thiamin (B-1)	Pork, legumes, peanuts, enriched or whole-grain products	Coenzyme used in energy metabolism	Nerve changes, sometimes edema, heart failure; beriberi	Generally nontoxic, but repeated injections may cause shock reaction

Source: Adapted from *Nutrition for Living*, 4th ed., by J. L. Christian and L. L. Greger, Copyright © 1994 by The Benjamin/Cummings Publishing Company.

FIGURE 5-11 Vitamin A Deficiency   Vitamin A deficiency causes the cornea of the eye to dry and become irritated. If the deficiency is not corrected, corneal ulcers may form and rupture, resulting in permanent blindness.

100,000 children worldwide each year. If not corrected, vitamin A deficiency causes the eyes to dry. Ulcers may form on the eyeball and can rupture, causing blindness (**FIGURE 5-11**).

Most people afflicted by vitamin deficiencies are those who fail to get enough to eat, although even apparently well-fed individuals may suffer from a vitamin defi-

Vitamin	Major Dietary Sources	Major Functions	Signs of Severe, Prolonged Deficiency	Signs of Extreme Excess
Riboflavin (B-2)	Dairy products, meats, eggs, enriched grain products, green leafy vegetables	Coenzyme used in energy metabolism	Skin lesions	Generally nontoxic
Niacin	Nuts, meats; provitamin tryptophan in most proteins	Coenzyme used in energy metabolism	Pellagra (multiple vitamin deficiencies including niacin)	Flushing of face, neck, hands; potential liver damage
B-6	High-protein foods in general	Coenzyme used in amino acid metabolism	Nervous, skin, and muscular disorders; anemia	Unstable gait, numb feet, poor coordination
Folic acid	Green vegetables, orange juice, nuts, legumes, grain products	Coenzyme used in DNA and RNA metabolism; single carbon utilization	Megaloblastic anemia (large, immature red blood cells); GI disturbances	Masks vitamin B-12 deficiency, interferes with drugs to control epilepsy
B-12	Animal products	Coenzyme used in DNA and RNA metabolism; single carbon utilization	Megaloblastic anemia; pernicious anemia when due to inadequate intrinsic factor; nervous system damage	Thought to be nontoxic
Pantothenic acid	Animal products and whole grains; widely distributed in foods	Coenzyme used in energy metabolism	Fatigue, numbness, and tingling of hands and feet	Generally nontoxic; occasionally causes diarrhea
Biotin	Widely distributed in foods	Coenzyme used in energy metabolism	Scaly dermatitis	Thought to be nontoxic
C (ascorbic acid)	Fruits and vegetables, especially broccoli, cabbage, cantaloupe, cauliflower, citrus fruits, green pepper, kiwi fruit, strawberries	Functions in synthesis of collagen; is an antioxidant; aids in detoxification; improves iron absorption; still under intense study	Scurvy; petechiae (minute hemorrhages around hair follicles); weakness; delayed wound healing; impaired immune response	GI upsets, confounds certain lab tests

ciency if they are not eating a well-rounded diet. According to the United Nations Food and Agricultural Organizations, about one of every seven people living in the non-industrialized nations of the world, or about 840 million people, go to bed hungry. They're classified as chronically malourished. Most of these people suffer from multiple vitamin deficiencies and exhibit many symptoms. One of the most common complaints is weakness and fatigue.

Children with insufficient vitamin intake fail to grow. All told, about 10 million children under the age of 5 suffer from extreme malnutrition in the less-developed nations of the world. Another 90 million under the age of 5 are moderately malnourished. In the United States, one of every five children is born into poverty and is a candidate for vitamin deficiency.

Before we move on to minerals, there's an important question we need to answer: How do you know if you should take vitamins?

The American Dietetic Association recommends the following strategy for promoting optimal health and reducing the risk of chronic disease: eat a wide variety of foods. Additional vitamins (and minerals, too) can be obtained from fortified foods, such as vitamin D-enriched milk, and from supplements.

If you don't eat a well-balanced diet, consider making the switch. Most people eat far too few fruits and vegetables, gorging instead on fat-rich meats (hamburgers) and desserts. While you make the shift, take a vitamin supplement.

Minerals. On average, an adult contains about 5 pounds of **minerals**, naturally occurring inorganic substances vital to many life processes. Humans require about two dozen minerals, such as calcium, sodium, iron, and potassium, to carry out normal body functions.

Minerals, like vitamins, are micronutrients and are derived from the food we eat and the beverages we drink. Minerals are divided into two groups: the major minerals and the trace minerals (**TABLE 5-5**). The **major minerals** are present in the body in amounts larger than 5 grams; the **trace minerals** are found in lesser quantities. Calcium and phosphorus, for example, are major minerals, and make up three-fourths of the total mineral content of the human body. These two minerals form part of the dense extracellular matrix of bone and are required in a much greater quantity than zinc or copper, two trace minerals that are components of some enzymes.

TABLE 5-5

Important Information on Minerals

Mineral	Major Dietary Sources	Major Functions	Signs of Severe, Prolonged Deficiency	Signs of Extreme Excess
Major minerals				
Calcium	Milk, cheese, dark green vegetables, legumes	Bone and tooth formation; blood clotting; nerve transmission	Stunted growth; perhaps less bone mass	Depressed absorption of some other minerals; perhaps kidney damage
Phosphorus	Milk, cheese, meat, poultry, whole grains	Bone and tooth formation; acid-base balance; component of coenzymes	Weakness; demineralization of bone	Depressed absorption of some minerals
Magnesium	Whole grains, green leafy vegetables	Component of enzymes	Neurologic disturbances	Neurologic disturbances
Sodium	Salt, soy sauce, cured meats, pickles, canned soups, processed cheese	Body water balance; nerve function	Muscle cramps; reduced appetite	High blood pressure in genetically predisposed individuals
Potassium	Meats, milk, many fruits and vegetables, whole grains	Body water balance; nerve function	Muscular weakness; paralysis	Muscular weakness; cardiac arrest
Chloride	Same as for sodium	Plays a role in acid-base balance; formation of gastric juice	Muscle cramps; reduced appetite; poor growth	High blood pressure in genetically predisposed individuals
Trace minerals				
Iron	Meats, eggs, legumes, whole grains, green leafy vegetables	Component of hemoglobin, myoglobin, and enzymes	Iron-deficiency anemia, weakness, impaired immune function	Acute: shock, death; Chronic: liver damage, cardiac failure
Iodine	Marine fish and shellfish; dairy products; iodized salt; some breads	Component of thyroid hormones	Goiter (enlarged thyroid)	Iodide goiter
Fluoride	Drinking water, tea, seafood	Maintenance of tooth (and maybe bone) structure	Higher frequency of tooth decay	Acute: GI distress; Chronic: mottling of teeth; skeletal deformation

SOURCE: Adapted from *Nutrition for Living*, 4th ed., by J. L. Christian and L. L. Greger. Copyright © 1994 by The Benjamin/Cummings Publishing Company.

Chapter 5 Nutrition and Digestion 117

The distinction between major and trace minerals is not meant to imply that one group is more important than the other. In fact, a daily deficiency of a few micrograms (a microgram is $\frac{1}{1000}$ of a gram, and a gram is $\frac{1}{454}$ of a pound) of iodine is just as serious as a deficiency of several hundred milligrams of calcium.

TABLE 5-5 lists some of the minerals, their function, and problems that arise when they are ingested in excess or deficient amounts.

Foods Also Contain Chemical Substances That Help Reduce Cholesterol Levels and Fight Cancer.

In recent years, scientists have discovered numerous chemicals in the foods we eat that help prevent disease. These chemicals are often classified as **neutraceuticals**, a name that combines *nutrients* with *pharmaceticals*, to indicate their healing role. Foods containing them are called **functional foods**. Functional foods are foods that may provide a health benefit beyond basic nutrition.

The number of neutraceuticals is mind boggling, and only limited information is available on them. Some substances are **antioxidants**. Antioxidants react with naturally occurring chemical oxidants, substances in the blood that are involved in cholesterol build-up in the walls of arteries as well as cancer. Eating a diet rich in antioxidants may reduce heart and artery disease as well as cancer.

In what is good news for chocolate lovers, chocolate and cocoa powder are produced from beans that contain large quantities of natural antioxidants. They're called **flavonoids**. (flay-vah-noids). Soy milk also contains flavonoids, as do tea and red wine.

Even commercially available chocolate products may contain significant amounts of these antioxidants. But you must shop carefully. Some chocolate production removes the flavonoids. At this writing, Mars is the only company that employs a process that preserves flavonoids. Other manufacturers will probably soon follow.

Flavonoids reduce atherosclerosis by limiting the oxidation of cholesterol-containing low density lipoproteins (LDLs) and very low-density lipoproteins. As discussed in the Health Note in this chapter, low density lipoproteins glom on to cholesterol and deliver it to the walls of the arteries. Oxidation of these molecules appears to be essential for plaque formation.

Chocolate's flavonoids not only reduce oxidation of LDLs, they help stimulate the relaxation of smooth muscle in arteries, which is important to maintaining healthy arteries. Flavonoid-rich foods may also benefit the heart by reducing the activity of blood platelets, the structures that stimulate blood clotting which, in arteries clogged by atherosclerotic plaque, can lead to heart attacks and strokes. As if that's not enough, dark chocolate and cocoa powder appear to raise the level of high density lipoprotein in the blood. Unlike its cohort, LDL, HDL gloms on to cholesterol and delivers it the liver for removal.

So does this mean you should load up on chocolate? Not really. Chocolates also contain a lot of saturated fat and calories (from sugars). Eat chocolate, but don't overindulge (as if that's possible!).

Fruits and vegetables also contain naturally occurring antioxidants, giving you yet another reason to eat a diet rich in these delicious, but often-overlooked foods. A recent study showed that each serving of salad consumed per day reduced the risk of stroke by 3 percent in women and 5 percent in men. A stroke occurs when an artery in the brain bursts or cholesterol-choked arteries develop blood clots that restrict the flow of blood to brain cells. Several foods seem to provide the most protection: broccoli, cabbage, cauliflower, green leafy vegetables, and vitamin C-rich foods such as oranges and orange juice. As noted earlier, black and green teas are also rich in antioxidants. Studies show that drinking black tea reduces one's risk of fatal heart attacks. One study showed that cholesterol build-up in arteries was the highest in those who drink the least amount of black tea.

Antioxidants have also been shown to reduce cancer. For example, one group of naturally occurring antioxidants, isoflaovones, which are found in soy products, have been shown to reduce prostate cancer in men.

The list of beneficial chemicals is growing larger every day. For example, researchers have found that a chemical found in dairy products and hamburgers called conjugated linoleic acid (CLA) is a potent anticancer agents in laboratory animals. The amount in our diets, however, is well below the amount that proved beneficial to lab animals. And who knows, CLAs may not be effective in humans at all.

Section 5-2

The Digestive System

The human digestive system consists of a tube opened at both ends (**FIGURE 5-12**). Food enters the mouth and is chemically and physically altered as it travels along this tube, called the gut. During its journey through the digestive system, food is absorbed through the wall of the gut, where it enters the bloodstream. Waste is excreted at the opposite end, the anus (EH-nuss). In the course of evolution, the various parts of the digestive tract have evolved to perform specific functions, as shown in the figure. Some regions grind and mix the food. Others store food. Still others play a role in digestion and ab-

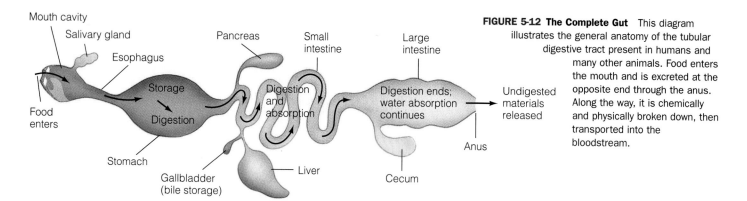

Mouth cavity
Salivary gland
Esophagus
Pancreas
Small intestine
Large intestine
Food enters
Storage
Digestion
Storage
Digestion and absorption
Digestion ends; water absorption continues
Undigested materials released
Anus
Stomach
Gallbladder (bile storage)
Liver
Cecum

FIGURE 5-12 The Complete Gut This diagram illustrates the general anatomy of the tubular digestive tract present in humans and many other animals. Food enters the mouth and is excreted at the opposite end through the anus. Along the way, it is chemically and physically broken down, then transported into the bloodstream.

sorption. In the mouth, for example, food is sliced, torn, and crushed by the teeth into smaller particles. This greatly increases the surface area presented to the digestive enzymes in the stomach and small intestine, which increases the efficiency of digestion. Enzymes participate in a chemical breakdown of food. In the small intestine, amino acids, monosaccharides, and other small molecules produced by enzymatic digestion are absorbed into the bloodstream for distribution to body cells.

The Physical Breakdown of Food Occurs in the Mouth

The mouth is a complex structure in which food is broken down mechanically and, to a much lesser degree, chemically. Food taken into the mouth is sliced into smaller pieces by the sharp teeth in front; it is then ground into a pulpy mass by the flatter teeth toward the back of the mouth. As the food is pulverized in the mouth, it is liquefied by **saliva** (sah-LIVE-ah), a watery secretion released by the salivary glands, three sets of exocrine glands located around the oral cavity (**FIGURE 5-13**). The release of saliva is triggered by the smell, feel, taste, and sometimes even by the thought of food.

Saliva performs at least five functions. It liquefies the food, making it easier to swallow. It kills or neutralizes some bacteria via the enzymes and antibodies it contains. It dissolves substances so they can be tasted. It begins to break down starch molecules with the aid of the enzyme **amylase** (AM-ah-lase). Saliva also cleanses the teeth, washing away bacteria and food particles. Because the release of saliva is greatly reduced during sleep, bacteria tend to accumulate on the surface of the teeth, where they break down microscopic food particles, producing some foul-smelling chemicals that give us "dragon breath," or "morning mouth."

Controlling the bacteria that live on the teeth by regular brushing is important because these organisms secrete a sticky material called **plaque**. Plaque adheres to the surface of the teeth, trapping bacteria. They release small

amounts of a weak acid that dissolves the hard outer coating of our teeth, the **enamel**. The acid forms small pits in the enamel, commonly referred to as **cavities.** Continued acid secretion may cause the cavities to deepen into the softer layer beneath the enamel. If the cavity is left untreated, an entire tooth can be lost to decay.

Brushing helps remove plaque and helps reduce the incidence of cavities. Most toothpastes also contain small amounts of fluoride, which hardens the enamel and helps reduce cavities. In most cities and towns, fluoride is added to drinking water as a preventive measure. Flossing your teeth also helps reduce cavities, by removing food particles between your teeth where toothbrushes can't reach.

One study showed that chewing sugarless gum increases the flow of saliva and cleanses the teeth. By

Parotid duct
Parotid gland
Masseter muscle
Submandibular duct
Submandibular gland
Sublingual gland

FIGURE 5-13 Salivary Glands Three salivary glands (parotid, submandibular, and sublingual) are located in and around the oral cavity and empty into the mouth via small ducts.

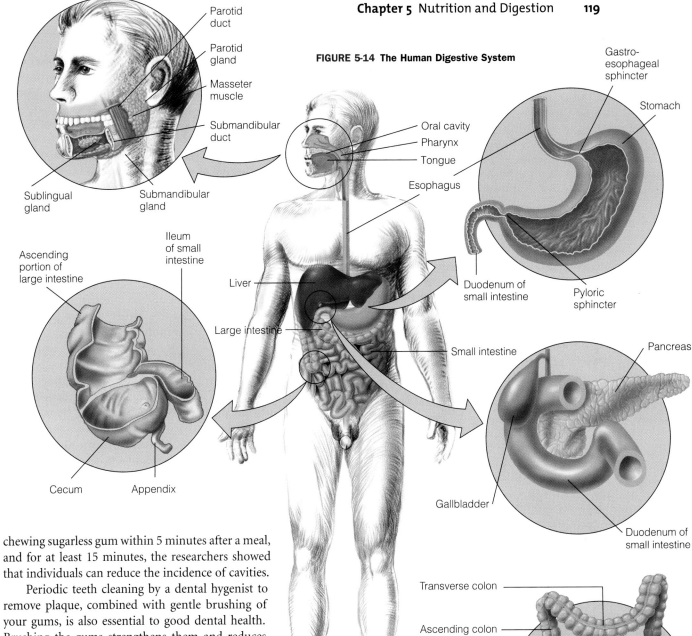

FIGURE 5-14 The Human Digestive System

chewing sugarless gum within 5 minutes after a meal, and for at least 15 minutes, the researchers showed that individuals can reduce the incidence of cavities.

Periodic teeth cleaning by a dental hygenist to remove plaque, combined with gentle brushing of your gums, is also essential to good dental health. Brushing the gums strengthens them and reduces the incidence of **gingivitis** (gin-je-VIE-tiss), a disease of the gums. In this disease, bacteria, plaque, mucus, and food particles accumulate between the swollen gums and the base of the teeth. The bacteria release an acid that gradually destroys the bone in which the teeth are embedded. Over time, the teeth may fall out.

How do you know if you've got gingivitis? You can tell by examining your gums in the mirror. Healthy gums are pale pink or brown. They are firm and may appear speckled. If you have gingivitis, your gums will be red, soft, shiny, and swollen. They also bleed easily, even from gentle brushing.

After food is chewed, it must be swallowed. The tongue plays a key role in swallowing by pushing food to the back of the oral cavity into the **pharynx** (FAIR-

inks), a funnel-shaped chamber that connects the oral cavity with the **esophagus** (ee-SOFF-ah-gus), a long muscular tube that leads to the stomach (**FIGURE 5-14**).

The **tongue**, which also aids in speech, contains taste receptors, or **taste buds**, on its upper surface (**FIGURE 5-15**). **Taste buds** are cocktail-onion-shaped structures lo-

FIGURE 5-15 Taste Buds   A photomicrograph of a taste bud.

cated in protrusions called **pappillae** (pah-pill-eye) on the upper surface of the tongue. They are stimulated by five basic flavors: sweet, sour, salty, bitter, and umami. Various combinations of these flavors (combined with odors we smell) give us a rich assortment of tastes.

Food propelled from the pharynx into the esophagus is prevented from entering the **trachea** (TRAY-key-ah), or windpipe, which carries air to the lungs and lies in front of the esophagus, by the **epiglottis** (ep-ah-GLOT-tis) (**FIG-URE 5-16**). The epiglottis is a flap of tissue that acts like a trapdoor, closing off the trachea during swallowing.

Swallowing begins with a voluntary act—the tongue pushing food into the back of the oral cavity. Once food enters the pharynx, however, the process becomes automatic. Food in the pharynx stimulates stretch receptors in the wall of this organ, which, in turn, trigger the **swallowing reflex**, an involuntary contraction of the muscles in the wall of the pharynx. This forces the food into the esophagus.

The Esophagus Transports Food to the Stomach Via Peristalsis

Involuntary contractions of the muscular wall of the esophagus propel food to the stomach. As **FIGURE 5-17** shows, the muscles of the esophagus contract above the swallowed food mass, squeezing it along. This involuntary muscular action is called **peristalsis** (pear-eh-STALL-sis). It is so powerful that you can swallow when hanging upside down. Peristalsis also propels food (and waste) along the rest of the digestive tract.

Scientists once thought that esophageal peristalsis could proceed in the opposite direction under certain conditions and called this process **reverse peristalsis**, or, more commonly, **vomiting**.

Vomiting is a reflex action that occurs when irritants are present in the stomach. It is, therefore, believed to be a protective adaptation that allows the body to rid the stomach of bad food and harmful viruses and bacteria with obvious survival benefits to humans and other vertebrates (back-boned animals). Vomiting may also be caused by (1) emotional factors, such as stress, (2) rotation or acceleration of the head, as in motion sickness, (3) stimulation of the back of the throat, and (4) elevated pressure inside the brain caused by injury. Today we know that during vomiting food is expelled from the stomach as a result of contractions of muscles in the abdomen and diaphragm (DIE-ah-fram) (the diaphragm separates the thoracic and abdominal cavities and plays an important role in breathing).

The Stomach Stores Food, Releasing It Into the Small Intestine in Spurts

In humans, the stomach (**FIG-URES 5-14** and **5-18**) lies on the left side of the abdominal cavity, partly under the protection of the rib cage. Food enters the stomach via the esophagus. The opening to the stomach, however, is closed off by the **gastroesophageal sphincter** (GAS-trow-eh-SOFF-a-gee-al SFINCK-ter), a thickened layer of smooth muscle at the juncture of the esophagus and stomach (**FIGURE 5-17B**). As food enters the lower esophagus, the gastroesophageal sphincter opens, al-

FIGURE 5-16 The Epiglottis   This trapdoor prevents food from entering the trachea during swallowing. As illustrated, the trachea is lifted during swallowing, pushing against the epiglottis, which bends downward.

Soft palate
Bolus of food
Tongue
Pharynx
Epiglottis
Glottis
Esophagus
Trachea

Esophagus closed; glottis open; food in mouth.

Esophagus open; glottis closed; food in pharynx.

Esophagus closed; glottis open; food in esophagus.

lowing the food to enter the stomach. The sphincter then promptly closes, preventing food and stomach acid from percolating upward. If the sphincter fails to close, acid rising in the esophagus causes irritation, a condition known as "heartburn."

Inside the stomach, food is liquefied by acidic secretions of tiny glands in the wall of the stomach, the **gastric glands**. These glands produce a watery secretion called **gastric juice,** which contains hydrochloric acid (HCl) and an enzyme precursor called pepsinogen (pep-SIN-oh-gen) (discussed below).

Inside the stomach, food is churned by peristalsis and mixed with gastric juice. The churning action of the stomach's muscular walls helps break down large pieces of food. Combined with the liquid from salivary glands and the gastric glands, the food becomes a rather thin, watery paste known as **chyme** (KIME). The stomach can hold 2–4 liters (2 quarts to 1 gallon) of chyme, which is gradually released into the small intestine at a rate suitable for efficient digestion and absorption.

Contrary to what many think, very little enzymatic digestion occurs in the stomach. The stomach's role is largely to prepare most food for the enzymatic digestion that will occur in the small intestine. There are some exceptions to this rule, however. Protein is one of them.

Proteins are denatured (coagulated) by HCl in the stomach. HCl also acts on **pepsinogen,** converting it to the active form pepsin. **Pepsin** is a proteolytic (pronounced pro-tee-oh-LIT-ic; protein-digesting) enzyme that catalyzes the breakdown of proteins into large fragments. These fragments are further broken down in the small intestine, the next stop in the digestive system.

Hydrochloric acid creates an acidic environment (pH 1.5–3.5) in the stomach. Besides activating pepsinogen and denaturing protein (rendering it digestible), HCl also breaks down connective tissue fibers in meat and kills most bacteria, thereby protecting the body from infection.

Also contrary to popular belief, the stomach does not absorb foodstuffs. Only a few substances, such as alcohol, actually penetrate the lining of the stomach to enter the bloodstream. Alcohol consumed on an empty stomach passes quickly into the blood, often producing an immediate dizzying effect. The presence of food in the stomach, however, slows alcohol absorption.

The stomach lining is protected from destruction by an alkaline secretion known as **mucus** (MEW-kuss), produced by certain cells in the lining. Mucus coats the epithelium, protecting it from acid and pepsin. Acid is further prevented from penetrating the lining of the stomach and reaching underlying tissues by tight junctions in the cells of the epithelium. These structures join the epithelial cells very tightly, creating a leakproof barrier.

Until recently, scientists believed that the stomach's protective mechanisms could be hampered by certain factors such as stress; excess coffee (caffeine); excess aspirin, nicotine, and alcohol; or combinations of them. These factors were thought to increase the levels of acid in the stomach, overwhelming the mucous layer and tight junctions. When this happened, scientists believed that

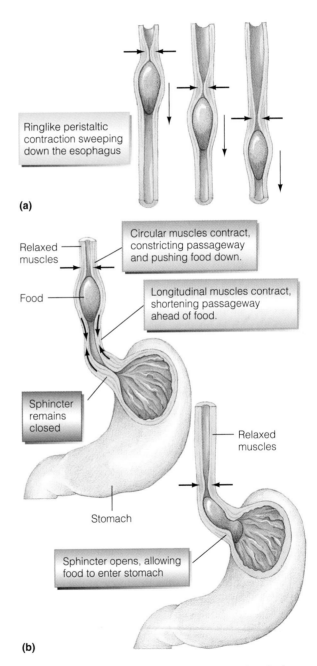

Ringlike peristaltic contraction sweeping down the esophagus

(a)

Relaxed muscles

Circular muscles contract, constricting passageway and pushing food down.

Food

Longitudinal muscles contract, shortening passageway ahead of food.

Sphincter remains closed

Relaxed muscles

Stomach

Sphincter opens, allowing food to enter stomach

(b)

FIGURE 5-17 Peristalsis *(a)* Peristaltic contractions in the esophagus propel food into the stomach. *(b)* When food reaches the stomach, the gastroesophageal sphincter opens, allowing food to enter.

Esophagus

Gastroesophageal sphincter

Pyloric sphincter

Duodenum

Longitudinal smooth muscle

Circular smooth muscle

Oblique smooth muscle

FIGURE 5-18 The Stomach The stomach lies in the abdominal cavity. In its wall are three layers of smooth muscle that mix the food and force it into the small intestine, where most digestion occurs. The gastroesophageal and pyloric sphincters control the inflow and outflow of food, respectively.

HCl and pepsin came in contact with the epithelial cells and digested parts of the wall of the stomach, forming painful **ulcers** (**FIGURE 5-19**). Accordingly, most ulcers that were detected early were treated by reducing stress and changing one's diet (eating smaller amounts of food and reducing coffee, aspirin, and alcohol) to reduce acid secretion in the stomach (see Health Note 1-1). When ulcers were not detected early and when damage was severe, parts of the stomach had to be removed surgically.

Now, once again, new research has thrown these beliefs into doubt. One researcher has discovered that most ulcers are caused by a fairly common bacterium, *Heliocobacter pylori*, or *H. pylori* for short. Numerous studies now support this once-improbable suggestion.

Thanks to efforts of the American Gastroenterological Association and other organizations, numerous physicians now routinely test for the presence of this bacterium in patients with stomach ulcers. Antibiotics are becoming a much more common and highly successful way to treat ulcers.

Chyme Leaves the Stomach and Enters the Small Intestine. Chyme is ejected from the stomach into the small intestine by peristaltic muscle contractions. When the wave of contraction reaches the pyloric (pie-LORE-ick) sphincter (a ring of smooth muscle at the juncture of the small intestine and stomach), it opens, and chyme squirts into the small intestine.

The stomach contents are emptied in 2–6 hours, depending on the size of the meal and the type of food. The larger the meal, the longer it takes to empty. Solid foods (meat) empty slower than liquid foods (milk shakes). Peristaltic contractions continue after the stomach is empty and are felt as hunger pangs.

As chyme and protein leave the stomach, gastric gland secretion declines and the stomach slowly shuts down its production of HCl until the next meal.

The Small Intestine Serves as a Site of Food Digestion and Absorption

The **small intestine** is a coiled tube in the abdominal cavity about 6 meters (20 feet) long in adults (**FIGURE 5-14**). So named because of its small diameter, the small intestine consists of three parts in the following order: the duodenum (DUE-oh-DEEN-um), jejunum (jeh-JEW-num), and ileum (ILL-ee-um).

Inside the small intestine, macromolecules are broken into smaller molecules (that is, digested) with the aid of enzymes. These molecules are then transported into the bloodstream and the lymphatic system. The **lymphatic system**, discussed more fully in Chapter 8, is a network of vessels that carries extracellular fluid from the tissues of the body to the circulatory system. In addition, tiny lymphatic vessels in the wall of the small intestine, known as **lacteals** (LACK-teels), absorb fats and transport them to the bloodstream.

Digestion in the Small Intestine Requires Enzymes From Two Major Sources. The digestion of food molecules inside the small intestine requires enzymes produced from two distinctly different sources:

FIGURE 5-19 Ulcers An ulcer in the lining of the stomach.

the pancreas, an organ that lies beneath the stomach, and the lining of the small intestine itself.

The **pancreas** is nestled in a loop formed by the first portion of the small intestine, the duodenum (**FIGURE 5-20**). The pancreas is a dual-purpose organ—that is, it has endocrine and exocrine functions. As an exocrine gland, it produces enzymes and sodium bicarbonate essential for the digestion of foodstuffs in the small intestine. Its endocrine function is fulfilled by special cells that produce hormones (insulin and glucagon) that help regulate blood glucose levels and thus assist in maintaining homeostasis.

The digestive enzymes of the pancreas flow through the large pancreatic duct into the duodenum. Each day, approximately 1200–1500 milliliters (1.0–1.5 quarts) of pancreatic juice is produced and released into the small intestine. This liquid is composed of water, sodium bicarbonate, and several important digestive enzymes (**TABLE 5-6**).

Sodium bicarbonate neutralizes the acidic chyme released by the stomach and thus protects the small intestine from stomach acid. It also gives the pancreatic juice a pH of about 8, creating an environment optimal for the function of the pancreatic enzymes.

The pancreatic enzymes released act on the large molecules in food (proteins, starches, and so on), as shown in **TABLE 5-6**. As a result of pancreatic enzymatic activity, fats are completely reduced to monoglycerides (glycerol attached to one fatty acid) and fatty acids, which can be absorbed without further action. Proteins are broken into small peptide fragments and some amino acids. Carbohydrates are broken down into disaccharides and some monosaccharides.

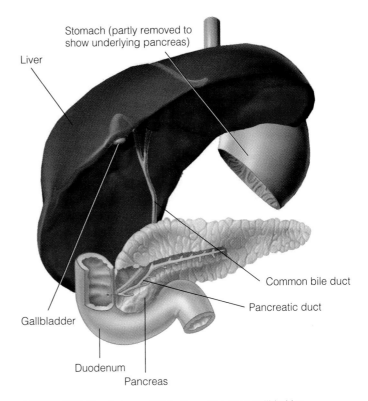

Liver
Stomach (partly removed to show underlying pancreas)
Common bile duct
Pancreatic duct
Gallbladder
Duodenum
Pancreas

FIGURE 5-20 The Organs of Digestion The liver, gallbladder, and pancreas all play key roles in digestion. All empty by the common bile duct into the small intestine, in which digestion takes place.

Like the stomach, the pancreas secretes its enzymes in an inactive form. This protects the gland from self-destruction. **Trypsinogen** (trip-SIN-oh-gin), for example, is the inactive form of the protein-digesting enzyme **trypsin** (TRIP-sin). Produced by the pancreas, trypsino-

---

TABLE 5-6

Digestive Enzymes

Site of Production	Enzyme	Action
Salivary glands	Amylase	Digests polysaccharides in oral cavity
Stomach	Pepsin	Breaks proteins into peptides
Pancreas	Trypsin	Cleaves peptide bonds of polypeptides and proteins
	Chymotrypsin	Same as trypsin
	Carboxypeptidase	Cleaves peptide bonds on carboxyl end of polypeptides
	Amylase	Breaks starch molecules into smaller units (maltose)
	Phospholipase	Cleaves fatty acids from phosphoglycerides to form monoglycerides
	Lipase	Cleaves two fatty acids from triglycerides
	Ribonuclease	Breaks RNA into smaller nucleotide chains
	Deoxyribonuclease	Breaks DNA into smaller nucleotide chains
Epithelium of small intestine	Maltase	Breaks maltose into glucose subunits
	Sucrase	Breaks sucrose into glucose and fructose subunits
	Lactase	Breaks lactose into glucose and galactose subunits
	Aminopeptidase	Breaks peptides into amino acids

gen is activated by a substance on the epithelial lining of the small intestine. Trypsin, in turn, activates other digestive enzymes.

The final stage of digestion occurs with the aid of enzymes produced by the epithelial cells of the small intestine. These enzymes are embedded in the membranes of the epithelial cells (**TABLE 5-6**). As a result, the final phase of digestion occurs just before the nutrient is absorbed into the cell.

The Liver Produces an Emulsifying Agent, Bile, Which Plays a Key Role in the Digestion of Fat.

The **liver** is one of the largest and most versatile organs in the body. By various estimates, the liver performs as many as 500 different functions. Situated on the right side of the abdomen under the protection of the rib cage, the liver is one of the body's storage depots for glucose (**FIGURE 5-3**). It also stores fats, iron, copper, and many vitamins. By storing glucose and lipids and releasing them as they are needed, the liver helps ensure a constant supply of energy-rich molecules to body cells. The liver also synthesizes some key blood proteins involved in clotting, and it is an efficient detoxifier of potentially harmful chemicals such as nicotine, barbiturates, and alcohol. These functions contribute significantly to homeostasis.

The liver also plays a key role in the digestion of fats through the production of a fluid called **bile**, which contains water, ions, and molecules such as cholesterol, fatty acids, and bile salts. **Bile salts** are steroids that emulsify fats, which means that they break fat globules into smaller ones. This process is essential for lipid digestion, because lipid-digesting enzymes in the small intestine do not work well on large fat globules. Unless fat globules can be broken into smaller ones, fat digestion is incomplete.

Produced by the cells of the liver, bile is first transported to the **gallbladder**, a sac attached to the underside of the liver (**FIGURE 5-20**). The gallbladder concentrates the bile by removing water from it. Bile is stored in the gallbladder until needed. When chyme is present in the small intestine, the gallbladder contracts and bile flows out through the duct system into the small intestine (**FIGURE 5-20**).

Bile flow to the small intestine may be blocked by **gallstones**, deposits of cholesterol and other materials that form in the gallbladder of some individuals. Gallstones may lodge in the ducts draining the organ, thus reducing—even completely blocking—the flow of bile to the small intestine. The lack of bile salts greatly reduces lipid digestion. Because lipid digestion is reduced, fat is not digested and absorbed.

Gallstones occur more frequently in older, overweight individuals, and the incidence in the elderly is about one in five. When they cause problems, gallstones are usually removed surgically. This procedure requires that the entire gallbladder be removed. Bile continues to be produced in these patients but is stored in the common bile duct, which becomes distended to accommodate the liquid bile. Scientists are now testing drugs that dissolve gallstones in many patients, hoping that they may someday eliminate or reduce the need for surgery.

The Intestinal Epithelium Is Specially Modified for Absorption.

Virtually all food digestion occurs in the duodenum and jejunum. Once food molecules are digested, they must be absorbed—that is, transported across the epithelial lining of the small intestine into the bloodstream or lymphatic system, a network of vessels that drains excess fluid from tissues into the bloodstream. In these regions, absorption is facilitated by three structural modifications of the small intestine. **FIGURE 5-21A** shows, for instance, that the lining of the small intestine is thrown into folds, which increase the overall surface area. On the surfaces of the folds are many fingerlike projections known as **villi** (VILL-eye), which also increase the surface area available for the absorption of food molecules. The intestinal surface area is further increased by **microvilli**, tiny protrusions of the plasma membranes of the epithelial cells lining the villi (**FIGURE 5-21D**). Each epithelial cell that functions in absorption contains an estimated 3000 microvilli. Two hundred million microvilli occupy a single square millimeter of intestinal lining. Together, the circular folds, villi, and microvilli result in a dramatic increase in the surface area of the lining of the small intestine, making it 600 times greater than if it were a flat layer. As shown in **FIGURE 5-21E**, each villus of the small intestine is endowed with a rich supply of blood and lymph capillaries. These tiny vessels absorb nutrients that have passed through the lining of the small intestine.

Numerous mechanisms are involved in absorption—too numerous to be discussed here. Three of the most common are diffusion, osmosis, and active transport (Chapter 3).

Although most nutrients diffuse from the epithelial cells into the blood capillaries, fatty acids and monoglycerides produced by the enzymatic digestion of triglycerides follow a different route. As shown in **FIGURE 5-22**, these molecules diffuse into the cells lining the villi; inside these cells they combine to reform triglycerides. The triglycerides form fat droplets, which are then coated with a layer of lipoprotein (lipid bound to protein), which is produced by the endoplasmic reticulum. This treatment renders the fat droplets, or **chylomicrons** (KIE-low-MIE-krons), water-soluble. They are released by the epithelial cells into the interstitial fluid by exocytosis (**FIGURE 5-22**). Because blood capillaries are relatively impermeable to chylomicrons, most of the lipid globules enter the more porous lymph capillaries in the villi. As shown in **FIGURE 5-22**, small- or medium-chain fatty acids not incorporated in triglycerides pass directly into blood capillaries in the villi.

The Large Intestine Is the Site of Water Resorption

The large intestine is about 1.5 meters (5 feet) long and consists of four regions. Starting at the small intestine, they are the cecum, appendix, colon, and rectum (**FIGURE 5-23**). The **cecum** (SEA-come) is a pouch that forms below the juncture of the large and small intestine. A small, wormlike structure, the **appendix**, attaches to the bottom of the cecum. Most of the large intestine consists of the **colon** (COE-lun). Unlike the small intestine, which is coiled and packed in a small volume, the colon consists of three relatively straight portions, the ascending colon, the transverse colon, and the descending colon. The colon empties into the **rectum** (WRECK-tum).

So named because of its large diameter, the large intestine receives materials from the small intestine. The material entering the large intestine consists of a mixture of water, undigested or unabsorbed food molecules, and undigestible food residues, such as cellulose. It also contains sodium and potassium ions.

The colon absorbs approximately 90% of the water and sodium and potassium ions that enter it. The undigested or unabsorbed nutrients feed a rather large population of *E. coli* bacteria. These bacteria synthesize

FIGURE 5-21 The Small Intestine
The small intestine is uniquely "designed" to increase absorption. *(a)* A cross section showing the folds. LN means lymph nodules (aggregation of lymphocytes); V means villi; PC means plica circulares (circular fold). *(b)* A light micrograph of folds and villi. *(c)* Higher magnification of villi. *(d)* An electron micrograph of the surface of the absorptive cells showing the microvilli. *(e)* Each villus contains a loose core of connective tissue; a lacteal, or lymph, capillary; and a network of blood capillaries. Nutrients pass from the lumen of the small intestine through the epithelium and into the interior of the villi, where they are picked up by the lymph and blood capillaries.

several key vitamins: B-12, thiamine, riboflavin, and, most importantly, vitamin K, which is often deficient in the human diet. These vitamins are absorbed by the large intestine.

The contents of the large intestine (after water and salt have been removed) are known as the feces. The **feces** consist primarily of undigested food, indigestible materials, and bacteria. Bacteria, in fact, account for about one-third of the dry weight of the feces.[3]

The feces are propelled by peristaltic contractions along the colon until they reach the rectum (**FIGURE 5-23**). As fecal matter accumulates in the rectum, it distends the organ. This action, in turn, stimulates stretch receptors in the wall of the rectum. These receptors stimulate the **defecation reflex** (DEAF-eh-KA-shun). In this reflex, nerve impulses from the stretch receptors in the rectum travel via nerves to the spinal cord. In the spinal cord, the nerve impulses stimulate nerve cells that supply the smooth muscle in the wall of the rectum, causing them to contract and expel the feces. Other nerve impulses from the spinal cord travel to the **internal anal sphincter**, a ring of smooth muscle, which normally keeps fecal matter from entering the anal canal. In the defecation reflex, however, the sphincter relaxes and the fecal matter can escape.

It is important to note that in adults and children, defecation does not occur until the **external anal sphincter** relaxes. This sphincter is composed of skeletal muscle and is under conscious control in all individuals except babies. If the time and place are appropriate, the external anal sphincter is relaxed, and defecation can occur. Defecation is usually assisted by voluntary contractions of the abdominal muscles and a forcible exhalation, both of which increase intraabdominal pressure.

If circumstances are inappropriate, voluntary tightening of the external anal sphincter prevents defecation, despite prior activation of the reflex. When defecation is delayed, the muscle in the wall of the rectum relaxes, and the urge to defecate subsides—at least until the next movement of feces into the rectum occurs.

FIGURE 5-22 Fat Digestion and Absorption

[3]The feces are about 30% dead bacteria, 10%–20% fat, 10%–20% inorganic matter, 2%–3% protein, and about 30% undigested roughage (cellulose).

FIGURE 5-23 The Large Intestine This organ consists of four basic parts: the cecum, appendix, colon, and rectum.

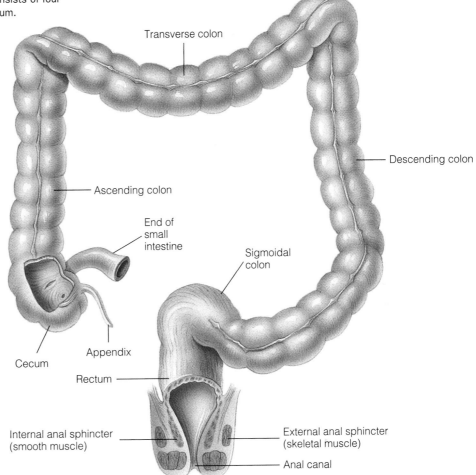

If defecation is delayed too long, additional water may be removed from the feces, making them hard and dry and difficult to pass. This condition is called **constipation.**

Besides being uncomfortable, constipation may result in a dull headache, loss of appetite, and depression. Constipation is generally caused by (1) ignoring the urge to defecate; (2) decreases in colonic contractions, which occur with age, emotional stress, or low-fiber diets; (3) tumors or colonic spasms that obstruct the movement of feces; (4) certain drugs like those containing codeine; and (5) nerve injury that impairs the defecation reflex.

Constipation is not only uncomfortable, it can result in serious problems. Hardened fecal material, for instance, may become lodged in the appendix. This, in turn, may lead to inflammation of the organ, a condition called **appendicitis** (ah-PEND-eh-SITE-iss). When this occurs, the appendix becomes swollen and filled with pus and must be removed surgically to prevent the organ from bursting and spilling its contents into the abdominal cavity. Fecal matter leaking into the abdominal cavity introduces billions of bacteria and can result in a deadly infection.

Section 5-3

Controlling Digestion

Digestion is a complex and varied process that is controlled largely by nerves and hormones. This section discusses some of the key events involved in the control of digestion.

Salivation Is Stimulated by a Nervous Reflex

Digestion begins in the oral cavity. As noted earlier, the sight, smell, taste, and sometimes even the thought of food like a hot fudge sundae stimulates the release of saliva. Chewing has a similar effect. The secretion of saliva via these routes is controlled by the nervous system and is largely a reflex response. For a discussion of the discovery of this phenomenon, see Scientific Discoveries 5-1.

Gastric Gland Secretion Is Controlled by a Variety of Different Mechanisms

Besides activating salivary production, the stimuli listed above also cause the brain to send nerve impulses along the **vagus nerve** (VAG-gus) to the stomach (**FIGURE 5-24**). These nerve impulses initiate the secretion of hydrochloric acid (HCl) and pepsinogen from cells of the gastric glands. Nerve impulses also stimulate the secretion of the hormone gastrin. As shown in **FIGURE 5-24**, gastrin is released into the blood and acts on the gastric glands, stimulating additional HCl and pepsinogen secretion.

The most potent stimulus for gastric secretion is the presence of protein in the stomach. Protein stimulates chemical receptors inside the stomach that activate networks of nerves in the stomach wall. These

Discovering the Nature of Digestion
Featuring the Work of van Helmont, Beaumont, and Pavlov

The foundation for the modern understanding of digestion was laid by a number of pioneering scientists. Two noteworthy contributors were a seventeenth-century Flemish physician, Jan Baptista van Helmont, and a nineteenth-century American, William Beaumont.

In van Helmont's time, most people thought that the digestion of food in the human was akin to cooking—that is, that food inside the stomach was broken down by body heat. Van Helmont, however, dismissed this theory with the simple observation that digestion occurs in cold-blooded animals such as fish. The lack of heat in such animals suggested to him that an alternative process was at work. But what was it?

The road to discovery began in a rather bizarre way. One day, a tame sparrow that often visited the scientist and would sit on his shoulder at-tempted to bite van Helmont's tongue. (We hope this was a playful gesture.) The physician detected a slight acidity in the bird's throat and hypothesized that acid must digest food.

To test this hypothesis, van Helmont tried to digest meat with a vinegar solution, but he could not. Consequently, he hypothesized that the body must contain "ferments," chemical substances in the stomach and small intestine that are specific for different types of food. Today, we know these "ferments" to be digestive enzymes.

Little insight into digestion was forthcoming in the period between van Helmont's work and the studies of the American scientist William Beaumont. Beaumont was the adventurous son of a Connecticut farmer who left his home in 1806. Soon thereafter, he became a schoolmaster in New York, where he studied medicine and associated sciences in his spare time. Several years later, he became an apprentice to a physician in Vermont, and 2 years later, he received a license to practice medicine. (Medical education was much less involved back then!)

Soon after becoming a licensed physician, Beaumont joined the army, where he would make his important discoveries about digestion. He owed his great work to an accident. In 1822, a French-Canadian porter and servant in the army was wounded in the abdomen by a musket that had accidentally discharged at close range. The servant, Alexis St. Martin, who was only 18, was brought to Beaumont for treatment. The doctor found that the bullet had ripped a hole in St. Martin's stomach, out of which poured food the man had eaten.

As was the custom of the time, Beaumont bled the victim. Despite

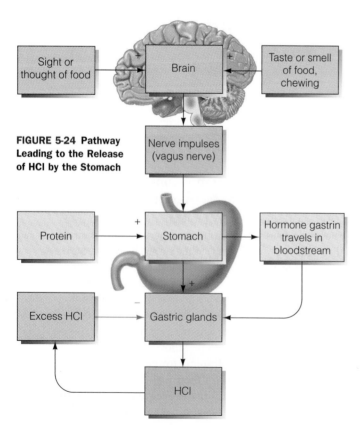

FIGURE 5-24 Pathway Leading to the Release of HCl by the Stomach

nerves, in turn, stimulate the gastric glands to secrete HCl and pepsinogen.

The concentration of HCl in the stomach is also regulated by a negative feedback mechanism, illustrated in **FIGURE 5-24.** If the acid content rises too high, HCl inhibits gastrin secretion, thus shutting off production by the gastric glands.

Pancreatic Secretions Released Into the Small Intestine Are Stimulated by Two Intestinal Hormones

Acidic chyme leaves the stomach and enters the small intestine, where it stimulates the release of the hormone **secretin** (se-CRETE-in), as shown in **FIGURE 5-25.** Secretin is produced by the cells of the duodenum and, like all hormones, travels in the bloodstream. In the pancreas, secretin stimulates the release of sodium bicarbonate. Sodium bicarbonate, in turn, is excreted into the small intestine, where it neutralizes the acidic chyme and creates an environment optimal for pancreatic enzymes. The release of pancreatic enzymes is triggered by yet another intestinal hormone with the tongue-twisting name **cholecystokinin** (COAL-ee-sis-toe-KIE-nin) or **CCK.** This hormone is produced by cells of the duodenum in the presence of chyme (**FIGURE 5-25**).

this treatment, the patient survived, but the wound was slow to heal. For over 8 months, Beaumont tried in vain to close the hole in the stomach. During this time, it dawned on the young physician that he had stumbled across a golden opportunity to study digestion.

Beaumont's experiments consisted of feeding the patient various types of food, then studying what took place inside the man's stomach. In the next 9 years, Beaumont studied St. Martin's stomach contents with a wide assortment of foods, looking at the rate and temperature of digestion and the chemical conditions that favored different stages of the process.

Beaumont's studies helped settle a controversy over the nature of digestion. Some of his contemporaries contended that gastric juice was a kind of chemical solvent. Others believed that it merely liquefied food and that di-gestion occurred as a result of a vital force present in living organisms. By showing that some digestion could take place outside the stomach in the presence of gastric juice, Beaumont demonstrated that gastric secretions did more than moisten food and that no "vital force" was at work. Digestion, Beaumont asserted, was a chemical phenomenon.

Beaumont did not address one question that could have been answered with existing techniques—that is, what caused gastric juice to be secreted? Was it the presence of food in the stomach or something else?

The answer came in 1889 from the work of Ivan Pavlov, a notable scientist whose experiments on behavior are legendary. In studies on dogs, Pavlov showed that the secretion of gastric juice was stimulated by the nervous system. How did he make this determination?

In one of many experiments, the Russian scientist surgically connected a fold of a dog's stomach to an opening in the animal's side; this permitted him to examine the production of gastric secretions. He next cut and tied off the esophagus of the dog, so that food the animal swallowed could not enter the stomach. Following the surgery, Pavlov gave the dog food and found that as soon as food entered the dog's mouth, gastric juice began to be secreted. These secretions continued as long as food was present, thus suggesting nervous system involvement.

Since that time, a great deal has been learned about digestion and its control. For example, as you learned in this chapter, hormones are also involved in the control of many digestive processes. But don't close the book on this subject; much more will inevitably be discovered.

CCK also stimulates the gallbladder to contract, releasing bile into the small intestine.

Interestingly, recent evidence links abnormally low secretion of CCK to **bulimia** (boo-LEEM-ee-ah), a disorder characterized by recurrent binge eating followed by intentional vomiting. Some researchers believe that CCK may trigger satiety, the feeling of being full. Approximately 4% of America's young women, and a far smaller fraction of men, suffer from bulimia. This disorder is thought to have both biological and psychological roots, but researchers had failed to identify a biochemical cause until recently. Although no single chemical is likely to control a complex behavior such as appetite, it appears that CCK plays an important role. Low secretion rates in people with bulimia may cause recurrent binging.

Health, Homeostasis, and the Environment

Eating Right/Living Right

There are few places where the relationship between homeostasis, human health, and the environment is as evident as in nutrition. Because cells and organs involved in homeostasis require an adequate supply of nutrients, nutritional deficiencies can have noticeable impacts on

FIGURE 5-25 Control of the Pancreas and Gallbladder

body functions and health. Supporting this idea, many studies show that an unhealthy diet can increase the risk of contracting certain diseases, including cancer, heart disease, and hypertension.

Consider an example. Magnesium (a major mineral) is routinely ingested in insufficient amounts. New research suggests that such deficiencies may underlie a number of medical conditions, including diabetes, high blood pressure, problems during pregnancy, and cardiovascular disease.

Research shows that adding magnesium to the drinking water of rats with hypertension can eliminate the disease. Studies in rabbits show that magnesium reduces lipid levels in the blood and also reduces plaque formation in blood vessels. Rabbits on a high-cholesterol, low-magnesium diet, for example, have 80%–90% more atherosclerotic (ah-ther-oh-skler-AH-tick) plaque than rabbits on a high-cholesterol, high-magnesium diet.

Studies have shown that magnesium deficiencies during pregnancy result in migraine headaches, high blood pressure, miscarriages, stillbirths, and babies with low birth weight. Research suggests that magnesium deficiency causes spasms in the blood vessels of the placenta, which reduce blood flow to the fetus. This can retard fetal growth and may even kill a fetus in utero. Magnesium supplements greatly reduce the incidence of these problems.

Researchers believe that 80%–90% of the American public may be magnesium deficient. One reason the American diet may be deficient in magnesium is that phosphates in many carbonated soft drinks bind to magnesium in the intestine, preventing it from being absorbed into the blood. Magnesium deficiencies can be reversed by eating more green leafy vegetables, seafood, and whole grain cereals and reducing consumption of carbonated soft drinks with high phosphate levels. Mineral supplements could help as well, but they should be used with extreme caution, because excess magnesium can cause neurological disorders.

Over the years, numerous dietary recommendations have been issued to help Americans live healthier lives and reduce the risk of cancer and heart attack. Nutritionists recommend that daily we consume (1) fruits and vegetables, especially cabbage and greens, (2) high-fiber foods, such as whole-wheat bread and celery, and (3) foods high in vitamins A and C. A healthy diet also minimizes the consumption of animal fat; red meat; and salt-cured, nitrate-cured, smoked, or pickled foods, including bacon and lunch meat.

A healthy diet results largely from habit and circumstance—that is, our social environment. How does our environment affect our nutrition and health?

In the hustle and bustle of modern society, many of us ignore proper nutrition, grabbing fat-rich foods because we haven't the time to sit down to a nutritionally balanced meal. Our fast-paced world places a high premium on saving time, often ignoring the importance of eating and living right. Fast food may allow us to hurry on to our next appointment, but unless it is nutritionally sound, it probably decreases the quality of our lives in the long run.

Summary

1. Studies suggest that iron levels in the body may affect heat production, a relationship that, if substantiated by additional research, illustrates the importance of diet to physiological processes.

A Primer on Nutrition

2. Humans acquire energy and nutrients from the food they eat. These nutrients fall into two categories: *macronutrients*, substances needed in large quantity, and *micronutrients*, substances required in much lower quantities.

3. The four major macronutrients are water, carbohydrates, lipids, and proteins.

4. Water is contained in the liquids we drink and the foods we eat. Maintaining adequate water intake is important, because water is involved in many chemical reactions in the body. It also helps maintain body temperature and a constant level of nutrients and wastes in body fluids, both vital to homeostasis.

5. Carbohydrates and lipids are major sources of energy; 70%–80% of all energy required by the body is for basic functions.

6. Glucose is a six-carbon sugar that is broken down in the body to produce energy. In the human diet, glucose comes primarily from the polymer, starch.

7. Glucose molecules are stored in the liver and muscle as glycogen.

8. Another important dietary carbohydrate is cellulose. Although not digested, cellulose facilitates the passage of fecal matter through the intestinal tract and reduces the incidence of colon cancer.

9. Dietary protein is chiefly a source of amino acids for building proteins, enzymes, and protein hormones.

10. Contrary to popular myth, protein is not a source of energy, except when lipid and carbohydrate intake is low or when protein intake exceeds daily requirements.

11. Protein is broken down into amino acids and absorbed into the bloodstream. However, the body can synthesize some amino acids. These are known as *nonessential amino acids*. Others cannot be synthesized in the

body and must be supplied in the food we eat. These are known as *essential amino acids.*

12. To ensure an adequate supply of all amino acids, individuals should eat *complete proteins,* such as those found in milk or eggs, or combine lower quality protein sources.

13. Lipids are a diverse group of organic chemicals characterized by their lack of water solubility. The biologically important lipids serve many functions.

14. Some lipids (triglycerides) provide energy. They also form layers of heat-conserving insulation. Other lipids (phospholipids and steroids) are part of the plasma membranes of cells.

15. Triglycerides are fats and oils.

16. Triglycerides with many double bonds in their fatty acid side chains (the polyunsaturated fatty acids) lower one's risk of developing atherosclerosis, a build-up of placque on arterial walls. Triglycerides low in saturated fatty acids tend to increase this disease; they are commonly found in animal fats.

17. Micronutrients are needed in much smaller quantities and include two groups: vitamins and minerals.

18. *Vitamins* are a diverse group of organic compounds that are required in relatively small quantities for normal metabolism. A deficiency or surplus of one or more vitamins may alter homeostasis, with serious effects on human health.

19. Human vitamins fit into two categories: water-soluble and fat-soluble. The *water-soluble vitamins* include vitamin C and the B-complex vitamins. The *fat-soluble vitamins* include vitamins A, D, E, and K.

20. *Minerals* fit into one of two groups: *trace minerals,* those required in very small quantity, and *major minerals,* those required in greater quantity. Deficiencies and excesses of both types of minerals can lead to serious health problems.

21. In recent years, scientists have discovered numerous chemicals in the foods we eat that help prevent disease. These chemicals are often classified as neutraceuticals. Foods containing them are called functional foods because that provide a health benefit beyond basic nutrition.

22. Numerous neutraceuticals have been discovered. One important group is known as antioxidants, chemicals that react with naturally occurring chemi-

cal oxidants, substances in the blood that are involved in cholesterol build up in the walls of arteries as well as cancer.

23. Eating a diet rich in antioxidants may reduce heart and artery disease as well as cancer.

The Digestive System

24. Food is physically and chemically broken down in the digestive system. Small molecules produced during digestion are absorbed by the intestinal tract into the bloodstream and circulated throughout the body for use by the cells.

25. Food digestion begins in the mouth. The teeth mechanically break down the food. *Saliva* liquefies it, making it easier to swallow. *Salivary amylase* begins to digest starch molecules.

26. Food is pushed by the tongue to the *pharynx,* where it triggers the swallowing reflex. *Peristaltic contractions* propel the food down the *esophagus* to the stomach.

27. The *stomach* is an expandable organ that stores and further liquefies the food. The churning action of the stomach, brought about by peristaltic contractions, mixes the food, turning it into a paste referred to as *chyme.*

28. The stomach releases food into the small intestine in timed pulses, ensuring efficient digestion and absorption. Very limited chemical digestion and absorption occur in the stomach.

29. The stomach produces *hydrochloric acid,* which denatures protein, allowing it to be acted on by enzymes. The stomach also produces a proteolytic enzyme called *pepsin,* which breaks proteins into peptides. The lining of the stomach is protected from acid by mucus.

30. The functions of the stomach are regulated by neural and hormonal mechanisms.

31. The *small intestine* is a long, coiled tubule in which most of the enzymatic digestion and absorption of food occur. Digestive enzymes come from the lining of the intestine and the pancreas.

32. Pancreatic enzymes break macromolecules into smaller fragments. The intestinal enzymes break these molecules into even smaller fragments that can be absorbed by the epithelial lining of the small intestine.

33. The pancreas also releases *sodium bicarbonate,* which neutralizes HCl entering the small intestine with the chyme and creates an environment suitable for pancreatic enzyme function.

34. The *liver* plays an important role in digestion. It produces a liquid called *bile* that contains, among other substances, bile salts. Bile is stored in the *gallbladder* and released into the small intestine when food is present. Bile salts emulsify fats, breaking them into small globules that can be acted on by enzymes.

35. Undigested food molecules pass from the small intestine into the *large intestine,* which absorbs water, sodium, and potassium, as well as vitamins produced by intestinal bacteria. It also transports the waste, or feces, to the outside of the body.

Controlling Digestion

36. Digestive processes are largely controlled by the nervous and endocrine systems. The release of saliva is stimulated by the sight, smell, taste, and the thought of food. These stimuli also cause the brain to send nerve impulses to the gastric glands of the stomach, initiating the secretion of HCl and gastrin, a hormone that also stimulates HCl secretion.

Health, Homeostasis, and the Environment: Eating Right/Living Right

37. Human health is dependent on good nutrition. Numerous studies suggest that a healthy, balanced diet can decrease the risk of cancer, heart disease, hypertension, and other diseases.

38. Nutritionists recommend the daily consumption of (a) fruits and vegetables, especially cabbage and greens; (b) high-fiber foods, such as whole-wheat bread and celery; and (c) foods high in vitamins A and C.

39. In addition, nutritionists recommend reducing the consumption of animal fat; red meat; and salt-cured, nitrate-cured, smoked, or pickled foods, including bacon and lunch meat.

40. Studies suggest, however, that Americans have not taken these recommendations to heart. Many of us ignore proper nutrition, because we don't take the time to sit down to a nutritionally balanced meal. Living fast-paced lives, we often ignore the importance of eating right.

Critical Thinking

Thinking Critically— Analysis

This Analysis corresponds to the Thinking Critically scenario that was presented at the beginning of this chapter.

To test this hypothesis, one might simply measure oxalate in the urine and blood of people eating both high- and low-calcium diets. If levels were highest in the people eating low-calcium diets, the hypothesis might very well be valid. Knowing that one study is not enough to validate a hypothesis, it might be wise to perform others.

This exercise illustrates the importance of questioning basic assumptions or popularly held beliefs. It shows how dead wrong popular wisdom can be and is a startling testimony to the need for scientific testing of beliefs. One has to wonder how many other assumptions are in error.

Test of Concepts

1. The body requires proper nutrient input to maintain homeostasis. Give an example, and explain how the nutrient affects homeostasis.
2. Describe the conditions during which protein provides cellular energy.
3. If you were considering becoming a strict vegetarian, eating no animal products, even milk and eggs, how would you be assured of getting all of the amino acids your body needs?
4. Describe how the different types of dietary fiber help protect human health.

5. What are vitamins, and why are they needed in such small quantities?
6. A dietary deficiency of one vitamin can cause wide-ranging effects. Why?
7. What organs physically break food down, and what organs participate in the chemical breakdown of food?
8. Describe the process of swallowing.
9. Describe the function of hydrochloric acid and pepsin in the stomach. How does the stomach protect itself from these substances?
10. How do ulcers form, and how can they be treated?

11. Describe the endocrine and nervous system control of the stomach function.
12. The small intestine is the chief site of digestion and absorption. Where do the enzymes needed for this process come from, and how is the release of these enzymes stimulated? What other molecules are needed for proper digestion?
13. Describe the functions of the large intestine.

www.jbpub.com/humanbiology

Connect to this book's web site: www.jbpub.com/humanbiology
The site features eLearning, an online review area that provides quizzes, chapter outlines, and other tools to help you study for your class. You can also follow useful links for in-depth information, research the differing views in the Point/Counterpoints, or keep up on the latest environmental and health news.

CHAPTER 6

The Circulatory System

Red blood cells in a small vein.

Thinking Critically

High blood pressure, or hypertension, is a disease that afflicts many people the world over. African Americans, however, are more prone to this disease than most people. In fact, they are twice as likely to contract the disease as Caucasians.

Some scientists believe that this anomaly may be the result of genetic differences in the population and that these differences arose when many blacks were captured in Africa and transported to plantations where they were held as slaves. According to this hypothesis, many African Americans are hypertensive today because of a rare genetic trait that helped a small subset of their ancestors survive the inhumane conditions of slavery. That trait is an inherited tendency to conserve salt within the body.

According to the hypothesis, the ancestors of African Americans that could conserve water were more likely to survive the grueling trip to the United States and the arduous conditions on the plantations. Conserving water meant they were less likely to die of dehydration. This trait, which proved to be an asset for slaves, may now be a deadly attribute among slavery's modern descendants. As a scientist how could you test this hypothesis? ■

David McMahon, a 48-year-old New York attorney, collapsed in his office one morning and was rushed to a nearby hospital. There a team of cardiologists discovered a blood clot lodged in a narrowed section of his right coronary artery, which supplies the heart. The physicians began immediate action to prevent further damage to the oxygen-starved heart muscle. Through a small incision in McMahon's groin, they inserted a tiny plastic catheter into the artery that carries blood to the leg. They then threaded the catheter up through the arterial system to his heart (**FIGURE 6-1**). Once they reached the heart, physicians guided the catheter into the coronary artery, where they injected

an enzyme, called *streptokinase* (strep-toe-KI-nace), through the catheter. Streptokinase dissolved the blood clot, restoring blood flow to McMahon's heart muscle.

Although David McMahon survived, many others who suffer similar attacks are not so lucky. They either arrive at the hospital too late or, if they do make it to the hospital, do not receive blood-clot-dissolving agents or other treatments in time to avoid extensive damage to their heart muscle.

Heart attacks strike thousands of Americans each year. They are one of a handful of diseases of the circulatory system caused by the stressful conditions of modern life, smoking, poor eating habits, and a host of other

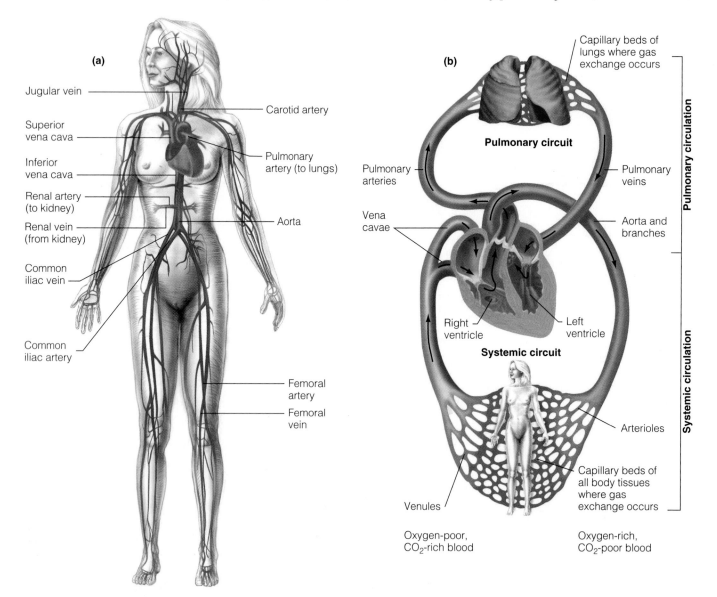

FIGURE 6-1 The Circulatory System   (a) The circulatory system consists of a series of vessels that transport blood to and from the heart, the pump. (b) The circulatory system has two major circuits, the pulmonary circuit, which transports blood to and from the lungs, and the systemic circuit, which transports blood to and from the body (excluding the lungs).

factors. This chapter examines the circulatory system—in sickness and in health. It also discusses the lymphatic system, which functions in both circulation and immune protection.

The Circulatory System's Function: An Overview

The human circulatory system consists of a muscular pump, the heart, and a network of vessels (**FIGURE 6-1**). These vessels transport blood throughout the body, ensuring the adequate distribution of oxygen, taken in via the respiratory system, and nutrients, absorbed by the digestive system, to the cells, tissues, and organs. The circulation of blood throughout the body also ensures the distribution of body heat. Besides transporting nutrients and heat, the circulatory system picks up waste from cells in the body's tissues and transports them to the organs of excretion such as the kidneys. Each of these functions serves a higher purpose: to maintain the relatively constant internal conditions (homeostasis) necessary for cellular function. For a review of these functions, see **TABLE 6-1**.

The Heart

The **heart** is a muscular pump in the thoracic (chest) cavity. Often referred to as the workhorse of the cardiovascular system, the heart propels blood through the 50,000 miles of blood vessels in the body. Each day, this tireless organ beats approximately 100,000 times, adjusting its rate to meet the changing needs of the body. If you had a dollar for every heartbeat, you would be a millionaire in 10 days. Over a 70-year lifetime, you would collect $2.5 billion for your heart's work!

The heart, shown in **FIGURE 6-2**, is a fist-sized organ whose walls are composed of three layers, the pericardium, the myocardium, and the endocardium. The **pericardium** (pear-ah-CARD-ee-um) forms a thin,

TABLE 6-1
Functions of the Circulatory System
Transports oxygen to body cells
Transports nutrients from the digestive system to body cells
Transports hormones to body cells
Transports wastes from body cells to excretory organs
Distributes body heat

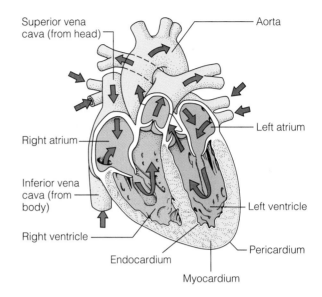

FIGURE 6-2 Blood Flow Through the Heart Deoxygenated (carbon-dioxide-enriched) blood (blue arrows) flows into the right atrium from the systemic circulation and is pumped into the right ventricle. The blood is then pumped from the right ventricle into the pulmonary artery, which delivers it to the lungs. In the lungs, the blood releases its carbon dioxide and absorbs oxygen. Reoxygenated blood (red arrows) is returned to the left atrium, then flows into the left ventricle, which pumps it to the rest of the body through the systemic circuit.

closed sac that surrounds the heart and the bases of large vessels that enter and leave the heart. The pericardial sac is filled with a clear, slippery aqueous fluid that reduces the friction produced by the heart's repeated contraction. The middle layer, the **myocardium** (my-oh-CARD-ee-um), is the thickest part of the wall and is composed chiefly of cardiac muscle cells (Chapter 4). The inner layer, the **endocardium** (end-oh-CARD-ee-um), is the endothelial layer, which lines the heart chambers.

The Circulatory System Has Two Distinct Circuits Through Which Blood Flows

To understand how the heart's anatomy relates to its function, it is important to first know a bit about circulation. As shown in **FIGURE 6-1B**, the circulatory system consists of two distinct circuits, the **pulmonary circuit,** which carries blood to and from the lungs, and the **systemic circuit,** which transports blood to and from the rest of the body.

As you shall soon see, the pulmonary circuit has one main function, to supply oxygen-rich blood that can then be distributed via systemic circulation and to get rid of carbon dioxide, a waste product of energy production in cells.

As shown in **FIGURE 6-1B**, the heart consists of four hollow chambers—two on the right side of the heart and two on the left. Blood is pumped through the pulmonary circuit by the right side of the heart—the right atrium and right ventricle. Blood is pumped through the systemic circuit by the left side of the heart—the left atrium and left ventricle.

FIGURE 6-2 illustrates the course that blood takes through the heart. Drawn in blue, blood low in oxygen (and rich in carbon dioxide) enters the right side of the heart from the **superior** and **inferior vena cavae** (VEEN-ah CAVE-ee), which are part of the systemic circulation. These veins empty directly into the **right atrium** (A-tree-um), the uppermost chamber of the heart. The vena cavae carry oxygen-poor, waste-filled blood to the heart. The blood is pumped from here into the **right ventricle** (VEN-trick-el), the lower chamber on the right side. When the right ventricle is full, the muscles in its wall contract, forcing blood into the pulmonary arteries, which lead to the lungs.

In the lungs, this blood is oxygenated, then returned to the heart via the pulmonary veins. The pulmonary veins, in turn, empty directly into the **left atrium,** the upper chamber on the left side of the heart. It's the first part of the systemic circuit.

Next, the oxygen-rich blood is pumped to the left ventricle. When it's full, the left ventricle's thick, muscular walls contract and propel the blood into the aorta (a-OR-tah). The **aorta** is the largest artery in the body. It carries the oxygenated blood away from the heart, delivering it to the cells and tissues of the body.

The flow of blood just described presents a slightly misleading view of the way the heart really works. As shown in **FIGURE 6-3**, both atria actually fill and contract simultaneously, delivering blood to their respective ventricles. The right and left ventricles also fill simultaneously, and when both ventricles are full, they too contract in unison, pumping the blood into the systemic and pulmonary circulations. The coordinated contraction of heart muscle is brought about by an internal timing device, or pacemaker (described later).

Heart Valves Are Located Between the Atria and Ventricles and Between the Ventricles and the Large Vessels into Which They Empty

The human heart contains four valves that control the direction of blood flow, ensuring a steady flow from the atria to the ventricles and from the ventricles to the large vessels that lead away from the heart (**FIGURE 6-4A**).

The valves between the atria and ventricles are known as **atrioventricular valves** (AH-tree-oh-ven-TRICK-u-ler). Each valve consists of two or three flaps of tissue anchored to the inner walls of the ventricles by slender tendinous cords, the **chordae tendineae** (CORD-ee ten-DON-ee-ee), resembling the strings of a parachute (**FIGURES 6-4A** and **6-4B**). The right atrioventricular valve, between the right atrium and right ventricle, is called the **tricuspid valve** (try-CUSS-pid), because it contains three flaps. The left atrioventricular valve is the **bicuspid valve** (bye-CUSS-pid).[1] To remember the valves, imagine you are wearing a jersey with the number 32 on the front. This reminds you that the *tri*cuspid valve is on the right side and the *bi*cuspid valve is on the left.

Between the right and left ventricles and the arteries into which they pump blood (pulmonary artery and aorta, respectively) are the **semilunar valves** (SEM-eye-

---

[1]The bicuspid valve is also called the *mitral valve,* because it resembles a miter, a hat worn by the Pope and Catholic bishops.

FIGURE 6-3 Blood Flow Through the Heart *(a)* Blood enters both atria simultaneously from the systemic and pulmonary circuits. When full, the atria pump their blood into the ventricles. *(b)* When the ventricles are full, they contract simultaneously, *(c)* delivering the blood to the pulmonary and systemic circuits.

Atria

Ventricles

(a)

(b)

(c)

Aorta

Superior vena cava

Right pulmonary veins

Right atrium

Right atrio-ventricular (tricuspid) valve

Inferior vena cava

Left pulmonary artery

Left pulmonary veins

Left atrium

Left atrio-ventricular (bicuspid) valve

Semilunar valves

Left ventricle

Chordae tendineae   Right ventricle   Septum

(a)

(b)

Aortic semilunar valve

Pulmonary semilunar valve

Tricuspid valve

Bicuspid valve

Fibrous connective tissue

(c)

(d)

FIGURE 6-4 Heart Valves *(a)* A cross section of the heart showing the four chambers and the location of the major vessels and valves. *(b)* Photograph of chordae tendineae.

(c) A view of the heart from above, with the major vessels removed to show the valves. *(d)* Pulmonary semilunar valve photographed from the ventricle.

LUNE-ir) (**FIGURES 6-4A** and **6-4C**). The semilunar valves (literally, "half moon") consist of three semicircular flaps of tissue (**FIGURES 6-4C** and **6-4D**).

The atrioventricular and semilunar valves are one-way valves that open when blood pressure builds on one side and close when it increases on the other, much like the purge valves in scuba diving masks, which allow divers to force water out of their masks, or the ball valves in snorkels, which operate similarly. When the ventricles contract, blood forces the semilunar valves open. Blood flows out of the ventricles into the large arteries. The backflow of blood causes the valve to close, preventing blood from draining back into the ventricles. The atrioventricular valves function in similar fashion.

Heart Sounds Result from the Closing of Various Heart Valves

When physicians listen to your heart, they are actually listening to sounds of the heart valves closing. The noises they hear are called the heart sounds and are often described as "LUB-dupp." The first heart sound (LUB) results from the closure of the atrioventricular valves. It is longer and louder than the second heart sound (dupp), produced when the semilunar valves shut.

Interestingly, the right and left atrioventricular valves do not close at precisely the same time. Nor do the semilunar valves. Thus, by careful placement of the stethoscope, a physician can listen to each valve individually to determine whether it is functioning properly.

For most of us, our heart valves function flawlessly throughout life. However, in some individuals, diseases alter the function of the valves. This, in turn, may dramatically decrease the efficiency of the heart and the circulation of blood. Rheumatic (RUE-mat-tick) fever, for example, is caused by a bacterial infection and affects many parts of the body, including the heart. Although it is relatively rare in the more affluent countries, rheumatic fever is still a significant problem in the less developed countries. Rheumatic fever begins as a sore throat caused by certain types of **streptococcus** (STREP-toe-COCK-iss) **bacteria.** The sore throat—known as **strep throat**—is usually followed by general illness. During this infection, the body forms **antibodies** (proteins made by cells of the immune system) to the bacteria. These antibodies circulate in the blood and can damage the heart valves, preventing them from closing completely. This causes blood to leak back into the atria and ventricles after contraction and results in a distinct "sloshing" sound, called a **heart murmur.** This condition reduces the efficiency of the heart and causes the organ to work harder to make up for the inefficient pumping. Increased activity, in turn, causes the walls of the heart to enlarge and in severe cases, can result in heart failure. To prevent heart failure, damaged valves can be replaced by artificial implants.

Tumors (benign and malignant) and scar tissue have an opposite effect—that is, they reduce blood flow through the heart valves. This condition is known as **valvular stenosis** (sten-OH-siss; from the Greek word steno, meaning "narrow"). Valvular stenosis prevents the ventricles from filling completely. As in valvular incompetence, the heart must beat faster to ensure an adequate supply of blood to the body's tissues. This acceleration also puts additional stress on the organ.

Heart Rate Is Largely Controlled by an Internal Pacemaker

The human heart functions at different rates under different conditions. At rest, it generally beats slowly. When one is excited or working hard, it beats much faster. This variation in heart rate helps the body adjust for differences in oxygen requirements by cells and tissues. Heart rate is controlled by a number of mechanisms.

One of the most important mechanisms is an internal pacemaker, the **sinoatrial (SA) node** (SIGN-oh-A-tree-ill noad) (**FIGURE 6-5**). Located in the wall of the right atrium, the SA node is composed of a clump of specialized cardiac muscle cells. These cells contract spontaneously and rhythmically. Each contraction produces a bioelectric impulse, akin to those produced by nerve cells. This impulse spreads rapidly from the SA node to the cardiac muscle, and then from muscle cell to muscle cell in both atria. Because cardiac muscle cells are tightly joined, and because the impulse travels quickly, the two atria contract almost simultaneously.

Left to their own devices, cardiac muscle cells would contract independently and in a disorderly way, creating an ineffective pumping action. The SA node, however, imposes a single rhythm on all of the atrial heart muscle cells. The SA node is therefore like the conductor of an orchestra.

The electrical impulse generated by the SA node and transmitted throughout the atria next passes to the ventricles. However, its passage is briefly slowed by a barrier of unexcitable tissue that separates the atria from the ventricles. The impulse is delayed approximately 1/10 second. This delay gives the blood-filled atria time to contract and empty their contents into the ventricles. It also provides the ventricles plenty of time to fill before they are stimulated to contract.

After this brief delay, the impulse is channeled through a second mass of specialized muscle cells, the **atrioventricular (AV) node,** shown in **FIGURE 6-5**. From the AV node, the impulse travels along a tract of specialized cardiac muscle cells, known as the **atrioventricular bundle**.

As **FIGURE 6-5** shows, the atrioventricular bundle divides into two branches (called the *bundle branches*) that travel on either side of the wall separating the ventricles. The bundle branches give off smaller branches that terminate on specialized muscle cells, **Purkinje fibers** (per-KIN-gee), named after the scientist who discovered them. These fibers terminate on the cardiac muscle cells in the walls of the ventricles, stimulating them to contract.

Unlike the muscle cells of the atria, the cardiac muscle cells of the ventricles do not contract in unison, in large part because the impulse is not transmitted as quickly and as uniformly through the ventricles as it is through the atria. Instead, contraction begins at the bottom of the heart and proceeds upward, squeezing the blood out of the ventricles into the aorta and pulmonary arteries.

The SA node of the human heart produces a steady rhythm of about 100 beats per minute when isolated from outside influences, but this is much too fast for most human activities. To bring the heart rate in line with body demand, the SA node must therefore be dampened. The SA node is curbed by impulses transmitted by nerves that connect the heart with a control center in the brain. At rest or during nonstrenuous activity, these impulses slow the heart to about 70 beats per minute, thus aligning heart rate with body demands. During exercise or stress, when the heart rate must increase to meet body demands, the decelerating impulses from the brain are reduced.

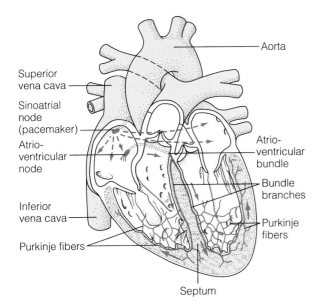

FIGURE 6-5 **Conduction of Impulses in the Heart** The sinoatrial node is the heart's pacemaker. Located in the right atrium, it sends timed impulses into the atrial heart muscles, coordinating muscle contraction. The impulse travels from cell to cell in the atria, then passes to the atrioventricular node and into the ventricles via the atrioventricular bundle and its two branches, which terminate on the Purkinje fibers.

Other nerves also influence heart rate. These nerves carry impulses that accelerate the heart rate even further, allowing the heart to attain rates of 180 beats or more when the cells' demand for oxygen is great.

Several hormones also play a role in controlling heart rate. One of these is **epinephrine** (EP-eh-NEFF-rin), also known as **adrenalin.** This hormone is secreted during stress or exercise by the adrenal glands located on top of the kidneys. Epinephrine increases the heart rate, increasing the flow of blood through the body.

The nervous and endocrine system mechanisms described above are important evolutionary adaptations that help us and other vertebrates cope with the changing demands of our lives.

Electrical Activity in the Heart Can Be Measured on the Surface of the Chest

When the electrical impulse that stimulates muscle contraction in the heart reaches a cardiac muscle cell, it causes the cell to contract. Normally, the outside surface of the cardiac muscle cell is slightly positive. The inside surface is slightly negative. When the impulse arrives, it causes a rapid change in the permeability of the cardiac muscle cell's plasma membrane to sodium ions. Sodium ions flow inward, changing the polarity of the membrane and temporarily making the

inside of the cell more positive than the outside. This change in polarity causes the release of calcium from internal storage depots, which, in turn, causes the cell to contract.

The shift in cardiac muscle cell polarity, or **depolarization,** can be detected by surface electrodes, small metal plates connected to wires and a voltage meter (**FIGURE 6-6A**). The electrodes are placed on a person's chest. The resulting reading on a voltage meter is called an **electrocardiogram** (**ECG** or, sometimes, **EKG**) (**FIGURE 6-6B**).

For a normal person, the tracing produced on the voltage meter has three distinct waves (**FIGURE 6-6B**). The first wave, the P wave, represents the electrical changes occurring in the atria of the heart. The second wave, the QRS wave, is a record of the electrical activity taking place during ventricular contraction, and the third wave, the T wave, is a recording of electrical activity occurring as the ventricles relax.

Diseases of the heart may disrupt one or more waves of the ECG. As a result, an ECG is often a valuable diagnostic tool for cardiologists. Bear in mind, though, that the ECG detects only those diseases that alter the heart's electrical activity.

P = atrial depolarization, which triggers atrial contraction.

QRS = depolarization of AV node and conduction of electrical impulse through ventricles. Ventricular contraction begins at R.

T = repolarization of ventricles.

P to R interval = time required for impulses to travel from SA node to ventricles.

FIGURE 6-6 **The Electrocardiogram** (a) This patient taking a treadmill test to check his heart's performance is wired to a meter that detects electrical activity produced by the heart. (b) An electrocardiogram.

Cardiac Output Varies from One Person to the Next, Depending on Activity and Conditioning

The total amount of blood pumped by the ventricles each minute is called the **cardiac output.** Cardiac output is a function of two factors: **heart rate,** the number of contractions the heart undergoes per minute, and **stroke volume,** the amount of blood pumped by each ventricle during each contraction. At rest, the heart beats approximately 70 times per minute, and the stroke volume is about 70 milliliters. This produces a cardiac output of 5000 milliliters, or 5 liters per minute.

Cardiac output varies among individuals, depending on their physical condition and their level of activity. The heart of a trained athlete, for example, can pump 35 liters of blood per minute (seven times the cardiac output at rest). Most nonathletes, however, can increase the cardiac output to only about 20 liters per minute.

Heart Attacks: Causes, Cures, and Treatments

Heart attacks come in several varieties. The most common heart attack is a **myocardial infarction** (my-oh-CARD-ee-al in-FARK-shun). Myocardial infarctions are caused by **thromboses** (throm-BOW-seas), blood clots that block one or more of the coronary arteries, usually those narrowed by atherosclerotic plaque (discussed next). A blood clot lodged in a coronary artery restricts the flow of blood to the heart muscle, cutting off the supply of oxygen and nutrients. This deprivation can damage and even kill the heart muscle cells. The damaged region is called an **infarct** (in-FARKT)—hence, the name myocardial infarction.

Myocardial Infarctions Usually Occur When Blood Clots Lodge in Arteries Narrowed by Atherosclerosis

As noted in Health Note 5-1, the formation of atherosclerotic plaque results from a combination of factors: stress, poor diet, lack of exercise, smoking, heredity, and several others. Narrowing of a coronary artery by plaque does not usually block the flow of blood enough to cause a heart attack, however, unless it is quite severe—around 80% or 90% blockage. Nonetheless, less severe narrowing does make the vessel more susceptible to blood clots. That is, clots often form in the vessel at the site of narrowing. Also, clots that form in other parts of the body can lodge in the narrowed vessels.

The outcome of heart attacks varies. If the size of the damaged area is small and if the change in electrical activity of the heart is minor and transient, a heart attack is usually not fatal. If the damage is great or electrical activity is severely disrupted, myocardial infarctions can prove fatal.

Getting help quickly also lessens the chances of severe damage to the heart. Giving a person an aspirin during a heart attack also lessens the damage, for reasons you'll soon understand.

Heart attacks can occur quite suddenly, without warning, or may be preceded by several weeks of **angina** (an-GINE-ah), pain that is felt when the supply of oxygen to the myocardium is reduced. Anginal pain appears in the center of the chest and can spread to a person's throat, upper jaw, back, and arms (usually just the left one). Angina is a dull, heavy, constricting pain that appears when an individual is active, then disappears when he or she ceases the activity.

Angina may also be caused by stress and exposure to carbon monoxide, a pollutant that reduces the oxygen-carrying capacity of the blood. Angina begins to show up in men at age 30 and is nearly always caused by coronary artery disease. In women, angina tends to occur at a much later age. Interestingly, about 90% of all "chest pain" patients report to physicians turns out to be unrelated to the heart. What causes it? Many people who are stressed feel pain in the wall of the chest, typically in the muscles between the ribs. The muscles become sore because they're constantly contracted when one is tense. Deep breathing, relaxation, and stress reduction are effective means of eliminating this pain.

Heart Muscle Cells Unleashed from Their Control Beat Independently, Greatly Reducing the Heart's Effectiveness

Another type of heart attack results from a kind of cardiac anarchy known as **fibrillation** (FIB-ril-LAY-shun). This occurs when the SA node loses control of the heart. With the SA node no longer in charge, the cardiac muscle cells beat independently. The lack of coordination converts the heart into an ineffective, quivering mass that pumps little, if any, blood. If the heart stops beating altogether, the condition is known as **cardiac arrest.**

Physicians treat fibrillation by applying a strong electrical current to the chest, a procedure known as **defibrillation.** The electrical current passes through the wall of the chest and is often sufficient to restore normal electrical activity and heartbeat. A normal heartbeat can also be restored by **cardiopulmonary resuscitation (CPR),** in which the heart is "massaged" externally by applying pressure to the sternum (breastbone).

Prevention Is the Best Cure, But in Cases Where Damage Has Already Occurred, Medical Science Has a Great Deal to Offer

Proper diet, exercise, and stress management can reduce the risk of heart problems, as noted in Health Notes 1-1 and 5-1. Research also shows that a daily dose of aspirin (half a tablet a day is enough) taken over long periods can substantially reduce an individual's chances of a heart attack. Studies suggest that aspirin reduces heart attacks by reducing the formation of blood clots.[2] Aspirin is said to thin the blood, although this is not really what it is doing. It's just reducing clotting.

Prevention should be the first line of attack against heart disease. It could save Americans hundreds of millions of dollars each year in medical bills, lost work time, and decreased productivity. But given human nature, the fast pace of modern life, and our inattentiveness to exercise and proper diet, heart disease will probably be around for a long time. To reduce the death rate, physicians therefore also look for ways to treat patients after they have had a heart attack.

One promising development is the use of blood-clot-dissolving agents such as **streptokinase**, mentioned at the beginning of this chapter. When administered within a few hours of the onset of a heart attack, streptokinase can greatly reduce the damage to heart muscle and accelerate a patient's recovery.

Ironically, streptokinase is an enzyme derived from the bacterium that causes rheumatic fever. Because streptokinase is a foreign substance, it evokes an immune reaction. In some people, the reaction is quite severe and may even cause death. The immune reaction to this drug has inspired a search for similar chemicals without the dangerous side effects. One promising clot-busting enzyme is **urokinase** (YOUR-oh-kine-ace), which is produced by human cells.

Scientists are also testing another naturally occurring clot dissolver, called **TPA (tissue plasminogen activator)**. Tests in humans suggest that TPA may also be free of the dangerous side effects of streptokinase. TPA has been approved for use in humans in the United States since 1987. Nevertheless, its use is not without problems. Two of the most significant are (1) the recurrence of blood clots in many patients and (2) the high cost of the drug.

In mild cases, physicians can open clogged blood vessels by inserting a small catheter with a tiny balloon attached to its tip. After chemical clot dissolvers are administered to a patient, the balloon is inflated, forcing the artery open and loosening the plaque from the wall. This procedure is called **balloon angioplasty** (AN-gee-oh-PLAST-ee). Scientists are also experimenting with lasers that burn away plaque in artery walls. Unfortunately, as in other techniques, cholesterol builds up again in the walls of arteries within a few months.

To avoid this problem, surgeons now insert a catheter into the coronary artery, as explained in the Health Note 6-1 in this chapter. At the tip of the catheter is a tiny device called a **stent** (**FIGURE 6-7**). This tubular wire structure is placed in the narrowed artery, then expanded with a tiny balloon. After the balloon is extracted, the stent remains expanded to hold the narrowed artery open.

In severe cases where the coronary arteries are completely blocked by atherosclerotic plaque, heart surgeons often perform coronary bypass surgery to restore blood flow to the heart muscle. In this procedure, surgeons transplant small segments of veins from the leg into the heart (**FIGURE 6-8**). These venous bypasses shunt blood around the clogged coronary arteries, restoring blood flow to the heart muscle. Once hoped to be a long-term answer to a widespread problem, it now appears that coronary bypass surgeries are only a temporary solution. Studies show that bypass patients have a significantly higher rate of survival in the 5 years following surgery than patients who just receive drugs. In the next 7 years, however, studies show that long-term survival from coronary bypass surgery is about the same as that of patients treated with diet and medications. In the long run, bypass surgery is only slightly more effective than nonsurgical medical treatments. Why?

Venous grafts often fill fairly quickly with plaque. The recurrence of plaque in grafts has led researchers to turn to marginally important arteries, such as the internal mammary artery, for this procedure. Many researchers believe that arteries will prove more resistant to plaque buildup than veins.

FIGURE 6-7 Stent

---

[2]You should consult your physician if you are thinking about taking aspirin as a preventive measure.

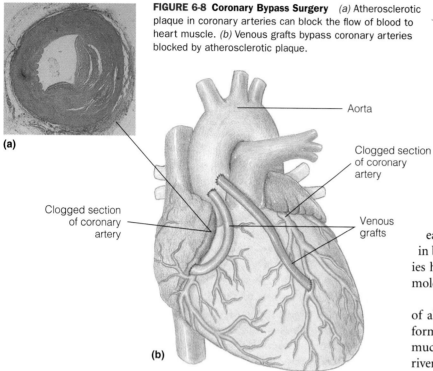

FIGURE 6-8 Coronary Bypass Surgery *(a)* Atherosclerotic plaque in coronary arteries can block the flow of blood to heart muscle. *(b)* Venous grafts bypass coronary arteries blocked by atherosclerotic plaque.

The Blood Vessels

The circulatory system can be divided into four functional parts. The first is the heart, which pumps blood throughout the body. The second is the arteries, which form a delivery system that transports blood from the heart to the body tissues. The third is an exchange system, consisting of networks of tiny vessels known as capillaries, found in body tissues. The fourth is the return system, consisting of veins that carry oxygen-depleted and waste-enriched blood back to the heart from the body tissues. (For a discussion of some of the discoveries that led to our understanding of circulation, see Scientific Discoveries 6-1.)

Arteries, which transport blood *away* from the heart, branch many times, forming smaller and smaller vessels. The smallest of all arteries is the **arteriole** (are-TEAR-ee-ol). As shown in **FIGURE 6-9**, arterioles empty into **capillaries** (CAP-ill-air-ees), tiny, thin-walled vessels that permit wastes and nutrients to pass through with relative ease. Capillaries form extensive, branching networks in body tissues, referred to as **capillary beds.** Capillaries have very thin walls that permit water and various molecules to pass through with ease.

Blood flows out of the capillaries into the smallest of all veins, the **venules.** Venules, in turn, converge to form small veins, which unite with other small veins, in much the same way that small streams unite to form a river. Blood in veins flows toward the heart.

FIGURE 6-10 shows a cross section of an artery and a vein. As illustrated, these two vessels are structurally different. Veins, for example, tend to be smaller and to have thinner walls. Despite their obvious differences, arteries and veins have a common architecture. Both consist of three layers: (1) an external layer of connective tissue, which binds the vessel to surrounding tissues; (2) a mid-

FIGURE 6-9 Capillary Network A network of capillaries between the arteriole and the venule delivers blood to the cells of body tissues (not shown).

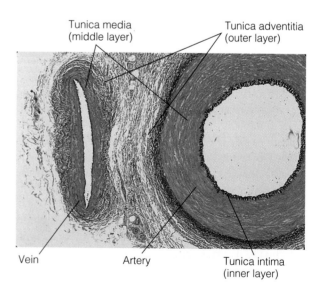

FIGURE 6-10 Artery and Vein A cross section through a vein shows that the muscular layer, the tunica media, is much thinner than it is in an artery. Veins typically lie alongside arteries and, in histological sections such as these, usually have irregular lumens (cavities).

Endothelium
Tunica intima
Tunica media
Tunica adventitia

FIGURE 6-11 General Structure of the Blood Vessel The artery shown here consists of three major layers, the tunica intima, tunica media, and tunica adventitia.

dle layer, which is primarily made of smooth muscle; and (3) an internal layer, which is composed of a layer of flattened cells, the endothelium, and a thin, nearly indiscernible layer of connective tissue, which binds the endothelium to the middle layer. **FIGURE 6-11** shows these layers and the fancy scientific names used to describe them.

Arteries and Arterioles Deliver Oxygen-Rich Blood to Tissues and Organs

The largest of all arteries is the aorta, a massive vessel that carries oxygenated blood from the left ventricle of the heart to the rest of the body. The aorta loops over the back of the heart, then descends through the chest and abdomen, giving off large branches along its way. These branches carry blood to the head, the extremities (arms and legs), and major organs, such as the stomach, the intestines, and the kidneys (**FIGURE 6-1**). The very first branches of the aorta are the coronary arteries.

The aorta and many of its chief branches contain numerous wavy elastic fibers interspersed among the smooth muscle cells of the wall. For this reason, they're called **elastic arteries.** As blood pulses out of the heart, these arteries expand to accommodate it. Like a stretched rubber band, the elastic fibers cause the arterial walls to recoil. This helps push the blood along the arterial tree, maintaining an even flow of blood through the capillaries.

The elastic arteries branch to form smaller vessels, the **muscular arteries.** Muscular arteries contain fewer elastic fibers, but still expand and contract with the flow of blood. You can feel this expansion and contraction in the arteries lying near the skin's surface in your wrist

and neck. It's the pulse that health care workers use to measure heart rate.

The smooth muscle of the muscular arteries responds to a number of stimuli, including nerve impulses, hormones, carbon dioxide, and lactic acid. These stimuli cause the blood vessels to open or close to varying degrees. This allows the body to adjust blood flow through its tissues to meet increased demands for nutrients and oxygen. Arterioles in muscles, for instance, dilate (DIE-late) when a person is threatened by danger. This increases blood flow to the muscle, allowing the person to flee or to meet the danger head on. At the same time, vessels in the digestive system constrict, reducing the digestive process and increasing the amount of blood available to the muscles. As you shall soon see, body temperature can also be regulated in part by regulating the flow of blood to body tissues.

Blood Pressure. The force that blood applies to the walls of a blood vessel is known as the **blood pressure.** Like many other physical conditions in the human body, blood pressure varies from time to time. For example, it changes in relation to one's activity and stress levels. When someone makes you angry, they really are raising your blood pressure! In a given artery, blood pressure rises and falls with each heart beat. Blood pressure also varies throughout the cardiovascular system, being the highest in the aorta and the lowest in the veins. Blood pressure is also rather low in the capillaries, a feature that enhances the rate of exchange between the blood and the tissues.

Blood pressure is measured by using an inflatable device with the tongue-twisting name of **sphygmomanometer** (SFIG-mo-ma-NOM-a-ter), or, more commonly, **blood pressure cuff** (**FIGURE 6-12A**, page 146). The blood pressure cuff is first wrapped around the upper arm. A stethoscope is positioned over the artery just below the cuff. Air is pumped into the cuff until the pressure stops the flow of blood through the artery (**FIGURE 6-12B**). The pressure in the cuff is then gradually reduced as air is released. When the blood pressure in the artery exceeds the external pressure of the cuff, the blood starts flowing through the vessel once again. This point represents the **systolic pressure** (sis-STOL-ick), the peak pressure at the moment the ventricles contract. Systolic pressure is the higher of the two numbers in a blood pressure reading (120/70, for example).[3] The pressure at the moment the heart relaxes to let the ventricles fill again is the **diastolic pressure** (DIE-ah-STOL-ick) and is the lower of the two readings. It is determined by continuing to release air from the cuff until

---

[3]Blood pressure is measured in millimeters of mercury (mm Hg; see **FIGURE 6-12B**).

Scientific Discoveries that Changed the World 6-1

The Circulation of Blood in Animals

Featuring the Work of Harvey and Hales

The seventeenth-century British physician William Harvey is generally credited with the discovery of the circulation of blood in animals (**FIGURE 1**). Harvey is known as a scientist with a short temper who wore a dagger in the fashion of the day, which he re-

FIGURE 1 William Harvey This flamboyant scientist greatly advanced our knowledge on circulation in animals.

portedly brandished at the slightest provocation. He was probably not the kind of professor you might "argue" with over grades.

Temperament aside, Harvey is generally honored for his work on the role of the heart and the flow of blood in animals and is often praised as a pioneer of scientific methodology. His application of quantitative procedures to biology, some say, ushered in the modern age of this science.

In Harvey's medical school days, anatomists thought the intestines produced a substance called *chyle*. Chyle, they thought, was a fluid derived from the food people ate. It was passed from the intestines to the liver. The liver, in turn, converted the chyle to venous blood, then distributed the blood through arteries and veins.

As a medical student, Harvey was told that blood oozing through arteries and veins supplied organs and tissues with nourishment. He was also told that the blood merely ebbed back to the heart and lungs, where impurities were removed. In other words, there was no form of circulation, just an ebb and flow similar to

the tides. These ideas had been proposed by the Greek physician Galen 14 centuries earlier and persisted nearly without challenge until Harvey's time.

As a teacher in the Royal College of Physicians in 1616, Harvey began to describe the circulation of blood, based on the results of his experiments and observations on animals. Apparently rebuked for his ideas by some of his colleagues, Harvey engaged in many years of research to provide supporting evidence. He described the muscular character of the heart and the origin of the heartbeat. He also demonstrated that the pulse felt in arteries resulted from the impact of blood pumped by the heart. Furthermore, he described the pulmonary and systemic circuits and proposed that blood flowed to the tissues and organs of the body via the arteries and returned via the veins.

A brief examination of one of his experiments illustrates that even though Harvey is a key figure in the history of biological science and played a key role in promoting quantitative study, some of his work was

---

no arterial pulsation is audible. At this point, blood is flowing continuously through the artery.

A typical reading for a young, healthy adult is about 120/70, although readings vary considerably from one person to the next. Thus, what is normal for one person may be abnormal for another. As a person ages, blood pressure tends to rise. Thus, a healthy 65-year-old might have a blood pressure reading of 140/90.

Hypertension is a prolonged elevation in blood pressure. Like other cardiovascular diseases, it has many causes, including kidney disease, high salt intake, obesity, and genetic predisposition. Nearly always a symptomless disease early on, hypertension is often characterized by a gradual increase in blood pressure over time. A person may feel fine and display no physical problems whatsoever for years. Symptoms, such as headaches, palpitations (rapid, forceful beating of the

heart), and a general feeling of ill health, usually occur only when blood pressure is dangerously high. Consequently, early detection and treatment are essential to prevent serious problems, including heart attacks.

Capillaries Permit the Exchange of Nutrients and Wastes Between Blood and Body Cells

As described above, the heart, arteries, and veins form an elaborate system that propels and transports blood to and from the capillaries. Capillaries form branching networks, the capillary beds, among the cells of body tissues. It is in these extensive networks of vessels that wastes and nutrients are exchanged between the cells of the body and the blood.

As shown in **FIGURE 6-13** (page 146), the walls of the capillaries consist of flattened endothelial cells. These cells permit dissolved substances to pass through them less than exceptional. It was sometimes based on poor assumptions and inaccurate observations. As an example, consider the work he used to rebut Galen's hypothesis that the blood was produced by the food people ate.

Harvey first approximated the amount of blood the heart ejected with each heartbeat (stroke volume), then determined the pulse rate. He called on earlier observations of a heart from a human cadaver to determine stroke volume. At that time, he had noted that the left ventricle contained more than 2 ounces of blood, and then, for reasons not entirely clear to historians of science, he hypothesized that the ventricle ejected "a fourth, a fifth, a sixth or only an eighth" of its contents. (Today, studies indicate that the heart ejects nearly all of its contents.) Based on this assumption, Harvey estimated that the stroke volume was about 3.9 grams of blood per beat. Modern estimates put it at 89 grams per beat.

Harvey also made a grave error in determining pulse. His value of 33 beats per minute is about half of the actual rate in humans. No one knows how he could have been so wrong. Armed with two erroneous measurements, Harvey derived a figure for the amount of blood that circulated through the body that was $\frac{1}{36}$ of the lowest value accepted today.

Regardless, Harvey "proved" his point—that each half-hour the blood pumped by the heart far exceeds the total weight of blood in the body. From this he concluded that blood must be circulated. It is not, as Galen proposed, produced by the food we eat. The amount of food one eats could not produce blood in such volume.

Harvey debunked another falsehood perpetrated through the centuries—the Galenic myth that blood flowed into the extremities in both arteries and veins. Harvey first wrapped a bandage around an extremity. This obstructed the flow of blood through the veins but not the arteries. He noted that the veins swelled because, as he conjectured, blood was being pumped into them via underlying arteries and there was nowhere for the blood to go. Tightening the bandage further cut the blood flow in the arteries as well and thus prevented the veins from swelling. From these observations, Harvey correctly surmised that the arteries deliver blood to the extremities and the veins return it to the heart.

Harvey's work laid the foundation for modern cardiovascular physiology but left many questions unanswered. Many of these were addressed by the highly industrious English biologist Stephan Hales, who was born a century after Harvey. In a long series of scientifically rigorous experiments on horses, dogs, and frogs, Hales explored many aspects of the cardiovascular system. Benefiting from more modern methods of study, he charted blood pathways and examined blood flow and blood pressure in different parts of the circulatory system. After settling many of the unanswered questions left by Harvey, Hales went on to study plant physiology and is perhaps best known for his work on the circulation of sap in plants.

---

with ease—and provide another example of the correlation between structure and function in the body.

If you could remove all of the capillaries from the body and line them up end to end, they would extend over 80,000 kilometers (50,000 miles)—enough to circle the globe at the equator two times. The extensive branching of capillaries not only brings them in close proximity to body cells, but also slows the rate of blood flow through capillary networks and decreases pressure, both of which increase the efficiency of capillary exchange.

As blood flows into a capillary bed, nutrients, gases, water, and hormones carried in the blood immediately begin to diffuse out of the tiny vessels. Meanwhile, water-dissolved wastes in the tissues, such as carbon dioxide, begin to diffuse inward.

The constriction and dilation of the arterioles that "feed" the capillaries also help regulate body temperature. On a cold winter day, for example, the arterioles close down, restricting blood flow through the capillaries and conserving body heat. Just the reverse happens on a warm day. The flow of blood through the skin increases, releasing body heat and often creating a pink flush. Capillaries are therefore a part of the body's system of homeostasis.

Veins and Venules Transport the Oxygen-Poor and Waste-Laden Blood Back to the Heart

Blood leaves the capillary beds stripped of its nutrients and loaded with cellular wastes. As it drains from the capillaries, the blood enters the smallest of all veins, the **venules**. Venules converge to form small veins, which join with others to form larger and larger vessels. Unlike the arteries, then, the veins start off small and converge with other veins, forming larger and larger vessels. Even-

Pressure-recording device

Inflatable cuff

(a)

FIGURE 6-12 Blood Pressure Reading *(a)* A sphygmomanometer (blood pressure cuff) is used to determine blood pressure. *(b)* As shown, the blood pressure (indicated by the red line) rises and falls with each contraction of the heart. When the pressure in the cuff exceeds the arterial peak pressure, blood flow stops ①. No sound is heard. Cuff pressure is gradually released. When pressure in the cuff falls below the arterial pressure, blood starts flowing through the artery once again. This is the systolic pressure ②. The first sound will be heard. Cuff pressure continues to drop. When cuff pressure is equal to the lowest pressure in the artery, the artery is fully open and no sound is heard ③. This is the diastolic pressure.

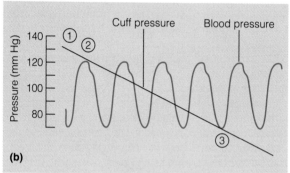

(b)

tually, all blood returning to the heart in the systemic circuit enters the superior or inferior vena cavae, the two main veins that drain into the right atrium of the heart (**FIGURE 6-2**). These vessels drain the upper and lower parts of the body, respectively.

Veins and arteries generally run side by side throughout the body. The arteries take blood away from the heart and toward body tissues, and the veins return blood to the heart.

As noted earlier, blood pressure in the veins is low, and veins have relatively thin walls with fewer smooth muscle cells than arteries (**FIGURE 6-10**). Because the veins' walls are so thin, obstructions can cause blood to pool in them, in much the same way that a tree down across a small stream can cause water to pool upstream. Blood pools in the obstructed veins, forming rather unsightly bluish bulges called **varicose veins** (VEAR-uh-cose) (**FIGURE 6-14**).

Some people inherit a tendency to develop varicose veins, but most cases can be attributed to various factors that reduce the flow of blood back to the heart: abdominal tumors, pregnancy, obesity, and even sedentary life-styles.

Varicose veins are not only unsightly, they can result in considerable discomfort. The restriction of blood

(a) Capillary

FIGURE 6-13 The Capillary *(a)* A light micrograph of a capillary showing the endothelial cells that make up the wall of this vessel. *(b)* A cross section of a capillary showing the nucleus of an endothelial cell and capillary lumen.

(b) Endothelial cell nucleus   Capillary lumen

FIGURE 6-14 Any restriction of venous blood flow to the heart causes veins to balloon out, creating bulges commonly known as varicose veins.

flow, for example, may result in muscle cramps and the buildup of fluid, **edema** (uh-DEEM-ah; swelling), in the ankles and legs.

Varicose veins may also form in the wall of the anal canal. The veins in this region are known as the **internal hemorrhoidal veins** (hem-eh-ROID-il). A swelling of the internal hemorrhoidal veins results in a condition known as **hemorrhoids** (hem-eh-ROIDS). Because the internal hemorrhoidal veins are supplied by numerous pain fibers, this condition can be quite painful.

How Do the Veins Work? FIGURE 6-15 shows that blood pressure is lowest in the veins. With such low pressure, how do the veins return blood to the heart?

For blood in veins above the heart, gravity is the chief means of propulsion. But for veins below the heart, return flow depends on the movement of body parts, which "squeezes" the blood upward. As you walk to class, for example, the contraction of muscles in your legs pumps the blood in the veins. This forces the blood upward, slowly and surely causing it to move against the force of gravity. Even the nervous muscle contractions that occur when you're studying help move the blood back to the heart.

Valves also facilitate the return of blood. Valves are flaps of tissue that span the veins and prevent the backflow of blood. The structure of the valves is shown in **FIGURE 6-16**. As illustrated, the semilunar flaps of the veins resemble those found in the heart. Just as in the valves of the heart, blood pressure, however slight, pushes the flaps open (**FIGURE 6-16**). This allows the blood to move forward. As the blood fills the segment of the vein in front of the valve, it pushes back on the valve flaps and forces them shut.

To locate a valve, hold your arm out in front of you and make a fist. The veins should stick out or at least be apparent beneath the skin of your forearm. To locate a valve in the superficial veins on your forearm, press gently on a vein, then run your finger toward your wrist. You will note that the vein collapses behind your finger until it crosses a valve.

Just as surgeons can fix damaged arteries in the body, they can also repair smaller vessels. Each year thousands of people lose fingers or toes or even ears in

unfortunate accidents. In many cases, the recovered body part can be reattached.

This procedure requires an enormous amount of time and skill. Nerves, bones, muscles, and blood vessels must be carefully reconnected. Severed arterioles and venules about the same diameter of a metal paper clip can be sewn back in place via microsurgery.

In many cases, blood flow is restored and all that remains of the injury is a nasty scar or some loss of sensation or movement. In other cases, however, blood flow does not return. If it is not re-established, the reattached part will die. Fortunately, there's a new tool that's helping doctors re-establish blood flow: leeches. They can be placed on the tip of a severed toe or finger and will begin

FIGURE 6-15 Blood Pressure in the Circulatory System
Blood pressure declines in the circulatory system as the vessels branch. Arterial pressure pulses because of the heartbeat, but pulsation is lost by the time the blood reaches the capillary networks, creating an even flow through body tissues. Blood pressure continues to decline in the venous side of the circulatory system.

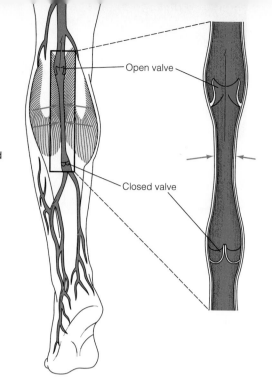

FIGURE 6-16 Valves in Veins The slight hydrostatic pressure in the veins and the contraction of skeletal muscles propel the blood along the veins back toward the heart. The one-way valves stop the blood from flowing backward.

sucking blood, so forcefully that circulation is restored. If you are interested in learning more, see Health Note 6-1.

Section 6-5

The Lymphatic System

The lymphatic system is an extensive network of vessels and glands (**FIGURE 6-17**). It is functionally related to two systems: the circulatory system and the immune system. This section examines the circulatory role of the lymphatic system.

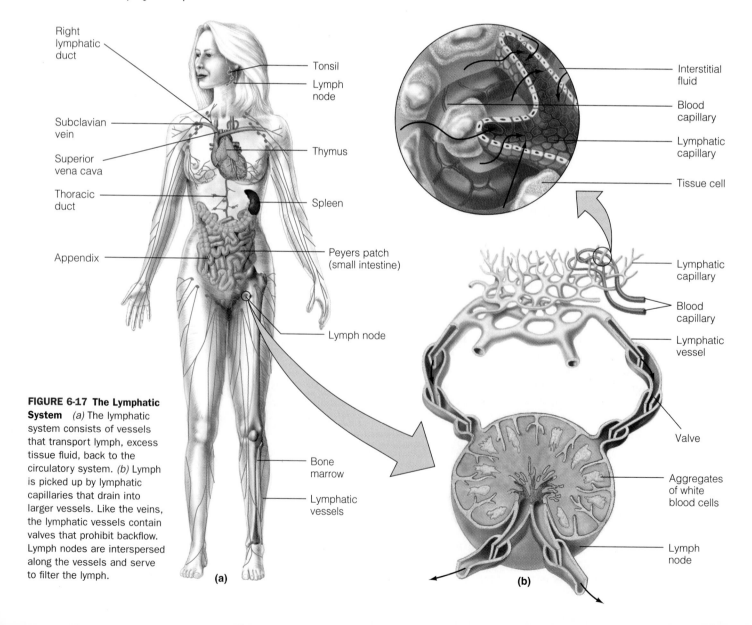

FIGURE 6-17 The Lymphatic System (a) The lymphatic system consists of vessels that transport lymph, excess tissue fluid, back to the circulatory system. (b) Lymph is picked up by lymphatic capillaries that drain into larger vessels. Like the veins, the lymphatic vessels contain valves that prohibit backflow. Lymph nodes are interspersed along the vessels and serve to filter the lymph.

FIGURE 6-18 Elephantiasis A parasitic worm that invades the body stimulates the production of scar tissue, which blocks the flow of lymph through the nodes, causing tissue fluid to build up. This condition is known as elephantiasis.

You may recall from Chapter 4 that the cells of the body are bathed in a liquid called **interstitial fluid** (in-ter-STISH-il). Interstitial fluid provides a medium through which nutrients, gases, and wastes can diffuse between the capillaries and the cells.

Tissue fluid is replenished by water that diffuses out of the capillaries. The flow of water out of the capillaries, however, normally exceeds the return flow by about 3 liters per day. The "excess" water is picked up by small **lymph capillaries** in tissues. Like the capillaries of the circulatory system, these vessels have thin, highly permeable walls through which water and other substances pass with ease.

Lymph drains from the capillaries into larger ducts. These vessels, in turn, merge with others, creating larger and larger ducts, which empty into the large veins at the base of the neck.

Lymph moves through the vessels of the lymphatic system in much the same way that blood is transported in veins. In the upper parts of the body, it flows by gravity. In regions below the heart, it is propelled largely by muscle contraction. Breathing pumps lymph out of the chest and walking pumps the lymph out of the extremities. Lymphatic flow is also assisted by valves similar to those in the veins.

The lymphatic system also consists of several lymphatic organs: the lymph nodes, the spleen, the thymus, and the tonsils. The lymphatic organs function primarily in immune protection and are discussed in Chapter 8. Lymph nodes, however, play a role worth considering here.

Varying in size and shape, lymph nodes are found in association with lymphatic vessels in small clusters in the armpits, groin, neck, and other locations (**FIGURE 6-17**). A lymph node consists of a network of fibers and irregular channels that slow down the flow of lymph and filter out bacteria, viruses, cellular debris, and other particulate matter transported in the lymph. Lining the channels are numerous cells (macrophages) that phagocytize microorganisms and other materials.

Normally, lymph is removed from tissues at a rate equal to its production. In some instances, however, lymph production exceeds the capacity of the system. A burn, for example, may cause extensive damage to blood capillaries, increasing their leakiness and overwhelming the lymphatic capillaries. This "flood" results in a buildup of fluid in tissues called edema.

Lymphatic vessels may also become blocked. One of the most common causes of blockage is an infection by tiny parasitic worms that are transmitted to humans by mosquitoes in the tropics. The worm larvae (an immature form) enter lymph vessels and take up residence in the lymph nodes. An inflammatory reaction causes the buildup of scar tissue in the nodes, which blocks the flow of lymph. After several years, the lymphatic drainage of certain parts of the body may be almost completely obstructed. A leg may swell so much, in fact, that it weighs as much as the rest of the body (**FIGURE 6-18**). This condition is known as **elephantiasis** (el-uh-FUN-TIE-ah-sis).

Health, Homeostasis, and the Environment

Cadmium and Hypertension

In recent years, scientists have discovered numerous chemical pollutants that are released into the environment and ingested in our food, air, and water, affecting our health by altering homeostatic mechanisms. Cadmium is one of those pollutants.

Cadmium is a heavy metal. In earlier times, cadmium was used to treat syphilis and malaria, a remedy soon abandoned when physicians learned of its toxic effects. Today, cadmium is used for many commercial purposes. One of the most common uses is as a chemical stabilizer in polyvinyl chloride, a compound used to make vinyl (found in children's toys such as beach balls). Cadmium is combined with gold and other metals to make jewelry and also used to make camera batteries, engine parts, and radio and television sets.

Cadmium is released into the air and water during the manufacture of many products. Incinerators that burn municipal garbage also release small amounts of cadmium once contained in rubber tires, plastic bottles, furniture, and other items. Recycling facilities that melt down radiators and scrap steel also emit cadmium. Together, these facilities emit over 4 million pounds of cadmium into the air each year in the United States alone.

Cadmium, which ends up in food, air, and water, is toxic to practically all the body systems of humans and other animals. It is absorbed into the body and retained, so its levels increase as we get older. The average American has 30 milligrams of cadmium in his or her body at death.

What are the effects of low-level cadmium exposure over a lifetime? One probable result is hypertension, a subject described more fully in Health Note 6-2. Cadmium acts on the smooth muscle of blood vessels,

Modern Medicine Turns to Leeches

Donna Amark is a college professor at a midwestern University. A few years ago, Donna lost her thumb in an unfortunate accident involving a neighbor's dog. Donna stopped by to visit the new neighbor. When no one answered the door, she went to the back yard. There she was confronted by the neighbor's dog, who was chained to a large maple tree. The dog seemed friendly, but as Donna approached he lunged toward her. She side-stepped the dog and grabbed the chain. Unfortunately, the chain had wrapped around her thumb. When the dog lunged at her, the sudden jerk of the chain severed her thumb, ripping it out, tendons and all.

Paramedics who rushed Donna to the hospital were unable to find the severed thumb, so she elected to have a new procedure. Doctors removed her big toe, tendons and all, and inserted it into the hand where her thumb had once been.

Her surgery went well. However, despite the tedious work of reconnecting blood vessels Donna's translocated thumb showed no signs of restored blood flow. Soon after, it became apparent that she was going to lose her new thumb. The surgeons in charge made what seemed at first to be a ludicrous suggestion: use leeches to restore the blood flow.

Leeches, it turns out, have become one of modern medicine's most effective tools. They're routinely used in Great Britain and the United States to re-establish blood flow in reattached ears, fingers, and toes.

Hypertension, Atherosclerosis, and Aneurysms: Causes and Cures

Hypertension, or high blood pressure, is one of the most common health problems of our time. Its causes vary widely. Hypertension can be hereditary—that is, passed from parent to offspring. It is also thought to result from stress and diet, especially high salt intake in some individuals. People who are overweight when they are young are more likely to suffer from hypertension when they reach adulthood. In others, it is caused by disorders such as kidney failure or hormonal imbalances. Pregnancy can lead to hypertension, as can the use of oral contraceptives. Cadmium in food, air, and water may also contribute to this disease, as noted in this chapter.

If hypertension is untreated, blood pressure rises steadily over the years. Unfortunately, hypertension is a nearly symptomless disease for many people. Individuals feel fine for many years, despite their gradually rising blood pressure. Many exhibit no signs of the disease until it has progressed to the dangerous stage. Because of this, it is important for people over the age of 40 to have their blood pressure checked each year.

Hypertension is more common in men than in women and is twice as prevalent in African Americans than Caucasians. The disease is dangerous because the increased pressure in the circulatory system forces the heart to work harder. Elevated blood pressure may also damage the lining of arteries, creating a site at which atherosclerotic plaque forms. Atherosclerosis increases the risk of heart attack: A hypertensive person is six times more likely to have a heart attack than an individual with normal blood pressure. Hypertension also increases the chances for an occlusion in the arteries supplying the brain, which can result in strokes.

Another common problem of modern times is **atherosclerosis**, the buildup of cholesterol plaque in the walls of arteries, discussed in previous chapters. Arteries clogged with cholesterol force the heart to work harder, putting strain on this organ. Perhaps the most significant problem arises from blood clots that lodge in narrowed coronary arteries, reducing the flow of blood to the heart muscle.

Arteries can not only clog, they can also rupture. Certain infectious diseases (such as syphilis), atherosclerotic plaque, and hypertension can all result in a weakening of the wall of arteries. This weakening causes arteries to balloon outward, a condition known as an **aneurysm** (**FIGURE 1**). Like a worn spot on a tire, an aneurysm can rupture when pressure builds inside or when the wall becomes too thin.

FIGURE 1 Aneurysm This X-ray shows a ballooning of one of the arteries in the brain. If untreated, an aneurysm can break, causing a stroke.

A leech has a wicked looking mouth with 100 teeth. When it attached to the skin, it bites in. But you don't feel any pain because the leech releases a tiny amount of natural anesthetic that deadens the sensory nerves in the area. The leech also releases a natural anticoagulant into the wound so blood flows uninterrupted into its mouth.

When placed on a reattached finger or toe, the germ-free leech gloms on rather quickly and begins sucking. The patient feels nothing, but in short order oxygen-rich blood begins to flow through the finger or toe, bringing the body part back to life better than any surgeon could. The leech is left in place for some time to ensure adequate flow. After it is removed, blood continues to flow through the reattached body part. If further treatment is needed, the leech is placed on the reattached part again.

Leeches are raised in captivity in sterile environments and rushed to hospitals when needed. In Donna's case, the leeches worked miracles. She's alive and well with functional hands thanks to the lowly leech, modern medicine's latest and greatest new tool.

Visit *Human Biology's* Internet site for links to web sites offering more information on this topic.

When an aneurysm breaks, blood pours out of the circulatory system. Because it happens so quickly, most aneurysms lead to death. An estimated 30,000 Americans die each year from ruptured aneurysms in the brain, and nearly 3000 die from ruptured aortic aneurysms.

As in most diseases, the first line of defense against aneurysms is prevention. By reducing or eliminating the two main causes—atherosclerosis and high blood pressure—individuals can greatly lower their risk.

Physicians recommend a number of steps to reduce your chances of developing atherosclerosis and hypertension. If you smoke, stop. If you are overweight, exercise and lose weight. If you're one of those people for whom salt raises your blood pressure, cut back. If you suffer from stress at work and at home, find ways to reduce your stress levels. If you drink alcohol, consume it in moderation, or quit altogether. If you are fond of foods that are rich in fats and cholesterol, cut down on them and consume foods containing water-soluble fiber such as apples, bananas, citrus fruits, carrots, barley, and oats. These reduce cholesterol uptake by the intestine, as explained in Chapter 5.

Studies show that fish oil also protects the cardiovascular system. Fish oil contains omega-3 fatty acids that have many beneficial functions. For example, it increases high density lipoprotein (HDL), the so-called "good cholesterol" that binds to cholesterol in the blood and transports it to the liver for removal. This may decrease plaque build-up in arteries. It has also been shown to reduce decrease platelet aggregation by making them less sticky. This reduces blood clots. Eating fatty fish once a week will provide minimal benefit. Three days a week provides maximum benefit. Although all fish, shell fish, and crustaceans contain omega-3 fatty acids, certain cold water species including salmon, macerel, lake trout, and sardines have the highest amounts. Fish oil capsules apparently provide the same benefit.

The second line of defense against cardiovascular disease is early detection and treatment. As noted earlier, hypertension can be detected by regular blood pressure readings. Atherosclerosis can be discovered by blood tests that measure cholesterol. Aneurysms can be detected by X-rays. Pain also alerts patients and physicians that something is wrong. Once any of these diseases is detected, physicians have many options.

In the event of an aneurysm, surgeons can remove the weakened section of the artery and replace it with a section of a vein. In cases where venous grafts are not practical (in the brain, for example), surgeons can clamp or tie off the artery just before the bulge, preventing blood flow through the damaged section. This works only when other arteries provide adequate blood flow to the area served by the damaged artery. In larger arteries, pieces of Dacron or other synthetic materials can be sewn into the wall of the artery, protecting it from breaking.

While medical science is finding new ways to detect and treat cardiovascular disease, we must never lose sight of the importance of preventing disease in the first place. A healthy diet and lifestyle can go a long way to avoid diseases that kill tens of thousands of people each year.

Visit *Human Biology's* Internet site for links to web sites offering more information on this topic.

causing hypertension. Laboratory animals that consume even small amounts of cadmium develop hypertension. Humans with hypertension secrete 40 times more cadmium in their urine than individuals with normal blood pressure.

No one knows how many people are suffering from hypertension caused by cadmium, but the number is probably fairly large. Given the rise in cadmium use and the increases in recycling and incineration of trash, exposure can only get worse unless concerted efforts are made to tighten controls on facilities that release this toxic element and, perhaps more importantly, to reduce the use of cadmium in the first place.

Summary

The Circulatory System's Function: An Overview

1. The *circulatory system* is one of the body's chief homeostatic systems. It helps maintain constant levels of nutrients and wastes, helps regulate body temperature, distributes body heat, protects against microorganisms, and, through clotting, protects against blood loss.

The Heart

2. The circulatory system consists of a pump, the *heart,* and two circuits, the *pulmonary circuit,* which transports blood to and from the lungs, and the *systemic circuit,* which delivers blood to the body and returns it to the heart.

3. The human heart consists of four chambers: two atria and two ventricles.

4. The right atrium and right ventricle service the pulmonary circuit. The left atrium and left ventricle pump blood into the aorta and are part of the systemic circuit.

5. The right atrium receives blood from the superior and inferior vena cavae. This blood, returning from body tissues, is low in oxygen and rich in carbon dioxide.

6. From the right atrium, blood is pumped into the right ventricle, then to the lungs, where it is resupplied with oxygen and stripped of most of its carbon dioxide. Blood returns to the heart via the pulmonary veins, which empty into the left atrium.

7. Blood is pumped from the left atrium to the left ventricle, then out the aorta to the body, where it supplies cells of tissues and organs with oxygen and picks up cellular wastes.

8. *Heart valves* help control the direction of blood flow. The *atrioventricular valves* permit blood to flow from the atria to the ventricles and then prevent it from flowing in the reverse direction when the ventricles contract. The *semi-lunar valves* in the base of the aorta and pulmonary artery prevent blood from flowing back into the ventricles.

9. The closing of the valves produces distinct *heart sounds,* which can be detected through the chest using a stethoscope. Irregularities in heart sounds indicate the presence of diseased or damaged valves.

10. Cardiac muscle cells contract rhythmically and independently; contraction is coordinated by the heart's pacemaker, the *sinoatrial node* located in the upper wall of the right atrium.

11. The cells of the SA node discharge periodically, sending impulses to all atrial muscle cells, which cause them to contract in unison.

12. The impulse next travels to the ventricles, but its passage is delayed, providing time for the ventricles to fill before contracting.

13. The impulse travels from the *atrioventricular node* down the *atrioventricular bundle* into the myocardium of the ventricles.

14. Contraction in the ventricles begins at the tip of the heart and proceeds upward.

15. Left on its own, the SA node would produce 100 contractions per minute. Nerve impulses, however, reduce the heart rate to about 70 beats per minute when a person is inactive. During exercise or stress, the heart rate increases to meet body demands.

16. Depolarization of the heart muscle produces weak electrical currents that can be detected by surface electrodes. The change in electrical activity is detected by a voltage meter.

17. The tracing produced on the voltage meter is called an *electrocardiogram (ECG)* and has three distinct waves. Diseases of the heart may disrupt one or more of the waves, making the ECG a valuable diagnostic tool.

Heart Attacks: Causes, Cures, and Treatments

18. The most common type of heart attack is a *myocardial infarction,* caused by a blood clot that either forms in an already narrowed *coronary artery* or arises elsewhere and breaks loose, only to become lodged in a coronary artery. The obstruction decreases the flow of blood and oxygen to heart muscle, sometimes killing the cells.

19. Heart attacks can occur quite suddenly without warning, or they may be preceded by several weeks of *angina,* pain felt when blood flow to heart muscle is reduced. Angina appears when an individual is active, then disappears when he or she rests.

20. The risk of heart attack can be reduced by proper diet, exercise, and daily doses of aspirin. Numerous treatments are available for patients who have had a heart attack.

The Blood Vessels

21. The heart pumps blood into the *arteries,* which distribute the blood to *capillary beds* in body tissues where nutrient and waste exchange occurs. Blood is returned to the heart in the *veins.*

22. The largest of all arteries is the *aorta.* It carries oxygenated blood from the left ventricle of the muscles, glands, and organs of the head and the rest of the body (except the lungs).

23. The aorta and many of its chief branches are *elastic arteries.* As blood pulses out of the heart, the elastic arteries expand to accommodate the blood, then contract, helping pump the blood and ensuring a steady flow through the capillaries.

24. As they course through the body, the elastic arteries branch to form *muscular arteries,* which also expand and contract with the flow of blood.

25. The smooth muscle in the walls of muscular arteries responds to a variety

of stimuli. These stimuli cause the blood vessels to open or close to varying degrees, controlling the flow of blood through body tissues.

26. Blood pressure and flow rate are highest in the aorta and drop considerably as the arteries branch. By the time the blood reaches the capillaries, its flow and pressure are greatly reduced. This dramatic decline enhances the rate of exchange between the blood and the tissues.

27. *Capillaries* are thin-walled vessels that form branching networks, or capillary beds, among the cells of body tissues. Cellular wastes and nutrients are exchanged between the cells of body tissues and the blood in capillary networks.

28. Blood flow through a capillary network is regulated by constriction and relaxation of the arterioles that empty into them.

29. Blood draining from capillary beds enters *venules,* which join to form veins.

Veins return blood to the heart and generally run alongside the arteries.

30. Because the walls of veins have very little smooth muscle, they are easily affected by obstructions, which cause the walls to balloon, forming bluish bulges called *varicose veins.*

31. In the veins above the heart, blood drains by gravity. Veins below the heart, however, rely on the movement of body parts to squeeze the blood upward and on *valves,* flaps of tissue that span the veins and prevent the backflow of blood.

The Lymphatic System

32. The *lymphatic system* is a network of vessels that drains excess interstitial fluid from body tissues and transports it to the blood.

33. The lymphatic system also consists of several lymphatic organs, such as the lymph nodes, the spleen, the thymus, and the tonsils, which function primarily in immune protection.

34. Along the system of lymphatic vessels are small nodular organs called *lymph nodes,* which filter the lymph.

35. Under normal circumstances, lymph is removed from tissues at a rate equal to its production, keeping tissues from swelling. In some cases, however, lymph production exceeds the capacity of the lymphatic capillaries, and swelling (edema) results.

Health, Homeostasis, and the Environment: Cadmium and Hypertension

36. Cadmium is a toxic heavy metal that is released into the air and water during the manufacture of numerous products, the incineration of municipal garbage, and the recycling of steel and other metals.

37. Cadmium ends up in food, air, and water and increases in humans and other organisms over time. Cadmium acts on the smooth muscle of blood vessels, causing hypertension.

Critical Thinking

Thinking Critically— Analysis

This Analysis corresponds to the Thinking Critically scenario that was presented at the beginning of this chapter.

This hypothesis suggests that a selective survival process was in operation—that is, that salt-retaining (dehydration-resistant) slaves were more likely to survive the rigors of slavery than those who lacked this trait. To test the validity of this idea, one might begin by looking at hypertensive African Americans to see whether they actually have the capacity to retain excess salt and, if so, whether this capacity leads to hypertension.

Another research study that might lead to useful results would require one to locate populations of blacks consisting of individuals of African and non-African heritage. By studying differences in blood pressure and the ability to retain salt, one might be able to draw some conclusions as to the validity of the salt-retention hypothesis. One such example is the Island of Barbados in the Caribbean. Its population contains some African blacks who were imported as slaves to work on the island's sugar plantations.

One set of researchers actually performed this analysis and found that blacks of African descent had a slightly higher incidence of high blood pressure than blacks of non-African descent. What does this suggest? The researchers thought that it helped support the salt-retention hypothesis.

Yet another study might involve tests of blacks who reside in the regions of Africa from which slaves were drawn. Finding a low rate of hypertension in this group would suggest that a selective survival mechanism was in effect. One such study showed that, in rural parts of Nigeria, blacks did not suffer from hypertension despite the fact that they consumed large amounts of salt. The researchers concluded that if these people are descendants of the ancestors of slaves, as are African American blacks, then the hypothesis supporting selective survival seems valid.

Critics of this hypothesis argue that this kind of evolutionary change in such a short period is unlikely. Critically analyze this argument. (You may want to read the chapter on evolution to form an argument.) Would it affect your view if you found out that 70% of African slaves died within 4 years of their capture?

Test of Concepts

1. List and describe several ways in which the circulatory system functions in homeostasis.

2. Describe how the pacemaker, the sinoatrial node, coordinates muscular contractions of the heart.

3. Define the pulmonary and systemic circuits.

4. Based on what you know about the heart, what would happen if the septum separating the two atria failed to form completely during embryonic development?

5. Describe how the valves control the direction of blood flow in the heart. What are valvular incompetence and valvular stenosis? What causes these conditions, and how do they affect the heart?

6. How does atherosclerosis of the coronary arteries affect the heart?

7. Describe the general structure of the arteries and veins. How are they different? How are they similar?

8. How do the elastic fibers in the major arteries help ensure a continuous blood flow through the capillaries?

9. Capillaries illustrate the remarkable correlation between structure and function. Do you agree with this statement? Why or why not?

10. Describe how the movement of blood through capillary beds is controlled. Why is this homeostatic mechanism so important? Give some examples.

11. Explain how the blood is returned to the heart via the veins.

12. Explain the role of the lymphatic system in circulation.

www.jbpub.com/humanbiology

Connect to this book's web site: www.jbpub.com/humanbiology
The site features eLearning, an online review area that provides quizzes, chapter outlines, and other tools to help you study for your class. You can also follow useful links for in-depth information, research the differing views in the Point/Counterpoints, or keep up on the latest environmental and health news.

CHAPTER 7

The Blood

7-1 Blood: Its Composition and Functions

Thinking Critically

High concentrations of a bloodborne chemical, lipoprotein(a) (LIE-po-PRO-teen), are a known risk factor of atherosclerosis. This molecule transports cholesterol in the blood and deposits it in arterial walls, causing a thickening of the walls. Studying muscle cells isolated from a normal human artery and grown in tissue culture, two researchers also found that lipoprotein(a) stimulates smooth muscle cells to proliferate. The researchers concluded that high concentrations of lipoprotein(a) have two effects—they deposit cholesterol and cause muscle cells to divide—which may account for the elevated risk of cardiovascular disease they present.

Analyze this assertion based on what little you know about the experiment. What critical thinking rules helped you analyze this matter?

Scanning electron micrograph of human red blood cells.

n 1966, Dr. Leland C. Clark of the University of Cincinnati's College of Medicine immersed a live laboratory mouse in a clear fluorocarbon solution saturated with oxygen. To the amazement of the audience, the mouse did just fine, "breathing" the oxygen-rich liquid as if it were air. Some time later, Clark extracted the mouse from the solution. After a moment, the rodent began to move about, apparently unharmed by the ordeal.

The point of this demonstration was not to show that an animal could "breathe" this fluid into its lungs and survive but, rather, to show that the solution held enormous amounts of oxygen, so much so that it could possibly be used as a substitute for blood. Clark and his colleagues hoped that their "artificial blood" would someday be a boon to medical science, helping paramedics keep accident victims who have lost substantial amounts of blood alive while they are being transported to hospitals.[1] In rural America, where a trip to a hospital takes considerable time, artificial blood could save thousands of lives a year.

---

[1]"Artificial blood" is, of course, a misnomer. The fluorocarbon solution takes over the role of the plasma and the red blood cells, which transport oxygen and carbon dioxide, but not the role of the white blood cells, which protect the body against infection, among other things.

Blood: Its Composition and Functions

Human blood is a far cry from Clark's artificial substitute. The blood in our circulatory system, for example, is a water-based fluid, not a fluorocarbon, and consists of two basic components: plasma and formed elements. **Plasma** is the liquid portion of the blood and is about 90% water. It contains many dissolved substances. Three types of **formed elements** are suspended in the plasma: (1) white blood cells (or leuko-cytes; LUKE-oh-sites), (2) red blood cells (or erythrocytes; eh-RITH-row-sites), and (3) platelets (or thrombocytes; THROM-bow-sites).

Blood accounts for about 8% of our total body weight. A man weighing 70 kilograms (150 pounds), has about 5.6 kilograms (12 pounds). That's equal to 5 to 6 liters (1.3 to 1.5 gallons) of blood. On average, women have about a liter less.

FIGURE 7-1 shows that the plasma makes up about 55% of the blood volume and formed elements about 45%. The volume of the blood occupied by blood cells is referred to as the **hematocrit** (he-MAT-o-krit).

The hematocrit varies in individuals living at different altitudes. In people living in Denver, a mile above sea level, for example, hematocrits are typically about 5% higher than in people living at sea level. The slight increase in the hematocrit (red blood cell [RBC] concentration) in Denver residents is the result of a physiological mechanism that compensates for the slightly lower level of oxygen in the

Withdraw blood

Centrifuge

Plasma
(55% of whole blood)

White blood cells and platelets
(<1% of whole blood)

Red blood cells
(45% of whole blood)

Hematocrit

White blood cells

Red blood cells   Platelets

FIGURE 7-1 Blood Composition Blood removed from a person can be centrifuged to separate plasma from the cellular component. Red blood cells constitute about 45% of the blood volume, except at higher altitudes where they make up about 50% of the volume to compensate for the lower oxygen levels.

atmosphere at the higher altitude. This homeostatic mechanism helps the body deliver the oxygen needed by body cells.

In this day of high-tech athletic competition, where trainers and athletes look for any competitive edge they can find, many athletes train at high altitudes. Some athletes sleep in specially designed chambers that expose them to air with slightly lower oxygen content. The rationale in both these strategies is that the higher hematocrit improves their performance at lower altitudes because their blood contains more oxygen-carrying hemoglobin. In fact, it is partly for this reason that the U.S. Summer Olympic team is headquartered in Colorado Springs, Colorado.

The Blood Plasma Is a Watery Transport Medium

Plasma is a light yellow (straw-colored) fluid. Dissolved in the plasma are (1) gases such as nitrogen, carbon dioxide, and oxygen; (2) ions such as sodium, chloride, and calcium; (3) nutrients such as glucose and amino acids; (4) hormones; (5) proteins; (6) various wastes; and (7) lipid molecules. Lipids are either suspended in tiny globules or bound to certain plasma proteins, which transport them through the bloodstream.

Proteins are the most abundant of all dissolved substances in the plasma. Blood proteins contribute to osmotic pressure (described briefly in Chapter 3). **Osmotic pressure** helps regulate the flow of materials in and out of capillaries. It is therefore essential to the proper distribution of wastes and nutrients in the body, so vital to homeostasis.[2]

Blood proteins also help to regulate the pH of the blood. They do so by binding to hydrogen ions, thus preventing the H^+ concentration in the blood from rising, which is also essential to homeostatic balance.

Some plasma proteins serve as carrier proteins. Human blood contains three types of protein: (1) albumins, (2) globulins, and (3) fibrinogen (**TABLE 7-1**). Albumins (al-BEW-mins) and two types of globulins (GLOB-u-lins), for example, are carrier proteins. They bind to hormones, ions, and fatty acids, and transport these molecules through the bloodstream. Carrier proteins are large, water-soluble molecules. Their binding to much smaller lipid molecules (which are not soluble

TABLE 7-1

Summary of Plasma Proteins

Protein	Function
Albumins	Maintain osmotic pressure and transport smaller molecules, such as hormones and ions
Globulins	Alpha and beta globulins transport hormones and fat-soluble vitamins; gamma globulins (antibodies) bind to foreign substances
Fibrinogen	Converted into fibrin network that form blood clots

in water) renders the lipids water-soluble. This, in turn, facilitates their transport through the largely aqueous bloodstream. Carrier proteins also protect smaller molecules from destruction by the liver. These proteins are therefore essential to maintaining chemical balance in the blood and tissue fluids.

Another group of globulins, known as the **gamma globulins,** are **antibodies,** proteins that "neutralize" viruses and bacteria or target them for destruction by phagocytic cells in body tissues known as macrophages (Chapter 8).

Still another important blood protein is **fibrinogen** (fie-BRIN-oh-gin). This unique protein is converted into **fibrin** (FIE-brin), which forms blood clots in the walls of injured blood vessels. Clots prevent blood loss and thus also help maintain homeostasis.

Red Blood Cells Are Flexible, Highly Specialized Cells That Transport Oxygen and Small Amounts of Carbon Dioxide in the Blood

The **red blood cell** is the most abundant cell in human blood. In fact, 20 drops of blood (equal to 1 milliliter) contain approximately 5 billion RBCs.[3] If RBCs were people, a single milliliter of blood would contain slightly more than 80% of the world population!

Human RBCs are highly flexible, biconcave disks that transport oxygen and, to a lesser degree, carbon dioxide in the blood (**FIGURE 7-2**; **TABLE 7-2**). The unique shape of the human RBC, shown in **FIGURE 7-2**, increases

---

[2]Osmotic pressure is the force responsible for the movement of water across a selectively permeable membrane; it is created by the difference in solute concentrations on either side of the membrane. The greater the concentration difference, the greater the osmotic pressure.

[3]Many texts state the concentration of RBCs per cubic millimeter, which is about 5 million RBCs. There are 1000 cubic millimeters in 1 cubic centimeter, or 1 milliliter.

FIGURE 7-2 Red Blood Cells *(a)* Transmission electron micrograph of human RBCs showing their flexibility. *(b)* Scanning electron micrograph of human RBCs.

(b)

(a)

its surface area. The greater the surface area, the more readily gases move in and out of RBCs. Like so many other structures encountered in biology, the human RBC is a remarkable example of the marriage of form and function forged during the evolution of life on Earth.

TABLE 7-2

Summary of Blood Cells

Name	Light Micrograph	Description	Concentration (Number of Cells/mm³)	Life Span	Function
Red blood cells (RBCs)		Biconcave disk; no nucleus	4–6 million	120 days	Transports oxygen and carbon dioxide
White blood cells Neutrophil		Approximately twice the size of RBCs; multi-lobed nucleus; clear-staining cytoplasm	3000 to 7000	6 hours to a few days	Phagocytizes bacteria
Eosinophil		Approximately same size as neutrophil; large pink-staining granules; bilobed nucleus	100 to 400	8–12 days	Phagocytizes antigen-antibody complex; attacks parasites
Basophil		Slightly smaller than neutrophil; contains large, purple cytoplasmic granules; bilobed nucleus	20 to 50	Few hours to a few days	Releases histamine during inflammation
Monocyte		Larger than neutrophil; cytoplasm grayish-blue; no cytoplasmic granules; U- or kidney-shaped nucleus	100 to 700	Lasts many months	Phagocytizes bacteria, dead cells, and cellular debris
Lymphocyte		Slightly smaller than neutrophil; large, relatively round nucleus that fills the cell	1500 to 3000	Can persist many years	Involved in immune protection, either attacking cells directly or producing antibodies
Platelets		Fragments of megakaryocytes; appear as small dark-staining granules	250,000	5–10 days	Play several key roles in blood clotting

FIGURE 7-3 Sickle-Cell Anemia Scanning electron micrograph of a sickle cell.

Swept along in the bloodstream, RBCs travel many times through the circulatory system each day. As they pass through the capillaries, the RBCs bend and twist. This permits them to pass through the many miles of tiny capillaries whose internal diameters are often smaller than the RBC's.

The flexibility of RBCs is an adaptation that serves us well. However, not all people are so fortunate. According to various estimates, approximately one of every 500–1000 African Americans suffers from a disease called **sickle-cell anemia** (ah-NEEM-ee-ah). This disease results in a marked decrease in the flexibility of RBCs and is caused by a genetic mutation—a slight alteration in the hereditary material (DNA) (Chapter 16). This mutation, in turn, results in the production of hemoglobin that contains one incorrect amino acid. This small defect dramatically alters the three-dimensional structure of the hemoglobin molecule, causing RBCs to transform from biconcave disks into sickle-shaped cells when they encounter low levels of oxygen in capillaries (**FIGURE 7-3**). Sickle-shaped cells are considerably less flexible than the biconcave discs and are unable to bend and twist. As a result, the sickle cells collect at branching points in capillary beds like logs in a logjam. This blocks blood flow, disrupting the supply of nutrients and oxygen to tissues and organs. This, in turn, results in a condition known as **anoxia** (ah-NOCKS-ee-ah). Anoxia is a condition in which there's an inadequate amount of oxygen in tissues and organs. It not only causes considerable pain, the lack of oxygen can kill body cells. Thus, blockages in the lungs, heart, and brain can be life-threatening. Blockages in the heart and brain often lead to heart attacks and serious brain damage. Many people who have sickle-cell anemia die in their late twenties and thirties; some die even earlier.

On average, RBCs live about 120 days. At the end of their life span, the liver and spleen remove the aged RBCs from circulation. The iron contained in the hemoglobin, however, is recycled by these organs and used to produce new RBCs in the red bone marrow. The recycling of iron is not 100% efficient, however, so small amounts of iron must be ingested each day in the diet. Loss of blood from an injury or, in women, during menstruation, increases the body's demand for iron. Without adequate iron intake, oxygen transport may become impaired.

Human RBCs are highly specialized "cells" that lose their nuclei and organelles during cellular differentiation (**FIGURE 7-2A**). Because of this, RBCs cannot divide to replace themselves as they age. In humans, new RBCs are produced in the bone marrow. In the blood-producing bone marrow, known as **red marrow**, RBCs are produced by **stem cells**, undifferentiated cells that trace back to embryonic development. These cells give rise to 2 million RBCs per second!

In infants and children, almost all of the bone marrow is involved in the production of RBCs. As growth slows, however, the red marrow of many bones becomes inactive and gradually fills with fat cells and becomes **yellow marrow**, a fat storage depot. By the time an individual reaches adulthood, only a few bones, such as the hip bones, sternum (breastbone), ribs, and vertebrae are still engaged in RBC production. In severe, prolonged anemia, however, yellow marrow can be converted back into active red marrow.

The number of RBCs in the blood remains more or less constant over long periods. Maintaining a constant concentration of RBCs is essential to homeostasis. This process is controlled by a hormone with a rather forbidding name, **erythropoietin** (eh-RITH-row-po-EAT-in) or **EPO**. As a side note, EPO is one of a dozen or more performance-enhancing chemical substances being used by athletes.

Erythropoietin is produced by cells in the kidney when blood oxygen levels decline—for example, when a person moves to high altitudes or loses a significant amount of blood in an accident. In the red bone marrow, this hormone stimulates the stem cells to divide and multiply, thus increasing RBC production. As the RBC concentration increases, oxygen supplies increase. When oxygen levels return to normal, erythropoietin levels fall, reducing the rate of RBC formation in a classical negative feedback mechanism so common among the body's homeostatic mechanisms.

Hemoglobin Is an Oxygen-Transporting Protein Found in RBCs. Hemoglobin (HEME-oh-GLOBE-in) is a large protein molecule composed of four subunits. It is found exclusively in the RBCs. As shown in **FIGURE 7-4**, each hemoglobin subunit contains a **heme group** consisting of a large, organic ring structure,

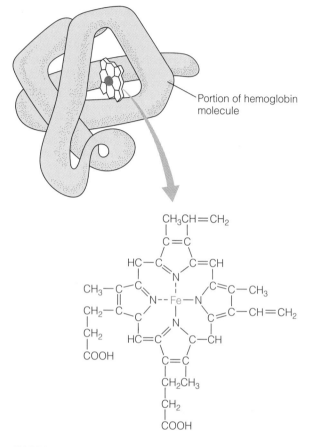

FIGURE 7-4 Porphyrin Ring The porphyrin ring of the hemoglobin molecule contains an iron ion that binds to oxygen and carbon monoxide.

called a **porphyrin ring** (POUR-for-in). In the center of the ring is an iron ion.[4]

When blood from the pulmonary arteries flows through the capillary beds of the lungs, oxygen diffuses into the plasma, then into the RBCs. Inside the RBC, oxygen binds to the iron in hemoglobin molecules for transport through the circulatory system. In fact, 98% of the oxygen in the blood is transported bound to iron in hemoglobin. Only 2% is dissolved in the blood plasma.

Carbon dioxide, a waste product of cellular respiration, also binds to hemoglobin, but to a much lesser degree. Most carbon dioxide molecules react with water in RBCs to form bicarbonate ions (HCO_3^-). This reaction is catalyzed by the enzyme **carbonic anhydrase** (car-BON-ick an-HIGH-drace) inside the RBCs. Most of the bicarbonate ions then diffuse out of the RBCs and are transported in the plasma.

[4]The iron is Fe^{++}, the ferrous ion. To be effective, iron supplements should contain ferrous iron.

Anemia Is a Condition Resulting in a Decrease in the Ability of Blood to Transport Oxygen. Homeostasis depends on the normal operation of the heart and blood vessels. It also requires that the blood be able to absorb a sufficient amount of oxygen as it passes through the lungs. Unfortunately, the oxygen-carrying capacity of the blood can be impaired by a number of conditions. A reduction in the oxygen-carrying capacity of the blood is known as **anemia** and may result from (1) a decrease in the number of circulating RBCs, (2) a reduction in the RBC hemoglobin content, or (3) the presence of abnormal hemoglobin in RBCs.

The causes of anemia are many. We will consider only a few. First, the number of RBCs in the blood may decline because of excessive bleeding or because of the presence of a tumor in the red marrow that reduces RBC production. Several infectious diseases (such as malaria) also decrease the RBC concentration in the blood. A reduction in the amount of hemoglobin in RBCs may be caused by iron deficiency or a deficiency in vitamin B-12, protein, and copper in the diet. Abnormal hemoglobin is produced in sickle-cell anemia and other genetic disorders.

Anemia generally results in weakness and fatigue. Individuals are often pale and tend to faint or become short of breath easily. People suffering from anemia often have an increased heart rate, because the heart beats faster to offset the reduction in the oxygen-carrying capacity of the blood. As a rule, anemia is not a life-threatening condition. However, it does weaken one's resistance to other diseases or injuries and also limits a person's productivity and energy level. Therefore, no matter what the cause, anemia should be treated quickly.

White Blood Cells Are a Diverse Group That Protects the Body from Infections

White blood cells (WBCs), or **leukocytes**, are nucleated cells that are part of the body's protective mechanism, a homeostatic system that combats harmful microorganisms such as bacteria and viruses. White blood cells are produced in the bone marrow and circulate in the bloodstream, but constitute less than 1% of the blood volume.

Interestingly, although WBCs are officially blood cells, they do most of their work *outside* of the bloodstream, in the tissues. The blood and circulatory system merely serve to transport the WBCs to sites of infection. When WBCs arrive at the "scene," they escape through the walls of the capillaries by "squeezing" between the endothelial cells (**FIGURE 7-5**).

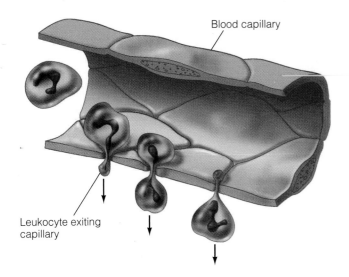

Blood capillary

Leukocyte exiting capillary

FIGURE 7-5 White Blood Cell Exit   White blood cells (leukocytes) escape from capillaries by squeezing between endothelial cells.

Aggregation of lymphocytes   Villi

Loose connective tissue

FIGURE 7-6 Lymphoid Tissue   The loose connective tissue beneath the lining of the large intestine and other sites is often packed with lymphocytes that have proliferated in response to invading bacteria.

TABLE 7-2 lists and describes the five types of WBCs found in the blood. The three most numerous, which are discussed here, are neutrophils, monocytes, and lymphocytes.

Neutrophils (NEW-trow-fills) are the most abundant of the WBCs. Approximately twice the size of the RBC, these cells are distinguished by their multi-lobed nuclei. So named because their cytoplasm has a low affinity for stains, neutrophils circulate in the blood like a cellular police force awaiting microbial invasion. Attracted by chemicals released by infected tissue, neutrophils escape from the bloodstream, then migrate to the site of infection by amoeboid movement. Neutrophils are usually the first WBCs to arrive on the scene. When they arrive, they immediately begin to engulf (phagocytize) microorganisms, thereby preventing the spread of bacteria and other organisms from the site of invasion. When a neutrophil's lysosomes are used up, the cell dies and becomes part of the yellowish liquid, or **pus,** that exudes from wounds. Pus is a mixture of dead neutrophils, cellular debris, and bacteria, both living and dead.

Monocytes (MON-oh-sites) are also phagocytic cells. Slightly larger than neutrophils, monocytes contain distinctive U-shaped or kidney-shaped nuclei. Like neutrophils, monocytes leave the bloodstream to do their "work" and migrate through body tissues via amoeboid motion. Once at the site of an infection, they begin phagocytizing microorganisms, dead cells, and dead neutrophils. Thus, while neutrophils are the "first-line" troops, monocytes constitute something of a mop-up crew.

Monocytes also take up residence in connective tissues of the body, where they are referred to as **macrophages** (MACK-row-FAY-ges). These cells remain more or less stationary, like watchful soldiers ever ready to attack and phagocytize invaders.

The second most abundant WBC is the **lymphocyte.** Although they are found in the blood, most lymphocytes exist outside the circulatory system in **lymphoid organs** (LIM-foid). This includes organs such as the spleen, thymus, and lymph nodes, and lymphoid tissue. Aggregations of lymphocytes also exist beneath the lining of the intestinal and respiratory tracts. It is in these locations that lymphocytes attack microbial intruders (**FIGURE 7-6**). Unlike neutrophils and monocytes, these cells are not phagocytic.

Two types of lymphocytes are found in the body. The first type is the **T lymphocyte,** or **T cell.** T cells attack foreign cells such as fungi, parasites, and tumor cells directly.[5] They are thus said to provide cellular immunity.

The second type is called the **B lymphocyte,** or **B cell.** When activated, B cells transform into another

[5]The T lymphocytes usually attack large eukaryotic cells such as fungi and parasites. Most bacteria are controlled by antibodies. Only the few bacteria that are intracellular parasites, such as *M. tuberculosis,* are attacked by T cells, but even then, the lymphocyte attacks the host cell, not the bacterium directly.

kind of cell, known as the plasma cells. **Plasma cells,** in turn, synthesize and release antibodies, proteins that circulate in the blood and bind to foreign substances. The binding of antibodies to "foreigners" coats them and neutralizes them. Or, it marks microorganisms and tumor cells for destruction by macrophages (Chapter 8).

Like the other formed elements of blood, the WBCs are involved in homeostasis. Their numbers can increase greatly during a microbial infection and other diseases. In fighting off a disease, they help return the body to normal function.

An increase in the number of WBCs, called **leukocytosis** (lew-co-sigh-TOE-siss), is a normal homeostatic response to intruders. It ends when the microbial invaders have been destroyed. Increases and decreases in various types of WBCs can be used to diagnose many medical disorders. For example, a dramatic increase in lymphocytes and lower abdominal pain are usually signs of appendicitis (Chapter 5). Because variations in the WBC count accompany many diseases, a blood test is a standard procedure for patients undergoing diagnostic testing.

Diseases Involving WBCs Also Affect the Body's Internal Balance. Like many other components of homeostasis, WBCs can go awry. For example, some WBCs can become cancerous, dividing uncontrollably in the bone marrow, then entering the bloodstream. A cancer of WBCs is called **leukemia** (lew-KEEM-ee-ah;

FIGURE 7-7 Rosy Periwinkle Many tropical plants contain chemicals that provide extraordinary medical benefits. One substance from the rosy periwinkle has helped physicians treat leukemia. Unfortunately, the tropical rain forests are being cut at an alarming rate, reducing our chances of finding other cures.

literally, "white blood"). The most serious type of leukemia is acute leukemia, so named because it kills victims quickly. Children are the primary victims of this disease.

In acute leukemia, WBCs fill the bone marrow, crowding out the cells that produce RBCs and platelets. This results in a decline in the production of RBCs, which leads to anemia. It also results in a reduction in platelet production, which reduces clotting and increases internal bleeding. Making matters worse, the cancerous WBCs produced in leukemia are often incapable of fighting infection. Leukemia patients typically succumb to infections and internal bleeding.

(a)

(b)

FIGURE 7-8 Forest Destruction *(a)* Rampant deforestation not only leaves the tropics denuded, but also robs humankind of many potential cures for disease. *(b)* The loss of forests and other habitats in the industrial countries is also of grave importance. The bark of this tree, the Pacific yew, contains a chemical that may prove effective in fighting breast cancer. However, each year thousands of acres of old-growth forest, where the tree lives, are cut down.

Leukemia can be treated by irradiating the bone marrow and by administering a drug called vincristine (VIN-chris-teen) that stops mitosis. Twenty-five years ago, only one of every four children with leukemia survived. Today, thanks to vincristine, three of every four children with the disease survive! Vincristine was discovered in a plant known as the rosy periwinkle found in tropical rain forests (**FIGURE 7-7**). Thousands of other drugs have come from other tropical plants, underscoring the importance of protecting the rain forests (**FIGURE 7-8**).

Another common disorder of the WBCs is **infectious mononucleosis** (MON-oh-NUKE-clee-OH-siss), commonly called "mono" or "kissing disease." Mono is caused by a virus transmitted through saliva and may be spread by kissing; by sharing silverware, plates, and drinking glasses; and possibly even through drinking fountains. The virus spreads through the body. In the blood, the virus infects only lymphocytes in the bloodstream; however, the number of monocytes and lymphocytes both increase rapidly during an infection. Individuals suffering from mono complain of fatigue, aches, sore throats, and low-grade fever. Physicians recommend that victims get plenty of rest and drink lots of liquids while the immune system eliminates the virus. Within a few weeks, symptoms generally disappear, although weakness may persist for two more weeks.

Platelets Are a Vital Component of the Blood-Clotting Mechanism

The capillaries are rather delicate structures. Even minor bumps and scrapes can cause them to leak. Fortunately, leakage is quickly halted by blood clotting, surely

one of the most intricate homeostatic systems to have evolved. A simplified version is discussed here.

Among the most important agents of blood clotting are the **platelets,** tiny formed elements produced in the bone marrow by fragmentation of a huge cell known as the **megakaryocyte** (MEG-ah-CARE-ee-oh-site) (**FIGURE 7-9**). Like RBCs, platelets lack nuclei and organelles and therefore are not true cells. Also like RBCs, platelets are unable to divide. Carried passively in the bloodstream, platelets are coated by a layer of a sticky material, which causes them to adhere to irregular surfaces such as tears in blood vessels or atherosclerotic plaque.

Clotting is a chain reaction stimulated by the release of a chemical called **thromboplastin** (THROM-bow-PLASS-tin) from injured cells lining damaged blood vessels (**FIGURE 7-10A**). Thromboplastin is a lipoprotein that acts on an inactive plasma enzyme in the blood known as **prothrombin** (produced by the liver). Thromboplastin causes prothrombin to be converted into its active form, **thrombin.** Thrombin, in turn, acts on another blood protein, **fibrinogen,** also produced by the liver. When activated, fibrinogen is converted into **fibrin,** long, branching fibers that produce a weblike network in the wall of the damaged blood vessel (**FIGURE 7-10B**). The fibrin web traps RBCs and platelets, forming a plug that stops the flow of blood to the tissue. Platelets captured by the fibrin web release additional thromboplastin, known as **platelet thromboplastin,** which causes more fibrin to be laid down, thus reinforcing the fibrin network. You may want to take a look at **FIGURE 7-10A** to review these steps.

Blood clotting occurs fairly quickly. In most cases, a damaged blood vessel is sealed by a clot within 3–6 minutes of an injury; 30–60 minutes later, platelets in the clot begin to draw the clot inward, stitching the wound together. How do they perform this remarkable task?

Platelets contain contractile proteins like those in muscle cells. Contraction of the protein fibers draws the fibrin network inward, pulling the edges of the cut or damaged blood vessel together. This closes the wound like a surgical stitch.

Blood clots do not stay in place indefinitely. If they did, the circulatory system would eventually become clogged, and blood flow would come to a halt. Instead, clots are dissolved by a blood-borne enzyme known as **plasmin** (PLAZ-min), which is produced from an inactive form, **plasminogen** (plaz-MIN-oh-gin). Plasminogen is incorporated in the clot as it forms. It is then gradually converted to plasmin by an activating factor secreted by the endothelial cells of the blood vessel. This ensures that the plasmin dissolves the clot after the blood vessel damage has been repaired.

Megakaryocyte   Platelets

FIGURE 7-9 Megakaryocyte A light micrograph of a megakaryocyte, a large, multinucleated cell found in bone marrow; the megakaryocyte fragments, giving rise to platelets.

Injured cells
in wall of vessel
release ①

Plasma

Thromboplastin

Prothrombin
converts to ②

Thrombin

Fibrinogen
converts to

Platelets release
platelet
thromboplastin ⑤

③

④

RBCs and platelets
trapped

Fibrin
network

(a)

(b)

FIGURE 7-10 Blood Clotting Simplified *(a)* Injured cells in the walls of blood vessels release the chemical thromboplastin (1). Thromboplastin stimulates the conversion of prothrombin, found in the plasma, into thrombin (2). Thrombin, in turn, stimulates the conversion of the plasma protein fibrinogen into fibrin (3). The fibrin network captures RBCs and platelets (4). Platelets in the blood clot release platelet thromboplastin (5), which converts additional plasma prothrombin into thrombin. Thrombin, in turn, stimulates the production of additional fibrin. *(b)* A scanning electron micrograph of a fibrin clot that has already trapped platelets and RBCs, plugging a leak in a vessel. The RBCs are red, and the fibrin network is turquoise.

As important as blood clots are in protecting the body, clotting can also cause problems. For example, blood clots can break loose from their site of formation, circulate in the blood, and become lodged in arteries, especially those narrowed by plaque. In such cases, the blood clots restrict blood flow, causing considerable damage to tissues served by the vessel. Blood clots typically lodge in the narrow vessels serving the heart muscle, brain, and other vital organs.

Clotting Disorders Not Only Upset the Homeostatic Balance, They Can Be Life-Threatening. In some individuals, blood clotting is impaired because of: (1) an insufficient number of platelets; (2) liver damage that hinders the production of clotting factors; or (3) mutations that reduce the production of clotting factors.

A reduced platelet count may result from leukemia (noted earlier). It may also result from an exposure to excess radiation, which damages bone marrow where the megakaryocytes reside. Liver damage, which impairs the production of blood-clotting factors, can be caused by hepatitis, liver cancer, or excessive alcohol consumption. The most common genetic defect is **hemophilia** (he-moe-FEAL-ee-ah), a disease in which the liver fails to produce the necessary clotting factors. Problems begin early in life, and even tiny cuts or bruises can bleed uncontrollably, threatening one's life. Because of repeated bleeding into the joints, victims suffer great pain and often become disabled; they often die at a young age.

Hemophiliacs can be treated by transfusions of blood-clotting factors. This therapy, however, is expensive and is required every few days. It has also put hemophiliacs at risk for AIDS, acquired immunodeficiency syndrome, which is caused by a virus transmitted primarily by sexual contact (Chapter 8). The AIDS virus invades certain white blood cells, known as **helper T cells,** resulting in a gradual deterioration of the immune function. For years, AIDS has been considered

100% fatal—that is, everyone who gets it eventually dies. Although it is too early to tell, new treatments may change the prognosis.

Unfortunately, testing for the AIDS virus began late, and many transfusions of whole blood, blood plasma, and clotting factors were contaminated by the virus. Clotting factors produced by genetic engineering, however, have eliminated the need for transfusions of clotting agents taken from whole blood, reducing the risk to hemophiliacs of contracting AIDS.

Health, Homeostasis, and the Environment

Carbon Monoxide

The blood is vitally important to homeostasis. It transports materials, especially oxygen, to and from the cells. It protects against changes in pH. It transports excess heat to the body's surface, where it is eliminated. It plays a key role in the body's defense system, and it seals injuries in blood vessels through clots.

It is no surprise then to learn that cells depend mightily on the proper functioning of blood. Anything that upsets this function can upset cellular function throughout the body. A good example is carbon monoxide gas, a pollutant produced from many sources in our society.

Carbon monoxide (CO) is a colorless, odorless gas produced by the incomplete combustion of organic fuels. It emanates from stoves and furnaces in our homes and spews out of the tailpipes of our automobiles, causing increased levels along streets and highways, in parking garages, and in tunnels. It pours out of power plants and factory smokestacks, polluting the air in our cities. It is even a major pollutant in tobacco smoke. According to estimates by the Environmental Protection Agency, over 40 million Americans (one of every six people) are exposed to levels of CO harmful to their health.

What makes CO so dangerous? Carbon monoxide, like oxygen, binds to hemoglobin. However, hemoglobin has a much greater affinity for CO than for oxygen (about 200 times greater). Consequently, CO "outcompetes" oxygen for the binding sites on the hemoglobin molecules and reduces the blood's ability to carry oxygen, which is essential for energy production.

For healthy people, low levels of CO in their blood do not create much of a problem. Their bodies simply produce more RBCs or increase the heart rate to augment the flow of oxygen to tissues. CO does create a problem, however, when levels are so high that the body cannot compensate, and at very high levels, CO becomes deadly.

New research suggests that CO levels currently deemed acceptable by federal standards can trigger chest pain (angina) in active adults with coronary artery disease. Chest pains result from a lack of oxygen in the heart muscle. Levels such as those once thought safe in many workplaces or levels in the blood encountered after 1 hour in heavy traffic cause angina and abnormal ECGs in these people.

In levels commonly found in and around cities, CO is also troublesome for the elderly. Carbon monoxide places additional strain on their hearts, making the already weakened organ work harder. Thus, the elderly and people suffering from cardiovascular disease are advised to stay inside on high-pollution days.

Carbon monoxide is just one of many pollutants we breathe. No one knows what, if any, long-term effects it might have on our health. In the short term, however, it is clear that CO upsets oxygen delivery, which is essential to homeostasis in all of us, and especially in the elderly and the infirm. It has become another risk factor in an increasingly risky society, but it is not an insolvable problem. Much more efficient automobiles, widespread use of mass transit, overall reductions in driving, and alternative automobile fuels (such as hydrogen) can all reduce the level of CO in and around the cities. More efficient factories, home furnaces, and power plants can also reduce CO levels in emissions. Passive-solar homes and improvements in insulation can also cut our demand for fossil fuel energy. Bans on smoking indoors could go a long way, too, in ridding our air of this transparent killer.

Summary

Blood: Its Composition and Functions

1. *Blood* is a watery tissue consisting of two basic components: the *plasma,* a fluid that contains dissolved nutrients, proteins, gases, and wastes, and the *formed elements,* red blood cells, white blood cells, and platelets, which are suspended in the plasma.

2. The functions of the formed elements are listed in **TABLE 7-2**.

3. The plasma constitutes about 55% of the volume of a person's blood, and the formed elements make up the remainder. The volume occupied by the blood cells and platelets is called the *hematocrit.*

4. *Red blood cells (RBCs)* are highly specialized cells that lack nuclei and organelles. Produced by the red bone marrow, RBCs transport oxygen in the blood.

5. The concentration of RBCs in the blood is maintained by the hormone *erythropoietin,* produced by the kidneys in response to falling oxygen levels.

6. *White blood cells (WBCs)* are nucleated cells and are part of the body's protective mechanism to combat microorganisms. WBCs are produced in the bone marrow and circulate in the bloodstream but do most of their work outside it, in the body tissues.

7. The most abundant WBCs are the *neutrophils,* which are attracted by chemicals released from infected tissue. Neutrophils leave the bloodstream and migrate to the site of infection by amoeboid movement.

8. Neutrophils are the first WBCs to arrive at the site of an infection, where they phagocytize microorganisms, preventing the spread of bacteria and other organisms.

9. The second group of cells to arrive are the *monocytes,* which phagocytize microorganisms, dead cells, cellular debris, and dead neutrophils.

10. *Lymphocytes* are the second most numerous WBCs and play a vital role in immune protection.

11. *Platelets* are fragments of large bone marrow cells and are involved in blood clotting.

12. Platelets are coated by a layer of a sticky material, which causes them to adhere to irregular surfaces such as tears in blood vessels. Blood clotting is summarized in **FIGURE 7-10**.

Health, Homeostasis, and the Environment: Carbon Monoxide

13. Carbon monoxide is produced by the incomplete combustion of organic fuels in our homes, automobiles, factories, and power plants.

14. Carbon monoxide binds to hemoglobin and reduces the oxygen-carrying capacity of the blood, which impairs cellular energy production, upsetting homeostasis.

15. At high concentrations, carbon monoxide can be lethal. At lower concentrations, it is harmful to people with cardiovascular disease and lung disease. For individuals with heart disease, it puts additional strain on the heart.

Critical Thinking

Thinking Critically— Analysis

This Analysis corresponds to the Thinking Critically scenario that was presented at the beginning of this chapter.

The researchers themselves freely admit that this study only looks at the effect of lipoprotein(a) on smooth muscle cells grown in laboratory culture dishes. They have not yet determined whether the effect occurs in the body itself.

Caution is advised when examining studies of cells and tissues in culture. Although studies in tissue culture are essential to medical science, it's important to remember that a culture dish is an artificial environment. Because of this, such studies may lead to erroneous conclusions. This exercise requires one to scrutinize the experimental method.

Test of Concepts

1. Describe the structure and function of each of the following: red blood cells, platelets, lymphocytes, monocytes, and neutrophils.

2. Define each of the following terms: leukemia, anemia, and infectious mononucleosis.

3. Explain how a blood clot forms and how it helps prevent bleeding.

4. Describe the many ways blood participates in homeostasis. How can these homeostatic mechanisms be upset?

www.jbpub.com/humanbiology

Connect to this book's web site: www.jbpub.com/humanbiology
The site features eLearning, an online review area that provides quizzes, chapter outlines, and other tools to help you study for your class. You can also follow useful links for in-depth information, research the differing views in the Point/Counterpoints, or keep up on the latest environmental and health news.

CHAPTER 8

The Immune System

Electron micrograph of a macrophage binding to three tumor cells.

Thinking Critically

You're the parent of a young child and are debating whether to have your child vaccinated. Some friends tell you that it's dangerous—that in the past some children have been paralyzed by vaccinations. They also tell you that vaccination damages the immune system and that there's no need to subject a child to this treatment because the truly dangerous infectious diseases have been eliminated.

After reading this chapter, how would you respond? Is there merit to the claim that a vaccination damages the immune system? Have the diseases been eliminated? Do you have enough information to make an informed decision? ■

Each day as you venture outside your home, you are entering a war zone. Floating in the air and circulating in the water are billions upon billions of microorganisms. Although the vast majority of the bacteria and viruses in our environment are innocuous, there are a few that are not, especially if you are traveling in a busy airport or walking on a crowded city street.

Why don't we succumb to this sea of potentially dangerous microorganisms? The answer is that humans come equipped with a rather elaborate armor (the skin and other protective layers) that protects us from potential intruders. If a microorganism breaks through this armor, there's an internal force ready to combat them. That's the immune system.

In this chapter, we'll examine the body's protective measures.. We will also see how the body's defense mechanisms work again cancer, AIDS, and tissue or organ transplants. To set the stage for understanding the body's protective mechanisms, we begin with a brief overview of infectious agents.

Section 8-1

Viruses and Bacteria: An Introduction

We humans live in a virtual sea of microorganisms. All around us are bacteria and viruses. But as noted, most of them are pretty harmless.

Viruses Are Nonliving Biological Agents That Consist of a Nucleic Acid Core and a Layer of Protein Molecules and Take Over Cells' Metabolic Machinery to Produce More of Their Kind.

Viruses are the simplest of the two. Viruses are composed of a nucleic acid core, consisting of either DNA or RNA (**FIGURE 8-1**). Surrounding the nucleic acid core is a protein coat known as the **capsid**. Some viruses have an additional protective layer, an outer envelope that lies peripheral to the capsid. This layer, the envelope, is structurally similar to the plasma membranes of eukaryotic cells.

Viruses are an enigma to scientists. They are not even considered to be living things because they do not possess many of the features we attribute to living organisms. For example, viruses cannot multiply and divide like cells on their own. They also have no metabolism. However, they can cause enormous problems.

Viruses have been likened to pirates because they invade cells and then commandeer their metabolic machinery in much the same way that pirates take over ships. Viruses have very simple demands, however.

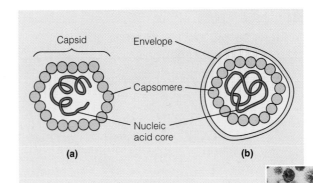

FIGURE 8-1 General Structure of a Virus *(a)* The virus consists of a nucleic acid core of either RNA or DNA. Surrounding the viral core is a layer of protein known as the capsid. Each protein molecule in the capsid is known as a capsomere. *(b)* Some viruses have an additional protective coat known as the envelope. *(c)* Electron micrograph of the Human Immunodeficiency Virus (HIV).

When they comandeer a cell, their sole purpose is to reproduce. Thus, viruses convert host cells into miniature virus factories. They use the cell's organelles and its biochemical reserves to make new protein and nucleic acid. Inside the host cell, hundreds of thousands of new viruses are formed. They soon begin to be released from the cell, spreading to other cells through the bloodstream and the lymphatic vessels. So completely spent is the host cell that it dies.

Viruses most often enter the body through the respiratory and digestive systems. However, other avenues of entry are also possible—for example, sexual contact.

Fortunately for us, the immune system (discussed more fully later) kills many viruses, but usually not until we've undergone considerable suffering. Influenza viruses, for example, result in the flu, which is characterized by fevers, chills, headaches, and muscle pains that can last up to two weeks (see **TABLE 8-1**: How Do I Know If I Have a Cold or the Flu?). During this time, the immune system mounts an attack, but it usually takes 10 to 14 days before it can eliminate the virus (unless you've been vaccinated for it). Colds are also caused by approximately 200 different viruses. Like the flu, colds cannot be treated with antibiotics.

Some viruses, like the two that cause fever blisters and genital herpes, evade the immune system. They take refuge in body cells, reemerging from time to time to cause problems, usually when we're under stress or some other influence. The virus responsible for genital herpes (HER-pees), for example, causes tiny sores that emerge periodically on the genitals, thighs, and buttocks of infected men and women

TABLE 8-1

How Do You Know If You Have A Cold or the Flu?

Symptoms	Cold	Flu
Onset	Gradual	Sudden
Fever	Rare	Common, may reach 101˚F; may last 3 to 4 days
Headache	Rare	Common and can be severe
Cough	Hacking	Dry cough
Muscle aches and pains	Slight	Typical, often severe
Tiredness and weakness	Mild	Common, often severe
Chest discomfort	Mild to moderate	Common
Stuffy nose	Common	Sometimes
Sneezing	Usual	Sometimes
Sore throat	Common	Sometimes; may last 3 to 4 days
Caused by	Any of 200 viruses	Influenza virus

Bacteria Are Prokaryotic Cells That Reproduce on Their Own; Many Bacteria Perform Useful Functions, While Others Cause Serious Diseases.

As noted earlier, viruses are not considered living organisms, because they cannot reproduce on their own,

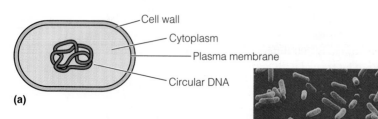

(a)

FIGURE 8-2 General Structure of a Bacterium
(a) Bacteria come in many shapes and sizes, but all have a circular strand of DNA, cytoplasm, and a plasma membrane. Surrounding the membrane of many bacteria is a cell wall.
(b) Electon micrograph of samonella bacteria.   **(b)**

and unless they've invaded a host cell, they cannot metabolize. In contrast, **bacteria** (singular, bacterium) are classified living organisms. They are capable of reproducing without taking over host cells. In fact, unlike viruses, bacteria do not enter cells. They proliferate outside of cells.

As pointed out in Chapter 3, bacteria are prokaryotes. As you may recall, the term prokaryotes refers to cells without nuclei. In these cells, the genetic material consists of a circular strand of DNA, not bound by any kind of membrane. Prokaryotes have cytoplasm, which is enveloped by a plasma membrane, but no cellular organelles like eukaryotic cells (**FIGURE 8-2**). Outside the plasma membrane of bacteria is a thick, rigid **cell wall**. Many bacteria also contain tiny circular pieces of extrachromosomal DNA, called **plasmids**.

Like viruses, bacteria enter the body through the respiratory tract and GI tract. They may also enter through the epithelium of the urinary system. Cuts and abrasions in the skin also permit bacteria to enter the body. Inside the body, bacteria proliferate, using nutrients to make more of their kind. Some bacteria produce toxins, substances that make us ill.

Bacteria Respond to Antibiotics Although Many Have Become Resistant to Commonly Used Antibiotics; Viruses Do Not, But New Antiviral Drugs May Help Flu Sufferers

Bacteria have proven to be easily manipulated by drugs. Antibiotics, a large group of chemical substances, for example, have proven to be quite effective in combatting bacterial infections. Antibiotics inhibit protein synthesis in bacteria selectively. That is, they are able to alter protein synthesis in bacteria, but not the cells of the body. These target-specific compounds, therefore, can be used to kill invading bacteria.

Unfortunately, the heavy use of antibiotics (often when they're not useful, as in a viral infection) has resulted in a growing problem: antibiotic resistance in bacteria. Many thousands of people die each year of infections caused by antibiotic-resistant bacteria they contract in hospitals or in other places. Nationwide, one out of every four bacterial infections today involves a resistant strain. Most of these infections occur in children under the age of five. To treat them, doctors must use stronger doses or newer antibiotics. Even then, bacteria may exhibit resistance. Because of this, some doctors in Great Britain and the United States are now using maggots to clean wounds and destroy bacteria as explained in Health Note 8-1.

Bacteria can become resistant to drugs in one of several ways. They can, for example, chemically alter antibiotics, rendering them ineffective. Bacteria also undergo chemical changes so that antibiotics no longer bind to them. Some resistance occurs when bacteria develop mechanisms that permit them to pump antibiotics out of their interior, lowering internal concentrations so much that the drugs are no longer effective.

Making matters worse, researchers are also finding antibiotics (and other drugs) in treated sewage released into our waterways. This exposure is resulting in additional antibiotic-resistant strains of bacteria.

The important lesson in all of this is not to overindulge in antibiotics. Individuals can help, and so can doctors. Thanks to educational campaigns waged by the Centers for Disease Control, state health agencies, and various medical groups, many doctors now are becoming much more reluctant to give antibiotics to patients suffering from viral infections, even though the patient clearly wants an antibiotic, which is ineffective against viruses.

For the flu, doctors prescribe medicines that reduce some of the symptoms, such as acetaminophen to reduce fever, muscle aches, and headaches. Bed rest helps you heal, too, and warm fluids like tea will reduce the feeling of congestion while your immune system battles the virus. Stay home, when sick, too. This reduces the chances that you'll spread the virus to others.

For colds, bed rest in a warm house is advised. Drink fluids and take over-the-counter remedies to reduce symptoms such as a cough. Mild pain relievers can rid you of muscle pain and headaches, if you have them. Decongestants can help you relieve the stuffy nose and will help you breathe better.

In recent years, pharmaceutical companies have released anti-viral drugs such as Tamiflu. The first of their kind, these drugs actually attack the influenza virus. To be effective, however, antiviral drugs must be taken early in the disease, within a day or two of the onset of symptoms.

Flu shots are helpful. They're used to prevent the flu in the first place. Flu shots are a vaccine that prevents the influenza virus from gaining a foothold. Vaccines are discussed in more detail later in the chapter.

Antibiotics are used for bacterial pneumonia, bronchitis, sinus infections, and sore throats. Because all of these diseases can be caused by viruses, too, a doctor should be consulted. She can usually tell whether the infection is viral or bacterial. If it is bacterial, she'll prescribe antibiotics.

Because so many bacteria are resistant to antibiotics, medical researchers are working on a new family of antibiotics called *ketolides*. Chemically different from currently used drugs, these substances will be given once a day for five days. Researchers and drug companies that support them hope that this will reduce the likelihood that bacteria will become resistant to them. Only time will tell, but I wouldn't bet on it.

Individuals can help in the battle against bugs, too. When a doctor says you have a viral infection and that an antibiotic won't work, don't insist on one. But be careful, if the viral infection persists for more than two weeks, secondary bacterial infections can set in. Antibiotics are needed to fight them off.

Because bacteria and viruses can cause illness, many people assume that the best way to keep a child healthy is to protect him from exposure. Over the years, manufacturers have fueled what scientists now think is a misconception, some even say even a dangerous one. Manufacturers have produced a variety of cleaning agents designed to keep our homes germ free. In recent years, antibacterial dish and hand soaps have emerged.

Unfortunately, research is suggesting that the best way to develop a healthy immune system is to use it when you're young. That is, the best way to ensure maximum health is not to protect a child from exposure to non-life-threatening microbes. Although this idea seemed preposterous when first proposed, more and more evidence is showing that children who've been sheltered from normal childhood illnesses develop more asthma and allergies—a lot more! In fact, a study released in 2000 showed that infants who go to day care centers or who have older siblings—both of which increase their risk of catching colds or the flu—are less likely to develop asthma later in childhood than those who stay at home. The reason for this is not known, but researchers believe that early exposure to common microbes, even nonpathogenic ones, may somehow start the immune system off on the right path of development.

Small families, good sanitation, and widespread use of antibiotics, say researchers, reduce childhood exposure to bacteria and viruses. This may be responsible for the dramatic increase in allergies and asthma in the United States and other developed countries. The advice given now is not to sterilize the worlds we live in and not to protect children from common microbes they'd pick up at day care or school.

Although best known for their role in causing sickness and death, most bacteria perform useful functions. Soil bacteria, for example, help recycle nutrients in rotting plants and animals. Although this may not seem like a glamorous occupation, it's absolutely essential to the continuation of life on Earth. Without these bacteria, biological systems would quickly grind to a halt. Some of the biologically useful bacteria will be discussed in Chapter 23.

This chapter concerns itself primarily with harmful bacteria that invade the human body and the body's defensive mechanisms. The mechanisms that evolved to protect multicellular organisms such as humans from the hordes of potentially harmful microorganisms fall into three categories—or three lines of defense.

Health Note 8-1

Maggots: The Latest in Medical Care?

Elainor Brocknor is a diabetic who for 30 years has been injecting the hormone insulin to regulate her blood sugar. Careful as she has been, she's developed serious medical problems. The blood vessels in her feet have been damaged by periodic high concentrations of glucose. The tissues in two of her toes has begun to die and rot. She's developed gangrene and doctors fear they may have to amputate two of her toes and perhaps even her foot if the infection does not stop. Making matters worse, the bacteria infecting the dying tissues in her feet don't seem to respond to antibiotics.

One day her doctor makes a bizarre recommendation. He says he may be able to save her foot by using maggots. Maggots are the immature form of common ordinary flies. They're called larvae. They develop from eggs laid by flies. They're voracious eaters.

Elainor and her husband are mortified, at first, by the doctor's seemingly crazy suggestion. What a preposterous idea! But the doctor explains that maggots, raised in a sterile environment have been used very successfully to remove dead tis-

sue in people with gangrene. They not only feed on dead tissue, they gobble up harmful bacteria, so the infection doesn't spread.

Reluctant, Elainor agrees to try the procedure. The next day, her doctor visits her in her hospital room. He's carrying a glass jar full of writhing maggots. He removes the bandages from her feet, then prepares a new one. On the surface of the gauze, the physician sprinkles 100 tiny maggots. He then places the bandage over her wound and tapes it shut.

Elainor watches in amazement and is surprised that she feels nothing at all. A day later, the doctor returns, removes the bandage, and applies another. In a few days, he announces that the wound is clean and infection free. They won't have to amputate.

Elainor is just one of thousands of people each year treated with maggots. In this day of high-tech medicine, such an approach may seem ridiculously primitive. Problem is, it works when high-tech solutions don't. And it is saving many people the agony of amputation.

The idea of using maggots to clean wounds is an old one. During the Civil War, doctors who treated wounded

soldiers noticed that wounds in men returning from the battlefields several days away were often infested with maggots. They'd come from eggs flies had laid in open wounds. Surprisingly, the maggot-filled wounds were remarkably clean.

In Africa, rural doctors noticed a similar phenomenon. In modern times, doctors have found that when they removed maggots from wounds and put a patient on antibiotics, the patients died–apparently from antibiotic-resistant bacteria that had been under control. Maggots aren't the only creepy cure. Some doctors are using leeches to restore blood flow in severed limbs or fingers that have been sewn back in place (see Health Note 6-1). Others are using bees and bee venom to treat patients with multiple sclerosis. Both leeches and bees are turning out to be valuable tools in the doctor's medical bag.

Visit *Human Biology's* Internet site for links to web sites offering more information on this topic.

Section 8-2

The First and Second Lines of Defense

In Humans, the First Line of Defense Consists of the Skin; Epithelial Linings of the Respiratory, Digestive, and Urinary Systems; and Body Secretions That Destroy Harmful Microorganisms

The human body is like a fort with an outer barrier that wards off potential invaders. One component of this outer wall is the skin, a protective layer that repels many potentially harmful microorganisms.

As noted in Chapter 4, the skin consists of a relatively thick and impermeable layer of epidermal cells overlying the rich vascular layer, the dermis. Epidermal cells are produced by cell division in the base of the epidermis. As the basal cells proliferate, they move outward, become flattened, and die. The dead cells contain a protein called **keratin** (CARE-ah-tin). Keratin forms a fairly waterproof protective layer that not only reduces moisture loss, but also protects underlying tissues from microorganisms. The cells of the epidermis are joined by special structures known as **tight junctions**, which impede water loss and microbial penetration.

The skin protects the outer surfaces of the human body, but the human body contains three passageways that penetrate into its interior, making protection difficult. The passages into the interior are the respiratory, digestive, and urinary tracts. All three of them are protected by epithelial linings, which usually keep potentially harmful microorganisms from invading the underlying tissues. A break in these linings, however, permits microorganisms to enter.

The body's first line of defense consists of more than passive physical barriers. It also actively engages in "chemical warfare." For instance, the skin produces slightly acidic secretions that impair bacterial growth. The stomach lining produces hydrochloric acid, which destroys many ingested bacteria. Tears and saliva contain an enzyme called **lysozyme** (LIE-so-zime) that dissolves the cell wall of bacteria, killing them. Cells in the lining of the respiratory tract produce mucus, which has antimicrobial properties. These protective mechanisms are all nonspecific. Like a castle wall, they operate indiscriminately against all invaders.

The Body's Second Line of Defense Combats Infectious Agents That Penetrate the First Line and Consists of Cellular and Chemical Responses

The first line of defense is not impenetrable. Even tiny breaks in the skin or in the lining of the respiratory, digestive, or urinary tracts permit viruses, bacteria, and other microorganisms to enter the body. Fortunately, a second line of defense exists. It involves a host of chemicals and cellular agents that work together to combat invaders. Like the first line, these mechanisms are nonspecific. This section discusses four components of the second line of defense: the inflammatory response, pyrogens, interferons, and complement.

The Inflammatory Response Is a Major Part of the Second Line of Defense and Involves Chemical and Cellular Responses. Damage to body tissues triggers a series of reactions collectively referred to as an **inflammatory response.** Not a string of expletives released in anger, the inflammatory response is a protective mechanism. The word *inflammatory* refers to the heat given off by a wound. The inflammatory response is also characterized by redness, swelling, and pain.

The inflammatory response is a kind of chemical and biological warfare waged against bacteria, viruses, and other microorganisms. It begins with the release of a variety of chemical substances by the injured tissue (**FIG-URE 8-3**). Some chemicals attract macrophages that reside in body tissues and neutrophils in the blood (Chapter 7). These cells phagocytize bacteria that have

entered the wound. Soon after these cells begin to work, a yellowish fluid begins to exude from the wound. Called **pus,** it contains dead white blood cells (mostly neutrophils), microorganisms, and cellular debris, which accumulate at the site of inflammation.

Other chemical substances released by injured tissues cause blood vessels to dilate (expand) and leak (**FIGURE 8-3**). One such substance is **histamine** (HISS-tah-mean). Histamine stimulates the arterioles in the injured tissue to dilate, causing the capillary networks to swell with blood.[1] The increase in the flow of blood through an injured tissue is responsible for the heat and redness around a cut or abrasion. Heat, in turn, increases the metabolic rate of cells in the injured area and accelerates healing.

Still other substances released by injured tissues increase the permeability of capillaries, augmenting the flow of plasma into a wounded region. Plasma carries with it oxygen and nutrients that facilitate healing. It also carries the molecules necessary for blood clotting. As noted in Chapter 7, the clotting mechanism walls off injured vessels and reduces blood loss.

As illustrated in **FIGURE 8-3**, plasma leaking into injured tissues causes swelling, which stimulates pain receptors in the area. Pain receptors send nerve impulses to the brain. Pain also results from chemical toxins released by bacteria and from chemicals released by injured cells themselves. One important pain-causing chemical is **prostaglandin** (PROSS-tah-GLAN-din). Aspirin and other mild painkillers work by inhibiting the synthesis and release of prostaglandins.

Although it evokes pain, the flow of fluid into body tissues is helpful. Injury to joints, for example, results in local swelling that helps immobilize joints. In effect, swelling is nature's way of protecting joints and allowing tissues to mend. Inflammation even comes equipped with its own cleanup crew in the form of late-arriving monocytes that phagocytize dead cells, cell fragments, dead bacteria, and viruses. Take a moment to study **FIGURE 8-3** to review the inflammatory response.

The Second Line of Defense Consists of Three Additional Chemicals. In a nuclear power plant, safety is ensured in part by redundant systems—that is, backup systems that kick in if the main systems fail. In the human body, redundant systems also exist, but not as a backup. In the body's protective mechanism, the redundant systems function as supplementary systems—that is, they operate in addition to the inflammatory re-

---

[1]Histamine is produced by mast cells, platelets, and basophils, a type of white blood cell. Mast cells are a connective tissue cell described later in the chapter.

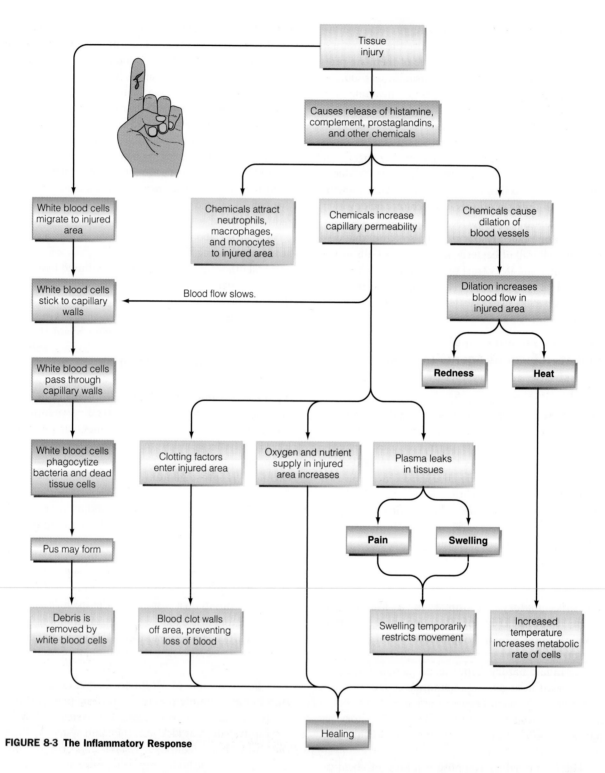

FIGURE 8-3 The Inflammatory Response

sponse. Three such systems are described in this section: pyrogens, interferons, and complement.

Pyrogens (PIE-rah-gins) are molecules released primarily by macrophages that have been exposed to bacteria and other foreign substances. Pyrogens travel to a region of the brain called the **hypothalamus**

(high-po-THAL-ah-mus). In the hypothalamus is a group of nerve cells that controls the body's temperature, in much the same way that a thermostat regulates the temperature of a room. Pyrogens turn the thermostat up, increasing body temperature and producing a fever.

Fever is actually an adaptation that helps combat bacterial infections. How? Mild fevers cause the spleen and liver to remove additional iron from the blood. Interestingly, many pathogenic bacteria require iron to reproduce. Fever therefore reduces the replication of bacteria. Fever also increases metabolism, which facilitates healing and accelerates cellular defense mechanisms such as phagocytosis. Important as it is, fever can also be debilitating, and a severe fever (over 105°F) is potentially life-threatening because it begins to denature (coagulate) vital body proteins, especially enzymes needed for biochemical reactions in body cells.

Another chemical safeguard is a group of small proteins known as the **interferons** (in-ter-FEAR-ons). Interferons are released from cells infected by viruses. They diffuse away from the site of production through the interstitial tissue and bind to receptors on the plasma membranes of noninfected body cells (**FIGURE 8-4**). The binding of interferon to uninfected cells, in turn, triggers the synthesis of cellular enzymes that inhibit viral replication. Thus when viruses enter the previously uninfected cells, they cannot replicate. They die.

Interferons do not protect cells already infected by a virus; they simply stop the spread of viruses from one cell to another. In essence, the production and release of interferon are the dying cell's last act to protect other cells of the body. Interferons are a remarkable adaptation that stops the spread of viruses while the immune response attacks and destroys the viruses outside the cells.

Another group of chemical agents that fight infection are the complement proteins. These blood proteins form the **complement system,** so named because it complements the action of antibodies, briefly described in Chapter 7.

The details of the complement system are very complex. A few points will demonstrate how this remarkable system works. Complement proteins circulate in the blood in an inactive state. When foreign cells such as bacteria invade the body, the complement protein is activated. This triggers a chain reaction in which one complement protein activates the next.

Five proteins in the complement system join to form a large protein complex, known as the **membrane-attack complex** (**FIGURE 8-5**). The membrane-attack complex embeds in the plasma membrane of bacteria, creating an opening into which water flows. The influx of water causes bacterial cells to swell, burst, and die.

Several of the activated complement proteins also function on their own and are part of the inflammatory response. Some of them, for example, stimulate the dilation of blood vessels in an infected area, described earlier. Others increase the permeability of the blood

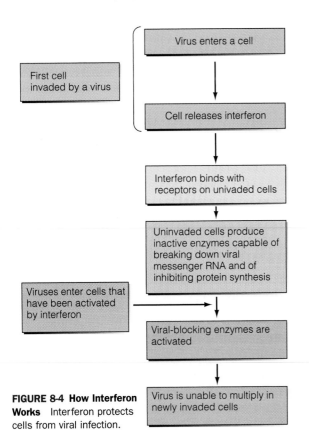

FIGURE 8-4 How Interferon Works Interferon protects cells from viral infection.

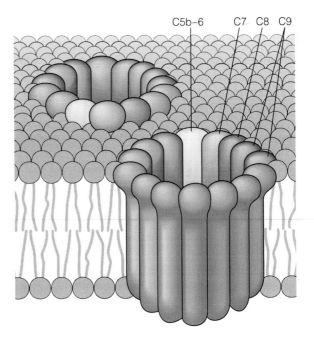

FIGURE 8-5 The Membrane-Attack Complex Five complement proteins combine and embed in a cell's membrane, causing it to leak, swell, and burst. (Source: By Dana Burns from John Ding-E Young and Zanvil A. Kohn, "How Killer Cells Kill." Copyright © January 1988 by *Scientific American, Inc.* All rights reserved.)

vessels, allowing white blood cells and nutrient-rich plasma to pass more readily into an infected zone. Certain complement proteins may also act as chemical attractants, drawing macrophages, monocytes, and neutrophils to the site of infection, where they phagocytize foreign cells. Yet another complement protein (C3b) binds to microorganisms, forming a rough coat on the intruders that facilitates their phagocytosis.

The Third Line of Defense: The Immune System

The immune system is the third line of defense. Unlike the respiratory or digestive systems, the immune system is rather diffuse—spread out and indistinct. Lymphocytes, for example, circulate in the blood and lymph and also take up residence in the **lymphoid organs** such as the spleen, thymus, lymph nodes, and tonsils, as well as other body tissues. The cells of the immune system selectively target foreign substances and foreign organisms. As a result, the immune system is said to be specific.

The immune system, like the first and second lines of defense, is an important homeostatic mechanism that eliminates foreign organisms—including bacteria, viruses, single-celled fungi, and many parasites. It comes into play when foreign organisms penetrate the outer defenses of the body. The immune system also helps prevent the emergence of cancer cells. Thus, in a world filled with infectious agents and natural mutagens (agents that cause mutation, some of which might lead to cancer), the immune system struggles to provide the internal constancy needed by body cells to carry out their functions and, as such, is an important evolutionary advance.

Lymphocytes Detect Foreign Substances in the Body and Mount an Attack on Them

One of the chief functions of the immune system is to identify what belongs in the body and what does not. Once a foreign substance has been detected, the immune system mounts an attack to eliminate it. Therefore, like all homeostatic systems, the immune system requires receptors to detect a change and effectors to bring about a response. In the immune system, the lymphocytes serve both functions.

Foreign Substances That Trigger an Immune Response Are Proteins and Polysaccharides with Large Molecular Weights

The immune response is triggered by large foreign molecules, notably proteins and polysaccharides. These molecules are called **antigens** (AN-tah-gins), which is an abbreviation for *anti*body-*gen*erating substances. The larger the molecule is, the greater its antigenicity (AN-tah-gen-ISS-eh-tee).

As a rule, small molecules generally do not elicit an immune reaction. In some individuals, however, small, nonantigenic molecules such as formaldehyde, penicillin, and the poison ivy toxin bind to naturally occurring proteins in the body, forming complexes. These large complexes are unique compounds that are foreign to the body and are therefore capable of eliciting an immune response.

The immune system reacts to viruses, bacteria, and single-celled fungi in the body. It also responds to parasites such as the protozoan that causes malaria. Viruses, bacteria, fungi, and parasites elicit a response because they are enclosed by membranes, or coats, that contain large-molecular-weight proteins or polysaccharides—that is, antigens.

Cells transplanted from one person to another also elicit an immune response, because each individual's cells contain a unique "cellular fingerprint," resulting from the unique array of plasma membrane glycoproteins (Chapter 3). The immune system is activated by these antigens on the foreign cells. Cancer cells also present a slightly different chemical fingerprint, making them essentially foreign cells within our own bodies to which the immune system responds. Although cancer cells evoke an immune response, it is often not sufficient to stop the disease.

Antigens stimulate two types of lymphocytes: **T lymphocytes**, commonly called **T cells**, and **B lymphocytes**, also called **B cells** (Chapter 7). The "T" and "B" in their names will be explained shortly. B cells and T cells respond to different antigens and function quite differently. As a rule of thumb, B cells recognize and react to microorganisms such as bacteria. They also react to **bacterial toxins**, chemical substances released by bacteria. B cells also respond to a few viruses. When activated, B cells produce antibodies to these antigens. In contrast, T cells recognize and respond to our own body cells that have gone awry. This includes cancer cells as well as body cells that have been invaded by viruses. T cells also respond to transplanted tissue cells and larger disease-causing agents, such as single-celled fungi and parasites. Unlike B cells, T cells attack their targets directly.

Immature B and T Cells Are Incapable of Responding to Antigens, but Soon Gain This Ability

Lymphocytes are produced in the red bone marrow and released into the bloodstream. These immature cells circulate in the blood and lymph, but are not able to function until they become immunologically competent.

This process occurs in specific organs in the body. Consider the T cell.

T Cells. T cells get their name from the place where they mature, the thymus. The **thymus** (THIGH-muss) is a lymphoid organ located above the heart. After they're formed in the bone marrow, immature (undifferentiated) lymphocytes enter the bloodstream and some of them end up in the thymus. Here, over the next few days, these lymphocytes mature and become functional T cells. **Immunologists**, scientists who study the immune system, say that the lymphocytes have developed **immunocompetence** (IM-you-know-COM-pahtense)—that is, they've developed the capacity to respond to antigens. But not just any antigens. In ways not completely understood, T lymphocytes leave the organ transformed to respond to very specific antigens.

As you may recall from the discussion of the plasma membrane in Chapter 2, the cells in each of us produce proteins and glycoproteins that reside in the plasma membrane, giving our cells a unique chemical fingerprint. When the T cells leave the thymus they have that same fingerprint, but each of their membranes also contain a unique type of membrane receptor that will bind to one—and only one—type of antigen.

Over an individual's lifetime, thousands upon thousands of antigens will be encountered. Thanks to the immunocompetence developed during fetal development, each of us is equipped with an army of uniquely programmed T cells that respond to the onslaught of antigens.

B Cells. B cells mature and differentiate in the bone marrow. The B in B cell, however, did not come originally from the bone marrow. It came from the bursa, an organ found in chickens. Early researchers used chickens to study lymphocytes.

After they mature, immunologically competent B cells circulate in the blood and take up residence in connective and lymphoid tissues. They therefore become part of the body's vast cellular reserve, stationed at distant outposts, awaiting the arrival of the microbial invaders.

By various estimates, several million immunologically distinct B and T cells are produced in the body early in life. Over a lifetime, only a relatively small fraction of these cells will be called into duty.

B Cells Provide Humoral Immunity Through the Production of Antibodies

The immune response consists of two separate but related reactions: humoral immunity, provided by the B cells, and cell-mediated immunity, involving T cells

TABLE 8-2

Comparison of Humoral and Cell-Mediated Immunity

Humoral	Cell-Mediated
Principal cellular agent is the B cell.	Principal cellular agent is the T cell.
B cell responds to bacteria, bacterial toxins, and some viruses.	T cell responds to cancer cells, virus-infected cells, single-cell fungi, parasites, and foreign cells in an organ transplant.
When activated, B cells form memory cells and plasma cells, which produce antibodies to these antigens.	When activated, T cells differentiate into memory cells, cytotoxic cells, suppressor cells, and helper cells; cytotoxic T cells attack the antigen directly.

(**TABLE 8-2**). Let's consider humoral immunity and the B cells first.

When a bacterium first enters the body, B cells programmed to respond to the unique proteins found in the bacterium's cell membrane bind to it (**FIGURE 8-6**). The B cells soon begin to divide, producing a population of immunologically similar cells known as **lymphoblasts**. As shown in **FIGURE 8-6**, some of the lymphoblasts differentiate to form another kind of cell, the **plasma cell**. Plasma cells then begin to produce copious amounts of antibody. **Antibodies** are proteins that help eliminate antigens, whether they're entire bacteria or bacterial toxins.

Released from plasma cells, antibodies circulate in the blood and lymph, where they bind to the antigens that triggered the response. Bacteria, bacterial toxins, and some viruses are the main targets of B cells. Because the blood and lymph were once referred to as body "humors," this arm of the protective immune response is called **humoral immunity**.

The Initial Reaction to an Antigen Is Slower and Weaker Than Subsequent Responses. The first time an antigen enters the body, it elicits an immune response, but the initial reaction—or **primary response**—is relatively slow (**FIGURE 8-7**). During the primary response, antibody levels in the blood do not begin to rise until approximately the beginning of the second week after the intruder was detected, partly explaining why it takes most people about 7–10 days to combat a cold or the flu. This delay occurs because it takes time for B cells to multiply and form a sufficient number of plasma cells. Antibody levels usually peak about the end of the second week, then decline over the next three weeks.

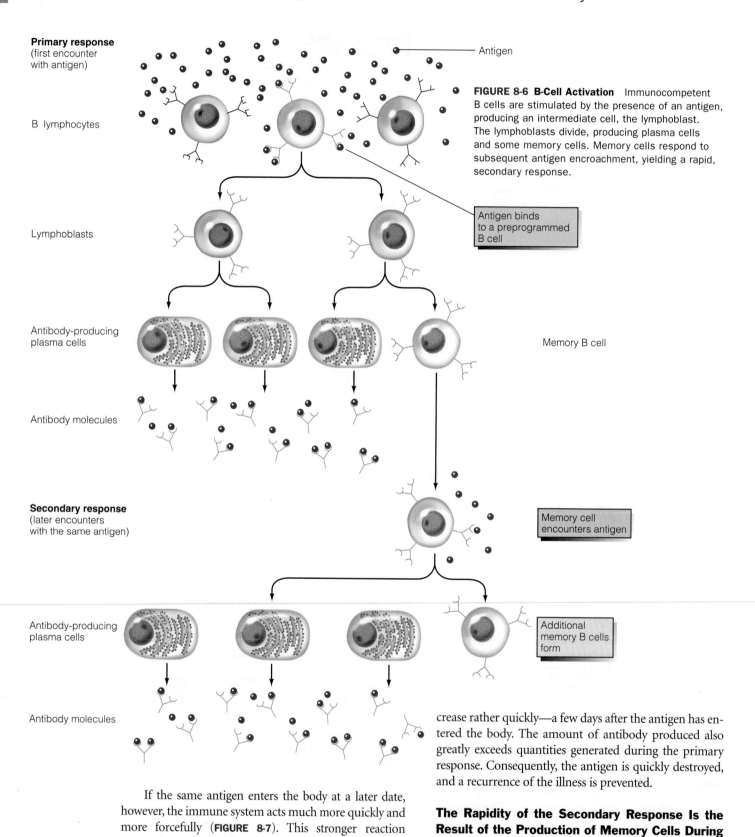

Primary response
(first encounter
with antigen)

Antigen

B lymphocytes

FIGURE 8-6 B-Cell Activation   Immunocompetent
B cells are stimulated by the presence of an antigen,
producing an intermediate cell, the lymphoblast.
The lymphoblasts divide, producing plasma cells
and some memory cells. Memory cells respond to
subsequent antigen encroachment, yielding a rapid,
secondary response.

Lymphoblasts

Antigen binds
to a preprogrammed
B cell

Antibody-producing
plasma cells

Memory B cell

Antibody molecules

Secondary response
(later encounters
with the same antigen)

Memory cell
encounters antigen

Antibody-producing
plasma cells

Additional
memory B cells
form

Antibody molecules

crease rather quickly—a few days after the antigen has entered the body. The amount of antibody produced also
greatly exceeds quantities generated during the primary
response. Consequently, the antigen is quickly destroyed,
and a recurrence of the illness is prevented.

If the same antigen enters the body at a later date,
however, the immune system acts much more quickly and
more forcefully (**FIGURE 8-7**). This stronger reaction
constitutes the **secondary response**. As **FIGURE 8-7** illustrates, during a secondary response, antibody levels in-

**The Rapidity of the Secondary Response Is the
Result of the Production of Memory Cells During
the Primary Response.** Why is the secondary response so different? **FIGURE 8-6** shows that during the

primary response, some lymphocytes divide to produce **memory cells.** Memory cells are immunologically competent B cells. Although they do not transform into plasma cells, they remain in the body awaiting the antigen's reentry. These cells are produced in large quantity and thus create a relatively large reserve of antigen-specific B-cells. When the antigen reappears, memory cells proliferate rapidly, producing numerous plasma cells that quickly crank out antibodies to combat the foreign invaders. Memory cells also generate additional memory cells during the secondary response. These remain in the body in case the antigen should enter the body at some later date. Immune protection afforded by memory cells can last 20 years or longer, which explains why a person who has had a childhood disease such as the mumps or chicken pox is unlikely to contract it again.

Antibodies Destroy Antigens in One of Four Ways.

Antibodies belong to a class of blood proteins called the **globulins** (GLOB-you-lynns), introduced in Chapter 7. Antibodies are specifically called **immunoglobulins** (im-YOU-know-GLOB-you-lynns).

Each antibody is a T-shaped molecule consisting of four peptide chains (**FIGURE 8-8**). The arms of the T bind to antigens. Like active sites on enzymes, these binding regions confer antibody specificity.

Antibodies destroy foreign organisms and antigens via one of four mechanisms: (1) neutralization, (2) agglutination, (3) precipitation, and (4) complement activation. Let's consider each one briefly.

FIGURE 8-7 Primary and Secondary Responses *(a)* The primary (initial) immune response is slow. It takes about 10 days for antibody levels to peak. Almost no antibody is produced during the first week as plasma cells are being formed. *(b)* The secondary response is much more rapid. Antibody levels rise almost immediately after the antigen invades. T cells show a similar response pattern.

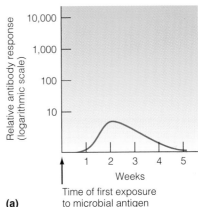

(a)

Neutralization. Some antibodies bind to viruses and bacterial toxins and form a complete coating around them. These antigens are said to be neutralized. This prevents viruses from binding to plasma membrane receptors of body cells. If a virus cannot bind to a plasma membrane receptor, it cannot get inside most cells (**FIGURE 8-9**, far right), and it is effectively neutralized. Toxins and viruses neutralized by their antibody coating are eventually engulfed by macrophages and other phagocytic cells (**FIGURE 8-9**).

Agglutination. Some antibodies eliminate antigens by a pro-

(b)

Light chains

Antigen binding site

Antigen binding site

(a)

Carbohydrate

Heavy chains

FIGURE 8-8 Antibody Structure *(a)* A three-dimensional model of an antibody showing the four chains. The molecule is T shaped before binding to an antigen. After it binds, it becomes Y shaped, as in *(b)*, a diagrammatic representation of the structure of an antibody molecule, which shows the four protein chains, two large (heavy chains) and two small (light chains). Note that the antigens bind to the arms of the molecule.

Antigen

Specific antigen binding sites

Light chain

Heavy chain

(b)

cess called **agglutination** (ah-GLUTE-tin-A-shun). Agglutination occurs when antibodies bind to numerous antigens, causing them to clump together. As shown in **FIGURE 8-9**, when the wrong type blood is transfused into a patient, antibodies in the recipient's blood bind several red blood cells together. The antigen-antibody complexes are then phagocytized by macrophages and other phagocytic cells. Bacteria may also be removed this way.

Precipitation.   Antibodies can also bind to soluble antigens (for example, a protein), forming much larger, water-insoluble complexes. These precipitate out of solution, where they are engulfed by phagocytic cells. The process is called **precipitation**.

Activation of the Complement System. Antibodies also help to rid the body of bacteria by activating the complement system. As noted earlier, the complement system is a family of blood-borne proteins that is part of the nonspecific immune response to antigens. The complement system is activated by the presence of antigen-antibody complexes (antibodies bound to antigens).

Macrophages in the Body's Tissues Play a Key Role in Activating B Cells. As you may recall from Chapter 7, macrophages are phagocytic cells found in connective tissue, lymphoid tissue, and the organs of the lymphatic system (for example, lymph nodes). As noted

FIGURE 8-9 How Antibodies Work

in that chapter, macrophages arise from monocytes that escape from the bloodstream and set up residence in body tissues.

Macrophages play several important roles in the immune response. When your skin is cut or abraded, for instance, macrophages engulf bacteria and other antigens at the site, thus lessening the initial assault. Those bacteria that do enter and begin to multiply and raise havoc may bind to antibodies produced by plasma cells. Macrophages phagocytize antigen-antibody complexes and they also engulf dead cells. Macrophages are therefore something of a mop-up crew.

Macrophages have another role, as well. They activate T cells and promote B cell differentiation. B cells, in fact, cannot differentiate into plasma cells and produce antibodies without macrophages.

FIGURE 8-10 is a simplified illustration showing the role of the macrophage in B-cell activation. As illustrated, macrophages first engulf invading bacteria. The macrophages then transfer antigens from the surface of the bacteria to their own plasma membrane. Next, macrophages cluster around B cells, "presenting" the bacterial antigen to them. B cells programmed to respond to the bacterial antigen concentrate on the surface of macrophages and

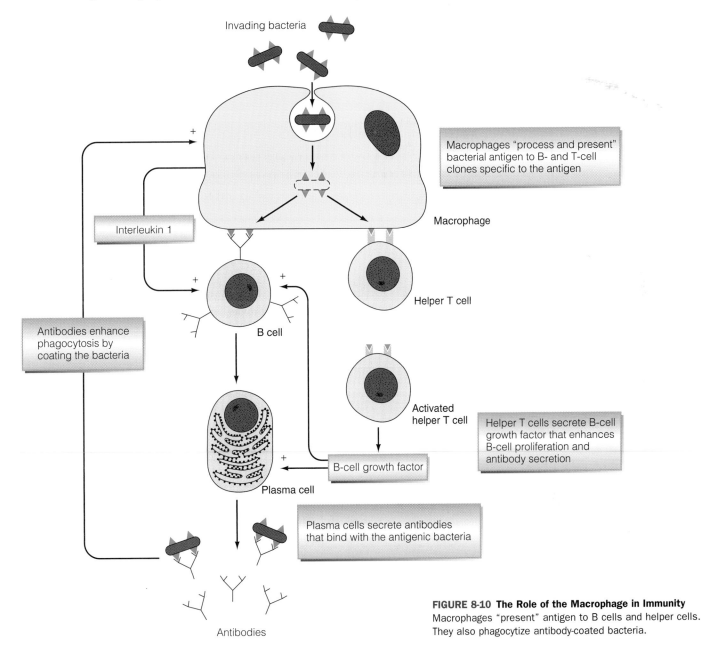

Invading bacteria

Macrophages "process and present" bacterial antigen to B- and T-cell clones specific to the antigen

Macrophage

Interleukin 1

Helper T cell

Antibodies enhance phagocytosis by coating the bacteria

B cell

Activated helper T cell

Helper T cells secrete B-cell growth factor that enhances B-cell proliferation and antibody secretion

B-cell growth factor

Plasma cell

Plasma cells secrete antibodies that bind with the antigenic bacteria

Antibodies

FIGURE 8-10 The Role of the Macrophage in Immunity
Macrophages "present" antigen to B cells and helper cells. They also phagocytize antibody-coated bacteria.

are activated. The B cells begin to divide and differentiate, forming antibody-producing plasma cells and memory cells. Also shown in the diagram, macrophages secrete a chemical substance known as **interleukin 1** (in-ter-LEW-kin). This substance enhances the proliferation and differentiation of B cells into plasma cells. In other words, it gives the process an additional boost.

Macrophages also present antigens to certain T cells, called **helper T cells** (described in detail shortly). As shown in **FIGURE 8-10**, the helper T cells are activated by this contact. They begin producing a chemical substance known as **B-cell growth factor.** It enhances the proliferation and differentiation of B cells into plasma cells. In other words, it provides an additional boost just like interleukin 1. B-cell growth factor, however, also enhances antibody production by the plasma cells (**FIGURE 8-10**).

FIGURE 8-11 How Cytotoxic T Cells Work Cytotoxic T cells, containing perforin-1 granules, bind to their target and release perforin-1, then detach in search of other invaders. Perforin-1 molecules congregate in the target plasma membrane, forming a pore that disrupts the plasma membrane, causing the cell to die. (Source: By Dana Burns from John Ding-E Young and Zanvil A. Kohn, "How Killer Cells Kill." Copyright © January 1988 by *Scientific American, Inc.* All rights reserved.)

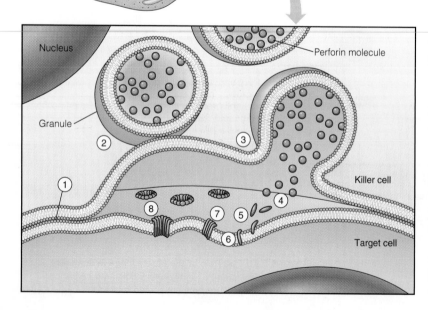

TABLE 8-3	
Summary of T Cells	
Cell Type	Action
Cytotoxic T cells	Destroy body cells infected by viruses, and attack and kill bacteria, fungi, parasites, and cancer cells
Helper T cells	Produce a growth factor that stimulates B-cell proliferation and differentiation and also stimulates antibody production by plasma cells; enhance activity of cytotoxic T cells
Suppressor T cells	May inhibit immune reaction by decreasing B- and T-cell activity and B- and T-cell division
Memory T cells	Remain in body awaiting reintroduction of antigen, at which time they proliferate and differentiate into cytotoxic T cells, helper T cells, suppressor T cells, and additional memory cells

T Cells Differentiate into at Least Four Cell Types, Each with a Separate Function in Cell-Mediated Immunity

T cells provide a much more complex form of protection than B cells. Like B cells, they respond to the presence of antigens by undergoing rapid proliferation. T cells, however, differentiate into at least four cell types: (1) cytotoxic T cells, (2) memory T cells, (3) helper T cells, and (4) suppressor T cells (**TABLE 8-3**).

Cytotoxic T cells are the principal functionaries of cell-mediated immunity. Some cytotoxic T cells attack and kill body cells infected by viruses. How does it know a cell is infected?

As noted earlier, when a virus infects a cell, the cell begins producing components needed to assemble new viruses. Some of the proteins that will be used to make new capsids or the virus's envelope, however, are incorporated in the plasma membrane of the host cell. Cytotoxic T cells recognize these foreign proteins. They bind to the antigen and destroy the host cell.

Other cytotoxic T cells attack and kill bacteria, parasites, single-celled fungi, cancer cells, and foreign cells introduced during blood transfusions or tissue or organ transplants. These organisms or cells have proteins in their membranes that identify them as foreign. How specifically do cytotoxic T cells work in these instances?

Cytotoxic T cells first bind to antigenic molecules in the membranes of cells they attack. They then release a chemical substance known as **perforin-1** (purr-FOR-in). As shown in **FIGURE 8-11**, perforin-1 molecules are housed in membranous sacs in the cytoplasm of the cytotoxic T cells. These structures bind to the membrane of the cytotoxic T cell. The membranes at the point of contact break down and the perforin-1 molecules are released into the space between the killer cell and its prey.

Perforin molecules then embed in the plasma membrane of the target cell. There, they join to form small pores, similar to those produced by the membrane-attack complex of the complement system. These pores cause the plasma membrane to leak, destroying the target cell within a few hours. After it has delivered its lethal payload, the cytotoxic cell detaches and is free to hunt down other antigens.

Memory T cells are also produced when antigens are present. As in B cells, the memory T cells form a cellular reserve. They exist to protect the body in the event of a further incursion at some other time.

Helper T cells are also produced from T cells. Helper T cells, already mentioned in the discussion of the B cells, play an important role in both humor and cell-mediated immunity. They enhance the immune response. As noted earlier, they are activated by the presence of certain antigens presented by macrophages. Helper T cells stimulate B cells, but also activate T cells via the release of a chemical known as **interleukin 2**.

Interleukin 2 increases the activity of cytotoxic T as well as that of suppressor T and other helper T cells. Its name *helper T cell* is therefore somewhat inaccurate. The cell "helps" just about all lymphocytes!

Helper T cells are the most abundant of all the T cells (comprising 60%–70% of the circulating T cells). Some immunologists liken helper T cells to the immune system's master switch. Without them, antibody production and T-cell activity are greatly reduced. In fact, without helper T cells, antigens would stimulate very few B and T cells and the process would come to a halt. We would have no immune protection.

On a side note, helper T cells are targeted by HIV, human immunodeficiency virus, which is responsible for AIDS (discussed later). Infection of helper T cells by HIV disables a person's immune system. Patients with AIDS therefore contract several infectious diseases to which they are unable to mount an effective immune response. Unless a cure can be found, all people infected with the AIDS virus will eventually die from these diseases.

The role of **suppressor T cells** is less understood. Research suggests that they "turn off" the immune reaction as the antigen begins to disappear—that is, as the antigen is phagocytized. The activity of suppressor T cells, therefore, increases as the immune system finishes its job. Suppressor cells release chemicals that reduce B- and T-cell division.

Two Types of Immunity Are Possible: Active and Passive

One of the major medical advances of the 1800s was the discovery of **vaccines** (vac-SEENS), used to prevent bacterial and viral infections. Vaccines contain inactivated or weakened viruses, bacteria, or bacterial toxins. When injected into the body, the "disabled" antigens in vaccines elicit an immune response just as if the real thing had entered the body. The immune system responds to the virus by producing antibodies or T cells.

Vaccines stimulate the immune reaction because the weakened or deactivated organisms (or toxins) they contain still possess the antigenic proteins or carbohydrates that trigger B- and T-cell activation. However, because the infectious agents have been seriously weakened or deactivated, viruses, bacteria, and bacterial toxins in vaccines do not cause disease. Some individuals may develop minor symptoms, but they're not life-threatening.

Problems may arise if the vaccines are given when a person is suffering from a cold, flu, other sicknesses. There's some evidence, although preliminary, that exposure to vaccines during these times may be connected to chronic illnesses, such as autism. Autism is a severe developmental disability characterized by withdrawal from social relations. Autistic children have reduced motor skills and are unable to or refuse to talk. Nationwide, autism has increased 300% between 1992 and 1997. Whether it is linked to vaccination during sickness is yet to be seen, but caution is advised. The new study showed that autism is four times more likely in vaccinated children than unvaccinated children.

Vaccination provides a form of protection that immunologists call **active immunity**—so named because the body actively produces memory T and B cells that will protect a person against future infections. The immune response is the same as the one that occurs when a pathogenic organism enters the body. Many vaccines provide immunity or protection from microorganisms for long periods, sometimes for life. Others give only short-term protection.

Vaccinations are vital in controlling deadly diseases such as polio, typhus, and smallpox—diseases that can kill people before their immune system mounts an effective response. In fact, in the wealthier nations of the world, such as the United States, vaccines have nearly eliminated many infectious diseases such as smallpox.

The second type of immunity, called **passive immunity,** is a temporary form of protection, resulting from the injection of **immunoglobulins** (antibodies to specific antigens). These antibodies are produced by injecting antigens in other animals such as sheep. The antibodies are then extracted from the blood for use in humans.

Passive immunity is so named because the cells of the immune system are not activated. T cells and B cells are not called into duty.

Immunoglobulins remain in the blood for a few weeks, protecting an individual from infection. Because the liver slowly removes these molecules from the blood, a person gradually loses protection.

Immunoglobulins are administered to prevent illnesses. Travelers to developing nations, for instance, are often given immunoglobulins to viral hepatitis (liver infection) as a preventive measure.

Immunoglobulins are also used to treat individuals who have been bitten by poisonous snakes (**FIGURE 8-12**). The venom in poisonous snakes is a mixture of proteins, enzymes, and polypeptides that attack body cells, especially nerve cells and heart muscle cells. In the United States, the most common poisonous snake-bites come from rattlesnakes.[2] Bites of poisonous snakes can be treated by antivenom, immunoglobulins that quickly destroy or deactivate the immunogenic molecules in snake venom before they can have adverse effects.

Passive immunity can also be conferred naturally—for instance, from a mother to her fetus (FEE-tuss). A fetus receives a dose of antibodies via the **placenta** (plah-SEN-tah), the organ that transfers nutrients from the mother's bloodstream to the fetal blood. Maternal antibodies transferred via the placenta remain in the blood of a newborn infant for several months, protecting the youngster from bacteria and viruses while its immune system is developing. Mothers also transfer antibodies to their babies in breast milk. The maternal antibodies in milk attack bacteria and viruses in the intestine, protecting the infant from infection. (For more on this topic, see Health Note 8-2.)

Vaccination Fears in the United States. Vaccines have lowered the incidence of many infectious diseases in the United States and other relatively affluent industrialized nations by 99% or more. Vaccines for diphtheria, tetanus, whooping cough, polio, measles, mumps, and congenital rubella (German measles) have all but eliminated these deadly or crippling disease organisms.

FIGURE 8-12 Poison and Antidote
Poisonous snakes like this rattler inject venom into their victims. Venom can be milked from the snake and used to produce antivenom, a serum containing immunoglobulins that neutralize the venom.

Despite the tremendous successes of vaccines, publicity concerning their rare side effects has created something of a medical dilemma in the United States, Japan, and Great Britain. In 1976 and 1977, for example, a mass-immunization program in the United States for the swine flu, one type of influenza, resulted in the paralysis of a number of people. As a result of public concern over this and other incidents, many parents have chosen *not* to have their children vaccinated. Proponents of vaccinations argue that the excessive media attention given to the rare but serious complications has harmed efforts to promote vaccination.

Another cause for the decline in vaccination stems from the success of previous immunization programs, which, as noted above, have greatly reduced the incidence of most infectious diseases. Parents who were reared in an environment free from such diseases are often unaware of the dangers of infectious disease. Having their children immunized seems unimportant. Some people, notably Christian Scientists, refuse to vaccinate children on religious grounds. Public health officials are quick to point out that pathogenic organisms that once took a huge toll on humans have not been eradicated. They fear that without widespread protection, epidemics could occur again.

Harmful side effects from conventional vaccines are often caused by reactions to certain "nonessential" antigens on the injected microorganism. These antigens frequently play little or no role in immunity. By eliminating them from vaccines, researchers hope to develop safer alternatives to the vaccines in use today.

Section 8-4

Practical Applications: Blood Transfusions and Tissue Transplantation

Although the immune system is important in protecting us from microorganisms, it presents something of a challenge to physicians during blood transfusions and tissue transplants—biological interventions unwitnessed in evolution. Let's consider blood transfusions first.

---

[2]In the United States, 15% of untreated rattlesnake bites and only about 1% of treated bites are fatal.

Blood Transfusions Require Careful Cross-Matching of Donors and Recipients

The surface of the red blood cell (RBC) membrane, like that of other cells, contains many glycoproteins that form a unique cellular fingerprint (Chapter 3). These glycoproteins are the basis of blood-typing. Four blood types exist: A, B, AB, and O. The letters refer to one type of glycoprotein (antigen) present on the plasma membrane of RBCs of an individual. As illustrated in **TABLE 8-4**, individuals with type A blood have RBCs whose plasma membranes contain the A antigen (glycoprotein). The RBCs in individuals with type B blood contain type B antigens. People with AB blood have both A and B antigens, and people with type O have neither antigen.

Physicians learned a long time ago that blood could be successfully transfused from one person to another, but only if their blood matched. In other words, an individual with type A blood could only receive type A blood, and individuals with type B blood can only receive type B blood.

Cross-matching blood is essential to prevent life-threatening immune reactions. These reactions result from antibodies found in the blood of most people. As shown in **TABLE 8-4**, each blood type carries a specific type of antibody. People with type A blood, for example, naturally contain antibodies to the B antigen. (This is why individuals with type A blood cannot receive type B blood.) People with type B blood contain antibodies to the A antigen. For reasons not well understood, these antibodies appear in the blood during the first year of life.

Serious problems arise when incompatible blood types are mixed. For example, consider what happens if an individual with type A blood is accidentally given type B blood (**FIGURE 8-13**, page 188). The antibodies to type B blood found in the recipient bind to the transfused RBCs (which contain type B antigens). This causes the type B RBCs to **agglutinate** (clump) and **hemolyze** (HEEM-oh-lize) (burst). Hemolysis and agglutination constitute the **transfusion reaction.**

RBC clumping restricts blood flow through capillaries, reducing oxygen and nutrient flow to cells and tissues. Massive hemolysis (heme-OL-eh-siss) results in the release of large amounts of hemoglobin into the blood plasma. Hemoglobin precipitates in the kidney, blocking the tiny tubules that produce urine. This can result in acute kidney failure, which can be life-threatening.

Because of the possibility of this potentially life-threatening reaction, successful transfusions require careful matching of the blood types of the donor and recipient. As **TABLE 8-4** shows, RBCs from individuals with type O blood have neither A nor B antigens. Therefore, type O blood can be transfused into individuals with all four blood types. Type O individuals are said to be **universal donors.** However, type O blood, while free of antigens, contains antibodies to both A and B antigens. Therefore, individuals with type O blood can receive only type O blood.

As shown in **TABLE 8-4**, individuals with type AB blood contain RBCs with both A and B antigens, but no antibodies related to the ABO system. People with AB blood can therefore *receive* blood from all others. Because of this, they are referred to as **universal recipients.**

Although AB blood permits one to be a universal recipient, AB blood can be safely transfused only into individuals with the same type. If it were given to people with Type A or Type B blood, the recipients would undergo a transfusion reaction, because they contain antibodies that would respond to the antigens on the RBCs.

TABLE 8-4

Summary of Blood Types

Blood Type	Antigens on Plasma Membranes of RBCs	Antibodies in Blood	Safe to Transfuse	
			To	*From*
A	A	b*	A, AB	A, O
B	B	a	B, AB	B, O
AB	A + B	—	AB	A, B, AB, O
O	—	a + b	A, B, AB, O	O

*Lowercase *b* indicates antibody to B antigen.

Health Note 8-2

Bringing Baby Up Right: The Immunological and Nutritional Benefits of Breast Milk

A baby is born into a dangerous world in which bacteria and viruses abound. Complicating matters, the immune system of a newborn child is poorly developed. Fortunately, the newborn is protected by passive immunity—antibodies that have traveled from its mother's blood. Antibodies also travel to the infant in breast milk (**FIGURE 1**).

Several immunoglobulins are present in breast milk. One of these is

FIGURE 1 Breast-Feeding Mother breast-feeding her newborn infant.

called secretory IgA. It is present in very high quantities in colostrum, a thick fluid produced by the breast immediately after delivery—before the breast begins full-scale milk production. Colostrum is so important, in fact, that some hospitals give "colostrum cocktails" to newborns who are not going to be breast-fed by their mothers. Nurses remove the colostrum from the mother's breast with a breast pump and feed it to the baby in a bottle.

Colostrum, said the late Sarah McCamman, a nutritionist at the University of Kansas Medical School, coats the lining of the intestines. The IgA antibodies in colostrum prevent bacteria ingested by the infant from adhering to the epithelium and gaining entrance. Breast milk also contains lysozyme, an enzyme that breaks down the cell walls of bacteria, destroying them.

Unfortunately, not all medical personnel agree on the benefits of breast milk. One problem is that breast milk has unusually low levels of iron. This fact has led many physicians to recommend iron supplements for newborns. A more careful

analysis, however, shows that breast-fed infants generally do not suffer from iron deficiency because the percentage of iron absorbed from breast milk is extraordinarily high. Thus, low levels of iron in breast milk are offset by the high absorption.

The wisdom of iron supplements for newborns has also been questioned on other grounds. Researchers have found that iron supplements increase the incidence of harmful bacterial infections in newborns. As noted earlier in the chapter, iron is a limiting factor in many pathogenic bacteria. Low levels of iron in breast milk, therefore, may reduce bacterial replication in an infant's intestinal tract.

In general, breast-fed babies are healthier than bottle-fed babies. The incidence of gastroenteritis (inflammation of the intestine), otitis (ear infections), and upper respiratory infections is lower in breast-fed babies. Studies also show that children breast-fed for at least 6 months contract fewer childhood cancers than their bottle-fed counterparts. The incidence of childhood lymphoma, a cancer of the lymph glands, in bottle-

The terms *universal donor* and *universal recipient* are somewhat misleading, however, because RBCs also contain other antigens that can cause transfusion reactions. The most important of these is the **Rh factor.** This antigen was first identified in rhesus (REE-suss) monkeys; hence the designation *Rh*. People whose cells contain the Rh antigen, or Rh factor, are said to be Rh-positive. Those without it are Rh-negative.

Unlike the ABO system, in which blood contains antibodies without exposure to other blood types, in the Rh system, the antibodies are produced only when Rh-positive blood is transfused into the bloodstream of a

person with Rh-negative blood. The first transfusion of Rh-positive blood into an Rh-negative person generally does not result in a transfusion reaction, but a second transfusion does. To reduce the likelihood of a transfusion reaction, Rh-negative people should receive only Rh-negative blood, and Rh-positive people should receive only Rh-positive blood.

The Rh factor becomes particularly important during pregnancy. Problems can arise if an Rh-negative mother has an Rh-positive baby (**FIGURE 8-14**, page 189). Even though the maternal and fetal bloodstreams are separate, small amounts of fetal blood usually enter the maternal bloodstream at birth. Rh antibodies form in fed babies is nearly double the rate in breast-fed children for reasons not yet understood.

Research also suggests that certain proteins in breast milk may stimulate the development of a newborn's immune system. In laboratory experiments, the proteins speed up the maturation of B cells and prime them for antibody production. These soluble proteins may also activate macrophages, which play a key role in the immune system.

Breast milk is also more digestible and more easily absorbed by infants than formula. Formula is a mixture of cow's milk, proteins, vegetable oils, and carbohydrates. It is only an approximation of mother's milk and is not broken down and absorbed as completely as breast milk.

Because of a growing awareness of the benefits of breast-feeding, virtually every national and international organization involved with maternal and child health supports breast-feeding, says McCamman. Breast-feeding can have a major health impact in this country. Unfortunately, the benefits are not as widely known as many people would like, even

among health care professionals. Fortunately, more and more health care workers are beginning to understand the benefits of breast-feeding and are promoting this option. As a result, many middle-class American women are now choosing to breast-feed.

Unfortunately, says McCamman, there is "a huge population of low-income, poorly educated . . . women who choose not to nurse." The federal government may be playing an unwitting role in their decision. A national program aimed at improving child nutrition provides free formula to needy women, perhaps discouraging mothers from breast-feeding.

Another reason is economic. Low-income women often work at jobs that do not provide maternity leave. Thus, these women must return to work soon after giving birth, and breast-feeding is difficult to do under these circumstances.

Still another reason for the low rate of breast-feeding among low-income women is that women need a lot of support to nurse. "People think nursing is innate, natural, and easy," says McCamman, "but this is not always the case." Getting started of-

ten requires guidance and education. Without such support, breast-feeding can be a difficult and painful experience. Breast-feeding among all women, rich and poor, may also be discouraged by cultural attitudes and fear of embarrassment. In fact, many otherwise open-minded people find breast-feeding in public or even semi-public settings embarrassing.

Given the many benefits of breast-feeding, McCamman recommends it to all mothers who can. Health care workers can help by educating their patients on the benefits of breast-feeding. "Doctors should present the information on breast- and bottle-feeding," says McCamman, "outlining the pros and cons of both methods. Then, let the woman choose. Too few doctors do that today, so women aren't making informed decisions."

Visit *Human Biology's* Internet site for links to web sites offering more information on this topic.

the maternal bloodstream, and the woman becomes sensitized to the Rh factor.

To prevent antibody production in Rh-negative women who give birth to Rh-positive babies, physicians routinely inject antibodies to fetal Rh-positive RBCs into the mother soon after she has given birth. (The antibody-containing serum is called *RhoGAM.*) These antibodies bind to Rh-positive RBCs from the fetus before a woman's immune system responds to them. This, in turn, prevents a woman from being sensitized. To be effective, however, the treatment must be given within 72 hours after the baby is born.

If the woman is not treated at the time and becomes pregnant again with an Rh-positive baby, mater-

nal antibodies to the Rh factor will cross the placenta. In the fetal circulation, these antibodies cause fetal RBCs to agglutinate, then break down, resulting in anemia and hypoxia (lack of oxygen to tissues). Unless the baby receives a blood transfusion (of Rh-negative blood) before birth and several after birth, it is likely to have brain damage and may even die.

Tissue Transplantation Often Evokes Cell-Mediated Immunity, Which Can Be Blocked by Certain Drugs

Organ and tissue transplantation is a much more complex matter. Only three conditions exist in which a person can receive a transplant and not reject it. One is if

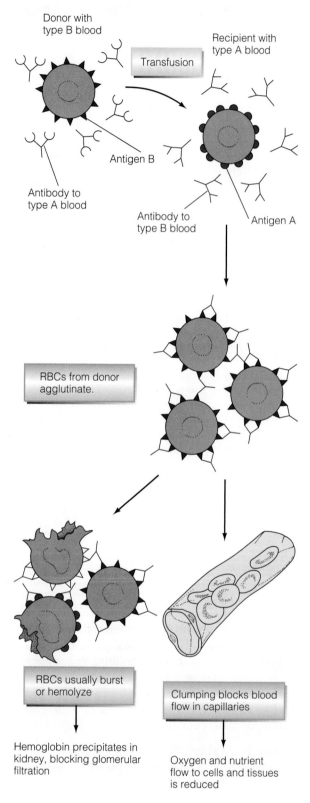

Donor with type B blood

Recipient with type A blood

Transfusion

Antigen B

Antibody to type A blood

Antibody to type B blood

Antigen A

RBCs from donor agglutinate.

RBCs usually burst or hemolyze

Clumping blocks blood flow in capillaries

Hemoglobin precipitates in kidney, blocking glomerular filtration

Oxygen and nutrient flow to cells and tissues is reduced

FIGURE 8-13 Transfusion Reaction Type B blood transfused into an individual with type A blood results in a transfusion reaction, characterized by agglutination and hemolysis.

the tissue comes from an individual's own body. For burn victims, surgeons might use healthy skin from one part of the body to cover a badly damaged region elsewhere. Hair transplants also qualify. In hair transplants, hair from the back of the head is often moved to balding spots up front or on top. The second instance is when a tissue is transplanted between identical twins—individuals derived from a single fertilized ovum that splits early in embryonic development to form two embryos. These individuals are genetically identical and have identical cellular antigens.

A third instance occurs when tissue rejection is inhibited by specific drugs. For example, heart, liver, and kidney transplants are successful only when recipients are treated with drugs that suppress the immune system. This treatment must be continued throughout the life of the patient. Unfortunately, most immune suppressants have numerous side effects and often leave the patient vulnerable to bacterial and viral infections. Without them, however, transplants from individuals not genetically identical to the recipient are quickly rejected.

In the 1980s, a new drug known as **cyclosporin** (SIGH-clow-SPORE-in) was introduced. This drug suppresses the formation of interleukin 2 by helper T cells, thus greatly reducing cell-mediated immunity without affecting B cells. Patients who receive the drug are therefore able to combat many bacterial infections with antibodies.

Section 8-5

Diseases of the Immune System

The immune system, like all other body systems, can malfunction. This section looks at two disorders: allergies and autoimmune diseases.

The Most Common Malfunctions of the Immune System Are Allergies

An **allergy** is an overreaction to some environmental substance, or antigen, such as pollen or a food (**FIGURE 8-15**). Antigens that stimulate allergic reactions are called **allergens** (AL-er-gens). Allergens cause the production of one class of immunoglobulins, the **IgE** antibodies, from plasma cells.[3] As **FIGURE 8-15** shows, these antibodies bind to mast cells, which are found in many tissues, but especially in the connective tissue surrounding blood vessels. Mast cells have large cytoplasmic vesicles containing the chemical histamine.

---

[3]Some allergies involve IgG or IgM, and some apparently do not involve antibodies at all.

FIGURE 8-14 **The Rh Factor and Pregnancy** *(a)* Rh-positive cells from the fetus enter the mother's blood at birth. If the mother is Rh-negative, her immune system responds, producing antibodies to the Rh-positive RBCs and destroying them. *(b)* Problems arise if the mother becomes pregnant again and has another Rh-positive baby. If the mother was not treated the first time, antibodies to Rh-positive RBCs cross the placenta and destroy fetal RBCs.

(a) First child. Rh⁺ red blood cells enter the maternal bloodstream during birth, evoking an immune reaction.

(b) Second child. Rh⁺ antibodies cross the placenta, destroying fetal red blood cells.

Allergens then bind to the IgE antibodies attached to the mast cells, triggering the release of histamine from the vesicles via exocytosis (**FIGURE 8-15**). Histamine, in turn, causes nearby arterioles to dilate. Histamine released in the lungs causes the bronchioles to constrict, reducing airflow and making breathing difficult. This condition is called **asthma** (AS-ma).

Allergic reactions usually occur in specific body tissues, where they create local symptoms that, while irritating, are not life-threatening. For example, an allergic response may occur in the eyes, causing redness and itching. Or, it may occur in the nasal passageway, causing stuffiness. However, the allergic response can also occur in the bloodstream, where it can be fatal if not treated quickly. For example, the presence of penicillin or bee venom in the bloodstream of certain people causes massive release of histamine and other chemicals. This, in turn, causes extensive dilation of blood vessels in the skin and other tissues. The blood pressure then falls precipitously, shutting down the circulatory system. Histamine released by mast cells also causes severe constriction of the bronchioles (the ducts in the lungs that open onto the alveoli), making breathing difficult. The decline in blood pressure and constriction of the bronchioles result in **anaphylactic shock** (ANN-ah-fah-LACK-tic). Death may follow if measures are not taken to reverse this catastrophic event. One such measure is an injection of the hormone epinephrine (commonly known as adrenalin), which rapidly reverses the constriction of the bronchioles.

Allergies are treated in three ways. First, patients are advised to avoid allergens—for instance, to avoid milk and milk products or stay clear of dogs and cats. Second, patients may also be given **antihistamines** (an-tea-HISS-tah-means), drugs that counteract the effects of histamine. Third, patients may also be given allergy shots, injections of increasing quantities of the offending allergen. In many cases, this treatment makes an individual less and less sensitive to the allergen. Desensitization results from the production of another class of antibod-

FIGURE 8-15 Allergic Reaction Antigen stimulates the production of massive amounts of IgE, a type of antibody produced by plasma cells. IgE attaches to mast cells. This is the sensitization stage. When the antigen enters again, it binds to the IgE antibodies on the mast cells, triggering a massive release of histamine and other chemicals. Histamine, in turn, causes blood vessels to dilate and become leaky. This triggers the production of mucus in the respiratory tract. In some people, the chemicals released by the mast cells also cause the small air-carrying ducts in the lungs to constrict, making breathing difficult.

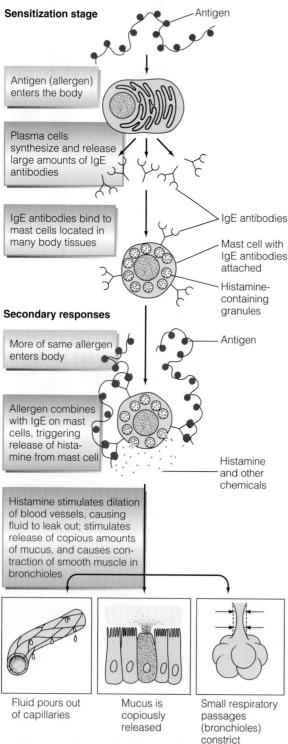

Sensitization stage

Antigen

Antigen (allergen) enters the body

Plasma cells synthesize and release large amounts of IgE antibodies

IgE antibodies bind to mast cells located in many body tissues

IgE antibodies

Mast cell with IgE antibodies attached

Histamine-containing granules

Secondary responses

More of same allergen enters body

Antigen

Allergen combines with IgE on mast cells, triggering release of histamine from mast cell

Histamine and other chemicals

Histamine stimulates dilation of blood vessels, causing fluid to leak out; stimulates release of copious amounts of mucus, and causes contraction of smooth muscle in bronchioles

Fluid pours out of capillaries

Mucus is copiously released

Small respiratory passages (bronchioles) constrict

ies, the **IgG antibodies,** which bind to allergens. This, in turn, prevents the allergen from binding to the plasma cells, thus reducing IgE production and reducing or eliminating the release of histamine and other chemical substances responsible for the allergic reaction.

Autoimmune Diseases Result from an Immune Attack on the Body's Own Cells

Occasionally, the immune system mounts an attack on the body's own cells. This unfortunate state of affairs is known as an **autoimmune disease.** Autoimmune diseases result from many causes. For example, in some instances, normal body proteins can be modified by environmental pollutants, viruses, or genetic mutations so that they are no longer recognizable by the body as self.

In other cases, normal body proteins usually isolated from the immune system enter the bloodstream and evoke an immune response. For example, a protein called *thyroglobulin* is produced by the thyroid gland in the neck. Thyroglobulin is stored inside the gland and not exposed to cells of the immune system. If the gland is injured, however, thyroglobulin may enter the bloodstream. Lymphocytes encountering this protein may then mount an immune response to it.

Yet another cause of autoimmune reaction is exposure to antigens that are nearly identical to body proteins. The bacterium that causes strep throat, for example, contains an antigen structurally similar to one of the proteins found in the plasma membranes of the cells lining the heart valves of some individuals. The body mounts an attack on the bacterium, but antibodies may also bind to the lining of the heart valve, causing a local inflammation and scar tissue to develop. This can damage the valve, resulting in valvular incompetence, discussed in Chapter 6.

Section 8-6

AIDS: The Deadly Virus

In 1985, Damion Knight, a bright, young cabinetmaker, began to lose weight and experience bouts of unexplained fever. His lymph nodes became swollen, and he felt weak and drowsy. A doctor found that Damion had acquired immunodeficiency syndrome, commonly known as **AIDS, acquired immune deficiency syndrome.** Like thousands of others, Knight died several years after his diagnosis. His doctor could not help him.

AIDS is caused by a virus that attacks and weakens the immune system. This virus is known as the **human immunodeficiency virus** or **HIV** for short (**FIGURE 8-16**).

HIV is an RNA virus that attacks helper T cells, severely impairing the immune system. AIDS patients grow progressively weaker and generally fall victim to other infectious agents. For example, many die from an otherwise rare form of pneumonia.

AIDS rose to infamy in the early 1980s. The first documented case was that of a young Missouri boy who died at age 15 in 1969. Studies of tissue samples of a British sailor revealed that he probably died of AIDS ten years earlier. In 1998, scientists announced the presence of HIV in a blood sample of a Bantu man from Africa's Democratic Republic of the Congo who died in 1959.

New research suggests that AIDS came to us via chimpanzees in west-central Africa. Chimpanzees contain a strain of simian immunodeficiency virus (SIV) that is very similar to HIV-1, one of the most common strains in humans. The virus was apparently transferred by exposure to blood of chimps killed by humans living the area. New studies also show that AIDS may have begun spreading among people as long ago as 1930.

The incidence of AIDS (number of cases) and the number of deaths from AIDS in the United States increased dramatically from 1981 to 1997.

The sharp increase in incidence and deaths prompted one researcher to liken AIDS to the bubonic plague that spread through Europe in the fourteenth and fifteenth centuries. In the 1300s, the plague killed one quarter of the adult population and numerous children. In some African villages today, AIDS runs rampant with as many as 50% of the residents testing HIV-positive. This fact suggests that, at least in some locations, predictions of a plaguelike scourge are not that far-fetched.

HIV infection is a global epidemic. In 1998, approximately 47 million people were been infected with HIV, up from 31 million only three years earlier. An estimated 25 million of those infected with HIV live in Africa.

As noted earlier, HIV is a rather lethal virus. Of the 47 million who have been infected, over 14 million have died.

AIDS affects virtually all countries. In the United States, nearly 775,000 cases of AIDS have been reported, including nearly 9,000 children (under age 13), since 1981. It is believed that as many as 900,000 people are infected with HIV. To date, 448,000 have died, including over 5,000 children. Although mortality from HIV infection has dropped dramatically in the United States due to new drugs that treat the virus and the infections that set in, better medical care, prevention, and other factors, an estimated 40,000 Americans will contract HIV this year alone.

The incidence of AIDS is increasing everywhere. Africa is one of the hardest hit nations. In a dozen coun-

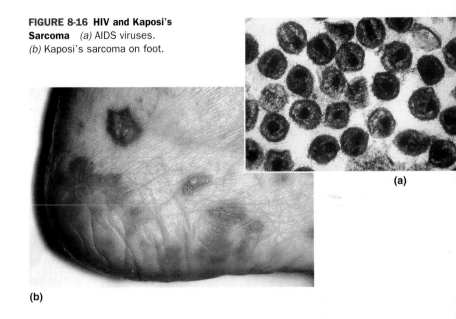

FIGURE 8-16 HIV and Kaposi's Sarcoma *(a)* AIDS viruses. *(b)* Kaposi's sarcoma on foot.

(a)

(b)

tries, 10% of the adult population carries the virus. In some African nations, such as Zimbabwe and Botswana, 25% of all adults are infected with HIV. AIDS is also on the rise in India, China, and southeast Asia.

In the United States, deaths from AIDS have fallen sharply, thanks to new drugs. But the number of HIV infections continues to rise. The hardest hit group is men; two-thirds of all new HIV infections occur in African American and Hispanic men. AIDS is now a leading killer of African American males. According to the U.S. Centers for Disease Control and Prevention, AIDS affects six times more African Americans and three times more Hispanics than Caucasians.

AIDS Is a Progressive Disease That Exhibits Three Distinct Phases

AIDS progresses through three distinct phases: asymptomatic, AIDS-Related Complex (ARC), and full-blown AIDS. Some individuals develop AIDS within 3 to 5 years of being infected. In others, the disease may take 10 to 12 years to manifest itself. Researchers have now isolated a group of genes in human chromosomes that apparently account for this difference.

No matter what the time until onset, all AIDS victims follow a similar progression, typically a three-phase process.

FIGURE 8-17 shows several key physiological parameters and symptoms during each phase. The top panel, for instance, plots the number of helper T cells, also called **T4 cells.** Symptoms are listed in the middle panel. The bottom panel shows the concentration of HIV and the HIV antibody levels.

(a)

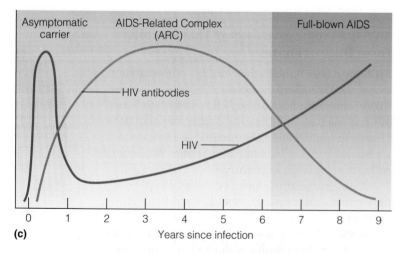

Symptoms of AIDS		
Asymptomatic Phase	**AIDS-Related Complex (ARC)**	**Full-Blown AIDS**
Lasts 9 months or more	10–63 months	64–83 months
Typically no symptoms	Fatigue	Swollen lymph nodes
	Persistent and recurrent fever	Persistent infections
	Persistent cough	Extreme loss of weight
	Diarrhea	Severe weakness
	Loss of memory	Persistent diarrhea
	Difficulty thinking	Persistent cough
	Depression	Kaposi's sarcoma
	Impaired judgement	

(b)

(c)

FIGURE 8-17 Tracking a Killer (a) T4 cell concentration, (b) symptoms, and (c) HIV and antibody levels (labeled immune system). (SOURCE: Data for parts a and c from R. R. Redfield and D. S. Burke, "HIV Infection: The Clinical Picture" in *Scientific American*, October 1988.)

As illustrated in **FIGURE 8-17**, most patients show no symptoms during the first few months after infection. A few, perhaps 1%–2%, may exhibit symptoms similar to those of infectious mononucleosis—that is, fever, chills, aches, and swollen lymph nodes. However, these symptoms vanish shortly thereafter, and individuals go on about their business, unaware that they have contracted a deadly disease—and unaware that they're transmitting it to others.

During the first phase, the T4-cell count is high (**FIGURE 8-17**). As the bottom panel in **FIGURE 8-17** shows, the number of viruses (blue line) rises rapidly during the first phase of AIDS. Antibodies to HIV begin to increase as a result.

During the second phase of this disease, T4-cell count begins to fall in response to the rise in HIV. Antibody levels rise initially, then fall as the immune system begins to falter. During the second phase, patients begin to show outward signs of the disease caused by the decline in the number of T4 cells. Severe fatigue and unexplained, persistent fever are two common symptoms. Some patients complain of a persistent cough and loss of memory, difficulty thinking, and depression. When recurring infections set in, the third and final phase of AIDS is about to begin.

The final phase, known as full-blown AIDS, is characterized by persistent infections, extreme loss of weight, and weakness. Most patients succumb to one of a handful of infectious organisms—microbes not ordinarily capable of producing infections. When a patient is in a state of extreme immune compromise, though, these organisms take hold and become life-threatening.

HIV Also Causes Cancer and Produces a Substance That May Cause Deterioration of Brain Function

HIV affects more than a person's immune system. AIDS patients, for example, often contract a rare form of skin cancer called **Kaposi's sarcoma** (kah-PO-sees sar-KOME-ah) (**FIGURE 8-16B**). Kaposi's sarcoma can also attack internal organs.

At one time, it was thought that Kaposi's sarcoma resulted from genetic engineering carried out by HIV itself. Studies suggested that HIV carries a gene (a segment of DNA) that's incorporated into the genetic material of body cells. This gene, they thought, caused skin cells to proliferate uncontrollably, forming a cancerous tumor. New research, however, suggests that Kaposi's sarcoma is caused by one strain of the herpes virus, herpes virus 8. It is believed to be transmitted by deep kissing, kissing that involves a lot of contact with saliva.

AIDS patients also experience a number of neurological disorders, beginning in the second phase. These include memory loss and progressive mental deterioration. A recent laboratory study may explain the cause of these symptoms.

Researchers have found that inside helper T cells, HIV produces several proteins that are incorporated into the viral capsid. One of those proteins is known as gp120. This protein kills fetal brain cells in culture. The researchers believe that gp120 travels in the blood to the brains of some patients, where it kills neurons, thus producing neurological defects.

Loss of mental function may also be caused by a single-celled parasite that is normally found in cats, but sets up residence in people whose immune systems are compromised by HIV. This parasite causes a brain infection (encephalitis) that leads to a loss of brain cells, seizures, and weakness.

HIV Is Transmitted in Many Ways, but Not by Casual Contact

Research has shown that HIV is passed primarily via three routes: (1) sexual contact, (2) blood transfusions, and (3) contaminated needles shared by intravenous drug abusers. Homosexual men, hemophiliacs, and drug addicts are the primary victims in the United States. But HIV is also transmitted among the heterosexual population and can even be transmitted from an infected mother to her baby through the placenta. An HIV infected mother who is nursing her infant can transmit the virus in her milk, too. A recent study showed that a man infected with AIDS is many times more likely to transmit the disease to a female partner than vice versa.

There's no evidence showing that HIV can be transmitted in saliva or by sharing utensils, plates, or cups. In fact, laboratory studies suggest that even though HIV can be found in saliva of infected individuals, saliva has natural components that reduce HIV's ability to infect cells. At this writing, researchers do not know whether deep kissing or oral sex increases the risk of infection.

Individuals with the genetic disorder hemophilia were once at risk for AIDS. Hemophiliacs are given clotting factors from pooled human plasma. Before 1984, blood donors were not screened for HIV. Consequently, many of the preparations were contaminated with HIV. As a result, a majority of the estimated 15,000 hemophiliacs in the United States who received clotting factors between 1975 and 1984 have HIV antibodies in their blood. Many of these people have died very unfortunate deaths.

To prevent the spread of AIDS through blood transfusions, blood is now routinely tested for HIV. Tissues and organs for transplantation are also tested. Improvements in screening have reduced the risk of HIV

infection from 1 in 2,500 units of blood in 1985 to 1 in 444,000 to 640,000 units in 1995. Thus, despite improvements in screening, blood transfusion is not a fail-safe proposition. Individuals who will need blood for an operation are therefore encouraged to donate blood ahead of time.

HIV, although lethal, does not spread as readily as the flu virus or cold viruses; individuals can protect themselves by practicing sexual abstinence before marriage, by engaging in safe sex (using condoms, for example), and by avoiding multiple sexual partners. To prevent the spread of HIV among intravenous drug users, some countries and some U.S. cities distribute clean hypodermic needles to addicts.

Pregnant women infected with HIV can be treated with AZT during pregnancy. If the baby is delivered by cesarean section (through an incision made in the lower abdomen), the chances of her baby contracting the disease can be reduced dramatically. Studies are underway on yet another drug treatment that's given to the mother during labor and the baby within three days of birth. Preliminary results show that it is even more more effective than AZT.

The Battle Against AIDS Has Been Facilitated by New Screening Tests and by Drugs That Slow Down the Development of the Disease

Health care workers determine the presence of HIV via an immunologic test, which detects antibodies to HIV in the blood. Scientists have also developed a new, more sensitive test that detects antigens—proteins in the HIV coat—that has greatly improved the screening of blood and tissue. There are even tests individuals can use at home, which require a pin prick to draw blood or a mouth swab to sop up antibodies to the HIV.

Although no cure has been discovered, a drug called **AZT** (zidovudine) may prolong the lives of people who have tested HIV-positive.[4] AZT inhibits viral replication and is effective in people with full-blown AIDS, or people who show early signs of HIV infection. It is now also used in people in who are infected, but who show no signs other than impaired immunity, and children. It is even used to prevent the transmission of HIV from mothers to fetuses and newborns (through breast milk). Unfortunately, AZT is costly and may be carcinogenic.

To date, 33 drugs are available to combat HIV and to treat infections, Kaposi's sarcoma, and other complications including weight loss. One of the newest

---

[4]This drug was first called *azidothymidine,* hence the name AZT.

treatments that has proved very useful in prolonging the lifespan of people infected with HIV is a three-drug regime. All three drugs are enzyme inhibitors.

The treatment consists of AZT, another similar drug, and a more recent drug known as a **protease inhibitor.** AZT blocks one of the key enzymes (reverse transcriptase) needed early on by HIV to make copies of itself. Reverse transcriptase allows the HIV to make DNA on its RNA. The DNA is then inserted into a host cell's chromosomes, and there successfully converts the cell to a virus-producing factory. Protease inhibitors block another enzyme (protease) that is also vital in the replication of HIV in infected cells.

AZT and other similar drugs slow the spread of HIV in the body and thus delay the onset of opportunistic infections. Because HIV can develop a resistance to AZT-type drugs and protease inhibitors, combination treatment is required to effectively suppress the virus.

The use of these and other drugs has resulted in a substantial decrease in deaths due to AIDS in the United States and other more developed nations where there's money to pay for the costly treatment. Even in such nations, drug costs can run as high as $15,000 a year. In less developed countries, most individuals cannot afford the treatment.

Although the three-drug treatment is greatly prolonging lives, it does present problems, other than its high cost. Researchers recently reported that long-term use of AIDS drugs, in particular, the protease inhibitors, can cause severe bone loss. It also causes other metabolic disorders, some very severe, when used over long periods of time. Some patients don't respond to the treatment or cannot tolerate the toxic effects of the drugs or have difficulty complying with the complex dosing schedules.

In good news, researchers have discovered two chemicals that could be added to the list of AIDS drugs. These two compounds, not named at this writing, sabotage yet another of the enzymes HIV needs to successfully reproduce. The enzyme is called *integrase* and it inserts DNA that is made on HIV's RNA into the host cell's chromosomes. Under direction of this integrated viral DNA, the cell switches gears, becoming an HIV factory. Complete takeover of the host cell requires about 24 hours.

Studies in the laboratory show that the new compounds, the only successful ones out of a group of 250,000 tested chemicals, stop the splicing of virally produced DNA into the host cell's DNA. They also prevent the spread of HIV in cell cultures and even stop strains of HIV that are resistant to other enzyme inhibitors.

AIDS will undoubtedly remain a significant public health threat in the world for many years. To bring this disease under control, more intensive efforts are needed to educate all people, especially individuals in high-risk groups, on ways to prevent the disease. Successes are occurring. In Thailand, Senegal, Tanzania, and Uganda, infection rates have slowed or declined thanks to sex education, the distribution of free condoms, needle exchange programs, and support from religious and civic leaders. (For a discussion of some of the social and political implications of efforts to control the spread of AIDS, see the Point/Counterpoint in this chapter.) Many scientists believe that a vaccine is the only way to ultimately bring this disease under control.

Although Some Researchers Are Optimistic About Finding a Vaccine for HIV, Not All Share Their View

HIV is notorious for its ability to mutate, a feature that is making the task of developing a vaccine extremely difficult, if not impossible.[5] Even within the body, HIV mutates fairly freely. In one study, for example, researchers analyzed viruses isolated from two infected patients. Over a 16-month period, they found 9–17 different varieties, all thought to have been formed from the original virus.

Making matters worse, HIV may be able to hide in the body. In 1988, a research team announced that out of 100 homosexual men studied, 4 initially showed antibodies to the AIDS virus, but slowly lost them. This process usually occurs only in the late stages of AIDS, when the immune system is too weak to produce antibodies. These men, however, had no overt symptoms of AIDS. Why?

Research suggests that HIV may take up residence in bone marrow stem cells that give rise to lymphocytes. If this is true, the virus can then be transmitted to new white blood cells by cell division. Thus, once the virus is in the body, it may be there forever. Eliminating the virus from the body may be virtually impossible. One of the upshots of these troubling findings is that if HIV can go into hiding, AIDS-infected blood donors may escape detection, even with the new genetic tests. AIDS-infected blood cells could unknowingly be passed to thousands of patients over the coming years. Despite

---

[5]The AIDS virus is a retrovirus, an RNA virus whose RNA is used to produce DNA after invading a cell. This process, called *reverse transcription*, is fairly inaccurate and results in many mutant forms of the virus.

these discouraging findings, researchers remain determined to find a cure for AIDS and a way to prevent it. At present, over two dozen vaccines are under study. Unfortunately, success has been elusive. In 2000, researchers studying a new vaccine for AIDS were dealt a major blow. The scientists had administered the vaccine to adult and juvenile rhesus monkeys. The monkeys were given an attenuated vaccine, that is, a vaccine containing HIV that had been deactivated. The researchers had stripped the genes from the virus that were required for it to multiply inside infected cells. Much to their surprise, they found that virtually all of the monkeys died or showed symptoms of AIDS. Somehow, the virus managed to replicate. A second study by a different group of researchers showed identical results. Although the mechanism responsible for the virus' ability to regain virulence is unknown, hopes for developing a vaccine appear even dimmer.

On another front, researchers have developed a genetically engineered weapon that could kill cells infected with HIV, possibly eliminating the disease after it has developed. As noted earlier, cells infected with the AIDS virus produce a protein known as gp120, which is part of the capsid (**FIGURE 8-18**). This protein also ends up in the plasma membrane of infected cells.

Researchers have genetically engineered a bacterium that binds to the gp120 protein. The bacterium carries with it a toxin that kills the HIV-infected cells. Preliminary studies indicate that noninfected cells are unharmed by this treatment. Although initial studies were disappointing, researchers hope that the technique can be improved or modified, making it possible to kill enough infected cells in AIDS patients to halt the disease. One question that must be answered before this procedure can be tried in people is whether AIDS-infected cells killed by this technique will degenerate and release active AIDS viruses that spread to other body cells.

Researchers are also looking into the DNA of chimpanzees for clues for a cure. Studies show that many wild chimps carry a virus very similar to HIV called SIV. Studies also suggest that the virus has been in the chimp population for over 10,000 years. Interestingly, though, chimps are not affected by it. Because chimps contain 98% of the genes we have, studying genetic differences of the two species could lead to a better understanding of why humans are so devastatingly affected by this virus. This, too, could help researchers develop a cure.

FIGURE 8-18 Duping the AIDS Virus The AIDS virus has a protein, gp120, in its capsid. When it infects cells, it produces more gp120 to make new capsids. However, some gp120 ends up in the infected cell's plasma membrane, thereby marking it. By genetically engineering a bacterium that can locate the infected cells through the gp120 marker, medical researchers may be able to hunt down and kill infected cells, stopping the spread of the virus.

Health, Homeostasis, and the Environment
Multiple Chemical Sensitivity

Human beings would not survive past early infancy without some means of protection against potentially harmful viruses and microorganisms that abound in our world. But what does protection have to do with homeostasis?

The answer is, plenty. Without the protective mechanisms you've studied in this chapter, homeostasis could not be maintained. Bacteria and viruses would take over. Therefore, the protective mechanisms of our bodies play a vital role in maintaining internal constancy. By regulating the concentration of viruses, bacteria, and other infectious agents, they help keep the cells of our tissues and organs alive so they can perform their specialized functions. Many of these cells, of course, help maintain homeostasis.

Despite its prowess, the immune system is not impenetrable. A growing body of evidence suggests that the chemically polluted world we live in may cause the immune systems of some people to run amuck. That is to say, chemical pollution in our world may be creating damaging physiological imbalances in people. Consider the case of Richard Sharp.

Richard Sharp was a physicist for a major aviation company in California. Today, he is confined to two stripped-down rooms equipped with special filters that remove all air contaminants. Why?

Sharp is one of many Americans who has developed a disease known as **multiple chemical sensitivity (MCS).** Much to his regret, Sharp has become a prisoner in his own home, unable to venture forth into modern society without suffering extreme discomfort, even debilitation.

Point/Counterpoint

Tracking People with AIDS

Anonymous Testing Is the Answer

Earl F. Thomas

Earl F. Thomas *has served on the Governor's AIDS Council and is on the boards of directors for the Colorado AIDS Project and the National Association of People with AIDS. Thomas was diagnosed as having AIDS in 1986.*

Confidential testing for HIV (in which the names and addresses of individuals who test positive are reported to health officials) versus anonymous testing continues to be a highly controversial topic. In today's society, the word *AIDS* still breeds fear in the general populace, which, for AIDS patients, translates into fear of discrimination. These fears, quite simply, are keeping people from being tested.

Health departments and AIDS organizations stress that persons who have reason to believe that they may have been infected with the HIV virus should be tested, for several reasons. First, the earlier a person knows he or she is HIV-positive, the earlier treatment can be started to slow the progression of the disease or simply to buy time while researchers explore better treatments. Second, knowledge of one's HIV status is crucial in determining what behavioral changes need to be made.

If the testing system discourages individuals from obtaining knowledge about their HIV status, however, no one benefits. Unfortunately, name reporting tends to create an atmosphere of distrust between health officials and those who wish to be tested. They believe that information

concerning their HIV status goes beyond the health department to others who may have a need to know, and they fear that the information will eventually find its way to persons who have no need to know. For instance, numerous links in the information chain (nurses, laboratory workers, therapists, and secretaries) all have access to a person's medical information. Confidential medical information is not so confidential after all. As a result of these concerns, many persons, even in high-risk groups, refuse to be tested at all.

In a survey conducted by the Educational Department of the Colorado AIDS Project in 1989, 32% of 1,112 respondents (homosexual and bisexual men) cited confidentiality concerns as their reason for not being tested. Despite the health department's insistence that fears of information leaks are poorly founded, they are very real to many individuals. More importantly, these fears prevent individuals who have engaged in high-risk behaviors from being tested.

Further information that supports anonymous testing comes from the state of Oregon. When anonymous HIV testing was offered along with confidential testing, there was a 50% increase in the demand to be tested during the first 4 months of the program. People from all segments of society sought out the anonymous test sites. Confidential testing sites reported no increase during the same period.

Fear of testing is justified. There is documented evidence of discrimina-

tion against people who are HIV-positive. Individuals have been denied housing and, in certain cases, have been evicted from their homes, lost their jobs, been denied access to public education, and have been shunned by families, friends, and co-workers.

Partner notification (contact tracing) may have a place when trying to control the spread of AIDS, but at what cost? Some feel that contact tracing is not a viable option due to the monetary cost. In 6 months in 1988, the state of Colorado spent $450,000 on partner notification. The result of this enormous expenditure was that 52 people were found.

The experiences of other health departments clearly show that partner notification can be carried out with reasonable success when testing is anonymous. If lists are being maintained, people shy away from testing and forfeit the possibility of early intervention treatment and partner notification information. When health officials act as contact tracers, they are perceived as police. In our society, police-state tactics will never work, and no one benefits.

Anonymous testing would reduce a serious impediment to a powerful, collective anti-AIDS effort. And most important, we could get an answer as to whether people are truly avoiding testing because of reportability.

Addendum: Anonymous testing began in Denver in September of 1990. It is a huge success with other Denver sites offering anonymous testing on request, along with the cities of Boulder, Longmont, and Lafayette.

MCS is a truly modern disease thought to be caused by exposure to a number of common household and industrial chemicals, including formaldehyde, solvents, acrylic resins, mercury compounds, and pesti-

cides. How do these chemicals create such debilitating symptoms?

The answer is, by acting through the immune system. Consider formaldehyde. Formaldehyde is a chemi-

Notification Works

John Potterat

The process of reporting people with the AIDS virus (HIV) by name to public health officers and in turn tracing their contacts should not be controversial. Such procedures have been standard public health practice for serious communicable diseases for nearly a century. Formal notification allows society to define the disease burden (surveillance) and to counterattack (control). You cannot control a communicable disease if you do not know who has it and who might be next to have it; moreover, you need to find those directly affected.

Notifying partners of people infected with sexually transmitted disease has been an effective control tool for 50 years. The fundamental reason that health officers are involved in this notification process is that STD patients are not good at referring their own sexual partners. Such "self-referral" fails more often than it succeeds: less than a third of STD partners are successfully referred for medical evaluation. Partner referral by HIV patients is even less successful (despite frequent assurances by patients that they "will take care of it!"). Part of this failure is due to the reluctance of HIV patients to face their partners (fear of anger or reprisal); part is due to selective notification (denial that "nice" partners can be infected); and part to failure to convince partners (partner denial). Trusting the notification process to infected people alone is a luxury that society can ill afford.

Those exposed to HIV have a right to know. Important sexual (safer practices) and reproductive (postponing pregnancy) decisions depend on knowledge of exposure and its outcome. Many persons are unaware that their partners have histories of needle exposures or of bisexuality. The duty to warn people has compelling moral, legal, and historical foundations. In free societies, notification is a straightforward, confidential process. Medical workers who detect HIV infection report the case by name and address to the local health officer who then discreetly contacts the patient to counsel him or her and to obtain identifying information on sexual and needle partners. People are persuaded, not coerced, into voluntary cooperation. Although counseling is "mandatory," blood testing is optional.

Even if "treatment" for partners were to consist solely of personal counseling to discourage behaviors that facilitate transmission or accelerate disease progression, partner notification would be worthwhile.

A disease control procedure should be acceptable to people. Partner notification by health officers has been well received by the affected populations. The majority (70%–80%) of notified partners accept blood testing, and almost all who decline testing accept counseling. Although organized gay advocacy groups have generally opposed both HIV reporting by name and partner notification by health officers, when approached individually and sympathetically, gay men have generally cooperated.

Health officers are responsible for maintaining the physical security of HIV records; such records are also immune from any discovery process. They cannot be subpoenaed or released to potentially adversarial agents like insurance, police, or employer investigators. Whatever discrimination is suffered by infected people, none of it stems from disease notification to, or by, public health officers.

Notification initiatives are affordable, acceptable to patients, and effective in reaching high-risk people. It is well known to health officers that those at highest risk are least inclined to appear for counseling and least likely to use safer practices. While notification is not a panacea, it is one of the most useful measures for containing this tragic epidemic.

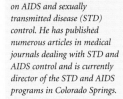

John Potterat *is an authority on AIDS and sexually transmitted disease (STD) control. He has published numerous articles in medical journals dealing with STD and AIDS control and is currently director of the STD and AIDS programs in Colorado Springs.*

Sharpening Your Critical Thinking Skills

1. Summarize Thomas's reasons for keeping AIDS testing anonymous.
2. Summarize Potterat's views in support of name reporting.
3. Do you agree or disagree with the following statement? Both writers believe that their approach will provide the greatest protection to the public health, but they differ in their approach. Explain.
4. Of the two basic approaches, which do you think would be most effective in reducing the spread of AIDS?

Visit *Human Biology's* Internet site for links to web sites offering more information on this topic.

cal found in embalming fluid. But is is also commonly found in adhesives in carpeting, plywood, furniture, and many other household products. It is also found in paints.

Formaldehyde is inhaled into the lungs. From there, it escapes into the bloodstream, where it is circulated throughout the body. In body tissues, formaldehyde binds to naturally occurring proteins in the body.

This process produces foreign substances that the immune system then attacks. In this process, a common household substance essentially turns the immune system against the body.

Over time, individuals exposed to formaldehyde become extremely sensitive to it, even very low levels of chemicals that initially caused them no harm.[6] This condition, referred to as **hypersensitivity**, can be debilitating. Moreover, individuals who have been sensitized to one chemical often react to other chemically similar substances.

The symptoms of MCS vary, ranging from life-threatening to mild. The most common symptoms are tension, memory loss, fatigue, sleepiness, headaches, confusion, and depression. Many victims of MCS experience gastrointestinal problems such as nausea, indigestion, and cramps. Some exhibit respiratory symptoms as well, including frequent colds, bronchitis, and shortness of breath. Skin rashes are not uncommon. Many people report allergylike symptoms such as nasal stuffiness and sinus infections.

MCS is puzzling to victims, their families, and physicians. Individuals often experience a sudden deterioration in their health and are often labeled "psychiatric cases." People suffering from MCS must often get rid of all cleaning agents, pesticides, perfumes, deodorants, and other household chemicals.

---

[6]Massive exposures to certain chemicals may also elicit a hypersensitivity reaction.

The National Research Council estimates that 15% of the U.S. population experiences some degree of chemical hypersensitivity. Studies show that 5% of the workers exposed to an agent used in the manufacture of plastics, TDI (toluene diisocyanate), develop asthmalike symptoms. TDI apparently binds to proteins in the respiratory tract, creating foreign substances that stimulate a hypersensitivity reaction. Individuals who have been hypersensitized have difficulty breathing when exposed to TDI, tobacco smoke, and air pollutants. In Japan, 15% of all cases of asthma in men have been attributed to industrial exposure to chemicals.

Other chemicals bind to proteins in the skin, creating foreign substances to which the immune system reacts. Formaldehyde, for example, results in a condition called contact dermatitis, characterized by a skin rash. T cells attack and destroy the cells of the skin. Even low levels of formaldehyde in newsprint dyes, some cosmetics, and photographic papers are sufficient to induce rashes.

Other chemicals apparently act by suppressing immune function, making individuals more susceptible to infectious agents. Dioxins, PCBs, ozone, certain pesticides, and a variety of other chemical pollutants suppress the immune response in laboratory animals and humans. However, the overall significance of immune suppression and hypersensitivity in human populations remains unknown. Nonetheless, there are subtle and potentially far-reaching effects of toxic chemicals, again underscoring how homeostasis and health are dependent on a healthy environment.

Summary

Viruses and Bacteria: An Introduction

1. Two of the most important common agents are viruses and bacteria. *Viruses* are submicroscopic structures that consist of a nucleic acid core, consisting of either DNA or RNA, and an outer protein coat, the *capsid*.

2. Viruses are not true living organisms and must invade other organisms to reproduce. Viruses most often enter the body through the respiratory and digestive systems and spread from cell to cell in the bloodstream and lymphatic system. However, other avenues of entry are also possible—for example, sexual contact.

3. *Bacteria* are single-celled microorganisms that consist of a circular strand of DNA and cytoplasm which is enclosed by a plasma membrane.

4. Unlike viruses, bacteria can be killed with antibiotics. Unfortunaely, overuse of antibiotics in medicine is a growing problem: antibiotic resistance in bacteria. Many thousands of people die each year of infections caused by antibiotic-resistant bacteria they contract in hospitals or in other places.

5. Antibiotic resistance is also created by antibiotics (and other drugs) in treated sewage released into our waterways. This exposure is resulting in additional antibiotic resistant strains of bacteria.

6. Although they are best known for their role in causing sickness and death, most bacteria perform useful functions.

The First and Second Lines of Defense

7. The first line of defense against viruses, bacteria, and other infectious agents is the skin and the epithelia of the respiratory, digestive, and urinary systems. Some epithelia also produce protective chemical substances that kill microorganisms.

8. The second line of defense consists of cells and chemicals that the body produces to combat infectious agents that penetrate the epithelia.

9. One of the chief combatants in the second line of defense is the *macrophage,* a cell derived from the monocyte. Macrophages are found in connective tissue beneath epithelia, where they phagocytize infectious agents, preventing their spread. Neutrophils and monocytes also invade infected areas from the bloodstream and destroy bacteria and viruses.

10. Another combatant in the second line of defense consists of the chemicals released by damaged tissue, which stimulate arterioles in the infected tissue to dilate. The increase in blood flow raises the temperature of the wound. Heat stimulates macrophage metabolism, accelerating the rate of the destruction of infectious agents. Heat also speeds up the healing process.

11. Still other chemicals increase the permeability of the capillaries, causing plasma to flow into the wound and increasing the supply of nutrients for macrophages and other protective cells.

12. The increase in blood flow, the release of chemical attractants, and the flow of plasma into the wound constitute the *inflammatory response.*

13. Another part of the secondary line of defense are the *pyrogens,* chemicals released primarily by macrophages exposed to bacteria, which raise body temperature and lower iron availability, thus decreasing bacterial replication.

14. *Interferons,* a group of proteins released by cells infected by viruses, are also part of the second line of defense. Interferons travel to other virus-infected cells, where they inhibit viral replication.

15. The blood also contains the *complement proteins,* which circulate in an inactive state, becoming activated only when the body is invaded by bacteria. They too are part of the second line of defense.

16. Some of the complement proteins stimulate the inflammatory response. Others embed in the plasma membrane of bacteria. There they combine to form *membrane-attack complexes,* which create holes in the bacterial plasma membranes, killing these pathogens. Another complement protein binds to the invader, making it more easily phagocytized by macrophages.

The Third Line of Defense: The Immune System

17. The *immune system* consists of billions of *lymphocytes* that circulate in the blood and lymph and take up residence in the *lymphoid organs* and *lymphoid tissues,* which are also part of the immune system.

18. The lymphocytes recognize *antigens*—foreign cells and foreign molecules, mostly proteins and large-molecular-weight polysaccharides.

19. *T and B cells* are two types of lymphocytes produced in red bone marrow. The T cells become immunocompetent—able to respond to a particular antigen in the thymus. B cells gain this ability in the bone marrow. During this process, the T and B cells produce membrane receptors that bind to specific antigens.

20. Immunocompetent B cells encounter antigens (often presented to them by macrophages) to which they are programmed to respond. They then begin to divide, forming *plasma cells* and *memory cells.* Plasma cells produce *antibodies.* The memory cells enable the body to respond more quickly to future invasions by the same antigen.

21. Antibodies are small protein molecules that bind to specific antigens, destroying them either by precipitation, agglutination, or neutralization, or by activation of the complement system.

22. When T and B cells first encounter an antigen, they react slowly. The initial response is called the *primary response.* Because the body responds slowly at first, there is often a period of illness before the pathogen is removed by the immune system.

23. Numerous memory cells produced during the first assault ensure that a reappearance of the antigen will elicit a much faster and more powerful reaction, the *secondary response.* Consequently, the pathogen is usually vanquished before symptoms of illness occur. The resistance created by a response to an antigen is called *immunity.*

24. When activated by an antigen, T cells multiply and differentiate, forming *memory T cells, cytotoxic T cells, helper T cells,* and *suppressor T cells* whose functions are summarized in **TABLE 8-3**.

25. A solution containing a dead or weakened virus, bacterium, or bacterial toxin that is injected into people to create *active immunity* is called a *vaccine.*

26. *Passive immunity* can be achieved by injecting antibodies into a patient or by the transfer of antibodies from a mother to her baby through the bloodstream or breast milk. Passive immunity is short-lived, lasting at most only a few months, compared to active immunity which lasts for years.

Practical Applications: Blood Transfusions and Tissue Transplantation

27. Blood transfusions require careful matching of donor and recipient blood types. Tissue transplantation requires similar matching. In such instances, only cells from the same individual or an identical twin will be accepted. All others are rejected by the T cells, unless the system is suppressed with drugs.

Diseases of the Immune System

28. The most common malfunctions of the immune system are *allergies,* extreme reactions to some antigens.

29. Allergies are caused by *IgE antibodies,* produced by plasma cells. IgE antibodies bind to mast cells, which causes them to release histamine and other chemical substances that induce the symptoms of an allergy—production of mucus, sneezing, and itching.

30. *Autoimmune diseases,* another immune system disorder, result from an immune attack on the body's own cells. Autoimmune diseases may occur when normal proteins are modified by chemicals or genetic mutations so that they are no longer recognizable as self. Other possible causes are the sudden presence of proteins that are normally isolated from the immune system and exposure to antigens that are nearly identical to body proteins.

AIDS: The Deadly Virus

31. *AIDS* is a disease of the immune system caused by *HIV,* a virus that attacks helper T cells (T4 cells), severely impairing a person's immune system.

32. AIDS progresses through three stages: asymptomatic carrier, AIDS-Related Complex, and full-blown AIDS.

33. During the first phase, no symptoms appear, although an individual is highly infectious—able to transmit the disease to others.

34. During the second phase, patients grow progressively weaker as their immune system falters. Lymph nodes swell and patients report persistent or recurrent fevers and a persistent cough. Mental deterioration may also occur.

35. During the last phase, patients suffer from severe weight loss and weakness. Many develop cancer and bacterial infections because of their diminished immune response.
36. AIDS is spread through body fluids during sexual contact and blood transfusions or through needles shared by drug users.
37. Stopping the virus has proved difficult, in large part because symptoms of AIDS do not appear until several months to several years after the initial HIV infection.
38. Numerous researchers are developing vaccines that they hope will protect people and eventually eradicate the virus, but so far efforts to develop a vac-cine have not proven successful. One reason is that HIV is highly mutable.
39. Although progress is being made in more developed nations, many poorer nations such as those in Africa, are witnessing an epidemic of AIDs. Lack of education and money to buy expensive treatments available in the West could result in the death of many millions of people in these nations.

Health, Homeostasis, and the Environment: Multiple Chemical Sensitivity

40. The immune system and protective mechanisms that constitute the first and second lines of defense protect the body from harmful viruses and mi-crobes. In a sense, they help maintain a constant internal state either directly, by warding off infectious agents, or secondarily, by protecting other body cells that are essential to homeostasis.
41. Chemicals can damage the immune system, upsetting homeostasis.
42. Many individuals suffer from *multiple chemical sensitivity*. Chronic exposure to low levels of pollutants or short-term exposure to high levels may alter the immune system, causing a wide range of symptoms.
43. Some toxic chemicals cause *hypersensitivity*, evoking allergylike symptoms. Others stimulate autoimmune responses, and still others cause immune suppression.

Critical Thinking

Thinking Critically—Analysis

This Analysis corresponds to the Thinking Critically scenario that was presented at the beginning of this chapter.

This chapter offers a brief overview of the topic of vaccination. The first conclusion that you might draw is that the text does not provide enough information to analyze the claims made by your friends about vaccination. You'd be advised to study an immunology book as well as the scientific literature. Once you've read some more, you will be better able to discern whether vaccination is worth the relatively small risk.

Despite the brief coverage, this chapter does point out that infectious diseases have not been eliminated. Vaccination has only kept them under control by reducing the potential population of hosts. Thus, if large numbers of people are unvaccinated against infectious disease, outbreaks could occur. The results could be quite dramatic because we're living on a crowded planet, and infectious organisms spread quickly in crowded environments.

Test of Concepts

1. Describe the structure of a typical virus.
2. Based on your previous studies (Chapter 3), in what ways are bacteria similar to human cells, and in what ways are they different?
3. The human body consists of three lines of defense. Describe what they are and how they operate.
4. Describe the inflammatory response, and explain how it protects the body.
5. Define each of the following terms, and explain how they help protect the body: pyrogen, interferon, and complement proteins.
6. The first and second lines of defense differ substantially from the third line of defense. Describe the major differences.
7. How does the immune system detect foreign substances?
8. Describe how the B cell operates. Be sure to include the following terms in your discussion: bone marrow, immunocompetence, plasma membrane receptors, primary response, plasma cell, antigen, antibody, and secondary response.
9. Describe the four mechanisms by which antibodies "destroy" antigens.
10. Describe the events that occur after a T cell encounters its antigen.
11. What is the difference between active and passive immunity?
12. A child is stung by a bee, swells up, and collapses, having great difficulty breathing. What has happened? What can be done to save the child's life?
13. What is an autoimmune disease? Explain the reasons it forms.
14. What is AIDS? What are the symptoms? What causes it?

The Vital Exchange

RESPIRATION

Thinking Critically

For years, representatives of the tobacco industry claimed that there was no proof that cigarette smoking caused cancer, despite the fact that over 40 epidemiological studies showed a strong correlation between smoking and lung cancer. Most of these studies correct for other factors that might cause lung cancer such as exposure to carcinogenic chemical pollutants in the workplace.

Why did representatives from the tobacco industry persist in claiming that there was no proof that smoking caused lung cancer? How would you have responded to their assertion? Can a study be devised to prove the connection? What critical thinking rules does this exercise rely on? ■

Air-conducting portion of the human lung.

George F. Eaton was a robust and handsome Irishman who grew up in eastern Massachusetts, married, and raised three children. To support his family, Eaton worked as a fire fighter for 30 years. Fire fighting is dangerous work, in part because it exposes men and women to smoke containing numerous potentially harmful air pollutants.

Upon retirement, Eaton moved to Cape Cod, but his retirement years were cut short by **emphysema**—a debilitating respiratory disease resulting from the breakdown of the air sacs, or **alveoli,** in the lungs, where oxygen and carbon dioxide are exchanged between the air and the blood. As the walls of the alveoli degenerate, the surface area for the diffusion of oxygen and carbon dioxide gradually decreases. Emphysema is irreversible and incurable. Patients suffer from shortness of breath; eventually, even mild exertion becomes trying, prompting one patient to describe the disease as a kind of "living hell."

The degeneration of the lungs in patients with emphysema creates a domino effect. One of the dominoes is the heart. Because oxygen absorption in the lungs declines quite substantially over time, the heart of an emphysemic patient must work harder and harder. This effort puts additional strain on this already hard-working organ and can lead to heart failure.

George Eaton died a slow death as his lungs grew increasingly more inefficient. Relatives mourning his death blamed it on the pollution to which he was exposed while working for the fire department. Fire fighting, however, was probably only part of the cause, for Eaton had smoked most of his adult life. Cigarette smoking is the leading cause of emphysema.

This chapter describes the respiratory system—its structure and function and the diseases that affect it, such as emphysema.

Structure of the Human Respiratory System

The human respiratory system functions automatically, drawing air into the lungs, then letting it out, in a cycle that repeats itself about 16 times per minute at rest—or about 23,000 times per day. If you got a dollar for each time you took a breath, you'd be a millionaire in a month and a half.

The respiratory system supplies oxygen to the body and gets rid of carbon dioxide. Oxygen, of course, is needed for cellular respiration; carbon dioxide is a waste product of this process. In its role as a provider of oxygen and a disposer of carbon dioxide waste, the respiratory system helps to maintain the constant internal environment necessary for normal cellular metabolism. Thus, like many other systems, it plays an important role in homeostasis.

The respiratory system consists of two basic parts: an air-conducting portion and a gas-exchange portion (**TABLE 9-1**). The air-conducting portion is an elaborate set of passageways that transports air to and from the **lungs,** two large, saclike organs in the thoracic cavity (**FIGURE 9-1A**). Like the arteries of the body, these passageways start out large, then become progressively smaller and more numerous, branching profusely in the lungs, where the exchange of oxygen and carbon dioxide between the air and the blood takes place.

The lungs are the gas-exchange portion of the respiratory system. Each lung has millions of tiny, thin-walled alveoli (singular, alveolus) (**FIGURE 9-1B**). The walls of the alveoli contain numerous capillaries that absorb oxygen from the inhaled air and release carbon dioxide (**FIGURE 9-1B**).

The Conducting Portion of the Respiratory System Moves Air In and Out of the Body and Also Filters and Moistens Incoming Air

Air enters the respiratory system through the nose and mouth, then is drawn backward into the **pharynx**

TABLE 9-1	
Summary of the Respiratory System	
Organ	Function
Air conducting	
Nasal cavity	Filters, warms, and moistens air; also transports air to pharynx
Oral cavity	Transports air to pharynx; warms and moistens air; helps produce sounds
Pharynx	Transports air to larynx
Epiglottis	Covers the opening to the trachea during swallowing
Larynx	Produces sounds; transports air to trachea; helps filter incoming air; warms and moistens incoming air
Trachea and bronchi	Warm and moisten air; transport air to lungs; filter incoming air
Bronchioles	Control air flow in the lungs; transport air to alveoli
Gas exchange	
Alveoli	Provide area for exchange of oxygen and carbon dioxide

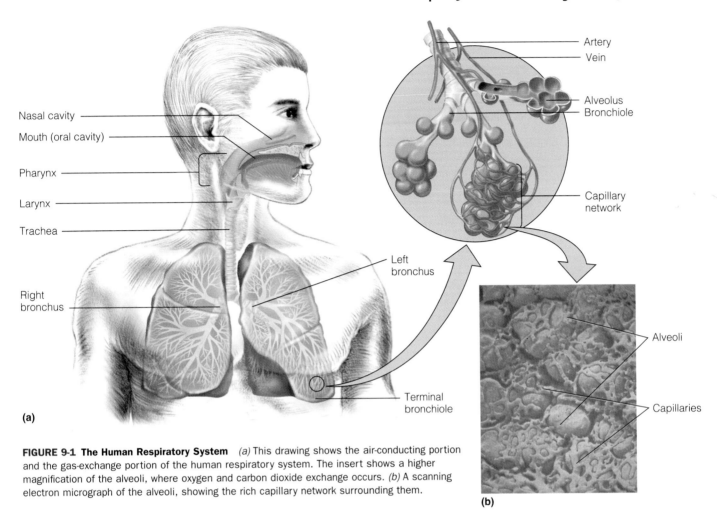

Nasal cavity

Mouth (oral cavity)

Pharynx

Larynx

Trachea

Right bronchus

Left bronchus

Terminal bronchiole

Artery

Vein

Alveolus

Bronchiole

Capillary network

Alveoli

Capillaries

(a)

(b)

FIGURE 9-1 The Human Respiratory System *(a)* This drawing shows the air-conducting portion and the gas-exchange portion of the human respiratory system. The insert shows a higher magnification of the alveoli, where oxygen and carbon dioxide exchange occurs. *(b)* A scanning electron micrograph of the alveoli, showing the rich capillary network surrounding them.

(FAIR-inks) (**FIGURE 9-2**). The pharynx is that portion of the respiratory system that opens into the nose and mouth in the front (anteriorly) and joins below with the larynx (LAIR-inks). The **larynx,** or voice box, is a rigid, hollow structure that houses the **vocal cords,** two folds of tissue that vibrate when we talk, sing, or hum, (**FIGURE 9-2**). To feel it, gently put your fingers alongside your throat, then swallow. The structure that moves up and down is the larynx.

The larynx opens into the **trachea** (TRAY-kee-ah) or windpipe below. You can feel the trachea beneath your Adam's apple, the protrusion of the laryngeal cartilage on your neck.

As explained in Chapter 5, food is prevented from entering the larynx by the **epiglottis** (ep-eh-GLOT-tis), a flap of tissue that closes off the opening to the larynx

during swallowing. Occasionally, however, food goes the wrong way, accidentally entering the larynx and trachea. This unfortunate event leads to violent coughing, a reflex that helps eject the food from the trachea. If the food cannot be dislodged by coughing, steps must be taken to remove it—and fast—or the person will suffo-

Nasal cavity

Tongue

Epiglottis

Larynx

Trachea

Pharynx

Vocal cords

Esophagus

FIGURE 9-2 Uppermost Portion of the Respiratory System Bony protrusions into the nasal cavity (not shown here) create turbulence that causes dust particles to settle out on the mucous coating. Notice that air passing from the pharynx enters the larynx. Food is kept from entering the respiratory system by the epiglottis, which covers the laryngeal opening during swallowing.

Health Note 9-1

First Aid for Choking That May Save Someone's Life

What do you do if you encounter a person who is choking? If the person can cough, speak, or breathe, do not interfere. Encourage the individual to continue coughing. If he or she cannot cough, speak, or breathe, **CALL OR HAVE SOMEONE CALL 911 OR YOUR LOCAL EMERGENCY NUMBER IMMEDIATELY.**

If the person is conscious:
- Stand behind him and wrap your arms around his waist.
- Make a fist with one hand (thumb outside the fist), and place the fist just above the navel in the

middle of the abdomen. Be sure that your fist is well below the lower tip of the sternum.
- Wrap the other hand around the fist and perform cycles of five quick inward and upward thrusts. After every five thrusts, check the person and repeat the cycles until the person begins to cough, speak, or breathe on his own.

If the person is unconscious:
- Carefully position her on her back.
- Open the airway by placing one hand on the forehead and one hand on the chin and gently tilt the head backward (head-tilt/chin-lift). Place your ear next to

the person's mouth, listening for air exchange; feel for air exchange with your cheek; and look to see the chest rise and fall during air exchange.
- If you do not see, hear, or feel air exchange, pinch the person's nose closed and seal your mouth around the victim's mouth and give two slow breaths. The chest should rise and fall gently.
- If the first breath did not go in, reposition the victim's head and attempt another breath.
- If the breaths did not go in, straddle the victim's thighs and place the heel of one hand just above the navel and place the other hand on top, interlocking your fingers.
- Give five quick inward and upward thrusts.
- Return to the victim's head; perform a finger sweep of her mouth, searching for a dislodged object; perform a head-tilt/chin-lift; and give one slow breath.
- If the breath will not go in, give five more abdominal thrusts, followed by a finger sweep, and one breath.

cate. Health Note 9-1 explains what to do when a person chokes.

The trachea is a short, wide duct. Starting in the neck below the larynx, it enters the thoracic cavity, where it divides into two large branches, the right and left **bronchi** (BRON-kee). The bronchi (singular, bronchus) enter the lungs alongside the arteries and veins. Inside the lungs, the bronchi branch extensively, forming progressively smaller tubes that carry air to the alveoli.

The trachea and bronchi are reinforced by hyaline cartilage, which is located in the walls of these structures. This cartilage reinforcement prevents the structures from collapsing during breathing, thus ensuring a steady flow of air in and out of the lungs.

The smallest bronchi in the lungs branch to form **bronchioles** (BRON-kee-ols). Bronchioles are small ducts that lead to the alveoli.

The smallest bronchi in the lungs branch to form **bronchioles** (BRON-kee-ols), which lead to the alveoli. Like the arterioles of the circulatory system, the walls of the bronchioles consist largely of smooth muscle. This permits them to open and close, and thus provides a means of controlling air flow in the lungs. During exercise or times of stress, the bronchioles open and the flow of air into the lungs increases. This homeostatic mechanism helps meet the body's need for more oxygen, in much the same way that the arterioles of capillary beds dilate to let more blood into body tissues in times of need.

- Continue this cycle until the victim begins to cough, speak, or breathe on his or her own.

Perform the same technique for children as you would for an adult. Children are considered those who are over one year of age and under the age of eight. The size of the child must also be a consideration.

For infants and very small children who cannot cough, speak, or breathe:

- Pick up the infant and place her face down on your forearm.
- Give the infant five back blows with the heel of your hand between the shoulder blades.

- Reposition the infant face up on the opposite forearm and give five chest thrusts using the pads of two or three fingers in the lower half of the sternum.
- Continue this cycle until the infant can breathe on his or her own or until the infant goes unconscious.

If the infant is unconscious:

- Perform a head-tilt/chin-lift and look, listen, and feel for air exchange.
- If no exchange is present, seal your mouth around the mouth and nose of the infant and give two slow breaths. The chest should rise and fall gently.

- If the first breath did not go in, reposition the infant's head and attempt another breath.
- If the breaths did not go in, position the infant for five back blows, five chest thrusts; then, check his mouth for an object and one give breath.
- Continue this cycle until the infant begins to breathe on his or her own.

In order to be skilled in these and other lifesaving skills, you should take a first aid and CPR class. Classes are offered in most communities through the National Safety Council. Call 1-800-621-7618 for information on classes in your area.

Source: Adapted by Jennifer Belcher, *EMT-B* from the guidelines of the American Red Cross, National Safety Council and the American Heart Association.

Visit *Human Biology's* Internet site for links to web sites offering more information on this topic.

The respiratory system is in direct contact with the external environment and is therefore quite vulnerable to infectious organisms and air pollutants present in the air all around us. The respiratory systems of animals have evolved several protective mechanisms. In humans and other animals, the conducting portion filters airborne particles such as dust and pollen from the air we breathe.

Airborne particles or particulates come in many sizes. The large and medium-sized particles are easily removed. They drop out of the air as it travels through the nasal passageways and the upper respiratory system. Smaller particles, also known as *fine particulates,* however, are so tiny that they remain in the air breathed into our lungs. As a result, they can penetrate deeply into the

lung. Some of these particles contain toxic metals such as mercury, which can cause lung cancer.

Particles that precipitate out of the inhaled air in the nose, trachea, and bronchi are trapped in a layer of **mucus** (MEW-kuss). Mucus is a thick, slimy secretion produced by certain cells, the **mucous cells**, in the epithelial lining of the nose, trachea, and bronchi (**FIGURE 9-3**)[1]

The epithelium of the respiratory tract also contains numerous ciliated cells. **Cilia**, you may recall from Chapter 2, are small organelles that extend from the surface of cells lining the respiratory tract and parts of the reproductive tract of women. The cilia in the respiratory

---

[1]You will notice that the adjective form is spelled "mucous" (as in mucous cell) and the noun form is spelled "mucus."

FIGURE 9-3 Mucous Trap
(a) Drawing of the lining of the trachea. Mucus produced by the mucous cells of the lining of much of the respiratory system traps bacteria, viruses, and other particulates in the air. The cilia transport the mucus toward the mouth. *(b)* Higher magnification of the lining showing a mucous cell and ciliated epithelial cells.

(b) Mucous cell   Cilia

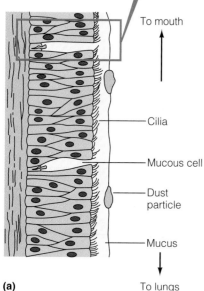

To mouth

Cilia

Mucous cell

Dust particle

Mucus

To lungs

(a)

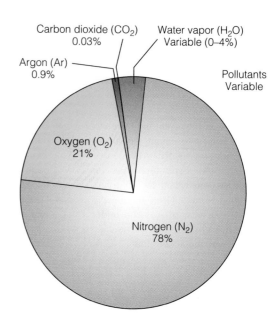

Carbon dioxide (CO_2) 0.03%   Water vapor (H_2O) Variable (0–4%)

Argon (Ar) 0.9%

Pollutants Variable

Oxygen (O_2) 21%

Nitrogen (N_2) 78%

FIGURE 9-4 Composition of Air

system beat upward, propelling mucus containing bacteria and dust particles toward the mouth. Operating day and night, they sweep the mucus toward the oral cavity, where it can be swallowed or expectorated (spit out). This protects the respiratory tract and lungs from bacteria and potentially harmful particulates. It is another of the body's homeostatic mechanisms.

Like all homeostatic mechanisms, the respiratory mucous trap is not invincible. Bacteria and viruses do occasionally penetrate the lining, causing respiratory infections. Making matters worse, sulfur dioxide, a pollutant in cigarette smoke and urban air pollution, temporarily paralyzes, and may even destroy, cilia. Sulfur dioxide gas in the smoke of a single cigarette, for instance, will paralyze the cilia for an hour or more, permitting bacteria and toxic particulates to be deposited on the lining of the respiratory tract, even enter the lungs. Ironically, the cilia of a smoker are paralyzed when they are needed the most!

Because smoking impairs a natural protective mechanism, it should come as no surprise that smokers suffer more frequent respiratory infections than nonsmokers. Research shows that alcohol also paralyzes the respiratory system cilia, explaining why alcoholics are prone to respiratory infections.

The conducting portion of the respiratory system also moistens and warms the incoming air. Beneath the epithelium of the respiratory tract is a rich network of capillaries that releases moisture and heat. Moisture protects the lungs from drying out, and heat protects them from cold temperatures. Except in extremely cold

weather, by the time inhaled air reaches the lungs, it is nearly saturated with water and is warmed to body temperature.

On the way out of the respiratory system, much of the water that was added to the air condenses on the lining of the nasal cavity, which was cooled by the evaporation of water as the air was drawn in. This mechanism is an adaptation that conserves water and also accounts for the reason our noses tend to drip in cold weather.

The Alveoli Are the Site of Gaseous Exchange

The air we breathe consists principally of nitrogen and oxygen, with small amounts of carbon dioxide and other gases (**FIGURE 9-4**). Oxygen in the atmosphere is generated by the photosynthetic activity of plants and photosynthetic single-celled organisms. Oxygen is vital to humans and virtually all other living organisms. A constant supply must be delivered to body cells to sustain cellular energy production. (Remember from Chapter 2 that the complete breakdown of glucose in body cells requires oxygen!)

Oxygen is delivered to the alveoli of the lungs by the conducting portion of the respiratory system, as noted above. Inside the lung are numerous small sacs, called alveoli, which give the lung the appearance of an angel food cake (**FIGURES 9-5A AND 9-5B**). The alveoli are the site of oxygen exchange with the bloodstream.

In humans, each lung contains an estimated 150 million alveoli. The surface area they create is about the size of a tennis court, that is, about 60 to 80 square meters. This provides ample area for the exchange of oxygen.

(a) Alveoli

FIGURE 9-5 Alveoli *(a)* A scanning electron micrograph of the lung showing many alveoli. The smallest openings are capillaries surrounding the alveoli. *(b)* A higher magnification scanning electron micrograph of lung tissue showing alveoli. *(c)* A transmission electron micrograph showing several alveoli and the close relationship of the capillaries containing RBCs (dark structures inside the capillaries). This close relationship between capillaries and alveoli ensures the rapid transport of oxygen and carbon dioxide.

As shown in **FIGURE 9-6**, the alveoli are lined by a single layer of flattened cells, called **Type I alveolar cells**. Aiding in the exchange of oxygen is an extensive network of capillaries, shown in **FIGURE 9-1B**. Each capillary is made of an equally thin layer of flattened cells. Together, the cells of the alveolar wall and the capillary present a fairly easy route for the passage of gases into and out of the alveoli.

(b) Alveoli

The large surface area of the lungs created by the alveoli and the relatively thin barrier between the blood and the alveolar air result in a rather rapid diffusion of gases across the alveolar wall. The alveoli therefore provide another example of the marriage of form and function produced by evolution.

Another important cell in the alveoli is the **alveolar macrophage**, sometimes known as the **dust cell**. Alveolar macrophages are the cellular equivalent of a janitorial staff. They wander freely through the alveoli, phagocytizing dust, bacteria, viruses, and other particulates that manage to escape filtration by the upper portions of the respiratory system (**FIGURE 9-6**). Once filled with particulates, they take up residence in the connective tissue surrounding the alveoli. Over time, numerous spent cells come to reside in this region. Because there are so many particulates in tobacco smoke, a smoker's lungs are often blackened by dust cells packed with particulates. The lungs of urban residents may also be blackened by the accumulation of smoke and dust particles.

Yet another important cell in the alveoli is the **Type II alveolar cell** (**FIGURE 9-6**). Type II alveolar cells are large, round cells located in the alveolar epithelium. These prominent cells produce a vital chemical sub-

(c) RBCs   Capillaries

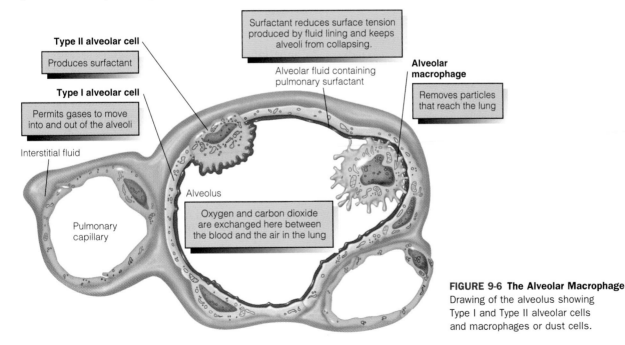

Type II alveolar cell
Produces surfactant

Type I alveolar cell
Permits gases to move into and out of the alveoli

Interstitial fluid

Surfactant reduces surface tension produced by fluid lining and keeps alveoli from collapsing.

Alveolar fluid containing pulmonary surfactant

Alveolar macrophage
Removes particles that reach the lung

Alveolus

Pulmonary capillary

Oxygen and carbon dioxide are exchanged here between the blood and the air in the lung

FIGURE 9-6 The Alveolar Macrophage
Drawing of the alveolus showing Type I and Type II alveolar cells and macrophages or dust cells.

FIGURE 9-7 Surface Tension Some insects can walk on water because of surface tension, the tight packing of water molecules along the surface of a pond.

stance known as **surfactant** (sir-FACK-tant). Surfactant is a general term that refers to any of dozens of detergentlike substances. The lung's surfactant dissolves in the thin layer of water lining the alveoli, where it plays an important role in keeping the tiny alveoli open. Let me explain.

The water covering the inside surface of alveolar epithelium produces surface tension. You've seen it many times before in the droplets of water that bead up on your car's windshield. Surface tension results from hydrogen bonds between water molecules. Discussed in Chapter 2, hydrogen bonds are intermolecular bonds. They form between the slightly charged oxygen atoms of water molecules with the slightly charged hydrogen atoms of others. These hydrogen bonds draw water molecules together. At the surface of a watery fluid, the hydrogen bonds pull water molecules together more tightly than elsewhere, creating a slightly denser region referred to as surface tension. Surface tension on a pond permits some insects such as water striders to walk on water and is the reason a drop of water beads up on your car's windshield (**FIGURE 9-7**).

In the alveoli, surface tension tends to draw the walls of the alveoli inward.

FIGURE 9-8 A Coyote Howls The vocal cords enable coyotes and many other species to create a wide assortment of sounds essential to communication.

In other words, it tends to make them collapse. Surfactant, however, reduces surface tension in the alveoli, decreasing forces that might otherwise cause the alveoli to close down.

Some premature babies lack sufficient surfactant. High surface tension in the alveoli causes the larger alveoli to collapse, resulting in a dramatic, life-threatening condition known as **respiratory distress syndrome** or **RDS**. Fortunately, children born with this problem are usually treated with an artificial surfactant that keeps the alveoli open until their lungs produce enough of their own to perform this small but important function.

<hr>

Section 9-2

Functions of the Respiratory System

The chief functions of the respiratory system are to (1) replenish the blood's oxygen supply and (2) rid the blood of excess carbon dioxide. However, the respiratory system serves other functions as well. The vocal cords, for example, located in the larynx, produce sounds that allow people to communicate. The respiratory system also houses the **olfactory membrane** (ol-FAC-tore-ee). This structure is a specialized patch of epithelium in the roof of the nasal cavity that contains sensors that detect odors. In addition, the respiratory system helps maintain pH balance by its influence on carbon dioxide levels (discussed shortly).

In Humans, Sound Is Produced by the Vocal Cords and Is Influenced by the Tongue and Oral Cavity

Phonation, the production of sounds, is critical to many members of the animal kingdom. The eerie cry of the coyote, for example, signals to the pack a member's whereabouts and helps the members of the pack stay in contact (**FIGURE 9-8**). The coyote's growl can signal to an intruder its intention to defend itself.

Except perhaps at sporting events, humans exhibit a much wider range of sounds for communication than do other animals. These sounds are produced by two elastic ligaments inside the larynx, the **vocal cords,** which vibrate as air is expelled from the lungs (**FIGURE 9-9**). The sounds generated by the vocal cords are modified by changing the position of the tongue and the shape of the oral cavity.

The vocal cords vary in length and thickness from one person to the next. They also vary between men and women. Most men, for example, have longer, thicker vocal cords than women as a result of testosterone, the male sex hormone produced by the testes. Men therefore tend to have deeper voices than most women.

The vocal cords are like the strings of a guitar or violin: they can be tightened or loosened, producing sounds of different pitch. The tighter the string on a guitar, the higher the note. In humans, muscles in the larynx that attach to the vocal cords make this adjustment possible. Relaxing the muscles lowers the tension on the cords, dropping the tone. Tightening the vocal cords has the opposite effect.

Bacterial and viral infections of the larynx result in a condition known as **laryngitis** (lair-in-JITE-iss). Lar-yngitis is an inflammation of the lining of the larynx and the vocal cords. This thickens the cords, causing a person's voice to lower. Laryngitis may also be caused by tobacco smoke, alcohol, excessive talking, shouting, coughing, or singing, all of which irritate the vocal cords. In young children, inflammation results in a swelling of the lining that may impede the flow of air and impair breathing, resulting in a condition called the **croup** (crewp).

Oxygen and Carbon Dioxide Diffuse Rapidly across the Alveolar and Capillary Walls

Deoxygenated blood entering the lungs arrives via the pulmonary arteries. This blood, as noted in Chapter 6, is laden with carbon dioxide picked up as it circulates through body tissues. In the capillary beds of the lungs, carbon dioxide is released, and oxygen is added, replenishing supplies depleted as blood flows through body tissues.

Carbon dioxide and oxygen readily diffuse across the capillary and alveolar walls, a process driven by the concentration difference between the alveoli and capillaries.[2] **FIGURE 9-10** illustrates the direction in which these gases flow. Oxygen in the alveolar air first diffuses through the alveolar epithelium, then into the extracellular fluid surrounding the capillaries. It then diffuses through the capillary wall and into the blood plasma (**FIGURE 9-11**). From here, oxygen molecules cross the plasma membrane of the red blood cells (RBCs) and bind to hemoglobin molecules in their cytoplasm. About 98% of the oxygen in the blood

[2]Physiologists actually speak of differences in partial pressure. The partial pressure of a gas is caused when gas molecules collide with a surface. The partial pressure of oxygen is proportional to the impact of all the oxygen molecules striking the alveolar wall. Thus, the partial pressure is proportional to the concentration of the gas molecules.

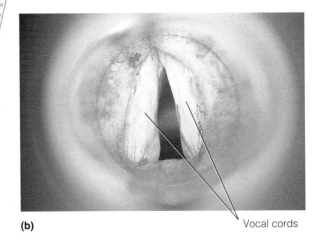

FIGURE 9-9 Vocal Cords
(a) Longitudinal section of the larynx showing the location of the vocal cords. Note the presence of the false vocal cord, so named because it does not function in phonation. (b) View into the larynx of a patient showing the true vocal cords from above.

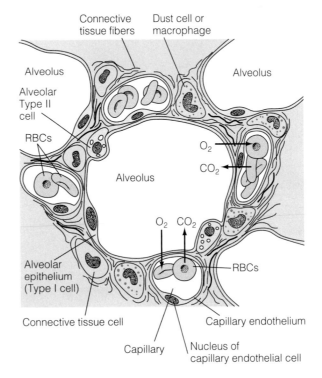

FIGURE 9-10 Close-Up of the Alveolus Oxygen diffuses out of the alveolus into the capillary. Carbon dioxide diffuses in the opposite direction, entering the alveolar air that is expelled during exhalation.

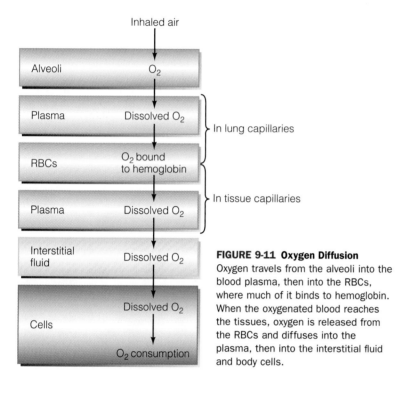

FIGURE 9-11 Oxygen Diffusion
Oxygen travels from the alveoli into the blood plasma, then into the RBCs, where much of it binds to hemoglobin. When the oxygenated blood reaches the tissues, oxygen is released from the RBCs and diffuses into the plasma, then into the interstitial fluid and body cells.

is carried in the RBCs bound to hemoglobin; the rest is dissolved in the plasma and cytoplasm of the RBCs.

In order to understand the details of carbon dioxide diffusion in the lung, we must go back to the body cells, where CO_2 is formed. As you may recall from Chapter 2, cells produce abundant CO_2 during cellular respiration, the chemical breakdown of glucose. In body tissues, carbon dioxide diffuses out of the cells and enters the blood plasma. Much of it then diffuses into the RBCs, where it is converted to carbonic acid, H_2CO_3 (**FIGURE 9-12**). This reaction is catalyzed by the enzyme carbonic anhydrase, found inside RBCs.

As shown at the top of **FIGURE 9-12**, carbonic acid molecules readily dissociate to form bicarbonate ions and hydrogen ions. Many of the bicarbonate ions then diffuse out of the RBCs into the plasma, where they are carried with the blood. Hydrogen ions stay behind. But not all carbon dioxide is transformed into bicarbonate. A small percentage (15%–25%) of it binds to hemoglobin of RBCs (but not at the oxygen binding site). Some carbon dioxide (7%) remains dissolved in the plasma (neither is shown in **FIGURE 9-12**).

When blood rich in carbon dioxide reaches the lungs, bicarbonate ions in the plasma reenter the RBCs, where they combine with hydrogen ions to form carbonic acid (**FIGURE 9-13**). Carbonic acid, in turn, reforms carbon dioxide. The CO_2 then diffuses out of the

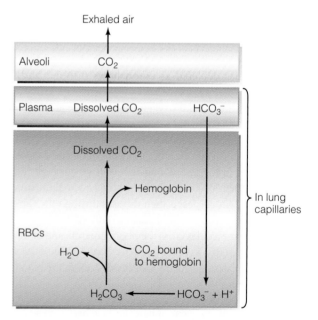

FIGURE 9-12 Bicarbonate Ion Production   Carbon dioxide (CO_2) diffuses out of body cells where it is produced and into the tissue fluid, then into the plasma. Although some carbon dioxide binds to hemoglobin and some is dissolved in the plasma, most is converted to carbonic acid (H_2CO_3) in the RBCs. Carbonic acid dissociates and forms hydrogen ions and bicarbonate ions. Hydrogen ions remain inside the RBCs, but most bicarbonate diffuses into the plasma where it is transported.

FIGURE 9-13 Carbon Dioxide Production from Bicarbonate
When the carbon dioxide-laden blood reaches the lungs, bicarbonate ions diffuse back into the RBCs and combine with hydrogen ions in RBCs forming carbonic acid, which dissociates, forming carbon dioxide gas. CO_2 diffuses out of the RBCs into the plasma, then into the alveoli.

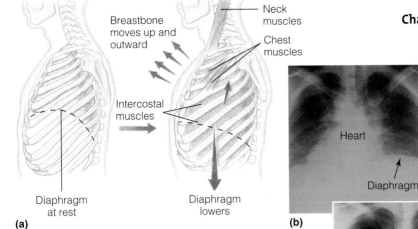

Breastbone moves up and outward

Neck muscles

Chest muscles

Intercostal muscles

Diaphragm at rest

Diaphragm lowers

(a)

(b)

Heart

Diaphragm

Heart

Diaphragm

FIGURE 9-14 The Bellows Effect *(a)* The rising and falling of the chest wall through the contraction of the intercostal muscles (muscles between the ribs) is shown in the diagram, illustrating the bellows effect. Inspiration is assisted by the diaphragm, which lowers. Like pulling a plunger out on a syringe, the rising of the chest wall and the lowering of the diaphragm draw air into the lungs. *(b)* X-rays showing the size of the lungs in full exhalation *(top)* and full inspiration *(bottom)*.

RBCs into the blood plasma. It then diffuses into the alveoli down a concentration gradient. Carbon dioxide is eventually expelled from the lungs during exhalation.

The uptake of oxygen and the discharge of carbon dioxide in the lungs "replenish" the blood in the alveolar capillaries. The oxygenated blood then flows back to the left atrium of the heart via the pulmonary veins. From here it empties into the left ventricle and is pumped to the body tissues via the aorta and its multitude of branches.

Section 9-3

Breathing and the Control of Respiration

Air moves in and out of the lungs in much the same way that it moves in and out of the bellows that blacksmiths

TABLE 9-2

Summary of Inhalation and Exhalation

Inhalation

Nerve impulses from the breathing center stimulate the muscles of inspiration—the diaphragm and intercostal muscles.

Contraction of the intercostal muscles causes the rib cage to move up and out.

Contraction of the diaphragm causes it to flatten.

Volume of the thoracic cavity increases.

Intrapulmonary pressure decreases.

Air flows into the lungs through the nose and mouth.

Exhalation

Nerve impulses from the breathing center feed back on it, shutting off stimuli to muscles of inspiration.

The intercostal muscles relax and the rib cage falls.

The diaphragm relaxes and rises.

The lungs recoil.

Air is pushed out of the lungs.

use to fan their fires. Breathing, however, is largely an involuntary action, controlled by the nervous system.

Air Is Moved In and Out of the Lungs by Changes in the Intrapulmonary Pressure

During breathing, air must first be drawn into the lungs. This process is known as **inspiration,** or **inhalation** (**TABLE 9-2**). Following inspiration, air must be expelled. This is known as **expiration,** or **exhalation**.

Inhalation is an active process controlled by the brain. Nerve impulses traveling from the brain stimulate the **diaphragm,** a dome-shaped muscle (unique to mammals) that separates the abdominal and thoracic cavities (**FIGURE 9-14A**). These impulses cause the diaphragm to contract. When it contracts, the diaphragm flattens and lowers. The contraction of the diaphragm draws air into the lungs much the same way that pulling the plunger of a syringe draws in air into the device.

Inhalation also involves the intercostal muscles, the short, powerful muscles that lie between the ribs. (They are the meat on barbecued ribs.) Nerve impulses traveling to these muscles cause them to contract as the diaphragm is lowered. When the intercostal muscles contract, the rib cage lifts up and out. Go ahead and try it right now. Place your hands on your chest, take a deep breath in and feel the chest wall expand and rise. Together, the contractions of the intercostal muscles and the diaphragm increase the volume of the thoracic cavity (**FIGURE 9-14B**, bottom). This, in turn, decreases the **intrapulmonary pressure,** the pressure in the alveoli. Air naturally flows in through the mouth and nose as the pressure inside the lungs decreases.

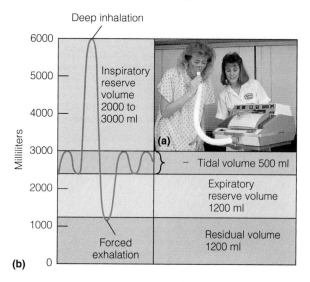

(b)

FIGURE 9-15 Measuring Lung Capacity (a) This machine allows health-care workers to determine tidal volume, inspiratory reserve volume, and other lung-capacity measurements to determine the health of an individual's lung. (b) This graph shows several common measurements.

At rest, each breath delivers about 500 milliliters of air to the lung. This is known as the **tidal volume.** Properly defined, the tidal volume is the amount of air inhaled or exhaled with each breath when a person is at rest. It is shown in **FIGURE 9-15.**

In contrast to inhalation, exhalation is a passive process—that is, it does not require muscle contraction in a person at rest. Exhalation begins after the lungs have filled with air. At this point in the cycle, the diaphragm and intercostal muscles relax. The relaxed diaphragm rises and resumes its domed shape. The chest wall falls slightly inward. These changes reduce the volume of the thoracic cavity, raising the internal pressure and forcing the air out in much the same way that squeezing an inflated beach ball forces air out of the opening. Try feeling after you've inhaled.

The lungs also contribute to passive exhalation of air due to the presence of numerous elastic fibers. During inspiration, the lungs fill like balloons. When inhalation ceases, the elastic fibers cause the lungs to recoil, forcing air out.

Although exhalation is a passive process in an individual at rest, it can be made active by contracting the muscles of the wall of the chest and abdomen. The forceful expulsion of air is called **forced exhalation.**

Inhalation can also be consciously augmented by a forceful contraction of the muscles of inspiration. (You can test this by taking a deep breath.) Forced inhalation increases the amount of air entering your lungs. Athletes often actively inhale and exhale just before an event to increase oxygen levels in their blood. A competitive swimmer, for example, may take several deep breaths before diving into the pool for a race. Deep breathing, while effective, can be dangerous, for reasons explained shortly.

The Health of a Person's Lungs Can Be Assessed by Measuring Air Flow In and Out of Them under Various Conditions

Children who are exposed to tobacco smoke at home experience a decrease in lung capacity—that is, a decrease in their ability to move air in and out of their lungs. Several measurements of lung capacity are routinely used to determine the health of a person's lungs.

Measurements of lung function are taken under controlled conditions. As shown in **FIGURE 9-15A**, patients breathe into a machine that measures and records the amount of air moving in and out of the lung at various times. **FIGURE 9-15B** shows a graph of some of the common measurements. The first is the tidal volume, which, as noted earlier, is the amount of air that moves in and out during passive breathing. After passive exhalation, however, the lungs still contain a considerable amount of air—about 2400 milliliters. Forced exhalation will expel about half of that air. This is known as the **expiratory reserve volume**. The remaining 1200 milliliters is known as the **residual volume**.

Another important measurement is the **inspiratory reserve volume (IRV)** This is the amount of air that can be drawn into the lungs during a deep inhalation. Deep inhalation draws in four to six times more air than the tidal volume, or 2000–3000 milliliters, depending on the size of the individual. So why learn all of this?

Lung diseases often result in changes in these measurements. Asthma, for example, reduces the inspiratory reserve volume—that is, the amount of air that can be inhaled during forced inspiration. Constriction of the brochioles and the build-up of mucus in these structures block air flowing into the lung, thus reducing IRV.

Breathing Is Controlled Principally by the Breathing Center in the Brain

Breathing is controlled by a region of the brain known as the breathing center. The **breathing center** is located in a region of the brain called the *brain stem* (or *medulla,* [meh-DEW-lah]).

The breathing center contains nerve cells that generate periodic bioelectric impulses. These impulses stimulate inhalation by causing the periodic contraction of the intercostal muscles and the diaphragm. When the lungs fill, however, the nerve impulses cease and the muscles relax. Air is forced out of the lungs.

Several mechanisms are responsible for the termination of the impulses to the diaphragm and intercostal muscles. The first is a negative feedback loop, shown on the right side of **FIGURE 9-16**. Here's how it works. As just noted, the breathing center sends nerve impulses to the diaphragm and intercostal muscles, causing them to contract. This results, as noted above, in inhalation.

However, the breathing center also sends nerve impulses to a nearby region of the brain stem. It transmits the impulses back to the breathing center. When they arrive, the impulses inhibit the activity of the neurons in the breathing center. This, in turn, temporarily terminates the signals traveling to the muscles of inspiration. These muscles relax and exhalation occurs.

Like many biological processes, this one has a second control mechanism. It consists of sensory nerve fibers that terminate inside the lung. The terminal ends of the nerve fibers are actually modified to become sensors, known as **stretch receptors** because they detect the level of distension in the lung. When the lung is full, nerve impulses from the stretch receptors are transmitted to the breathing center. These impulses turn off the breathing center. Important as they are, stretch receptors probably function only during exercise, when large volumes of air are moved in and out of the lungs.

Breathing is controlled by other processes, too. As shown in **FIGURE 9-16**, chemical receptors inside the

brain and arteries send bioelectric impulses via nerve cells to the breathing center. The chemical receptors detect the concentrations of carbon dioxide, hydrogen ions, and oxygen in the body. When levels of carbon dioxide are high, for instance, during vigorous exercise, chemical receptors send impulses to the breathing center causing an increase in the depth and rate of breathing. Next time you run up a flight of stairs and start breathing hard, you'll know why.

Although respiration is controlled by all three chemicals, the most important is carbon dioxide. As shown in **FIGURE 9-17**, carbon dioxide levels are monitored by chemical receptors in the **aorta** and the **carotid arteries** (kah-raw-tid). As you may recall from Chapter 6, the aorta is the large artery that carries oxygenated blood out of the heart. The carotid artery carries oxygenated blood from the aorta to the brain.

Carbon dioxide also diffuses into the **cerebrospinal fluid (CSF),** a clear liquid found in cavities in the brain known as the *ventricles*. In the CSF, carbon dioxide is converted into carbonic acid, which then dissociates to form bicarbonate and hydrogen ions. A rise in carbon dioxide in the blood, therefore, results in an increase in the H^+ concentration of the CSF. The in-

FIGURE 9-16 Breathing Center The breathing center controls respiration. It sends periodic impulses along the nerves to the muscles of inspiration, causing them to contract. The center also sends impulses along another route to a relay center in the brain stem. Impulses from here travel back to the breathing center, shutting off the impulses that stimulate inspiration. Stretch receptors in the lung also send signals to the breathing center to shut it off when the lungs are fully inflated. Chemical receptors in the brain and certain arteries and stretch receptors in the lung also alter the activity of the breathing center.

FIGURE 9-17 Chemical Control of Breathing CO_2 and hydrogen ions are the chief chemical controls of breathing. CO_2 stimulates chemoreceptors in the aorta and the carotid arteries. It also diffuses into the cerebrospinal fluid where it is converted to bicarbonate ions and hydrogen ions. Hydrogen ions stimulate receptors that send impulses to the breathing center, causing the depth and rate of breathing to increase.

crease in H$^+$, in turn, is detected by chemical receptors, or **chemoreceptors** (KEY-moe-ree-CEP-ters), in the brain. These receptors send impulses to the breathing center, triggering an increase in the rate and depth of breathing **(FIGURE 9-17).**

The chemoreceptors in the brain and arteries allow the body to adjust respiration to cellular demands. During exercise, for example, cellular respiration increases to meet rising demands for energy. As it increases, oxygen demand also escalates. But so does carbon dioxide production. As just noted, the carbon dioxide produced during exercise increases the depth and rate of breathing. As you breathe harder, carbon dioxide levels fall and oxygen concentrations in the blood increase.

The body also contains oxygen receptors. However, these receptors are not as sensitive as the H$^+$ or carbon dioxide receptors. In fact, oxygen levels must fall considerably before these receptors begin generating impulses that alter our breathing. This fact can have profound consequences for divers and swimmers. Many divers and swimmers hyperventilate before they take the plunge. Hyperventilation is repeated deep and rapid breathing that makes it possible for one to hold his breath under water longer. But how?

Hyperventilation works because it decreases carbon dioxide levels in the blood and H$^+$ concentrations in the CSF. This reduces the urge to breathe. Like many good things, there's a slight catch. When a diver enters the water after hypderventilating, low levels of carbon dioxide and H$^+$ concentrations suppress the urge to breathe, but oxygen levels in the blood may fall so low that the brain is deprived of oxygen. The diver may lose consciousness. This happens because levels of hydrogen ions and carbon dioxide aren't high enough to stimulate breathing; moreover, blood oxygen levels are not low enough to stimulate breathing. The diver blacks out well before the H$^+$ concentration in the CSF reaches the level needed to stimulate breathing. So be careful.

Section 9-4

Diseases of the Respiratory System

The respiratory tract is "home" to many diseases and illnesses. With its close proximity to the external environment, it will "host" numerous bacterial and viral infections throughout your life. Some will cause considerable discomfort, and some could be fatal if you don't seek medical attention.

Microbial infections may occur in many different locations in the respiratory system and are named by their site of residence. An infection in the bronchi is therefore known as **bronchitis** (bron-KITE-iss). An infection of the sinuses is known as **sinusitis** (sigh-nu-SITE-iss). (Bacterial and viral infections were discussed in the previous chapter; a few of the more common ones are listed in **TABLE 9-3.**)

Once inside the respiratory tract, bacteria, viruses, and other microorganisms can spread to other organ systems. For example, **meningitis** (MEN-in-JITE-iss) is a bacterial or viral infection of the **meninges** (meh-NIN-jees), the fibrous layers surrounding the brain and spinal cord. This potentially fatal disease usually starts out as an infection of the sinuses or the lungs. That's why you're advised to see a doctor if these infections last more than a few weeks.

The lungs are also susceptible to airborne materials, among them asbestos fibers. **Asbestos** is a naturally occurring fiber that has been used in thousands of products from pipe and sound insulation to car brake pads. Inside the lung, asbestos can cause enormous damage. Workers exposed to asbestos, for example, develop two types of lung cancer. Others have developed a debilitating disease known as **asbestosis** (ass-bes-TOE-sis). Asbestosis is a build-up of scar tissue that reduces the lung capacity. Because asbestos is believed to be dangerous, virtually all of its uses have been banned in the United States, and asbestos used for insulation and decoration is either being removed from buildings or stabilized so it won't flake off.

Another common disease of the respiratory system is **asthma.** Characterized by periodic episodes of wheezing and difficult breathing, asthma is a chronic disorder—that is, it's a disease that persists for many years.

Most cases of asthma are caused by allergic reactions (abnormal immune reactions) to common stimulants such as dust, pollen, and skin cells (dander) from pets. In some individuals, it is brought on by certain foods, such as eggs, milk, chocolate, and food preservatives. Still other cases are triggered by drugs, such as antibiotics. Vigorous exercise and physiological stress are known to trigger asthma attacks, too.

In asthmatics, irritants such as pollen and dander cause a rapid increase in the production of mucus by the bronchi and bronchioles. Irritants also stimulate the constriction of the bronchioles. Mucus production and constriction of the bronchioles make breathing difficult. Asthmatics also suffer a chronic inflammation of the lining of the respiratory tract.

Although asthma is fairly common in school children, it often disappears as they grow older. But that may be changing. Studies show that the incidence of asthma in adults is on the rise. Many more children suffer from the disease, too. In fact, the number of Americans now suffer-

TABLE 9-3

Common Respiratory Diseases

Disease	Symptoms	Cause	Treatment
Emphysema	Breakdown of alveoli; shortness of breath	Smoking and air pollution	Administer oxygen to relieve symptoms; quit smoking; avoid polluted air. No known cure.
Chronic bronchitis	Coughing, shortness of breath	Smoking and air pollution	Quit smoking; move out of polluted area; if possible, move to warmer, drier climate.
Acute bronchitis	Inflammation of the bronchi; yellowy mucus coughed up; shortness of breath	Many viruses and bacteria	If bacterial, take antibiotics, cough medicine; use vaporizer.
Sinusitis	Inflammation of the sinuses; mucus discharge; blockage of nasal passageways; headache	Many viruses and bacteria	If bacterial, take antibiotics and decongestant tablets; use vaporizer.
Laryngitis	Inflammation of larynx and vocal cords; sore throat; hoarseness; mucus buildup and cough	Many viruses and bacteria	If bacterial, take antibiotics, cough medicine; avoid irritants, like smoke; avoid talking.
Pneumonia	Inflammation of the lungs ranging from mild to severe; cough and fever; shortness of breath at rest; chills; sweating; chest pains; blood in mucus	Bacteria, viruses, or inhalation of irritating gases	Consult physician immediately; go to bed; take antibiotics, cough medicine; stay warm.
Asthma	Constriction of bronchioles; mucus buildup in bronchioles; periodic wheezing; difficulty breathing	Allergy to pollen, some foods, food additives; dandruff from dogs and cats; exercise	Use inhalants to open passageways; avoid irritants.

ing from asthma is estimated to be about 17.3 million, up from 6.7 million in 1980.

Public health officials are concerned about the growing epidemic of asthma because periodic attacks can be quite disabling. Some even lead to death. By one estimate, 5000 Americans die each year from severe asthma attacks. Victims are generally elderly individuals who suffer from other diseases as well.

The severity of asthma attacks can be greatly lessened by proper medical treatment. One of the most common treatments is an oral spray (inhalant) containing the hormone epinephrine, which stimulates the bronchioles to open. Anti-inflammatory drugs (steroids) can be administered to treat chronic inflammation. Screening tests can help a patient find out what substances trigger an asthmatic attack so they can be avoided. One of the most prevalent respiratory diseases is lung cancer caused by smoking, a topic discussed in Health Note 9-2.

Health, Homeostasis, and the Environment

Air Pollution

The respiratory system plays a vital role in homeostasis. It helps regulate oxygen and carbon dioxide levels in the blood and in body tissues. It helps maintain the pH (acidity) of extracellular fluid by controlling the rate at which acid-forming carbon dioxide is removed from the blood. Furthermore, the respiratory system helps to protect us from infectious disease. Like other body systems, the respiratory system can be thrown out of kilter by chemical contaminants in the environment. This, in turn, alters homeostasis.

The air of the industrialized world contains a multitude of potentially harmful chemical pollutants that damage human health by upsetting homeostasis. In fact, air pollutants generated in our homes, factories, and cities now claim the lives of thousands of Americans each year.

Health Note 9-2

Smoking and Health: The Deadly Connection

Urban air pollution worries many Americans, and with good reason. However, city air that many of us breathe is benign compared with the "air" that 54 million Americans over the age of 18 voluntarily inhale from cigarettes. Loaded with dangerous pollutants in concentrations far greater than those of our cities, cigarette smoke takes a huge toll on citizens of the world. In the United States, for example, an estimated 419,000 people—about 1150 every day—die from the many adverse health effects of tobacco smoke, including heart attacks, lung cancer, and emphysema. Making matters worse, smoking is addictive. Nicotine, one of the many components of tobacco smoke, hooks many people in a dangerous activity.

Smoking costs society a great deal in medical bills and lost productivity. According to the Worldwatch Institute, every pack of cigarettes sold in the United States costs our society about $1.25–3.17 in medical costs, lost wages, and reduced productivity—that's about $125–$400 billion a year!

Smoking is a principal cause of lung cancer, claiming the lives of an estimated 144,000 men and women in the United States each year. Smokers are 11–25 times more likely to develop lung cancer than nonsmokers. The more one smokes, the more risk one suffers.

Unfortunately, nonsmokers are also affected by the smoke of others. Nonsmokers inhale tobacco smoke in meetings, in restaurants, at work, and at home. Research has shown that nonsmokers—sometimes referred to as "passive smokers" because they "smoke" involuntarily—are more likely to develop lung cancer than those nonsmokers who manage to steer clear of smokers. In a study of Japanese women married to men who smoked, researchers found that the wives were as likely to develop lung cancer as people who smoked half a pack of cigarettes a day!

A report by the U.S. Environmental Protection Agency estimates that passive smoking causes 500–5000 cases of lung cancer a year in the United States. Passive smokers who are exposed to tobacco smoke for long periods also suffer from impaired lung function equal to that seen in light smokers (people who smoke under a pack a day).

Cigarette smoke in closed quarters can cause angina (chest pains) in smokers and nonsmokers afflicted by atherosclerosis of the coronary arteries. Carbon monoxide in cigarette smoke is responsible for angina attacks.

Smokers are also more susceptible to colds and other respiratory infections. And smoking affects children. One study showed that children from families in which both parents smoked suffered twice as many upper respiratory infections as children from nonsmoking families. Recently, researchers from the Harvard Medical School reported finding a 7% decrease in lung capacity in children raised by mothers who smoked. The researchers believe that this change may lead to other pulmonary problems later in life.

For years, passive smokers have had little power when it came to their exposure to other people's smoke. Today, however, as a result of a growing awareness of the dangers, new regulations ban or restrict smoking in many public places and in the workplace.

The effects of smoking extend way beyond respiratory disease. Recent studies, for instance, show that smoking even decreases fertility in women. For example, women who smoke more than a pack of cigarettes a day are half as fertile as nonsmokers. Smoking may also affect the outcome of pregnancy. According to the 1985 U.S. Surgeon General's Report, women who smoke several packs a day during pregnancy are much more likely to miscarry and are also more likely to give birth to smaller children. On average, the children of these women are 200 grams (nearly 0.5 pounds) lighter than children born to nonsmoking mothers. Finally, children of women who smoke heavily during pregnancy generally score lower on mental aptitude tests during early childhood than children whose mothers do not smoke.

Numerous studies also show that smoking is a major contributor to impotence in men. In fact, smokers are 50% more likely to be impotent than nonsmokers. Smoking also causes arterial changes that restrict blood flow to the penis. Changes be-

Air pollution upsets the homeostatic balance in our bodies and affects millions of us on a daily basis. Unfortunately, most people are unaware of the dangers of air pollution because the line between cause and effect is not always clear. Consider, for instance, the headache you experienced in traffic going home from school or work. Was it caused by tension, or could it have been caused by carbon monoxide emissions from cars, buses, and trucks? And what about the runny nose and sinus condition you experienced last winter? Were they caused by a virus or bacterium or by pollution?

One classic study of air pollution in New York City in the 1960s illustrates the relationship between air pollution and respiratory problems. Researchers found that gin to occur early in life. Teenage smokers could have problems in their thirties if they continue to smoke.

Tobacco smoke contains numerous hazardous substances that damage the lining of the respiratory system. Nicotine and sulfur dioxide, for example, paralyze the cilia lining the respiratory tract.

Tobacco smoke is also laden with microscopic carbon particles. These carbon particles penetrate deeply into the lungs, where they accumulate in the alveoli and alveolar walls, turning healthy tissue into a blackened mass that often becomes cancerous (**FIGURE 1**). Tobacco smoke may also paralyze the alveolar macrophages, making a bad situation even worse.

Toxic chemicals in cigarette smoke, many of which are known carcinogens, attach to carbon particles. Toxin-carrying particles adhere to the lungs, larynx, trachea, and bronchi. Virtually any place they stick, they can cause cancer, explaining why smokers are five times more likely than nonsmokers to develop laryngeal cancer and four times more likely to develop cancer of the oral cavity.

Nitrogen dioxide and sulfur dioxide in tobacco smoke penetrate deep into the lungs, where they dissolve in the watery layer inside the alveoli. Nitrogen dioxide is converted to nitric acid; sulfur dioxide is converted to sulfuric acid. Both acids erode the alveolar walls, leading to emphysema.

If tobacco smoke is so dangerous, why don't we ban smoking or discontinue generous government subsidies to tobacco growers? Surely, an air pollutant or food contaminant that killed hundreds of thousands of Americans each year would be prohibited immediately.

Part of the answer lies in the fact that tobacco use has a long history in the United States. Furthermore, many people think that because smoking is a voluntary act, individuals should have the right to make their own decision. Government, they say, has no right to regulate their pleasure. Furthermore, smoking supports a $30-billion-a-year tobacco industry that employs about 2 million people, including tobacco farmers, advertisers, and retailers. The tobacco industry lobbies diligently to protect the rights of smokers.

The dangers of smoking are becoming well known. As a result of widespread publicity and public pressure, smoking has dropped substantially in the United States. In 2000, for example, only 25% of American adults smoked, down from 34% in 1985 and down substantially from the 1950s and 1960s, when well over half of all men and over one-third of all women engaged in this potentially lethal habit.

Despite the downturn in smoking, 50 million American adults (over the age of 18) still smoke. An estimated six million teenagers and 100,000 children under the age of 13 smoke. Smoking occurs in greatest proportion in certain minority groups—particularly African American men, Native Americans, and Native Alaskans.

(a)   (b)

— Tumor

FIGURE 1 The Normal and Cancerous Lung *(a)* The normal lung appears spongy. *(b)* The cancerous lung from a smoker is filled with particulates and a large tumor.

On a global level, smoking is skyrocketing—increasing about 3% a year. A 3% growth rate means that the number of smokers will double in about 23 years. By one estimate, the number of deaths related to smoking could increase from 2.5 million per year today to about 12 million per year by 2050.

Visit *Human Biology's* Internet site for links to web sites offering more information on this topic.

as the level of sulfur dioxide, a pollutant produced by automobiles, power plants, and factories, increased due to certain weather conditions, the number of people reporting upper respiratory tract illnesses skyrocketed (**FIGURE 9-18**). Colds, coughs, nasal irritation, and other symptoms increased fivefold in just a few days. Soon after the pollution levels returned to normal, the symp-

toms subsided. Few people knew they'd been poisoned by the air they were breathing. Most thought they had been stricken by some infectious agent.

Air pollution is partly responsible for other long-term diseases. One of these is **chronic bronchitis,** a persistent irritation of the bronchi. Characterized by excess mucus production, coughing, and difficulty in breath-

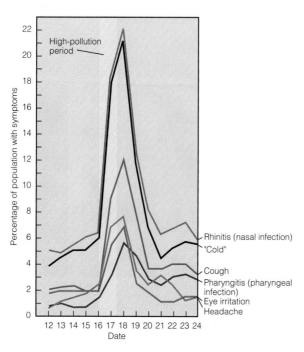

FIGURE 9-18 Air Pollution and Health Graph of respiratory illnesses associated with an air pollution episode in New York City in 1962. Sulfur dioxide levels rose on days 16 and 17 from 0.2 ppm to 0.8–0.9 ppm. (SOURCE: Redrawn from J. R. McCarroll, E. J. Cassell, W. T. Ingram, and D. Wolter, "Health and the Urban Environment: Health Profiles versus Environmental Pollutants," in *American Journal of Public Health* 56(1966): 266–75.)

ing, chronic bronchitis afflicts one out of every five American men between the ages of 40 and 60.

Although the leading cause of chronic bronchitis is cigarette smoking, urban air pollution also contributes to this disease. Three air pollutants have been identified as causative agents: sulfur dioxide, nitrogen oxides, and ozone. Each of these irritates the lung and bronchial passages and arises directly or indirectly from the combustion of fossil fuels by cars, buses, power plants, factories, and homes.

A far more troublesome disease is emphysema. Emphysema, discussed earlier in the chapter, is one of the fastest growing causes of death in the United States. Resulting principally from smoking and air pollution, emphysema afflicts over 1.5 million Americans. This condition, which is more common among men, is a progressive and incurable disease. As it worsens, lung function deteriorates, and victims eventually require supplemental oxygen to perform even routine functions, such as walking or speaking.

The leading cause of emphysema is smoking, a habit of 47 million American adults. Emphysema is also caused by urban air pollution. Not surprisingly, smokers who live in polluted urban settings have the highest incidence of the disease. Like chronic bronchitis, emphysema is caused by ozone, sulfur dioxide, and nitrogen oxides.

No one knows the exact role of urban air pollution. It is not something that can be determined easily, if at all, because people are exposed to many different pollutants over their lifetimes. However, some rersearchers estimate that 50,000 to 60,000 Americans die each year from lung disease caused by urban air pollution, illustrating once again that human health is clearly dependent on a clean environment. This statistic also illustrates that the respiratory system of humans is not well adapted to the physical environment we have made for ourselves. Cultural evolution has progressed in ways that are overwhelming biological evolution.

Connect to this book's web site: www.jbpub.com/humanbiology
The site features eLearning, an online review area that provides quizzes, chapter outlines, and other tools to help you study for your class. You can also follow useful links for in-depth information, research the differing views in the Point/Counterpoints, or keep up on the latest environmental and health news.

Summary

Structure of the Human Respiratory System

1. The respiratory system consists of an air-conducting portion and a gas-exchange portion.
2. The air-conducting portion transports air from outside the body to the alveoli in the *lungs,* the site of gaseous exchange.
3. The *alveoli* are tiny, thin-walled sacs formed by a single layer of flattened epithelial cells that facilitate diffusion. Surrounding the alveoli are capillary beds that pick up oxygen and expel carbon dioxide.
4. The lining of the alveoli is kept moist by water. *Surfactant,* a chemical substance produced in the lung, reduces the surface tension inside the alveoli and prevents their collapse.

Functions of the Respiratory System

5. The respiratory system conducts air to and from the lungs, exchanges gases, and helps produce sounds. Sound is generated as air rushes past the *vocal cords,* causing them to vibrate. The sounds are modified by movements of the tongue and changes in the shape of the oral cavity.
6. Oxygen and carbon dioxide diffuse across the alveolar wall, driven by concentration differences between the blood and alveolar air. Oxygen diffuses into the blood plasma, then into the RBCs, where most of it binds to hemoglobin. Carbon dioxide diffuses in the opposite direction.
7. Carbon dioxide, a waste product of cellular respiration, is picked up by the blood flowing through capillaries. Some carbon dioxide is dissolved in the blood. Most of it, however, enters the RBCs in the bloodstream, where it is converted into carbonic acid. Carbonic acid dissociates, forming hydrogen and bicarbonate ions. The latter diffuse out of the RBCs and are transported in the plasma.

Breathing and the Control of Respiration

8. Breathing is an involuntary action with a conscious override. It is controlled by the *breathing center* in the brain stem. Nerve cells in the breathing center send impulses to the *diaphragm* and *intercostal muscles,* which contract. This increases the volume of the thoracic cavity, which draws air into the lungs through the nose or mouth.
9. When the impulses stop, inspiration ends. Air is then expelled passively as the chest wall returns to the normal position, and the diaphragm rises. The recoil of the lungs also assists in expelling the air.
10. The breathing center is regulated by a negative feedback loop that it generates itself. It is also regulated by outside influences—notably, levels of carbon dioxide in the blood.
11. Expiration can be augmented by enlisting the aid of abdominal and chest muscles, as can inspiration.
12. The rate of respiration can be increased by rising blood carbon dioxide levels or falling oxygen levels and by an increase in physical exercise.

Diseases of the Respiratory System

13. Bacterial and viral infections of the respiratory tract can cause considerable discomfort, and some can be fatal.
14. Once inside the respiratory tract, bacteria, viruses, and other microorganisms can spread to other organ systems.
15. The lungs are also susceptible to airborne materials, among them asbestos fibers, which can cause two types of lung cancer and a debilitating disease called *asbestosis.*
16. Another common disease of the respiratory system is asthma, an allergy (abnormal immune reaction) to dust, pollen, and other common substances. It is characterized by periodic episodes of wheezing and difficult breathing.

Health, Homeostasis, and the Environment: Air Pollution

17. The respiratory system contributes mightily to homeostasis by regulating concentrations of oxygen and carbon dioxide in the blood and body tissues. It also helps control the pH of the blood and tissues. Proper functioning of the respiratory system is therefore essential for health.
18. Respiratory function can be dramatically upset by microorganisms as well as by pollution from factories, automobiles, power plants, and even our own homes.
19. *Chronic bronchitis,* a persistent irritation of the bronchi, is caused by sulfur dioxide, ozone, and nitrogen oxides, lung irritants sometimes found in dangerous levels in urban air.
20. *Emphysema* is a breakdown of the alveoli that gradually destroys the lung's ability to absorb oxygen. It is also caused by lung irritants. Despite the role of air pollution in causing emphysema and chronic bronchitis, smoking remains the number one cause of these diseases.

Critical Thinking

Thinking Critically— Analysis

This Analysis corresponds to the Thinking Critically scenario that was presented at the beginning of this chapter.

For years, the tobacco industry persisted in claiming there was no link between smoking and lung cancer because, they said, there was no positive proof. Semantically, they were quite correct. Science does not *prove* anything. Sure, scientists have performed many studies on people that show *correlations* between lung cancer and smoking. In other words, they've shown that smokers are much more likely to develop lung cancer than nonsmokers and that the more one smokes, the higher his or her chances are of developing this disease. Technically, they haven't proved anything, they've shown a correlation.

The tobacco industry was being a bit deceptive, though, for when a correlation like that between smoking and lung cancer shows up again and again or when the correlation is high, you can have a fair amount of confidence in the cause-and-effect relationship under study.

Can a study be devised to prove the connection? It's unlikely. As I mentioned earlier, science is in the business of supporting hypothesis and generating theory, not providing proof positive.

This exercise requires one to look at definitions (what constitutes proof and the difference between proving something and showing a correlation). It also shows that one usually needs to dig deeper to understand controversies. In this instance, the tobacco industry is hanging its argument on semantics. This exercise also suggests the importance of looking at who's talking—and what their hidden biases are. The tobacco industry clearly has a vested interest in assuring people that smoking is not harmful.

Test of Concepts

1. Trace the flow of air from the mouth and nose to the alveoli, and describe what happens to the air as it travels along the various passageways.

2. Draw an alveolus, including all cell types found there. Be sure to show the relationship of the surrounding capillaries. Show the path that oxygen and carbon dioxide take.

3. Trace the movement of oxygen from alveolar air to the blood in alveolar capillaries. Describe the forces that cause oxygen to move in this direction. Do the same for the reverse flow of carbon dioxide.

4. Why would a breakdown of alveoli in emphysemic patients make it difficult for them to receive enough oxygen?

5. Describe how sounds are generated and refined.

6. A baby is born prematurely and is having difficulty breathing. As the attending physician, explain to the parents what the problem is and how it could be corrected.

7. Smoking irritates the trachea and bronchi, causing mucus to build up and paralyzing cilia. How do these changes affect the lung?

8. Describe inspiration and expiration, being sure to include discussions of what triggers them and the role of muscles in effecting these actions.

9. How does the breathing center regulate itself to control the frequency of breathing?

10. Exercise increases the rate of breathing. How?

11. Turn to **FIGURE 9–15** on page 212. Explain each of the terms.

12. What is asthma? What are its symptoms? How does it affect one's inspiratory reserve volume?

13. Debate this statement: Urban air pollution has very little overall impact on human health.

14. Do you agree or disagree that the single most effective way of reducing deaths in the United States would be to ban smoking? Explain.

The Urinary System

RIDDING THE BODY OF WASTES AND MAINTAINING HOMEOSTASIS

Color-enhanced X ray of human urinary system showing ureters and kidneys.

Thinking Critically

Each year, 24,000 new cases of kidney cancer are diagnosed in the United States. About 10,000 people a year die from this disease. Chemotherapy is virtually the only treatment available for patients whose cancers have spread to other locations, but it helps fewer than 10% of the patients. Patients receiving chemotherapy survive about 9 months after initial diagnosis.

Recently, a new treatment was introduced that holds some promise. The treatment, known as autolymphocyte therapy (ALT), is marketed by a company in Massachusetts. Costing about $22,000 per patient, ALT is designed to strengthen the immune system of patients. Here's how it works: Blood is withdrawn from patients with kidney cancer. Lymphocytes are extracted, then treated with monoclonal antibodies (antibodies to the kidney tumor). This process activates the lymphocytes, causing them to produce a chemical substance known as cytokines, natural compounds that boost the activity of lymphocytes. The cytokines are divided into six batches and stored for later use. Once a month, for the next six months, patients donate more of their own lymphocytes. The cells are treated with cytokines, then reinjected, where they apparently go to work on the tumors.

Results of one study on the effectiveness of ALT were published in April 1990 in the British medical journal *Lancet*. This study of 90 individuals showed that patients who had undergone the procedure survived 22 months after diagnosis, two and a half times longer than patients treated with chemotherapeutic agents. Less than a year after the publication of this clinical trial, a treatment center opened in Boston.

Assume that you are considering investing in the company that markets ALT. Using your critical thinking skills and your knowledge of scientific method, what concerns do you have, and what questions would you ask before investing in this company? ■

Leon Markowitz is lowered into a large pool of warm water in a special room in the hospital (**FIGURE 10-1**). Physicians position a large, cylindrical device in the water in front of one of his kidneys, the organs that filter the blood. In so doing, the kidneys help to remove wastes and also maintain optimal concentrations of nutrients and wastes in the blood. Over the next few hours, as Markowitz listens to tapes of the Beastie Boys, ultrasound waves, undetectable by the human ear, will smash the kidney stones that are obstructing the flow of urine and causing excruciating pain.

A decade earlier, surgeons would have had to cut an incision 15–20 centimeters (6–8 inches) long in Markowitz's side to remove the stone. Leon would have spent 7–10 days recovering in the hospital and another 8 weeks at home recuperating before returning to work. With this new technique, known as **ultrasound lithotripsy** (LITH-oh-TRIP-see) ("stone crushing"), patients usually return home within a day.

In this chapter, we will examine the kidneys and other portions of the urinary system, which function to rid our bodies of potentially harmful wastes. We will briefly examine other excretory organs, too, like the skin and liver. Throughout the chapter, you will see how these systems contribute to homeostasis. We'll end with a discussion of common diseases, such as kidney stones, that disturb the function of this important organ system. And of course, we'll examine yet another example of the manner in which environmental pollutants affect human health.

Section 10-1

Organs of Excretion: a Biological Imperative

Ralph Waldo Emerson once said that as soon as there is life, there is risk. A biologist might say, as soon as there is life, there is waste. All living things produce waste and humans are no exception. Fortunately for life on Earth, elaborate systems of recycling have evolved to put this waste to good use. As many a TV nature show reminds us, in ecosystems, the waste of one organism is frequently the food of another.

Even though wastes are often recycled, they cannot accumulate in organisms without causing harm. Thus, all organisms face a common challenge—how to get rid of internally produced wastes such as carbon dioxide. **TABLE 10-1** lists the major metabolic wastes and other chemicals excreted from the body. The first three entries are nitrogen-containing wastes—ammonia (ah-MOAN-ee-ah), urea (yur-EE-ah), and uric acid (YUR-ick).

FIGURE 10-1 Lithotripsy   Ultrasound waves, undetectable to the human ear, bombard the kidney stones in this man, smashing them into sandlike particles that can be passed relatively painlessly in the urine.

Ammonia (NH_3), is a product of the breakdown of amino acids in the liver. Amino acid breakdown generally occurs when there's excess protein in the diet or a shortage of carbohydrate, in our diets. This causes the

TABLE 10-1		

Important Metabolic Wastes and Substances Excreted from the Body

Chemical	Source	Organ of Excretion
Ammonia	Deamination (removal of amine group) of amino acids in liver	Kidneys
Urea	Derived from ammonia	Kidneys, skin
Uric acid	Nucleotide breakdown in liver	Kidneys
Bile pigments	Hemoglobin breakdown in liver	Liver (into small intestine)
Urochrome	Hemoglobin breakdown in liver	Kidneys
Carbon dioxide	Breakdown of glucose in cells	Lungs
Water	Food and water; breakdown of glucose	Kidneys, skin, and lungs
Inorganic ions*	Food and water	Kidneys and sweat glands

*Ions are not a metabolic waste product like the other substances shown in this table. Nonetheless, ions are excreted to maintain constant levels in the body.

body to break down protein to acquire amino acids. The amino acids are further catabolized to produce energy. During the breakdown of amino acids, the amino groups (NH_2) are stripped from the molecules. The reaction is called *deamination* (dee-AM-in-A-shun). The amino groups are converted into ammonia. Ammonia is a highly toxic chemical. In the liver, most of it is converted to **urea** (**FIGURE 10-2**).

Another by-product of metabolism in humans is uric acid. Produced by the liver, **uric acid** derives not from the breakddown of amino acids, but rather from the breakdown of nucleotides. Nucleotides are the building blocks of DNA and RNA. Uric acid, like urea and ammonia, is excreted in the urine.

In adults, excess production may result in the deposition of uric acid crystals in the bloodstream and in joints, where they cause considerable pain. This condition is known as **gout** (gowt). Uric acid may also appear in the urine of some babies as orange crystals. Although alarming to a parent, their presence is generally not a problem.

Another metabolic waste of great importance are the bile pigments. Derived from the breakdown of hemoglobin in RBCs in the liver, bile pigments are not excreted in the urine like the nitrogen-containing wastes we've just studied. Rather, bile pigments are transferred from the liver to the gallbladder. The gallbladder empties into the small intestine, so bile pigments are excreted with the feces.

The liver produces another water-soluble pigment during the breakdown of hemoglobin. It is known as **urochrome** (YUR-oh-chrome). This yellow pigment is dissolved in the blood and passes to the kidneys, where it is excreted with the urine. In fact, urochrome gives urine its yellowish color.

TABLE 10-1 also lists inorganic ions excreted from the body. Even though they are not end-products of metabolism, inorganic ions are removed from the body by various excretory organs like the skin and kidneys. This is essential to maintain optimal levels in the blood, tissue fluids, and the cytoplasm of cells.

FIGURE 10-2 **Structure of Urea, Uric Acid, and Ammonia** These three waste products are released by cells.

portant, for they rid the body of the greatest variety of dissolved wastes. In so doing, the kidneys also play a key role in regulating the chemical constancy of the blood.

As **FIGURE 10-3A** shows, humans come equipped with two kidneys, They're part of the **urinary system**, one of the body's most important excretory systems. The kidneys don't work alone, however. They're aided by the (1) ureters (YUR-eh-ters), (2) the urinary bladder, and (3) the urethra (you-REETH-rah). The functions of these organs are described in more detail below and are listed in **TABLE 10-2**.

The Urinary System Consists of the Kidneys, Ureters, Bladder, and Urethra

The kidneys lie on either side of the backbone, the vertebral column. About the size of a person's fist, the kidneys are surrounded by a layer of fat. They are located high in the posterior (back) abdominal wall beneath the diaphragm.

The human kidneys are oval structures, slightly indented on one side, much like kidney beans (**FIGURE 10-3B**). (In fact, kidney beans get their name because they're shaped like this excretory organ.) As illustrated, each kidney is served by a renal artery, which enters at the indented region. The renal arteries are major branches of the abdominal aorta, a large blood vessel that delivers blood to the abdominal organs and lower limbs.

The Urinary System

Evolution has "provided" several avenues by which animals get rid of, or excrete, wastes. In humans, excretion of wastes occurs in the lungs, the skin, the liver, the kidneys, and even the intestines. These organs are consequently classified as excetory organs.

Of all the organs that participate in removing waste, however, the kidneys rank as one of the most im-

TABLE 10-2

Components of the Urinary System and Their Functions

Component	Function
Kidneys	Eliminate wastes from the blood; help regulate body water concentration; help regulate blood pressure; help maintain a constant blood pH
Ureters	Transport urine to the urinary bladder
Urinary bladder	Stores urine; contracts to eliminate stored urine
Urethra	Transports urine to the outside of the body

(a)

(b)

FIGURE 10-3 The Urinary System *(a)* Anterior view showing the relationship of the kidneys, ureters, urinary bladder, and urethra. *(b)* A cross section of the human kidney showing the cortex, medulla, and renal pelvis.

As you shall soon see, the kidneys filter wastes and excess chemicals from the blood entering via the renal arteries. After the blood has been filtered, it leaves the kidneys via the **renal veins,** which drain into the inferior vena cava, a vessel that transports venous blood to the heart.

Wastes extracted from the blood are eliminated in the urine (YUR-in), a yellowish fluid produced by the kidneys. It contains water, nitrogenous wastes (such as urea), small amounts of hormones, ions, and other substances.

Dissolved wastes are removed from the blood by numerous microscopic filtering units in the kidney, the

nephrons (NEFF-rons). The urine produced by the nephrons is drained from the kidney by the **ureters.** They transport urine to the urinary bladder with the aid of peristaltic contractions, which you may recall from Chapter 5 are smooth muscle contractions. The **urinary bladder** lies in the pelvic cavity just behind the pubic bone. With walls made of smooth muscle that stretch as the organ fills, the bladder serves as a temporary receptacle for urine. When the bladder is full, its walls contract, forcing the urine out through the urethra.

The **urethra** is a narrow tube, measuring approximately 4 centimeters (1.5 inches) in women and 15–20 centimeters (6–8 inches) in men. The additional

- Ureter
- Smooth muscle
- Ureteral openings
- Prostate gland
- Internal sphincter
- Cowper's glands
- Pelvic diaphragm
- External sphincter
- Urethra

(a)   External urethral orifice

- Urethra
- External urethral orifice

(b)

FIGURE 10-4 The Urinary Bladder and Urethra   These drawings show the differences in the urethras of men *(a)* and women *(b)*. The smooth muscle at the juncture of the urinary bladder and urethra forms the internal sphincter. The pelvic diaphragm is a flat sheet of muscle covering the lower boundary of the pelvic cavity. It forms the external sphincter and is under voluntary control.

The Human Kidney Consists of Two Zones, an Outer Cortex and Inner Medulla

Each kidney is surrounded by a connective tissue capsule, appropriately called the **renal capsule.** Immediately beneath the capsule is a region known as the **renal cortex.** This region contains many nephrons. The inner zone is the **renal medulla.** As shown in **FIGURE 10-3B**, the medulla consists of cone-shaped structures (renal pyramids) and intervening tissue (renal columns). The cone-shaped sections contain small ducts that transport urine from the nephrons into a central receiving chamber, the **renal pelvis** (**FIGURE 10-3B**). It joins with the ureters.

Nephrons Consist of Two Parts, a Glomerulus and a Renal Tubule

Each kidney contains 1–2 million nephrons, visible only through a microscope. One of the marvels of evolution, each nephron consists of a tuft of capillaries, the **glomerulus** (glom-ERR-you-luss),[2] and a long, twisted tube, the **renal tubule** (**FIGURE 10-5B**). The renal tubule consists of four segments: (1) Bowman's capsule, (2) the proximal convoluted tubule, (3) the loop of Henle, and (4) the distal convoluted tubule (**TABLE 10-3**). You may want to take a moment to study **FIGURE 10-5B** to acquaint yourself with these structures.

As illustrated in **FIGURE 10-5B**, the glomerulus is surrounded by a saclike portion of the renal tube, called **Bowman's capsule** (after the scientist who first described it). It is a double-walled structure; the inner wall fits closely over the glomerular capillaries and is separated from the outer wall by a small space, **Bowman's space.**

length in men largely results from the fact that the urethra travels through the penis (**FIGURE 10-4**).

The difference in the length of the urethra between men and women has important medical implications. The shorter urethra in women, for example, makes women more susceptible to bacterial infections of the urinary bladder.[1] Bladder infections may result in an itching or burning sensation and an increase in the frequency of urination. They may also cause blood to appear in the urine. Urinary tract infections can be treated with antibiotics. Untreated infections may spread up the ureters to the kidneys, where they can seriously damage the nephrons and impair kidney function.

---

[1]Sexual intercourse increases the frequency of urinary bladder infections in many women. To reduce chances of developing an infection, women are advised to empty their bladders soon after intercourse.

---

[2]Glomerulus is the Latin word for "ball of yarn."

FIGURE 10-5 The Nephron *(a)* A cross section of the kidney showing the location of the nephrons. *(b)* A drawing of a nephron.

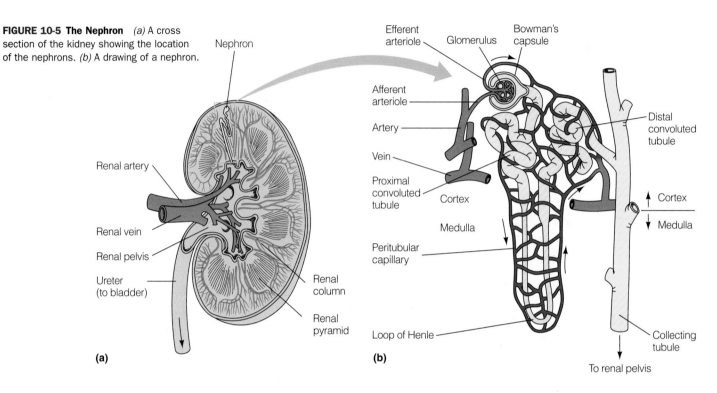

(a)

(b)

To understand the relationship between the glomerulus and Bowman's capsule, imagine that your fist is a glomerulus. Then imagine that you are holding a balloon in your other hand. If you push your fist (glomerulus) into the balloon, the layer immediately surrounding your fist would be the inner layer of Bowman's capsule. It is separated from the outer layer of the capsule by Bowman's space.

TABLE 10-3

Components of the Nephron and Their Function

Component	Function
Glomerulus	Mechanically filters the blood
Bowman's capsule	Mechanically filters the blood
Proximal convoluted tubule	Reabsorbs 75% of the water, salts, glucose, and amino acids
Loop of Henle	Participates in countercurrent exchange, which maintains the concentration gradient
Distal convoluted tubule	Site of tubular secretion of H^+, potassium, and certain drugs

The outer wall of Bowman's capsule is continuous with the **proximal convoluted tubule (PCT),** a contorted section of the renal tubule. The PCT soon straightens, then descends a bit, makes a sharp hairpin turn, and ascends. In the process, it forms a thin, U-shaped structure known as the **loop of Henle** (HEN-lee). The loops of Henle of some nephrons extend into the medulla.

The loop of Henle drains into the fourth and final portion of the renal tubule, the **distal convoluted tubule (DCT),** another contorted segment. This structure, shown in **FIGURE 10-5B,** empties into a straight duct called a **collecting tubule**. The collecting tubules, in turn, merge to form larger ducts that course through the cone-shaped renal pyramids and eventually empty their contents into the renal pelvis.

The nephrons filter enormous amounts of blood and produce from 1 to 3 liters of urine per day, depending on how much fluid a person ingests. **TABLE 10-3** summarizes the functions of each segment of the nephron.

Section 10-3

Function of the Urinary System

With the basic anatomy of the kidney and urinary system in mind, let us turn our attention to the function of the urinary system, focusing first on the nephron.

Blood Filtration in Nephrons Involves Three Processes: Glomerular Filtration, Tubular Reabsorption, and Tubular Secretion

Glomerular Filtration. The first step in the purification of the blood is **glomerular filtration** (**FIGURE 10-6**). It's a rather straightforward physical filtration not unlike what occurs when you filter coffee grinds. Here's how it works. As noted earlier, the glomerulus is a ball of capillaries. As blood flows through the glomerular capillaries, water and dissolved materials are forced through the walls of the capillaries. This liquid, called the **glomerular filtrate,** travels through the inner layer of Bowman's capsule. Red blood cells and large proteins in the blood can't escape because of the barrier formed by the inner layer of Bowman's capsule. From here, the filtrate passes into the proximal convoluted tubule, then into the loop of Henle, and finally out the distal convoluted tubule. Along its path, much of the water is absorbed back into the bloodstream. Good nutrients, such as glucose, are also absorbed, as you shall soon see.

Glomerular Filtration Is Controlled by Regulating the Flow of Blood and Blood Pressure in the Glomerulus.

Glomerular filtration is, as noted above, a pretty straightforward process. It can be increased by increasing the blood pressure within the glomerulus. Blood pressure inside the glomerulus can be increased by dilating (opening) the **afferent arterioles**, the small vessels that lead into the glomerulus. They're shown in **FIGURES 10-5B** and **10-6**. Increasing the diameter of the afferent arterioles permits more blood to flow into the glomerulus. Blood pressure in the glomerulus rises as it would in a hose after the faucet is opened. Glomerular filtration increases as a result.

FIGURE 10-6 Physiology of the Nephron The nephron carries out three processes: (1) glomerular filtration, (2) tubular reabsorption, and (3) tubular secretion. All contribute to the filtering of the blood.

The **efferent arterioles** drain blood from the glomerular capillaries, as illustrated in **FIGURES 10-5B** and **10-6**. The efferent arterioles are slightly smaller than the afferent arterioles, which results in a slight elevation in the blood pressure. If the body requires greater filtration, the efferent arterioles constrict a little more. This increases blood pressure within the glomerular capillaries, which increases the rate of filtration.

Tubular Reabsorption Helps Conserve Valuable Nutrients and Ions.

Each day, approximately 180 liters (45 gallons) of filtrate is produced in the glomeruli. However, the kidneys produce only about 1–3 liters of urine each day. Thus, only about 1% of the filtrate actually leaves the kidneys as urine. What happens to the rest of the fluid filtered by the glomerulus?

Most of the fluid filtered by the glomeruli is reabsorbed—it passes from the renal tubule *back* into the bloodstream. The movement of water, ions, and molecules from the renal tubule to the bloodstream is referred to as **tubular reabsorption.**

During tubular reabsorption, water containing valuable nutrients and ions that leaves the renal tubule enters the networks of capillaries that surround the nephrons. As shown in **FIGURE 10-5**, these capillaries are branches of the efferent arterioles. They will eventually empty into the renal veins, returning nutrients to the body.

Tubular reabsorption is valuable because it conserves water and important ions and nutrients indiscriminately filtered out in the glomerulus. Waste products like urea and uric acid, however, remain in the glomerular filtrate and will eventually be excreted in the urine. **TABLE 10-4** shows the reabsorption rates of various molecules.

TABLE 10-4

Fate of Various Substances Filtered by Kidneys

| Substance | Filtered Substance (Average %) | |
	Reabsorbed	*Excreted*
Water	99	1
Sodium	99.5	0.5
Glucose	100	0
Waste products		
Urea	50	50
Phenol	0	100

Tubular Secretion Is the Transport of Waste Products from the Peritubular Capillaries into the Renal Tubule. Waste disposal is supplemented by a third process, **tubular secretion**. It eliminates wastes not filtered out of the blood in the glomerulus the first time around. In other words, it catches wastes that might otherwise have escaped filtration. You can follow the steps in **FIGURE 10-6.**

As blood passes through the glomerular capillaries, much of it is filtered. The blood that isn't filtered passes from the efferent arterioles into the peritubular (pear-ee-TUBE-you-ler) capillaries surrounding the nephron. Some of the wastes pass through the capillary walls, then into the nephron. This is called *tubular secretion.* Tubular secretion not only helps rid the blood of wastes, it helps regulate the H^+ concentration of the blood. If you'd like to know exactly where tubular secretion and tubular reabsorption occur, check out **TABLE 10-3.**

Blood draining from the capillaries surrounding the nephrons is fairly well cleansed by the time it empties into the nearby veins. These veins converge to form the **renal vein**, which transports the filtered blood out of the kidney and into the inferior vena cava, which carries it to the heart.

As for the urine, it flows out of the nephron into the collecting tubules. The urine leaving the nephron consists mostly of water and a variety of dissolved waste products. The collecting tubules descend through the medulla and converge to form larger ducts that empty their contents into a central chamber known as the *renal pelvis.* As the collecting tubules descend through the medulla, much of the remaining water escapes by osmosis, further concentrating the urine and conserving body water.

Superior wall of
distended bladder

Section 10-4

Urination: Controlling a Reflex

Urine is produced continuously by the kidneys and flows down the ureters to the urinary bladder. Leakage out the bladder and into the urethra is prevented by two

Superior wall of
empty bladder

FIGURE 10-7 Urination in Babies
The bladder before and after it fills, showing how much this organ can expand to accommodate urine.

sphincters—muscular "valves" similar to those found in the stomach (**FIGURE 10-4**).

The first sphincter, the **internal sphincter,** is formed by a smooth muscle in the neck of the urinary bladder at its junction with the urethra. The second valve, the **external sphincter,** is a flat band of skeletal muscle that forms the floor of the pelvic cavity. When both sphincters are relaxed, urine is propelled into the urethra and out of the body. How is urination stimulated?

Urination is stimulated by the accumulation of urine inside the bladder. You need about 200-300 milliliters to start the process. When the bladder fills, the walls of the bladder stretch (**FIGURE 10-7**). Special sensors in the walls, called stretch receptors, detect the distension of the bladder and begin sending impulses via sensory nerves to the spinal cord. In the spinal cord, the incoming nerve impulses stimulate other nerve cells. Nerve impulses generated in these cells leave the spinal cord and travel along nerves that terminate on the muscle cells in the wall of the bladder. These impulses stimulate the smooth muscle cells to contract. Muscular contraction forces the internal sphincter to open, letting urine enter the urethra. Urination won't occur in adults, however, until the external sphincter is consciouly relaxed.

In babies and very young children, urination is entirely reflex. Once the bladder expands to a certain size, it empties. Not until children grow older (2–3 years) can they begin to control urination. In older children and adults, the external sphincter is under conscious control. It will not relax until you consciously permit it to do so.

Unfortunately, adults sometimes lose control over urination, resulting in a condition referred to as **urinary incontinence** (in-KAN-teh-nance). Urinary incontinence may be caused by a traumatic injury to the spinal cord that disrupts neural pathways from the brain that allow us to suppress urination. In such instance, then, the urinary reflex operates without conscious override, and the bladder empties as soon as it reaches a certain size, much as it does in a baby or young child.

Mild urinary incontinence is much more common. It is characterized by the escape of urine when a person sneezes or coughs. This is most common in women and usually results from damage to the external sphincter during childbirth. Childbirth stretches the skeletal muscles of the external sphincter, reducing their effectiveness and making such accidents embarrassingly common. To avoid this, many women undertake exercise programs to strengthen these muscles before and after childbirth. Urinary incontinence may also occur in men whose external sphincters have been injured in surgery on the prostate gland, which surrounds the neck of the urinary bladder.

FIGURE 10-8 ADH Secretion ADH secretion is under the control of the hypothalamus. When the osmotic concentration of the blood rises, receptors in the hypothalamus detect the change and trigger the release of ADH from the posterior lobe of the pituitary. Detectors in the heart also respond to changes in blood volume. When it drops, they send signals to the brain, causing the release of ADH.

ADH secretion is regulated by two receptors, one in the brain and one in the heart (**FIGURE 10-8**).

The first sensor is a group of nerve cells in a region of the brain called the **hypothalamus** (HIGH-poe-THAL-ah-muss). It is located just above the pituitary gland. The cells that regulate ADH actually monitor the osmotic concentration of the blood, as you shall soon see. The second sensor is, as noted above, located in the heart. It detects changes in blood volume, which is a reflection of water levels.

To understand how ADH secretion is controlled, let's imagine that you're out in the hot sun. Your body's sweating and you haven't got a thing to drink. Under these conditions, the body begins to lose water. As a result, the blood volume decreases and the osmotic concentration increases. The decrease in blood volume is detected by the heart receptors. The rise in osmotic concentration is detected by sensors in the brain. As shown in **FIGURE 10-8**, both of these stimuli trigger the release of ADH from the pituitary gland. ADH circulates in the blood. In the kidney, this hormone stimulates and increases the rate of tubular reabsorption of water. In other words, it stimulates the passage of water from the nephron into the peritubular capillaries. This reduces urinary output and restores the volume and osmotic concentration of the blood.

Excess water intake, on the other hand, has just the opposite effect. As you can imagine, drinking excess water will increase the blood volume and decrease its osmotic concentration. The sensors in the brain and heart note these changes and cause a reduction in ADH secretion. As ADH levels in the blood fall, tubular reabsorption decreases and more water is lost in the urine. As a consquence, blood volume and osmotic concentration are restored.

The Hormone Aldosterone Also Stimulates Water Reabsorption in the Kidney. Water balance is also regulated by the hormone **aldosterone** (al-DOS-ter-own). Aldosterone is a steroid hormone produced by the adrenal glands, which sit atop the kidneys like loose-fitting stocking caps (**FIGURE 14-1A**). Aldosterone levels in the blood are controlled by three factors: (1) blood pressure, (2) blood volume, and (3) osmotic concentration.

Controlling Kidney Function and Maintaining Homeostasis

The kidneys help the body control the chemical composition of the blood and maintain homeostasis. This section briefly describes the kidney's role in maintaining water balance (that is, proper levels of water).

Water Balance Is Maintained by Conserving Water When Intake Falls or by Ridding the Body of It When Intake Is Excessive

As noted earlier, much of the water filtered by the glomeruli is passively reabsorbed by the renal tubules and returned to the bloodstream. The rate of water reabsorption can be increased or decreased to alter urine production. The ability to adjust water reabsorption and urine output allows the body to rid itself of excess water or to conserve water when an individual is becoming dehydrated. Two hormones play a major role in this important homeostatic process.

The Hormone ADH Increases Water Reabsorption and Conserves Body Water. Water reabsorption is controlled in part by **antidiuretic hormone** (ANN-tie-DIE-yur-eh-tick) or **ADH.** ADH is released by an endocrine gland at the base of the brain known as the **pituitary** (peh-TWO-eh-TARE-ee) (Chapter 14).[3]

---

[3]ADH is manufactured by the hypothalamus and transported to the posterior lobe of the pituitary gland via modified nerve cells, called *neurosecretory cells,* which are described in Chapter 14.

FIGURE 10-9 Aldosterone Secretion Aldosterone is released by the adrenal cortex. Its release, however, is stimulated by a chain of events that begins in the kidney.

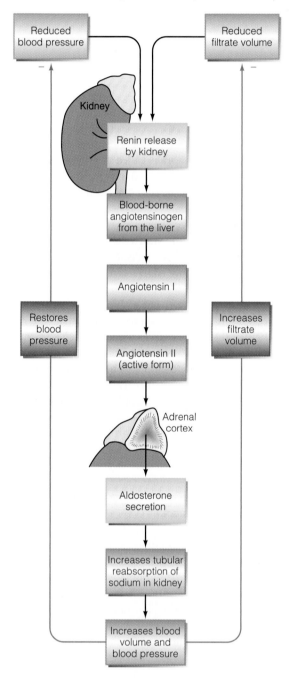

tubule triggers a series of changes that lead to the release of aldosterone. When blood pressure and the volume of filtrate in the nephrons declines, certain cells in the kidney produce an enzyme called **renin** (REE-nin). In the blood, renin cleaves a segment off a large plasma protein called **angiotensinogen** (AN-gee-oh-TEN-SIN-oh-gin). The result is a small peptide molecule called **angiotensin I**. Angiotensin I is inactive. It must be converted into the active form, **angiotensin II**, by enzymes it encounters as blood flows through the lungs.

Angiotensin II stimulates aldosterone secretion by the adrenal glands. Aldosterone released from the glands circulates in the blood. In the kidney, it stimulates cells of the nephron to increase the amount of sodium they reabsorb. In other words, it increases tubular reabsorption of sodium. Water follows sodium ions out of the nephron into the peritubular capillaries. This, in turn, increases blood volume and blood pressure, shutting down this complex series of events.

Water balance is also affected by several chemicals in many people's daily diet, two of the most influential being caffeine and alcohol.

Caffeine Increases Urine Output without Affecting ADH Secretion. Caffeine is a **diuretic** (DIE-yur-ET-ick), a chemical that increases urination. Found in coffee, (most nonherbal) teas, and many soft drinks, caffeine increases urine production in two ways.[4] First, it increases glomerular blood pressure, which, in turn, increases glomerular filtration. (As a result, more filtrate is formed.) Second, caffeine decreases the tubular reabsorption of sodium ions. As noted earlier, water follows sodium ions out of the renal tubule during tubular reabsorption. Thus, a decrease in sodium reabsorption results in a decline in the amount of water leaving the renal tubule and an increase in urine output.

Ethanol Inhibits the Secretion of ADH by the Pituitary. Ethyl alcohol or ethanol, for short, is also a diuretic. As you know, ethanol is found in a variety of beverages, including beer, wine, wine coolers, and hard liquor. After being absorbed by the stomach and small intestine, ethanol enters blood and circulates freely throughout the body. When it reaches the brain, it inhibits the cells that secrete ADH. When ADH levels fall, water reabsorption declines. The result is a marked increase in water loss by the kidneys, giving credence to the quip that you don't buy wine or beer, you rent it!

As illustrated in **FIGURE 10-9**, aldosterone release from the kidneys is controlled by a fairly complex sequence of events involving several chemical intermediaries.

To understand this process, begin at the top of **FIGURE 10-9**. Here you see that a reduction in blood pressure or a reduction in the volume of filtrate in the renal

---

[4]Part of the increase is due to the fluid contained in these drinks.

Kidney stone   Spine

(a)   Hip bone   Pelvic cavity

FIGURE 10-10 Kidney Stones *(a)* An X-ray of a kidney stone. *(b)* Kidney stones removed by surgery. (See nail for size.)

(b)

Section 10-6

Diseases of the Urinary System

Like other body systems, the urinary system can malfunction, creating a homeostatic nightmare in the body, not unlike the situation that might exist in a factory if its wastes could not be released or shipped elsewhere. This section discusses three disorders: kidney stones, kidney failure, and diabetes insipidus.

Kidney Stones Can Block the Outflow of Urine and Cause Severe Kidney Damage

Urine contains numerous ions and dissolved wastes. Ninety percent of the dissolved waste consists of three substances: urea, sodium ions, and chloride ions. Varying amounts of other chemical substances are also present, but in minute amounts.

In many ways, the urine provides a window to the chemical workings of the body. Thus, increases or decreases in the level of substances in the urine may signal underlying problems—upsets in homeostasis and possible health problems. Consequently, physicians routinely analyze the urine of their patients to test for metabolic disorders. One of the most common is **diabetes mellitus** (DIE-ah-BEE-tees mell-EYE-tus), or sugar diabetes. This disease results in a defect in glucose uptake

by cells in the body. Because body cells cannot absorb glucose, blood levels and urine levels are elevated.

Excess chemicals and ions in the urine not only signal problems elsewhere, they can be damaging to the kidney itself. For instance, higher than normal concentrations of calcium, magnesium, and uric acid in the urine, often caused by inadequate fluid intake, may crystallize inside the kidney, most often in the renal pelvis. Small deposits enlarge by a process called accretion (ah-CREE-shun)—the deposition of materials on the outside of the stone, which causes them to grow in much the same way that a pearl grows in an oyster (**FIGURE 10-10**). These small crystals, or **kidney stones,** eventually grow into fairly large deposits. Unlike pearls, however, kidney stones are a health threat and an economic liability.

Fortunately, many kidney stones are flushed out of the kidney on their own. They enter the ureter and are passed to the urinary bladder. Small stones that enter the urinary bladder are often excreted in the urine. The sharp edges of the stone often dig into the walls of the ureters and urethra, causing considerable pain.

Problems arise when stones become lodged inside the kidney or the ureters and obstruct the flow of urine. This causes internal pressure to increase, resulting in considerable damage to the nephrons if left untreated.

For years, kidney stones were removed surgically. Today, however, the relatively new medical technique of **ultrasound lithotripsy** is generally used. In this technique, mentioned in the opening paragraph of this chapter, physicians bombard kidneys with ultrasound waves, which shatter the stones, producing fine, sand-like grains that are passed in the urine without incident. The procedure is nearly painless and much safer than surgery. **TABLE 10-5** lists additional urinary system disorders.

TABLE 10-5

Common Urinary Disorders

Disease	Symptoms	Cause
Bladder infections	Especially prevalent in women; pain in lower abdomen; frequent urge to urinate; blood in urine; strong smell to urine.	Nearly always bacteria
Kidney stones	Large stones lodged in the kidney often create no symptoms at all; pain occurs if stones are being passed to the bladder; pains come in waves a few minutes apart.	Deposition of calcium, phosphate, magnesium, and uric acid crystals in the kidney, possibly resulting from inadequate water intake
Kidney failure	Symptoms often occur gradually; more frequent urination, lethargy, and fatigue; should the kidney fail completely, patient may develop nausea, headaches, vomiting, diarrhea, water buildup, especially in the lungs and skin, and pain in the chest and bones.	Immune reaction to some drugs, especially antibiotics; toxic chemicals; kidney infections; sudden decreases in blood flow to the kidney resulting, for example, from trauma
Pyelonephritis	Infection of the kidney's nephrons; sudden, intense pain in the lower back immediately above the waist, high temperature, and chills	Bacterial infection

Renal Failure May Occur Suddenly or Gradually and Can be Treated by Dialysis, a Mechanical Filtering of the Blood

The importance of the kidneys is most obvious when they stop working, a condition known as **renal failure.** Renal failure generally results from one of four causes. In some instances, it is caused by the presence of certain toxic chemicals in the blood. In others, it results from immune reactions to certain antibiotics. In still other cases, it is caused by severe kidney infections. In accidents where huge amounts of blood are lost, a sudden decrease in blood flow to the kidneys will result in renal failure.

Renal failure may occur suddenly, over a period of a few hours or a few days. This is referred to as **acute renal failure.** Kidney function may also deteriorate slowly over many years, resulting in **chronic renal impairment** (so named because the kidney function declines over time). Chronic renal impairment may lead to a complete or nearly complete shutdown, known as **end-stage failure.**

Kidney failure (whether acute or end stage) is life-threatening, for when the kidneys stop working, water and toxic wastes begin to accumulate in the body. This disrupts homeostasis. If untreated, a patient will die in 2–3 days. Patients usually die from an increase in the concentration of potassium ions in the blood and tissue fluids. Why? Although potassium is essential for the function of heart muscle, excess potassium destroys the rhythmic contraction of the heart, causing fibrillation.

As you may recall from Chapter 6, fibrillation is the uncoordinated contraction of heart muscle that may render the heart ineffective as a pumping organ. Patients most often die of heart attack.

Treating renal failure depends on the underlying cause. If the problem is caused by an acute loss of blood, transfusions may be required. Patients whose kidneys have shut down, even temporarily, may require **renal dialysis** (DIE-AL-eh-siss). In this procedure, blood is drawn out of a vein and passed through a piece of tubing that transports the blood to a filter that removes wastes. After filtration, the blood is pumped back into the patient's bloodstream. Dialysis requires several hours and must be repeated every 2 or 3 days. Some patients have dialysis units at home and simply hook themselves up each night before they go to bed.

Another more recent method is **continuous ambulatory peritoneal dialysis** or **CAPD.** In this procedure, 2 liters of dialysis fluid are injected into a person's abdomen through a permanently implanted tube or catheter (CATH-eh-ter). Waste products diffuse out of the blood vessels into the abdominal cavity across a thin membrane that lines the organs and wall of abdominal cavity, the **peritoneum** (PEAR-eh-tah-KNEE-um). The fluid, containing waste products, is drained from the abdominal cavity a couple of times a day.

This form of dialysis is much simpler. Patients can take care of it themselves. In addition, it allows for more frequent filtering of the blood and permits patients to continue their daily activities without having to strap themselves to a machine.

Complete kidney failure can be treated by kidney transplants. Transplants are generally most successful when they come from closely related family members, for reasons explained in Chapter 8.

For years, the complete or nearly complete destruction of kidney function was almost always fatal. Thanks to renal dialysis and kidney transplantation, many patients today can live normal, healthy lives. These procedures, especially transplants, are costly, however. The public currently picks up the tab for individuals without insurance—or they go without needed treatments and die. For a debate on prioritizing medical expenditures, see this chapter's Point/Counterpoint.

Diabetes Insipidus Is a Rare Disease Caused by a Lack of ADH

Hormonal imbalances can also lead to disruptions in the urinary system. Severe head injuries, for example, may halt the production of ADH, leading to a disease known as **diabetes insipidus** (DIE-ah-BE-teas in-SIP-eh-duss). This condition is not to be confused with diabetes mellitus (commonly called *sugar diabetes*), a disorder involving the hormone insulin. (You can remember these if you remember that insipid means tasteless, which describes the urine of those with diabetes insipidus, and mellitus refers to honey-like or sweet, which describes the taste, I'm told, of urine from people with sugar diabetes.[5])

Diabetes insipidus is characterized by frequent urination and excessive liquid intake. Diabetes insipidus results from insufficient ADH output. Remarkably, patients with this disease produce up to 20 liters (5 gallons) of colorless, dilute urine per day—fluid that must be replaced by frequent consumption of liquids. Sleeping through the night is impossible, for patients are continually awakened by thirst or the urge to urinate.

Diabetes insipidus can be treated in a variety of ways, depending on the severity of the disorder and the cause. In patients whose urine output is only slightly elevated, dietary salt restrictions and antidiuretics (drugs that reduce urine output) work. In severe cases, patients must receive synthetic ADH, which is administered by injections or nose drops. If the disease is caused by a head injury, treatment may be required only for a year or so. If the damage is permanent, however, treatment will be required for the rest of the person's life.

---

[5]The Latin word for "honey" is *mellifer.*

Health, Homeostasis, and the Environment

Mercury Poisoning

The kidneys are elaborate biological filters that help maintain the proper levels of nutrients. They also help us eliminate various cellular wastes and potentially harmful substances we ingest such as food additives, pesticides, and toxic chemicals in the food we eat and the water we drink.

Unfortunately, the kidneys can be seriously damaged by a variety of environmental contaminants. As the previous section showed, damage to the kidney has severe physiological repercussions, resulting from homeostatic imbalance.

One of the most toxic by-products of the modern world are heavy metals, such as mercury and cadmium. Heavy metals are used in large quantities in many manufacturing processes and in many products. As a group, the heavy metals are potent **nephrotoxins** (NEFF-row-TOX-ins)—toxic chemicals that affect the nephrons. Even relatively low doses of heavy metals can damage the kidneys.

Fortunately, the nephrons possess several protective mechanisms to reduce the impact of heavy metals. Lysosomes inside the cells of the renal tubule, for example, engulf heavy metals, decreasing their cytoplasmic concentration. As blood levels of these toxins increase, however, the protective mechanisms are overwhelmed, and the cells of the kidney begin to die.

Exposure to low levels of various heavy metals increases urinary output and increases the concentrations of amino acids and glucose in the urine. Both of these symptoms are good indicators that tubular reabsorption is not working properly. At higher levels, heavy metals can cause renal failure and death. The proximal convoluted tubule is the part of the nephron most sensitive to heavy metals.

One of the most common and hence more troublesome heavy metals is mercury. Found in the water we drink and occasionally even in the food we eat, mercury in high concentrations produces acute renal failure. This condition results from vasoconstriction of the afferent arterioles, which reduces the flow of blood into the glomeruli. Mercury also produces cellular deterioration.

In the 1950s, Japan announced an outbreak of mercury poisoning in residents who had consumed fish and shellfish taken from Minimata Bay, which had been contaminated by a nearby plastics factory. Over 100 people developed numbness of the limbs, lips, and tongue and lost muscular control, becoming clumsy. Most suffered from blurred vision, deafness, and mental derangement. All told, 17 people died and

Point/Counterpoint

Prioritizing Medical Expenditures

We Need to Learn to Prioritize Medical Expenditures

Richard D. Lamm

Richard D. Lamm is the director of the Center for Public Policy and Contemporary Issues at the University of Denver, where his primary research and teaching interests have been in the area of health policy. Before assuming his present position, he served three terms as governor of Colorado, from 1975 until 1987.

Heath care in the United States finds itself in (to paraphrase Dickens) "the best of times and the worst of times." It is the epoch of medical miracles, yet at the same time millions go without even basic health care.

The basic dilemma of American medicine is that we have invented more health care than we can afford to deliver. Health care costs are rising at three times the rate of inflation. They are absorbing funds desperately needed elsewhere in our system to educate our kids, rebuild our infrastructure, and revitalize our industries.

Health care costs are rising for many reasons. One major reason is that no one prioritizes the myriad of procedures that health care can deliver. No one asks, "How do we buy the most health for the most people with our limited funds?" Recent policy decisions in Oregon and California, relating to the public funding of transplant operations, illustrate how two states attempted to deal with a crisis in health care.

Oregon recently received adverse publicity for its decision not to publicly fund soft tissue transplant operations. As is often the case, much of the focus has been on the handful of individuals who have been adversely af-

fected by the policy rather than the numerous, but anonymous, people who will benefit. The Oregon policy sparked a public outcry over society's lack of compassion for individuals who desperately need transplants. Yet, when Oregon policymakers weighed the needs of a few transplant patients against the basic health care needs of the medically indigent, they decided against the former in favor of the latter. They have now set up a process that sets priorities throughout the health care system.

California took a contrary approach. Policymakers in California decided to publicly fund transplant operations. Then, one week later, they removed 270,000 low-income people from their state's medical assistance program.

Which was the wiser decision? The answer seems clear. Oregon bought more health for more of its citizens for its limited funds. Some say Oregon should have raised its taxes and funded transplants. That is very easy for nonpoliticians to say. Polls show people believe all Americans should have access to quality health care. But the polls also show that most are unwilling to accept even modest tax increases to provide the care they say they favor.

Illinois recently passed legislation giving "universal access to major organ transplants," but appropriated less than one-third of the funds needed. Politically, of course, Illinois played it far safer than Oregon but, in doing so, failed to confront one of the most pressing social issues of our time. Avoidance may be a politically expedient tactic, but sooner or

later our society will be forced to allocate scarce health resources.

Clearly, medical science is inventing faster than the public is willing or able to pay. Realistically, no system of health care can avoid rationing medicine. In fact, rationing already exists. But instead of rationing medicine according to need or a patient's prospects for recovery, we ration by seniority and ability to pay. Those who pretend that we do not ration medicine forget that 31 million Americans do not have full access to health care in America. Most states have staggering numbers of medically indigent, yet they provide a small percentage with a full program of coverage. Oregon is the first state to cover 100% of the people living under the federal poverty line with basic health care.

I suggest this yardstick: Which state best asked itself, "how do we buy the most health for the most people?" Which state tried to maximize limited resources? Which state benefited the greatest number of people and which state harmed the greatest number of people?

Oregon attempted to weigh the basic health needs of the medically indigent against other programs for which the state paid. It recognized that the money the state paid for transplants and other high-cost procedures for a few people could buy more health care elsewhere, providing basic low-technology services to people not covered at that time.

Prioritizing health care does not abandon the poor; it seeks to serve the largest number with the more effective procedures.

Medical Prioritization Is a Bad Idea

Arthur L. Caplan

The American health care system, the experts say, is going bust at a rapid rate. Efforts to contain our burgeoning $1 trillion-plus tab have been a total failure.

The dilemma of how to pay for health care is forcing some public officials to think the unthinkable. The state of Oregon instituted rationing policies for health care. But, before you applaud the realism, consider that the Oregon rations access to health care only for the poor. Those eligible for Medicaid in Oregon are required by law to forego life-saving medical care.

Officials in Oregon note that the poor have always had less access to health care than the rich. This is true. But, our society's failure to meet the health care needs of the poor hardly justifies a public policy that asks the poor to bear the burden of rationing as a matter of law.

Who concocted this blatantly unethical scheme? Incredibly, the inspiration for the Oregon plan for pocketbook triage comes in part from those in my line of work—medical ethicists.

A California bioethics consulting firm was paid by Oregon state officials to provide moral rationales for dropping the poor out of the health care lifeboat. The consultants appeared to approach their task with gusto.

"You have to draw the line somewhere," one moralist-for-hire said in a newspaper article about rationing for the poor. "We'll provide all services to a diminishing segment of the population, and literally we'll throw the rest of the people overboard."

No hint is given of the theoretical position that would justify aiming all rationing efforts at the poor. But it is hard to think of an ethic that holds that when a nation cannot pay its doctor bills, it is the poor and only the poor who should be denied the right to see a doctor.

It is hard to understand how any ethicist could become involved in a scheme so blatantly unfair as that of rationing necessary health care only for the poor. What is worse is that the same ethicists and the officials taking their advice are not asking whether it is really necessary to institute the rationing of necessary medical care for anyone.

Before saying goodbye to the indigent, why aren't public officials in Oregon thinking about cracking down on practices that add tens of millions of dollars to state-financed health care costs each year? Before saying no to a bone marrow transplant for a three-year-old whose mother is on Medicaid, couldn't county and state legislators insist that every licensed hospital and physician be required by law to provide a fixed percentage of care for those who cannot pay?

Before creating laws that would send some of the poor to a premature demise, county and state officials ought to require private health insurers to charge subscribers an additional premium that could be used to supplement the pitifully small budgets of Medicaid and public hospitals. And would it not make some sense to in-

sist on a luxury tax, which could be used to help meet the crucial health care needs of the poor, from the rich who avail themselves of psychotherapy, vitamins, Viagra, cosmetic surgery, diet clinics, and stress-management seminars?

Arthur L. Caplan *is director of the Center for Bioethics at the University of Pennsylvania.*

It is wrong to make the poor and only the poor bear the burden of rationing. It is unethical to institute rationing of necessary health services for any group of Americans unless we have made every effort to be as efficient as we can be in spending our health care dollars.

At a time when some can indulge their wants by buying a face-lift, it seems extraordinarily hard for ethicists or legislators to convincingly argue that they have no other option but to condemn the poor to die for want of money.

Sharpening Your Critical Thinking Skills

1. Summarize Lamm's and Caplan's key points. List supporting information given for each position or main point.
2. Do you agree with the views of Lamm or Caplan? Explain why.

Visit *Human Biology's* Internet site for links to web sites offering more information on this topic.

23 were permanently disabled, in large part due to the inability of their kidneys to cope with the mercury and subsequent nervous system effects. The tragedy was deepened by the discovery of birth defects in 19 babies born to women who had eaten contaminated seafood. Many of their mothers showed no signs of mercury poisoning, illustrating a general principle of toxicology: the younger an organism, the more sensitive it is to toxins.

The Minimata Bay incident was not an isolated event. A similar tragedy occurred on the Japanese island of Honshu. In Sweden in the early 1960s, mercury poisoning killed large numbers of birds that had been feeding on seeds treated with a mercury fungicide, a coating that retards mildew. Swedes who ate pheasant and other birds were also poisoned.

Fortunately, incidents of overt mercury poisoning are rare. However, mercury is one of the more common water pollutants in the industrialized world, and people are continually exposed to low levels from a variety of sources. For example, mercury is a by-product of the production of the plastic polyvinyl chloride (commonly called PVC plastic). PVC is used to manufacture children's toys, beach balls, car seats, and other products. Chances are you have some PVC nearby. Mercury is emitted into waterways by a variety of chemical manufacturers and also released by coal-fired power plants and garbage incinerators that burn batteries thrown out in our trash.

Many sources of mercury production are on the rise. Without tighter controls on emissions, low-level mercury poisoning may become more and more common in the years to come.

www.jbpub.com/humanbiology

Connect to this book's web site: www.jbpub.com/humanbiology
The site features eLearning, an online review area that provides quizzes, chapter outlines, and other tools to help you study for your class. You can also follow useful links for in-depth information, research the differing views in the Point/Counterpoints, or keep up on the latest environmental and health news.

Summary

Organs of Excretion: A Biological Imperative

1. All organisms produce waste and all organisms face the same challenge: getting rid of internally generated wastes.

2. Fortunately, humans have excretory organs that remove waste and help regulate internal concentrations of ions and water vital for homeostasis.

3. **TABLE 10-1** lists the major metabolic wastes and other molecules excreted from the body.

4. These wastes are removed by the skin, lungs, liver, kidneys, and intestines.

The Urinary System

5. One of the most important organs of excretion in humans (and other vertebrates) is the *kidney.* Kidneys remove impurities from the blood and also help regulate the water levels and ionic concentrations of the blood.

6. Blood enters the kidneys in the *renal arteries* whose branches deliver it to the millions of nephrons located in the kidney.

7. The nephrons produce urine, which drains from the kidneys into the *ureters,* slender muscular tubes that lead to the urinary bladder. Urine is stored in the *urinary bladder,* then voided through the *urethra.*

8. Each *nephron* consists of a *glomerulus,* a tuft of highly porous capillaries, and a *renal tubule,* where urine is produced.

9. The renal tubule consists of four parts: (a) *Bowman's capsule,* (b) the *proximal convoluted tubule,* (c) the *loop of Henle,* and (d) the *distal convoluted tubule.* The distal convoluted tubules of nephrons drain into *collecting tubules,* which converge and empty urine into the *renal pelvis.*

Function of the Urinary System

10. Blood filtration is accomplished by: glomerular filtration, tubular reabsorption, and tubular secretion.

11. *Glomerular filtration* occurs in the glomerulus, producing a liquid called the *filtrate.*

12. The filtrate is processed as it flows along the renal tubule. Water, ions, and nutrients are largely reabsorbed as they travel along the tubule. This process is called *tubular reabsorption.* Water and reabsorbed nutrients and ions pass into a network of capillaries, the *peritubular capillaries,* surrounding each nephron. What is left is a concentrated liquid, the *urine.*

13. Not all wastes are filtered from the blood in the glomerulus. Those that remain pass into the peritubular capillaries with the blood. These substances may be transported out of the peritubular capillaries into the renal tubule in a process known as *tubular secretion.* Hydrogen and potassium ions, for example, are secreted into the renal tubule.

Urination: Controlling A Reflex

14. *Urination* is a reflex in babies and very young children. In older children and adults, the urination reflex still operates, but it is overridden by a conscious control mechanism.

Controlling Kidney Function and Maintaining Homeostasis

15. Each drop of blood in your body flows through the kidneys many times in a single day. This flow allows for a thorough filtering of the blood and also helps the body control the chemical composition of the blood and extracellular fluid.

16. The concentration of water and dissolved substances in the blood is controlled by two hormones: ADH and aldosterone.

17. *ADH* or *antidiuretic hormone* is secreted by the posterior lobe of the pituitary gland. It is released when the osmotic concentration of the blood increases or when blood volume decreases.

18. ADH increases the permeability of the distal convoluted tubules and the collecting tubules to water. When ADH is present, water reabsorption increases.

19. *Aldosterone* is produced by the adrenal cortex. Aldosterone stimulates the reabsorption of sodium ions by the nephron. Water follows the sodium out of the renal tubule, increasing blood pressure and blood volume.

Diseases of the Urinary System

20. Calcium, magnesium, and other materials can precipitate out of the urine in the renal pelvis, forming *kidney stones.*

21. Smaller stones may be passed along the ureters to the bladder and are often eliminated during urination. Larger stones that remain in the kidney must be removed surgically or via *ultrasound lithotripsy.*

22. Renal failure is a disease in which the kidneys stop working. Renal failure may occur suddenly or gradually and is a life-threatening disorder. It can be treated by dialysis, a mechanical filtering of the blood.

23. Diabetes insipidus is a rare but troublesome disease resulting from a lack of ADH. The disease is characterized by frequent urination and excessive fluid intake.

Health, Homeostasis, and the Environment: Mercury Poisoning

24. The kidneys help regulate the levels of nutrients and toxins produced by the cells of the body. They also help eliminate toxins taken into the body from air, water, and food.

25. Unfortunately, the kidneys are not immune to many harmful substances. Heavy metals, for example, can destroy cells of the renal tubule and can restrict blood flow to the glomeruli. As a result, heavy metals can damage the kidney, impairing the function of this important homeostatic organ.

Critical Thinking

Thinking Critically— Analysis

This Analysis corresponds to the Thinking Critically scenario that was presented at the beginning of this chapter.

After preparing your list, compare your concerns and questions with mine to see how we match.

- Concern: A clinical trial on 90 patients is extremely small. With so few patients, the reliability of the results is in question.
- Question 1: Are more clinical tests under way?
- Question 2: Does the treatment have any adverse impacts?
- Question 3: Is the marketing company unbiased?

- Question 4: Is it promoting a product that may turn out to be ineffective, opening the company to lawsuits for fraud? In other words, is it letting financial concerns outweigh the need for good scientific research and carefully controlled experiments?

Now suppose that you have kidney cancer and have the $22,000 to pay for ALT. Would you do it? Are any of the issues above still relevant? How would you go about determining whether you should try the procedure?

To be fair to all parties concerned, let me point out that approximately two-thirds of the insurance companies in the United States pay for ALT treatment. As a rule, most companies do not pay for experimental procedures. In other words, they must be satisfied that ALT is an effective treatment before reimbursing clients.

Test of Concepts

1. Draw the various parts of the urinary system, and describe what each one does.
2. Draw a nephron, then label its parts. Explain what happens to the filtrate in each section of the nephron.
3. Trace the flow of blood into and out of the kidney. Be sure to include details of the pathway once it reaches the afferent arteriole.
4. Describe the three ways in which the kidney filters the blood.
5. A drug inhibits the uptake, or reabsorption, of water by the distal convoluted tubules and collecting tubules.

What effect would this drug have on urine output, urine concentration, blood pressure, blood volume, and the concentration of the blood?

6. Describe how ADH controls blood pressure and the water content of the body. Describe the hormonal and physiological changes in the body that take place when excess liquid is ingested. Do the same for dehydration.
7. How does urination differ between newborns and adults? Explain what is meant by this statement: In older

children and adults, urination is a reflex with a conscious override.

8. Aldosterone helps regulate blood pressure and water content. In what ways is this hormone different from ADH?
9. You have just finished your residency in family medicine. A patient comes to your office complaining that he drinks water all day long and spends much of the rest of the day in the bathroom urinating. What tests would you order? What diagnosis would you suspect?

CHAPTER 11

The Nervous System

INTEGRATION, COORDINATION, AND CONTROL

Light micrograph of the cerebellum of the human brain.

Thinking Critically

Researchers at the Washington University School of Medicine in St. Louis recently published a report in the *Journal of Neuroscience* on brain activity in people with severe depression. They compared brain activity in normal individuals with that in people suffering from severe depression, which is characterized by dreary moods, apathy, and hopelessness.

The scientists injected the subjects with radioactive oxygen, which is taken up by metabolically active brain cells. Inside the brain, radioactive oxygen molecules emit gamma rays; these are picked up by a special device that sends signals to a computer. The computer then maps brain cell metabolic activity.

In the study under discussion, researchers compared 6 patients with depression to 18 control subjects. To compare the results, they used a computer program that combines the "brain maps" of each group to produce a composite—sort of an average of the entire group.

The scientists found that a region of the brain known as the left prefrontal cortex was extremely active in patients suffering from depression. None of the controls showed a similar response. How would you interpret this data? What further studies would you perform? ■

Ernest Hemingway was one of America's most celebrated writers. His novels like *The Old Man and the Sea* and short stories won him the Nobel Prize in literature. Despite success and widespread popularity, Hemingway was a troubled man who eventually committed suicide. What ultimately caused him to take his life no one can know, but some believe that one contributing factor was a rare and painful nervous system disorder known as **trigeminal neuralgia** (try-GEM-in-al ner-AL-gee-ah). People suffering from this disease complain of periodic, unexplained flashes of pain along the course of the **trigeminal nerve,** which supplies the face. A slight breeze or the pressure of a razor can set off this intense pain, which lasts a minute or more. In some patients, the pain reappears for no apparent reason every few minutes for weeks on end. Some people believe that the pain Hemingway felt may have become unbearable. Combined with personal conflict, it may have caused the writer to take his life.

Today, physicians treat mild cases of trigeminal neuralgia with drugs. In extreme cases, however, they may elect to sever the nerve as it leaves the brain. This procedure ends the pain, but because it cuts off the inflow of other sensory information, it leaves half of the victim's face, tongue, and oral cavity numb—a little like the feeling you get when a dentist injects novocaine into your gums.

This chapter describes the anatomy and physiology of the human nervous system. You will briefly study the nerve that may have caused Hemingway so much trouble and will also examine ways in which the nervous system contributes to homeostasis.

An Overview of the Nervous System

The human nervous system governs the functions of the body, exerting control over muscles, glands, and organs. It also controls heartbeat, breathing, digestion, and urination. It helps regulate blood flow as well as the osmotic concentration of the blood. As such, it plays a major role in maintaining homeostasis.

The nervous system receives input from a large number of sources in the body. This input helps the nervous system "manage" body functions in much the same way that letters from citizens help elected officials govern society.

The human nervous system provides functions not seen in other animal species. For example, the brain is the site of ideation—the formation of ideas. Our brain allows us to think about and plan for the future. It en-

ables us to reason—that is, to judge right from wrong, logical from illogical. Although some species display a rudimentary ability to reason, this function is best expressed in humankind.

The nervous system also allows us to manipulate our environment to our own liking. Much more than any other species alive today, we humans are reshaping the planet. We level tropical forests to make room for cattle, drain and fill swamps to build homes and factories, split atoms to generate energy, and catapult men and women into space. Joan McIntyre, an author and critic, once wrote, "The ability of our minds to imagine, coupled with the ability of our hands to devise our images, brings us a power almost beyond control."

Today, many of the advances we humans have made, in our unrelenting pursuit of progress now threaten our very existence (Chapter 24). Pollution, resource depletion, and other troubles stand in the way of our own success. The human brain gives us the power to create yet also an incredible power to destroy. Numerous examples in this book show that the by-products of many activities and technologies are overwhelming environmental and human physiological systems involved in homeostasis and are consequently threatening our health and well-being. Fortunately, our hope of survival itself also depends on our brain, an evolutionary by-product unrivaled in the biological world.

The Nervous System Consists of Two Main Anatomical Subdivisions, the Central and Peripheral Nervous Systems

The human nervous system consists of three components: the brain, the spinal cord, and nerves (**FIGURE 11-1**). The brain and spinal cord constitute the **central nervous system (CNS)** and are housed in the skull and vertebral canal, respectively. Three layers of connective tissue, known as the **meninges** (men-IN-gees), surround the brain and spinal cord (**FIGURE 11-2**). The outer layer consists of fibrous connective tissue and is known as the **dura mater** (DURE-ah MAH-ter; meaning "hard mother"). The middle covering is the **arachnoid layer** (ah-RACK-noid), so named for its spider-weblike appearance. (Spiders belong to a group known as arachnids.) The innermost layer is the **pia mater** (PEE-ah MAH-ter; literally, "tender mother"). The pia mater is a delicate, vascular layer that adheres closely to the brain and spinal cord. The space between the arachnoid layer and pia mater is filled with a liquid called **cerebrospinal fluid (CSF)** (sir-REE-bro-SPIE-nal).

Nerves consist of bundles of nerve fibers. Each fiber is part of a nerve cell, or **neuron** (NER-on). Nerves transport messages to and from the CNS. These nerves end on receptors. These structures respond to a variety of inter-

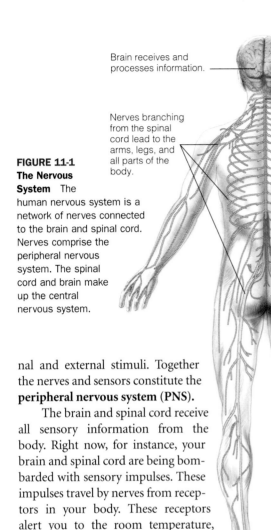

Brain receives and processes information.

Spinal cord, the main nerve trunk to and from the brain.

Nerves branching from the spinal cord lead to the arms, legs, and all parts of the body.

FIGURE 11-1 The Nervous System The human nervous system is a network of nerves connected to the brain and spinal cord. Nerves comprise the peripheral nervous system. The spinal cord and brain make up the central nervous system.

nal and external stimuli. Together the nerves and sensors constitute the **peripheral nervous system (PNS).**

The brain and spinal cord receive all sensory information from the body. Right now, for instance, your brain and spinal cord are being bombarded with sensory impulses. These impulses travel by nerves from receptors in your body. These receptors alert you to the room temperature, traffic sounds, and the touch of the page. They transmit visual images of words and figures on the pages.

This massive inflow of information is managed by the CNS. Some information is stored in memory. Some incoming information is ignored, and some elicits responses. A particularly interesting and exciting section you read, for example, might accelerate your heart rate.

The brain processes incoming stimuli and often responds by sending nerve impulses to muscles and glands (effectors) via the nerves. The nerves carry two types of information: (1) **sensory impulses** traveling to the CNS from sensory receptors in the body, and (2) **motor impulses** traveling away from the CNS to muscles and glands.

Sensory information entering the CNS is integrated with information stored in memory. Thus, a new fact may trigger memories of previous knowledge, causing you to think about a problem in a new way. Memory also influences the way we respond to stimuli. A pet cat brushing against your leg, for example, may elicit a smile. The stimulus is not startling, because your memory reminds you of the cat's presence. If you didn't own a cat, the stimulus might send you through the roof!

The Peripheral Nervous System Is Divided into Two Subdivisions: The Somatic and Autonomic

As **FIGURE 11-3** shows, the peripheral nervous system consists of the somatic nervous system and the autonomic nervous system. The **somatic nervous system**

Scalp
Cerebrum
Cerebellum

Cranium
Muscles
Meninges
Vertebra
Spinal cord

Skin of scalp
Bone of skull
Dura mater
Arachnoid layer } **Meninges**
Pia mater
Cortex of brain

FIGURE 11-2 The Meninges Consisting of three layers, the meninges are the connective tissue covering the brain.

(so-MAA-tick) is that portion of the PNS that controls voluntary functions of the body, such as the muscle contractions that cause the limbs to move. It also controls certain involuntary reflex actions, such as the knee-jerk response.

That part of the PNS that controls the rest of the involuntary functions such as heart rate and breathing is the **autonomic nervous system** (au-toe-NOM-ick) or ANS (**FIGURE 11-3**). Many other functions are under the control of the autonomic nervous system, including digestion and body temperature regulation. These are controlled by negative feedback loops.

The ANS is absolutely essential to survival. To understand why, imagine how much more difficult our lives would be if we had to consciously control our breathing and other automatic functions.[1] We'd have very little time for anything else.

---

[1]Note that breathing can be controlled voluntarily, but for the most part, it is an involuntary action.

FIGURE 11-3 Subdivisions of the Nervous System The nervous system is divided into two parts, the central nervous system (CNS) and the peripheral nervous system (PNS). The PNS consists of autonomic and somatic divisions. The activities of the autonomic and somatic divisions often overlap.

FIGURE 11-3 shows that each branch of the peripheral nervous system consists of two types of neurons. The first are **sensory,** or **afferent, neurons** (A-fair-ent), which transmit information to the CNS. The second are **motor,** or **efferent, neurons** (EE-fair-ent), which transmit information away from the CNS to the effectors such as muscles.

Structure and Function of the Neuron

Before we examine the structure and function of the nervous system in more detail, let us look at the neuron, or nerve cell. The **neuron** is the fundamental structural unit of the nervous system. This highly specialized cell generates bioelectric impulses and transmits them from one part of the body to another. Such signals alert us to a variety of internal and external stimuli and permit us to respond to them.

All Neurons Consist of a Cell Body and Two Types of Processes That Transmit Impulses

Neurons come in several shapes and sizes. Despite these differences, nerve cells share several characteristics. All neurons, for example, consist of a more or less spherical central portion, the **cell body** (**FIGURE 11-4**). It houses the nucleus, most of the cell's cytoplasm, and numerous organelles. Metabolic activities in the cell body sustain the entire neuron, providing energy and synthesizing materials necessary for proper cell function. Two organelles of particular interest are microtubules and microfilaments. These structures form the cytoskeleton that gives rise to the neuron's characteristic shape.

All nerve cells contain two types of processes that transmit bioelectric impulses. Those that transmit impulses *to* the cell body are **dendrites** (DEN-drights). Those that transmit impulses away from the cell body are **axons** (AXE-ons).

Neurobiologists classify neurons by their structure—notably, the type of processes they contain. Accordingly, three distinct types of neuron are found in the human nervous system. Shown in **FIGURE 11-5**, they are the unipolar, the bipolar, and the multipolar.

The **unipolar neuron** (you-nee-POLE-er) has a single cellular process that splits into an axon and a dendrite soon after it leaves the cell body. The **bipolar neuron** has two cellular processes, one axon and one dendrite, on opposite sides of the cell body. The **multipolar neuron** contains a single long axon and numerous short, branching dendrites that are attached to the cell body. Multipolar neurons are the most abundant and will be the focus of our discussion.[2] In multipolar neurons, the dendrites transmit impulses to the cell body. Axons transmit the impulses away from the cell body. Axons occasionally also give off side branches, **axon collaterals** (**FIGURE 11-4B**). When an axon reaches its destination, it often branches profusely, giving off many small fibers. These fibers terminate in tiny swellings called **terminal boutons** (boo-TAWNS; *boutons* is the French word for buttons). Terminal boutons serve as a

communication link with other neurons, muscle fibers, or glands.

Axons in the CNS and PNS Contain an Insulating Layer, the Myelin Sheath, Which Greatly Increases the Rate of Transmission of Nerve Impulses. The axons of many multipolar neurons in both the central and peripheral nervous systems are coated with a protective layer called the **myelin sheath** (MY-eh-lin) (**FIGURE 11-6A**). The myelin sheath is formed by nonconducting cells of the nervous system known as

---

[2]Multipolar neurons are involved in the efferent pathways of the PNS and carry motor information to effector organs such as glands and muscles.

FIGURE 11-4 A Neuron *(a)* A scanning electron micrograph of the cell body and dendrites of a multipolar neuron. The multipolar neuron resides within the central nervous system. Its multiangular cell body has several highly branched dendrites and one long axon. *(b)* Collateral branches may occur along the length of the axon. When the axon terminates, it branches many times, ending on individual muscle fibers.

(a)

(b)

(a) Unipolar   **(b) Bipolar**   **(c) Multipolar**

FIGURE 11-5 Three Types of Neurons

great speed down the axons, "jumping" from node to node like a stone skipping along the surface of the water (**FIGURE 11-6A**). In the CNS, a single oligodendrocyte produces myelin for several axons (**FIGURE 11-6E**).

Destruction of the myelin sheath of nerve cells in the central nervous system results in a condition known as **multiple sclerosis** (skler-OH-siss). The damaged myelin results in nerve cell death that leads to numbness, slurred speech, and paralysis. Thought to be an au-

glial cells (GLEE-al). In the PNS, the glial cells that form the myelin sheath are the **Schwann cells,** named after the German cytologist Theodore Schwann. In the CNS, the myelin sheath is laid down by glial cells known as **oligodendrocytes** (oh-LEE-go-DEN-drow-SITES).

During embryonic development, Schwann cells in the PNS attach to growing axons, then begin to encircle them (**FIGURE 11-6D**). As they do, they leave behind a trail of plasma membrane that wraps around the axon, forming many concentric layers—a little like an elastic bandage wrapped around your wrist (**FIGURES 11-6B** and **11-6C**).

The entire myelin sheath of an axon is formed by numerous Schwann cells that align themselves along the length of the axon. Each lays down a separate patch of myelin. Because the plasma membrane of the Schwann cell is about 80% lipid, the myelin sheath is mostly lipid (mostly triglyceride) and appears glistening white when viewed with the naked eye. As shown in **FIGURE 11-6A**, each segment of myelin is separated by a small unmyelinated segment known as a **node of Ranvier** (RON-vee-A). Although the term *node* implies a bump, the nodes are actually regions of axon that contain no myelin.

For reasons explained later, the myelin sheath permits nerve impulses to travel with

FIGURE 11-6 The Myelin Sheath and Saltatory Conduction   *(a)* The myelin sheath allows impulses to "jump" from node to node, greatly accelerating the rate of transmission. *(b)* A drawing showing the arrangement of Schwann cell membrane in the myelin sheath. *(c)* A transmission electron micrograph of an axon in cross section showing a myelin sheath. Drawings show how the myelin sheath is formed in the PNS *(d)* and CNS *(e).*

toimmune disease, multiple sclerosis can affect any part of the CNS. Early symptoms are generally mild weakness or a tingling or numb feeling in one part of the body. Temporary weakness may cause a person to stumble and fall. Some people report blurred vision, slurred speech, and difficulty controlling urination. In many cases, these symptoms disappear, never to return. Other individuals suffer repeated attacks. Because recovery after each attack is incomplete, patients gradually deteriorate, losing vision and becoming progressively weaker. Fortunately, many treatments are available, and only a small number of multiple sclerosis patients are crippled by the disease.

Although most axons are covered with myelin, some are unmyelinated. Found in both the central and peripheral nervous systems, unmyelinated axons conduct impulses much more slowly than their myelinated counterparts. The reduced rate of transmission in unmyelinated axons results from the fact that the impulse must travel along the entire membrane of the axon—more like a wave moving along the surface of a pond than a stone skipping across it. As a rule, the most urgent types of information are transmitted via myelinated fibers; less urgent information is transmitted via unmyelinated fibers.

Neurons Lose the Ability to Divide. During development, nerve cells lose the ability to divide. That's bad news for people, because it means that nerve cells that die as a result of injury or old age cannot be replaced by cell division. But not all damage leads to nerve cell death and not all nerve cell death leads to irreversible damage. Why?

Consider what happens in a stroke. Strokes or cerebrovascular accidents result from one of three causes: (1) cerebral hemorrhages, breaks in arteries of the brain; (2) cerebral thromboses (throm-BOW-sees), blood clots that form in brain arteries narrowed by atherosclerosis; and (3) cerebral embolisms (EM-bow-LIZ-ims), blood clots from other sources that lodge in arteries of the brain (**FIGURE 11-7**).

All three problems have the same end result: They terminate blood flow to brain cells, often killing them. But this doesn't mean a person is always left permanently impaired. If a person survives a stroke, undamaged neurons in the brain can take over the function of damaged brain cells, thus permitting partial to complete recovery. Recovery also occurs when cells that were injured but not killed by the injury regain their function. This generally takes a long time and explains why stroke patients require long-term rehabilitation.

Nerves can be severed in accidents or other injuries. The fate of a severed axon depends in large part on its

FIGURE 11-7 Brain Damage Caused by Stroke PET (positron emission tomography) scan of brain revealing damaged region of the cerebral cortex following a stroke. This color image was generated by a computer that converts readings of the rate of emission from radioactive glucose molecules injected into the patient. Damaged (dark region) areas show the lowest glucose uptake. Highest glucose uptake and highest emissions are in red.

location in the nervous system. In the brain and spinal cord, for example, severed axons *cannot* be repaired. Spinal cord injuries that sever nerve tracts result in paralysis and loss of sensation in the region below the damage. Although the prognosis for spinal cord injury victims is generally poor, new procedures are being tested that could reduce damage in such instances, so that people who would have been paralyzed will walk again.

One procedure currently being tested in Israel involves the injection of macrophages from a person's own body (skin and bone marrow) into the site of injury. Early results are quite promising. But in order to be effective, treatment must occur within nine days of the accident. Doctors treating a young college woman in Colorado whose back was fractured in a car accident recently reported voluntary movement in her feet four months after the treatment. Only time will tell if she can regain full use of her lower limbs.

In the peripheral nervous system, nerve regeneration is possible because severed axons can regrow. As **FIGURE 11-8** illustrates, a severed axon in the PNS generally degenerates from the point of injury to the muscle or gland it supplied. The segment of the axon still attached to the cell body may elongate and replace the degenerated section. During regeneration, the axon extends along the hollow tunnel left in the myelin sheath by the degenerated part. Eventually, the axon reestablishes connections with the muscles or glands it once supplied, making partial or nearly complete recovery of control possible.

Neurosurgeons can facilitate axonal regeneration in the PNS by **microsurgery**—surgery performed under a dissecting microscope. With painstaking care, surgeons sew the severed ends of nerves together after they've

(a) Nerve severed   Skeletal muscle

(b) Axon degenerates   Loses connections with muscles

(c) Axon regenerates   Reestablishes connections

FIGURE 11-8 Axonal Regeneration *(a)* A severed axon can regenerate in the peripheral nervous system. *(b)* The segment from the cut to the effector organ degenerates (white section). The myelin sheath remains, providing a tunnel *(c)* through which the axonal stub can regrow, often reestablishing previous contacts and restoring motor function.

lined up the empty myelin sheaths with those of the regenerating nerve fibers.

Neurons Have a High Metabolic Demand, Making Them Highly Susceptible to Loss of Oxygen and Glucose. Besides being unable to divide, nerve cells have an extraordinarily high metabolic rate. Consequently, they require a constant supply of oxygen for energy production. Making matters worse, neurons cannot generate ATP in the absence of oxygen via fermentation (glucose breakdown to lactic acid) the way most other cells can. Thus, if the amount of oxygen flowing to the brain is drastically reduced, neurons begin to die within minutes.

To prevent brain damage from occurring in someone who has collapsed with a severe heart attack or has drowned or suffered an electric shock, rescuers must start resuscitating the victim within 4–5 minutes. Although victims may be revived after this crucial period, the lack of oxygen in the brain often results in brain damage. Generally, the longer the deprivation, the greater the damage.

If one's "lucky" enough to drown in cold water, though, resuscitation may be successful if begun within an hour. In most cases, victims recover without any

detectable brain damage. Recovery is possible in such instances because cold water greatly slows brain metabolism. This, in turn, dramatically reduces oxygen demand. As a result, brain cells are preserved, and brain damage is minimized or avoided. In one exceptional case, a young boy from Fargo, North Dakota, was allegedly underwater for 5 hours before he was resuscitated. Much to his parents' delight, the boy not only survived the incident but also has no apparent ill effects.

Nerve cells are also highly dependent on glucose for energy production. Unlike most other body cells, they cannot use fatty acids to generate energy. Neither can they store glucose as liver and muscle cells do. As a result, when blood glucose levels fall, nerve cells are first to "feel" the ill effects.

A decline in blood glucose is normally prevented by homeostatic mechanisms described in Chapter 4. Serious problems can result in people whose glucose homeostasis is not working properly. In diabetics, for instance, blood glucose levels can fall dangerously low if too much insulin is taken or if not enough glucose is ingested. Deprived of glucose, brain cells begin to falter. Individuals can become dizzy and weak. Vision may blur. Speech may become awkward. Diabetics are sometimes mistakenly considered drunk. Chronic low blood glucose often results in severe headaches. Some diabetics become aggressive when blood sugar levels fall. In extreme cases, low blood sugar triggers convulsions and death. Other body cells are not adversely affected by a decline in blood glucose because they switch to alternative fuels, fats and proteins.

Bioelectric Impulses in Nerve Cells Result from the Flow of Ions Across Their Plasma Membranes

Nerve impulses are not like the electric current that powers computers or light bulbs, which is formed by the flow of electrons. Rather, nerve impulses are small ionic changes in the membrane of the neuron that move along the plasma membrane of a nerve cell.

To understand the nerve cell impulse, or **bioelectric impulse,** we begin by examining the plasma membrane of a neuron. If you placed tiny electrodes on the outside and inside of the plasma membrane of a neuron and hooked them up to a voltmeter, you would measure a small voltage, much like that produced in a battery. Voltage is a measure of the tendency of charged particles to flow from one pole of the battery to the other. The higher the voltage, the greater the tendency for electrons to flow through a wire connected to the poles. In the nerve cell, however, electrons do not flow from one side of the membrane to another; sodium and potassium ions do.

Axon

FIGURE 11-9 Resting Potential
Electrodes placed on both sides of the plasma membrane of a neuron measure a tiny potential difference, roughly −70 millivolts (mV). This is the resting potential.

In neurons, the potential difference, or voltage, is a measure of the force that can drive sodium ions from one side of the membrane to the other. For now, it is important just to remember that a small voltage exists across the plasma membrane of the neuron. It is so small, in fact, that it is measured in millivolts (MILL-ee-volts). A millivolt is 1/1000 of a volt.

As **FIGURE 11-9** shows, the potential difference in a typical neuron is about −70 millivolts. This is known as the **membrane potential,** or **resting potential**—so named because it is the membrane potential of a nerve cell at rest. The minus sign is added because the plasma membrane is positively charged on the outside and negatively charged on the inside, for reasons beyond the scope of this book.

To understand the bioelectric impulse, it is important to know that sodium ions are found in greater concentration *outside* the neuron. Potassium ions are found in greater concentration *inside* the cell. In fact, neurons expend a great deal of energy to maintain this concentration imbalance, so essential to the production of nerve impulses. The energy fuels the active transport pumps (proteins) in the plasma membrane of neurons, which pump sodium ions that have leaked into the cytoplasm of the neuron back out into the surrounding fluid and transport potassium ions that have leaked into the extracellular fluid back into the cell.

After a Nerve Cell Is Stimulated, the Membrane Undergoes Dramatic Changes in Permeability to Various Ions, Resulting in Sudden Shifts in Membrane Potential. The plasma membrane of a nerve cell has a built-up charge. The charge consists of sodium ions concentrated on the outside of the cell. When the neuron is stimulated, the membrane undergoes a rapid change, "discharging" the load. The first change occurring in the membrane is a rapid increase in its permeability to sodium ions. Neurophysiologists believe that

stimulating the nerve cell causes protein pores in the plasma membrane to open. Sodium ions flow *into* the cell through these pores.

Electrodes implanted in a nerve cell like those used to measure resting potential detect the sudden influx of positively charged sodium ions when the neuron is activated. The electrodes then register a shift in the resting potential from −70 millivolts to +30 millivolts. The change in voltage occurs at the site of stimulation and is called **depolarization.**[3] The membrane is said to be depolarized. Immediately after depolarization, the membrane returns to its previous state, which is referred to as **repolarization.**

The depolarization/repolarization of the membrane is shown graphically in **FIGURE 11-10A**. This tracing is an **action potential.** The action potential consists of (1) a brief upswing, depolarization, as the voltage goes from −70 millivolts to +30 millivolts, and (2) a rapid downswing, repolarization, the return to the resting potential.

The depolarization occurs so rapidly and the membrane returns to the resting state so quickly (in about 3/1000 of a second) that neurons can be stimulated in rapid succession. Such brisk recovery allows us to respond swiftly and forcefully to danger and to perform rapid muscle movements. Nerve cells can also transmit many impulses in sequence—one after another—because only a small number of sodium ions are exchanged with each impulse.

As noted above, depolarization results in the rapid inflow of sodium ions. But what causes repolarization, the shift from +30 millivolts back to −70 millivolts? Repolarization results from two factors. The first is a sudden decrease in the membrane's permeability to sodium

---

[3]Depolarization means that the membrane loses its previous polarization.

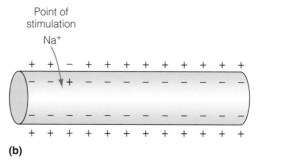

(a)

FIGURE 11-10 Action Potential *(a)* Stimulating the neuron creates a bioelectric impulse, which is recorded as an action potential. The resting potential shifts from −70 millivolts to +30 millivolts. The membrane is said to be depolarized. This graph shows the shift in potential and the change in the permeability of sodium (Na^+) and potassium (K^+) ions, which is largely responsible for the action potential. *(b)* The influx of sodium ions and the depolarization that occur at the point of stimulation. *(c)* The impulse travels along the membrane as a wave of depolarization (gray area). *(d)* The efflux of potassium ions restores the resting potential, allowing the neuron to transmit additional impulses almost immediately.

ions. This stops the influx of sodium ions. Repolarization also results from a rapid efflux of positively charged potassium ions (**FIGURE 11-10D**). Potassium ions flow out of the axon down a concentration gradient. Because the outside of the membrane becomes negatively charged during depolarization, an electrical gradient also facilitates repolarization. The net outward movement of potassium ions reestablishes the resting potential.

When a neuron is no longer stimulated, it quickly reestablishes the sodium- and potassium-ion concentrations inside and outside the cell. It does this by pumping sodium ions that flowed into the cell during activation out of the axon and by pumping potassium ions that flowed out of the neuron during repolarization back in. As noted earlier, the reestablishment of the chemical disequilibrium results from the action of numerous sodium-potassium active transport pumps in the plasma membranes of nerve cells. (You may recall from Chapter 3 that active transport pumps require energy in the form of ATP.) The sodium-potassium pumps, in fact, consume about 30% of the energy your body needs.[4]

Depolarization in One Region Stimulates Depolarization in Adjacent Regions and Allows Nerve Impulses to Move Along the Membrane of the Neuron. Researchers who have explored the neuron's mode of impulse conduction have found that a change in membrane permeability in the stimulated region, which results in depolarization, causes a change in the sodium permeability in adjacent regions. Thus, depolarization in one location on the axon stimulates depolarization in adjacent regions. This process continues along the length of the axon.

In unmyelinated fibers in the human nervous system, nerve impulses travel like waves in water from one region to the next. In myelinated fibers, however, the depolarization "jumps" from one node of Ranvier (the section between adjacent Schwann cells) to another. Shown in **FIGURE 11-6A**, impulse jumping greatly in-

Point of stimulation

Na^+

(b)

Na^+

Depolarization and generation of the action potential

Na^+

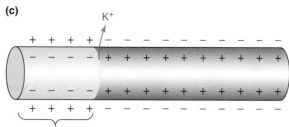

Propagation of the action potential

(c)

K^+

+ + + + / − − − − − − − − − − −
− − − − − / + + + + + + + + + +
− − − − − / + + + + + + + + + +
+ + + + / − − − − − − − − − − −

Repolarized membrane

(d)

---

[4]The sodium-potassium pump is found in all cells, not just neurons.

creases the rate of transmission. In fact, a nerve impulse travels along an unmyelinated fiber at a rate of about 0.5 meter per second (1.5 feet per second). In a myelinated neuron, the impulse travels 400 times faster or about 200 meters per second. That's about 400 miles per hour! The difference in the rate of transmission of these two modes is largely due to a difference in the total amount of membrane that must be depolarized and repolarized.

Nerve Impulses Travel from One Neuron to Another Across Synapses

Nerve impulses travel from one neuron to another across a small space that separates them (**FIGURE 11-11B**). This juncture is called a **synapse** (SIN-apse). A synapse consists of (1) a terminal bouton (or some other kind of axon terminus), (2) a gap between the adjoining neurons, the **synaptic cleft,** and (3) the membrane of the

dendrite or postsynaptic cell (**FIGURE 11-11B**). The neuron that transmits the impulse is the **presynaptic neuron;** the one that receives the impulse is the **postsynaptic neuron.**

How does a nerve impulse get across the synapse? Quite frankly, it doesn't. The nerve impulse ends at the terminal bouton of the presynaptic neuron. However, when it reaches the terminal bouton, the nerve impulse triggers a series of chemical changes that can stimulate an impulse in the postsynaptic neuron. Let me explain.

When an impulse reaches a terminal bouton, depolarization of the plasma membrane of the bouton stimulates a rapid influx of calcium ions into the bouton from the extracellular fluid. Calcium ions, in turn, stimulate the release (by exocytosis) of a chemical substance stored in small vesicles in the terminal bouton. These chemicals are known as **neurotransmitters.**

At least 30 chemicals serve as neurotransmitters. Produced and packaged in vesicles in the cell body of the neuron, neurotransmitters move down the axon along the microtubules to the terminal bouton, where they are stored until needed. When the bioelectric impulse arrives, calcium flows in, and the vesicles bind to the presynaptic membrane and release the neurotransmitter into the synaptic cleft.

Neurotransmitters are chemical messengers that travel from nerve cell to nerve cell—or from nerve cell to effector (such as muscle). Neurotransmitters diffuse across the synaptic cleft between adjoining nerve cells and bind to receptors in the plasma membrane of the postsynaptic neuron. The binding of most neurotransmitters to the post-

Cell body of postsynaptic neuron

Terminal boutons of presynaptic boutons

Axon terminals

(a)

FIGURE 11-11 The Terminal Bouton and Synaptic Transmission *(a)* A scanning electron micrograph showing the terminal boutons of an axon ending on the cell body of another neuron. *(b)* The arrival of the impulse stimulates the release of neurotransmitters held in membrane-bound vesicles in the axon terminals. Neurotransmitter diffuses across the synaptic cleft and binds to the postsynaptic membrane, where it elicits another action potential that travels down the dendrite to the cell body. *(c)* A transmission electron micrograph showing the details of the synapse.

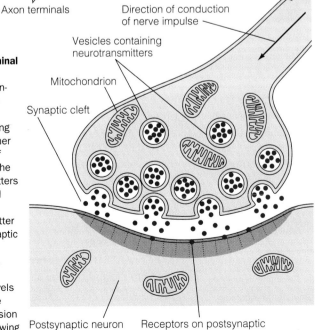

Presynaptic neuron

Direction of conduction of nerve impulse

Vesicles containing neurotransmitters

Mitochondrion

Synaptic cleft

Postsynaptic neuron

Receptors on postsynaptic membrane bound to neurotransmitter

(b)

Synaptic vesicles

Presynaptic neuron

(c) Postsynaptic neuron

Synaptic cleft

synaptic membrane stimulates a rapid increase in the permeability of the membrane of the postsynaptic cell to sodium ions. Do they stimulate another nerve impulse? Not necessarily.

Neurotransmitters May Excite or Inhibit the Postsynaptic Membrane. In the brain, a single nerve cell may have as many as 50,000 synapses. In some of these synapses, neurotransmitters stimulate the uptake of sodium ions, which slightly depolarizes the postsynaptic neuron. Synapses that depolarize the postsynaptic neuron are known as **excitatory synapses.** In other synapses, however, neurotransmitters hyperpolarize the membrane—that is, increase the voltage difference across the membrane, making it less excitable. These neurotransmitters cause chloride channels to open in the postsynaptic membrane. Because the chloride-ion concentration outside the cell is higher than it is inside, the opening of the chloride channels results in an influx of chloride ions, making the interior of the postsynaptic cell and hence the resting potential more negative, which renders the neuron less excitable. Such synapses are called **inhibitory synapses.**[5]

Whether a neuron fires (generates an action potential) depends on the summation of excitatory and inhibitory impulses. If the number of excitatory impulses exceeds the number of inhibitory impulses, a nerve impulse will be generated. If not, the neuron will not fire. This phenomenon provides the nervous system with a way of integrating incoming information—determining a response by the kinds of input it receives.

Because only terminal boutons contain neurotransmitters and because receptors for these substances are found only in the postsynaptic membrane, transmission across a synapse occurs only in one direction.

Neurotransmitters Are Quickly Removed from the Synaptic Cleft. Transmission across the synapse is remarkably fast, requiring only about 1/1000 of a second, or 1 millisecond. Synaptic transmission is also a transitory event. A short burst of neurotransmitter is released each time an impulse reaches the terminal bouton. It binds to the postsynaptic membrane, elicits a change, and is then removed from the synaptic cleft by three routes: (1) enzymatic destruction, (2) reabsorption by the terminal bouton or absorption by glial cells in the brain, and (3) diffusion away from the synapse.

Many Chemical Substances, Including Drugs and Insecticides, Exert Their Effect by Altering Synaptic Transmission. The synapses are vital links in the body's system of internal communication. As such, they are vulnerable to outside influences. Certain drugs and common environmental chemicals (for example, insecticides) impair the removal of neurotransmitters from the synaptic cleft. As long as neurotransmitters remain bound to the receptors on the postsynaptic membrane, the postsynaptic neuron remains activated.

Many insecticides inhibit the removal of the neurotransmitter **acetylcholine** (a-SEA-tol-KO-leen), the main excitatory neurotransmitter in the neurons that supply skeletal muscle cells. Insecticides kill insects by disrupting nerve transmission—creating a nervous system overload. Unfortunately, insecticides have the same effect on people such as farm workers and pesticide applicators exposed to high levels of the pesticides at work. Low doses can cause blurred vision, headaches, rapid pulse, and profuse sweating; higher doses can be fatal.

Each year, hundreds of Americans (mostly farm workers) are poisoned by pesticides. By various estimates, 200–1000 of them die. Worldwide, an estimated 500,000 people are poisoned, and 5000–14,000 people die each year from pesticides.

These problems and the widespread contamination of the environment have led some farmers to reduce pesticide use and to rely on other, nonpolluting methods of pest control. Crop rotation, insect-resistant crops, natural predators (ladybugs and praying mantises), and a variety of alternatives are available. Most are quite practical and cost-effective. Such strategies also benefit the soil and surrounding environment.

Anesthetics (an-es-THET-icks) are chemicals used to deaden pain or to put people to sleep for surgery. Some anesthetics may alter synaptic transmission, decreasing the transmission of pain impulses. Others seem to operate on the nerve cell itself. They apparently alter protein pores in the plasma membrane of neurons that regulate the flow of sodium ions into and out of the nerve cells. By blocking the flow of sodium, these anesthetics "paralyze" sensory nerves carrying pain messages to the brain.

Many antidepressant drugs such as Prozac and Paxil decrease the uptake of the neurotransmitter, serotonin, in the brain. Known as *serotonin selective reuptake inhibitors,* or SSRIs, these drugs elevate serotonin levels in the brain that "lifts" depression.

Caffeine and cocaine also affect synaptic transmission. Caffeine increases synaptic transmission, thus increasing overall neural activity. It is no wonder that coffee makes some people so jittery. Cocaine, on the

---

[5]Inhibitory neurotransmitters may also stimulate the opening of potassium channels. Potassium ions flow out of the postsynaptic cell, making the interior more negative.

other hand, blocks the uptake of neurotransmitters by terminal boutons in the brain. Because the neurotransmitter remains in the synaptic cleft for a longer time, neural activity is greatly increased. This increase results in a heightened state of alertness and euphoria, commonly known as a "high," which lasts for 20–40 minutes. Euphoria, however, is followed by a period of depression and anxiety, which causes the user to seek another high. Excessive cocaine use can result in serious mental derangement—in particular, paranoid delusions that others are out to get the user. In this state, heavy users may become violent.

For a discussion of the effect of recreational drug use see Health Note 11-1.

Nerve Cells Can Be Grouped Into Three Functional Categories

As noted earlier, nerve cells can be categorized by structure. For our purposes, though, a functional classification is more useful. According to this system, nerve cells fall into three groups: (1) sensory neurons, (2) motor neurons, and (3) interneurons.

Sensory neurons carry impulses from sensory receptors in the body to the CNS. Sensory receptors come in many shapes and sizes and respond to a variety of stimuli such as pressure, pain, heat, and movement (Chapter 12).

Motor neurons carry impulses from the brain and spinal cord to the muscles and glands of the body. Sensory information entering the brain and spinal cord via sensory neurons often stimulates motor neurons directly. Impulses leaving via the motor neurons then initiate a desired response.

In some cases, intervening neurons called **interneurons** (or association neurons) transmit impulses between sensory and motor neurons and represent a kind of neuronal bridge. Interneurons may also transmit impulses from sensory neurons to various parts of the CNS. The importance of interneurons is underscored by the fact that they make up 99% of the nerve cells in the human CNS. Interneurons form a neural communication network that transmits impulses from one part of the CNS to another and coordinates complex activities. They are also essential to many body reflexes.

Section 11-3

The Spinal Cord and Nerves

With these basics in mind, we can now turn our attention to some important aspects of the nervous system of humans, beginning with the spinal cord and nerves.

The Spinal Cord Transmits Information to and from the Brain and Also Houses Many Reflexes

The **spinal cord** is a long, ropelike structure about the diameter of a person's little finger. It connects to the brain and courses downward through the **vertebral canal** (VER-teh-brill) formed by the bones of the spine, the **vertebrae** (ver-tah-BREE) (**FIGURE 11-12**). The spinal

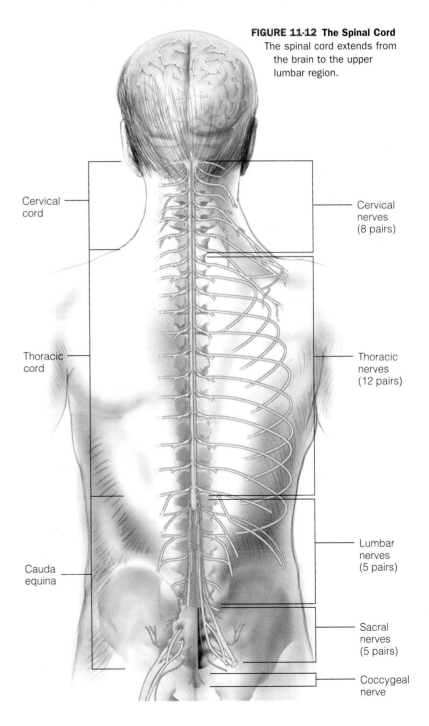

FIGURE 11-12 The Spinal Cord The spinal cord extends from the brain to the upper lumbar region.

Cervical cord

Thoracic cord

Cauda equina

Cervical nerves (8 pairs)

Thoracic nerves (12 pairs)

Lumbar nerves (5 pairs)

Sacral nerves (5 pairs)

Coccygeal nerve

Health Note 11-1

Recreational Drug Use: Is it a Good Idea?

Jason Wiley was a popular young man in his college dormitory. He was friendly, generous, and fun to be with. Like others of his age, Jason partied long and hard, often using recreational drugs like Special K or ecstasy. He'd started using drugs recreationally in high school. But then one day, Jason didn't return from his night of partying. When his friends found him, he was dead in the back seat of another friend's car. Jason, the coroner later told them, had died from an overdose of Special K and methamphetamine.

Jason is just one of millions of youths the world over who uses a small, but powerful assortment of

FIGURE 1 A rave

recreational drugs. The most commonly used are (1) methamphetamine, also known as meth, crystal meth, speed, ice, and crystal; (2) phencyclidine, also called PCP, angel dust, supergrass, killer weed, embalming fluid, and rocket fuel; (3) ecstasy, with a complex chemical name shortened to MDMA; (4) ketamine, alternatively referred to as Special K or simply k; (5) cocaine; (6) LSD; (7) gamma hydroxybutyrate or GHB, liquid x, Georgia home boy, goop, gamma-oh, and grievous body harm; and (8) Ritalin, also known as Vitamin R.

Many of these drugs, such as methamphetamine, ketamine, ecstasy, GHB, cocaine, and Ritalin are stimulants. They give the user a sense of euphoria, increased well being. These drugs increase heart rate, blood pressure, body temperature, and rate of breathing.

Some are stimulants and hallucinogens, substances that cause the user to perceive sites, sounds, and objects that are not present. Ketamine, ecstasy, Ritalin, and GHB are examples.

Some recreational drugs are addictive. Cocaine and Ritalin are examples.

All of these drugs have a dangerous side to them. Methamphetamine, the recreational drug whose use is

growing the fastest, is smoked, snorted, injected, or taken orally. This drug produces a state of hyperactivity, euphoria, and increased energy. It also causes tremors. High doses or chronic use of methamphetamine may cause increased nervousness, irritability, and psychosis, an altered state of mind. Chronic abusers, for instance, may become paranoid and may suffer auditory and visual hallucinations, as well as erratic and violent behavior. Withdrawal from the drug can cause severe depression.

PCP is considered by many to be the most dangerous of all recreational drugs. PCP use results in frequent bad trips, psychotic reactions, and extreme violence in its users. Moderate doses cause a person to feel detached, distant, and estranged from his or her surroundings. Loss of coordination, slurred speech, and numbness are commonly observed. Auditory and visual hallucinations, severe mood disorders, and amnesia may occur. Some users of PCP report acute anxiety and feelings of impending doom. In others, severe mental disorders are observed.

Ecstasy, which is frequently used with other drugs, is often distributed at late-night parties called raves, night clubs, and rock concerts. This drug produces very profound positive

---

cord gives off nerves along its course that supply the skin, muscles, bones, and organs of the body. The spinal cord ends at the lower back (at about the level of the second lumbar vertebra), at which point it gives off a series of nerves forming the **cauda equina** (CAW-dah eh-QUINE-ah; meaning "horse's tail"), which supply the lower sections of the body.

As **FIGURE 11-13** shows, the central portion of the spinal cord is an H-shaped zone of gray matter. **Gray matter** consists of nerve cell bodies of interneurons and motor neurons and is so named because it appears gray to the naked eye. Surrounding the gray matter are fiber tracts consisting of axons and a much smaller number of dendrites that travel up and down the spinal cord,

carrying information to and from the brain. The fiber tracts form the white matter, whose characteristic color comes from the myelin sheaths of the axons coursing through it.

The Nerves of the PNS Contain Motor and Sensory Fibers

As noted earlier, nerves are part of the peripheral nervous system. They carry sensory information to the spinal cord and brain and motor information out. Some nerves are strictly motor and some are strictly sensory, but many are mixed, having both motor and sensory fibers.

Nerves arising from the brain are **cranial nerves** (CRAY-knee-al) (**FIGURE 11-14**). The cranial nerves supfeelings, empathy for others, and relaxation, both physical and mental. Ecstasy suppresses the need to eat, drink, or sleep, so individuals can participate in two- to three-day parties. But ignoring these basic needs can result in severe dehydration and exhaustion. Ecstasy also produces nausea, hallucinations, chills, sweating, increased body temperature, tremors, muscle cramping, and blurred vision. After-effects include anxiety, paranoia, and depression.

Overdoses of ecstasy result in high blood pressure, faintness, and panic attacks. In severe cases, it may cause loss of consciousness, seizures, and a drastic increase in body temperature. Death may occur from heart failure or extreme heat stroke. Although it less addictive than cocaine and heroin, the drug does ensnare users in a cycle of dependency. New studies show that chronic use causes brain damage and may impair memory.

Cocaine, which produces a euphoric state, is addictive. It has destroyed families and careers. Overdoses cause respiratory failure, heart failure, and cerebral hemorrhages, bleeding into the brain.

GHB, also commonly used at rave parties with ketamine and ecstasy, can cause seizures, severe respiratory depression, and coma. It is also called the date rape drug, because men have used it to incapacitate women, leaving them vulnerable to sexual assault.

Ketamine causes intense but short-lived hallucinations; it is stronger and more profound than LSD but its effects last only an hour or so. Users commonly report experiences of the mind leaving the body and floating in space, or even death. Heavy use results in serious danger, including suicide. Ketamine is commonly sold in rave clubs, especially in Europe, and is frequently mixed with several other drugs, including heroin, cocaine, or ecstasy. Combining ketamine with these drugs produces an extremely dangerous mix.

Ritalin is one of the newest recreational drugs that is being used in schools and colleges throughout the nation. Ritalin is normally prescribed to children with attention deficit disorder. Such children are fidgety and full of energy. They cannot concentrate their attention on tasks for very long and can be quite disruptive in classes. Because of this, many doctors prescribe the drug Ritalin. It's taken by tens of thousands of American children.

But Ritalin is also ground into a powder and snorted. Because it is a stimulant, like many other recreational drugs, those who snort the drug can stay alert and active for long periods, partying all night if the desire strikes them. Ritalin's stimulant effect also reportedly maintains alertness, so students in college or high school can study all night long to cram for tests.

Generally considered much safer than other drugs such as cocaine, Ritalin has a dark side. Overdoses of Ritalin can be fatal because they cause heart attacks and strokes. Some health care workers warn that Ritalin tablets contain additives that were not meant to be snorted; because of this, they say the drug may be even more dangerous than cocaine.

The list of impacts of recreational drugs could go on, but the point should be well made: no matter how strong the allure, they're potentially dangerous, even life-threatening. Intentional and unintentional contaminants in these drugs could have lethal effects.

Visit *Human Biology's* Internet site for links to web sites offering more information on this topic.

ply structures of the head and several key body parts such as the heart and diaphragm. The trigeminal nerves mentioned in the introduction are one of the 12 pairs of cranial nerves.

Nerves associated with the spinal cord are known as **spinal nerves.** Each spinal nerve has two roots, the dorsal (back side) and ventral (belly side), which attach to the spinal cord (**FIGURE 11-13**). The **dorsal root** is the inlet for sensory information traveling to the spinal cord. On each dorsal root is a small aggregation of nerve cell bodies, the dorsal root ganglion (GANG-lee-on). The **dorsal root ganglia** house the cell bodies of sensory neurons. As **FIGURE 11-13** shows, the dendrites of these bipolar nerve cells conduct impulses from receptors in the body to the dorsal root ganglia; the axons, in turn, carry the impulse into the spinal cord along the dorsal root.

As noted earlier, sensory fibers entering the spinal cord often end on interneurons (**FIGURE 11-13**). Interneurons receive input from many sensory neurons and process this information, acting like a receptionist in a busy corporate office. Interneurons transmit the impulses to nearby multipolar motor neurons, whose axons leave in the **ventral root** of the spinal nerve, carrying impulses to muscles and glands. This anatomical arrangement of neurons allows information to enter and leave the cord quickly and forms the basis of the **reflex arc,** a neuronal pathway by which sensory impulses from receptors reach effectors without traveling to the

White matter

Sensory fiber

Cell body of afferent neuron

Motor fiber

Cell body of efferent neuron

Spinal nerve

Dorsal roots

Dorsal root ganglion

Interneuron

Gray matter

Ventral roots

FIGURE 11-13 The Spinal Cord and Dorsal Root Ganglia   Spinal nerves are attached to the spinal cord by two roots, the dorsal and ventral roots. The dorsal root carries sensory information into the spinal cord. The ventral root carries motor information out of the spinal cord. The spinal nerve often contains both sensory and motor fibers.

brain (**FIGURE 11-15**). Some reflex arcs contain interneurons, and some do not.

When a physician taps a rubber hammer on the tendon just below your kneecap (patellar tendon), he or she is testing one of your body's many reflex arcs. The tapping stimulates stretch receptors in the tendon. These receptors generate nerve impulses that travel to the spinal cord via sensory neurons. In this reflex, each sensory neuron ends directly on a motor neuron, which supplies the muscles of the thigh. Thus, a quick tap on the tendon results in a motor impulse sent to the anterior thigh muscles (quadriceps), causing them to contract and the knee to jerk.

Reflexes are mechanisms that protect the body from harm. Touching a hot stove, for example, elicits the withdrawal reflex. Sensory impulses stimulate the muscles of your arm to contract so that you pull your hand away from the stove before your brain is aware of what is happening.

Babies come equipped with a number of important reflexes. Rub your finger on the cheek of a newborn, and it immediately turns its head toward your finger. This reflex helps babies find the mother's nipple. Crying is also a reflex. When a baby is hungry, thirsty, wet, or uncomfortable, it cries, a reflex sure to get attention.

The spinal cord also transmits sensory information to the brain. Sensory impulses travel to the brain along special tracts lying outside the gray matter of the spinal cord. Although the incoming sensory information may elicit a reflex, the brain is still informed of the problem, allowing for appropriate follow-up action.

Damage to the Spinal Cord Can Cause Permanent Damage

The Severity of the Injury Depends on Its Location and the Extent of the Damage. An automobile crash, a bullet wound, or even a bad fall can damage or sever the fiber tracts of the spinal cord. Injury to the cord usually results in permanent damage because, as noted previously, axons of the CNS do not usually regenerate.

The amount of damage depends on where the cord is injured and the severity of the injury. Sensory and motor fibers traveling to and from the brain, respectively, run in separate tracts in the white matter in the spinal cord. If both tracts are severed—for example, by a severe vertebral fracture—all of the sensory and motor functions below the level of the injury are lost. That is, muscles supplied by nerves below the injury be-

Olfactory (I)

Olfactory tract

Oculomotor (III)

Trigeminal (V)

Facial (VII)

Glossopharyngeal (IX)

Spinal accessory (XI)

Optic (II)

Optic tract

Trochlear (IV)

Abducens (VI)

Vestibulocochlear (VIII)

Vagus (X)

Hypoglossal (XII)

FIGURE 11-14 Cranial Nerves   The 12 pairs of cranial nerves arise from the underside of the brain and brain stem.

FIGURE 11-15 Reflex Arc   When you accidentally touch a hot pan on the stove, you withdraw your hand before your brain even knows what's happening. This occurs because of a reflex arc. Sensory fibers send impulses to the spinal cord. The sensory impulses stimulate motor neurons in the spinal cord. This causes muscle contraction in the flexor muscles (+) and inhibits muscle contraction in the extensor muscles (−), allowing you to withdraw your hand. Nerve impulses also ascend to the brain to let it know what is happening.

come paralyzed and unable to contract voluntarily and the portion of the body below the injury loses all sensation. If the spinal cord injury occurs high in the neck (above the fifth cervical vertebra), it cuts the nerve fibers traveling to the muscles that control breathing. These muscles become paralyzed, and the person dies quickly. This is how a hangman's noose kills its victim.

Damage to the cord just below the fifth cervical vertebra does not affect breathing, but it does paralyze the legs and arms. This condition is known as **quadriplegia** (QUAD-reh-PLEE-gee-ah). If the spinal cord injury occurs below the nerves that supply the arms, the result is **paraplegia** (PEAR-ah-PLEE-gee-ah), paralysis of the legs.

New studies show that the administration of large doses of an anti-inflammatory steroid drug shortly after a head or neck injury stops swelling of the spinal cord. Swelling is thought to greatly increase the amount of damage resulting from such injuries. This treatment may therefore greatly reduce paralysis in such cases. Research is also under way to find ways to stimulate the regeneration of axons in the CNS. Some early results are promising, suggesting that physicians may one day be able to "repair" spinal cord damage.

<hr>

Section 11-4

The Brain

About the size of a cantaloupe, the human brain is an extraordinary organ, the product of many millions of

years of evolutionary trial and error. Our brains have given us art and music, remarkable feats of engineering, and abstract reasoning, not to mention the ability to ponder right and wrong and remember a vast amount of information.

The Cerebral Hemispheres Function in Integration, Sensory Reception, and Motor Action

The brain is housed in the skull, a bony shell that protects it from injury. **FIGURE 11-16** shows some of the ex-

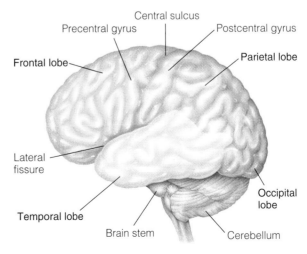

FIGURE 11-16 The Brain   The cerebral cortex consists of the lobes shown here. The lobes, in turn, can be divided into sensory, association, and motor areas (not shown).

FIGURE 11-17 Structures of the Brain   A cross section through the brain showing the gray and white matter of the cortex and deeper structures, notably the thalamus and hypothalamus.

ternally visible parts of the human brain. The largest and most conspicuous is the **cerebrum** (sir-EE-brum), a convoluted mass of nervous tissue that constitutes about 80% of the total brain mass.

The cerebrum is divided into two halves, the right and left **cerebral hemispheres.** Each hemisphere has a thin outer layer of gray matter, the **cerebral cortex** (**FIGURE 11-17**). It contains glial cells and the cell bodies of numerous multipolar neurons. Lying beneath the cerebral cortex is a thick central core of white matter containing bundles of myelinated axons that give it a white appearance. The axons of the white matter carry impulses from the cerebral cortex to the spinal cord, enabling information to flow from the brain to motor neurons that control many of the body muscles. Some axons also transmit impulses from one part of the cerebral cortex to another, permitting the integration of the activities of various parts of the cortex.

As shown in **FIGURE 11-17**, the cerebral cortex is thrown into numerous folds, called **gyri** (JI-reye; singular, gyrus, JI-russ). The gyri are separated by numerous valleys, known as **sulci** (SUL-see; singular, sulcus, SUL-kuss).

The Cerebrum Is Divided into Four Major Lobes, and Each Lobe Contains Areas That House Specific Functions. The cerebral hemispheres are divided into four major lobes, shown in **FIGURE 11-16**. They are the frontal lobe, the parietal lobe, the occipital lobe, and the temporal lobe. Within each of these lobes are areas that house specific functions. These functional areas (**FIGURE 11-18**) can be broadly classified into three types: motor cortex, sensory cortex, and association cortex. The **motor cortex** stimulates muscle activity. The **sensory cortex** receives sensory stimuli, and the **association cortex** integrates information, bringing

about coordinated responses. Let's examine the key regions, beginning with the primary motor cortex.

The Primary Motor Cortex Controls Voluntary Movement. The **primary motor cortex** occupies a single gyrus (ridge) on each hemisphere, just in front of the central sulcus (**FIGURE 11-18**). This area controls voluntary motor activity—for example, the muscles in your hand that are turning the pages of your book.

The neurons in the primary motor cortex are arranged in a very specific way, so that each region of the motor cortex controls a specific body part. As **FIGURE 11-19A** illustrates, the neurons that control the muscles of the toes are located in the uppermost region of the primary motor cortex. Hip muscle control occurs below that. Muscles of the hand are controlled by neurons located even lower.

To bring about a voluntary movement, a conscious thought stimulates the neurons of the primary motor cortex to generate an impulse. It travels from the brain down the spinal cord to the motor neurons in the spinal cord. The axons of these neurons exit the spinal cord and terminate on the muscles.

In front of the primary motor area is the **premotor cortex.** The premotor cortex is also involved in controlling muscle contraction. However, the movements that it controls are fairly complex, such as the fingering required to play a musical instrument, or type on a computer keyboard.

The Primary Sensory Cortex Receives Sensory Information from the Body. Just behind the central

FIGURE 11-18 Functional Regions of the Cortex (a) The cerebral cortex has three principal functions: receiving sensory input, integrating sensory information, and generating motor responses. Special sensory areas handle vision, smell, taste, and hearing. (b) A pet scan reveals the locations of increased blood flow in the brain during performance of certain tasks.

Key
M. Motor cortex
A. Association cortex
S. Sensory cortex

M. Supplementary motor area (on inner surface—not visible; programming of complex movements)

M. Premotor cortex (coordination of complex movements)

A. Prefrontal association cortex (planning for voluntary activity; decision making; personality traits)

M. Broca's area (speech formation)

S. Primary auditory cortex surrounded by higher-order auditory cortex (hearing)

A. Limbic association cortex (mostly on inner and bottom surface of temporal lobe; motivation and emotion; memory)

M. Primary motor cortex (voluntary movement)

Central sulcus

S. Primary sensory cortex (sensation)

A. Posterior parietal cortex (integration of somatosensory and visual input; important for complex movements)

A. Wernicke's area (speech understanding)

A. Parietal-temporal-occipital association cortex (integration of all sensory input; important in language)

S. Primary visual cortex surrounded by higher-order visual cortex (sight)

(a)

GENERATING WORDS   HEARING WORDS   SEEING WORDS

Min   Max

(b)

sulcus is a ridge of tissue running parallel to the primary motor area. Known as the **primary sensory cortex,** it is the destination of many sensory impulses traveling to the brain. As in the primary motor area, different parts of this ridge correspond to different parts of the body (**FIGURE 11-19B**).

The Association Cortex Is the Site of Integration and Complex Intellectual Activities. The **association cortex** consists of large expanses of cerebral cortex where integration occurs. In the frontal lobe is a region of the association cortex (prefrontal association cortex) that houses complex intellectual activities such as planning and ideation. This region also modifies behavior, conforming human actions with social norms.

Another important association area lies posterior to the primary sensory cortex (posterior parietal cortex). It interprets sensory information and stores memories of past sensations. Other association areas interpret language in written and spoken form.

Hearing, Vision, Taste, and Smell Are Also Housed in Specific Cortical Regions. **FIGURE 11-18** shows patches of sensory cortex for hearing (primary auditory

cortex) and vision (primary visual cortex). Separate regions (not shown) exist for taste and smell.

Unconscious Functions Are Housed in the Cerebellum, Hypothalamus, and Brain Stem

Consciousness resides in the cerebral cortex. However, many body functions occur at an unconscious level, among them heartbeat, breathing, and many homeostatic functions.[6] One region of the brain that controls

---

[6]Conscious control is possible for many automatic functions, but for the most part, breathing and swallowing are controlled automatically in lower brain centers.

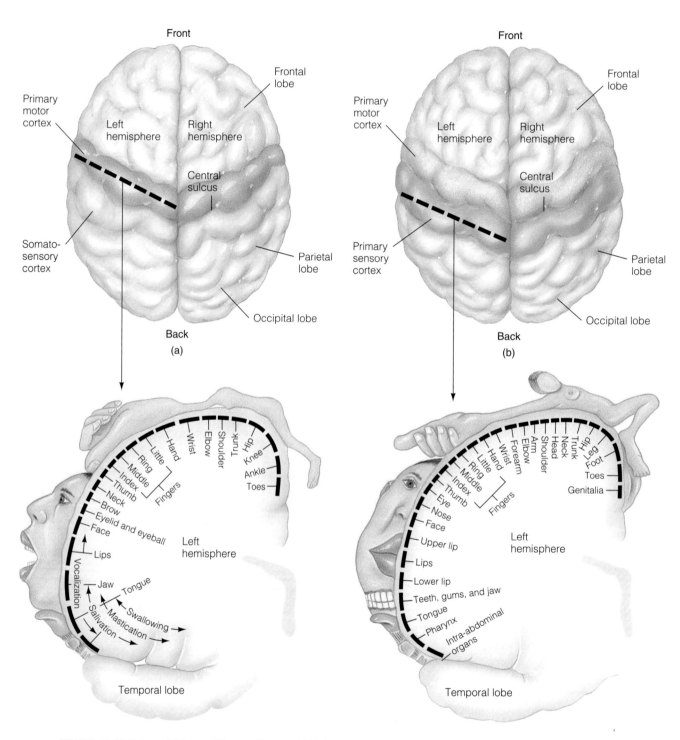

FIGURE 11-19 Primary Motor and Sensory Areas *(a)* Top view of the brain showing the primary motor cortex. Below is a map of the location of motor functions within the primary motor cortex. *(b)* The primary sensory cortex (somatosensory cortex). Below is a map of the location of regions within the primary sensory cortex.

unconscious actions is the **cerebellum** (sar-ah-BELL-um), the second largest structure of the brain. As **FIGURE 11-16** shows, it sits below the cerebrum on the brain stem.

The Cerebellum Controls Muscle Synergy and Helps Maintain Posture. The cerebellum plays several key roles. One of them is synergy. Neurophysiologists define **synergy** as the coordination of skeletal muscle contraction and the movement of body parts to create smooth, efficient motion. To understand this concept, hold your arm straight out, then bring your hand to your chest. To perform this simple action, your biceps (muscles in the front of the upper arm) contracted while your triceps (muscles in the back of the upper arm) relaxed. For smooth, coordinated movement, some muscles must contract while others relax. The cerebellum ensures that opposing sets of muscles work together to create a smooth motion.

Like most body functions, synergy is not something we think about unless it goes wrong. Commonly, dysfunction arises when the cerebellum is damaged during childbirth—for example, if the baby's blood supply is interrupted, which sometimes happens when the umbilical cord is wrapped around the baby's neck. The ensuing lack of oxygen to the brain can permanently damage the cerebellum, resulting in a loss of synergistic control of the skeletal muscles. Mild damage generally causes a slight rigidness (called *spasticity*) and moderately jerky motions. More severe damage causes serious impairment, with body motions becoming extremely jerky and simple tasks requiring several attempts. This condition is known as **cerebral palsy** (PALL-zee).[7]

---

[7]Cerebral palsy is also caused by abnormal brain development, possibly due to exposure to harmful chemicals (e.g., alcohol) during embryonic development.

Besides ensuring the smooth, coordinated contraction and relaxation of muscles, the cerebellum maintains posture. It receives impulses from sense organs in the ear that detect body position. It then sends impulses to the muscles to maintain or correct posture.

The Thalamus Is a Relay Center. Just beneath the cerebrum is a region of the brain called the **thalamus** (**FIGURE 11-17**). The thalamus is a relay center. It receives all sensory input, except for smell, then relays it to the sensory and association cortex.

The Hypothalamus Controls Many Autonomic Functions Involved in Homeostasis. Beneath the thalamus is the **hypothalamus** (high-poe-THAL-ahmuss; hypo = under). It consists of many aggregations of nerve cells. These are known as the *nuclei,* which should not to be mistaken for the nuclei in cells (**FIGURE 11-20**). Hypothalamic nuclei control a variety of autonomic functions, all of which are aimed at maintaining homeostasis. Appetite and body temperature, for example, are controlled by hypothalamic nuclei, as are water balance, blood pressure, and sexual activity.

The hypothalamus is a primitive brain center. One of its best-known functions is the control of the pituitary gland, an endocrine gland that regulates many body functions through the hormones it releases (Chapter 14).

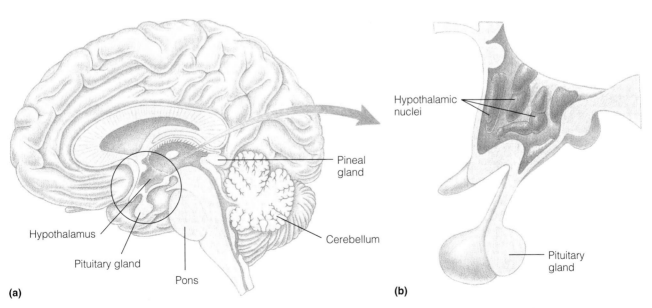

(a)   **(b)**

FIGURE 11-20 The Hypothalamus *(a)* The hypothalamus is clearly visible in a cross section of the brain. *(b)* The hypothalamus is at the base of the brain, just above the pituitary gland. It regulates many autonomic functions and plays a particularly important role in controlling the release of hormones by the pituitary.

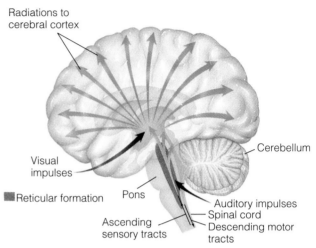

FIGURE 11-21 The Limbic System The odd assortment of structures shown in green is the limbic system. The limbic system is the seat of our emotions and instincts, among other functions.

FIGURE 11-22 The Reticular Activating System The reticular formation resides in the brain stem, where it receives input from incoming and outgoing neurons. Fibers projecting from the reticular formation to the cortex constitute the reticular activating system.

The Limbic System Is the Site of Instinctive Behavior and Emotion. Instincts, among other functions, reside in a complex array of structures called the **limbic system** (LIM-bick), shown in **FIGURE 11-21**. The limbic system operates in conjunction with the hypothalamus.

Instincts are among the most fundamental responses of organisms. They include the protective urge of a mother, the territorial assertions of a male, and the fight-or-flight response an animal experiences in the face of adversity.

The limbic system also plays a role in emotions—fear, anger, and so on. Electrodes placed in some areas of the limbic system elicit primitive rage and in other areas, placidity. Stimulation of specific regions within the limbic system of humans may elicit sensations patients describe as joy, pleasure, fear, or anxiety, depending on the site of stimulation. For a discussion of depression and its effects on emotions, see Health Note 11-2.

Many Basic Body Functions Are Controlled by the Brain Stem. The brain stem connects the brain to the spinal cord and gives rise to most of the cranial nerves. Like the hypothalamus, the brain stem contains aggregations of nerve cells that control many basic body functions such as heart rate, blood pressure, and breathing. It also regulates swallowing, coughing, vomiting, and many digestive functions. The hypothalamus and brain stem therefore often work in concert.

Besides containing control regions (nuclei), the brain stem is a main thoroughfare for information traveling to and from the brain. Nerve fibers passing through the brain stem, however, frequently give off branches that terminate in a special region of the brain stem known as the reticular formation (reh-TICK-you-ler) (**FIGURE 11-22**).

The **reticular formation** runs through the entire brain stem into the thalamus. It receives all incoming and outgoing information, monitoring activity much like a security guard at a doorway. Nerve impulses are then projected to the cerebral cortex via special nerve fibers. These impulses activate cortical neurons. These nerve fibers comprise the **reticular activating system (RAS)** and are like the alarm clock of the central nervous system, for they help maintain wakefulness or alertness. Consider what happens when you're asleep.

During sleep, the flow of information through the RAS is greatly reduced, and the cortex "sleeps." However, this sleep may be disturbed by a loud noise. Noise is picked up by the ear, which sends sensory impulses to the auditory cortex of the brain. But the cortex doesn't perceive the sound because it's asleep. To rouse the brain, nerve impulses branch off into the RAS. These fibers then send signals that awaken the cortex and the sleeper.

The RAS not only awakens us and keeps us alert, but it also prevents us from falling asleep from time to time. Pain from a bad sunburn, for example, prevents many people from falling asleep. Why? Pain impulses traveling to the brain from sensors in the skin enter the RAS. It, in turn, generates impulses that travel to the cortex and keep the cells active despite one's fatigue.

Cerebrospinal Fluid Cushions the CNS

The brain and spinal cord are housed in the skull and spinal column, respectively. These bony fortresses protect those vital and delicate organs. But as anyone who's ever packed a fragile object in a box knows, to provide true protection, you must supply some added cushion.

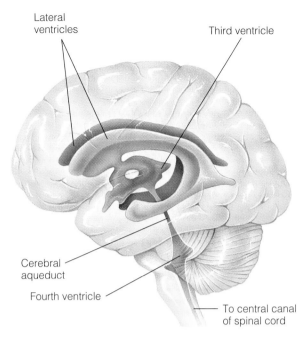

Lateral ventricles

Third ventricle

Cerebral aqueduct

Fourth ventricle

To central canal of spinal cord

FIGURE 11-23 Ventricles The brain contains four internal cavities, called *ventricles,* which are filled with a plasmalike fluid known as cerebrospinal fluid.

FIGURE 11-24 Hydrocephalus This birth defect results from a blockage in the ventricles, which causes CSF to build up, thinning the cortex and causing severe brain damage.

Evolution "solved" this dilemma by surrounding the brain with a watery liquid, called **cerebrospinal fluid (CSF).** Similar in composition to blood plasma and interstitial fluid, CSF is found in the arachnoid space, which lies between the inner and outer layers of the meninges. CSF also fills internal cavities (ventricles) in the brain and spinal cord (**FIGURE 11-23**). CSF cushions these organs and protects them from injury.

Cerebrospinal fluid is produced by the lining of two large cavities, the **lateral ventricles,** which are located in the cerebral hemispheres (**FIGURE 11-23**). CSF is continuously generated and slowly drains out of the brain and into the bloodstream. As a rule, the amount of CSF produced by the ventricles equals the amount removed.

If the circulation of CSF is blocked in a newborn, the accumulation of fluid causes the brain and head to enlarge and produces a condition known as **hydrocephalus** (HIGH-drow-CEFF-eh-luss; literally, "water on the brain") (**FIGURE 11-24**). As the ventricles fill with fluid, the cortex thins, which damages brain cells. If detected early, surgeons can insert a plastic tube in the brain to drain the fluid from the ventricles (upstream from the blockage) into the thoracic cavity. This permits the brain to develop normally. If not detected early and the damage is severe, the child will be permanently impaired and may die.

Because CSF bathes the CNS, examining fluid provides a means of detecting infections in the brain, spinal cord, and meninges. Samples of CSF are obtained by inserting a needle between the third and fourth lumbar vertebrae. The needle projects into the space between the dura mater and pia mater. CSF is then withdrawn.

One dangerous condition detected by this method is **meningitis** (men-in-JI-tiss), an infection of the meninges caused by certain viruses or bacteria. As noted in Chapter 9, meningitis usually begins with an infection in the respiratory system. In adults, meningitis is characterized by fever, headache, and nausea. Patients often vomit and complain of a stiff neck and an inability to tolerate bright light (photophobia). These symptoms develop over the course of a few hours. In babies and children, the symptoms are often less obvious, causing parents to overlook a potentially fatal condition until it is too late. In both cases, meningitis requires immediate attention because it can be fatal.

Electrical Activity in the Brain Varies Depending on Activity Level or Level of Sleep

Electrodes applied to different parts of the scalp detect underlying electrical activity in the brain and produce a tracing known as an **electroencephalogram** (ee-LECK-trow-en-CEFF-eh-low-GRAM) or **EEG.** Some sample tracings of the electrical activity at different times are shown in **FIGURE 11-25** on page 264; note that the type of brain wave recorded depends on the level of cortical activity. The waves often appear irregular, but distinct patterns can sometimes be observed, especially during the different phases of sleep.

Because diseases or injuries of the cerebral cortex often give rise to altered EEG patterns, EEGs are used to diagnose brain dysfunction. Perhaps the most common disorder is epilepsy (EP-eh-LEP-see). **Epilepsy** is characterized by periodic seizures that occur when a large number of neurons fire spontaneously. The seizures can be accompanied by involuntary spasms of skeletal muscles and alterations in behavior. Research has shown that in about two-thirds of the cases, patients have no identifiable structural abnormality in the brain. In the remaining cases, the seizures can usually be traced to

Health Note 11-2

Feeling Blue: Understanding and Treating Depression

All people feel sad from time to time. There are many causes: the death of a family member or a friend; the death of a pet; the loss of a job; divorce; the loss of a valuable friendship; or poor performance on an exam. All of these adversities—and a great many more—can bring on feelings commonly called *depression.* However, to psychologists, occasional and transient feelings of sadness are a normal part of life.

Psychologists reserve the term *depression* for a condition characterized by one of several symptoms, including feelings of intense sadness that are evoked by even minor stimuli, things that people who are not depressed seem to cope with quite well. People suffering from depression may not feel sad, but rather experience persistent numbness or emptiness. And, they often complain of feeling little or no pleasure in things that once brought them happiness. Depression can be manifested in anxiety, feelings of hopelessness, pessimism, and a general sense of worthlessness. People suffering from depression may feel irritable and restless. They may have difficulty concentrating and making decisions. Depressed individuals may feel helpless and often suffer from sleep disorders—waking up in the middle of the night or oversleeping (see Health Note 4-2 for a discussion of sleep disorders). Some people can't eat. Others overeat. They may complain of physical symptoms such as chronic pain and headaches that do not respond to treatment. Thoughts of suicide become prevalent.

Depression varies in intensity from mild to severe, and in duration from short term to long term. In its most extreme forms, depression can be life-threatening because severe depression can lead to suicide. Depression also comes in many forms. In this Health Note, we examine two of the many clinically recognizable forms: major depression and a less severe type called dysthymia (dis-THIGH-me-ah).

Major depression is so severe that it often incapacitates a person. Individuals suffering from depression are unable to work, sleep, eat, or enjoy anything. Dysthymia is less serious because it tends only to impair work, sleep, eating, and other functions. In other words, it does not "cripple" a person; it just keeps him or her from functioning at full capacity.

The causes of depression are something of a mystery to medical science. Researchers know that it results from a change in brain chemistry—involving the level of certain neurotransmitters such as serotonin or acetylcholine. The same changes occur during periodic bouts of sadness. But in patients suffering from depression, the changes are not reversed, even after the triggering event or stimulus is eliminated. In other words, the changes become self-sustaining. New stresses then emerge. A person may become stressed about feeling unhappy all of the time. Lack of sleep may put emotional stress on an individual. Depression can tax relationships, creating an additional stimulus for depression. Feeling down often kills the impulse to get outside for fresh

---

brain damage at birth, severe head injury, or inflammation of the brain. In some instances, epileptic seizures are caused by brain tumors.

Headaches Have Many Causes, But Are Rarely the Result of Life-Threatening Anomalies

No discussion of the brain would be complete without considering something we've all had experience with, headaches. **Headaches** are the most common form of pain. Many headaches are caused by tension—sustained tightening of the muscles of the head and neck when a person is nervous, stressed, or tired. Headaches also commonly result from swelling of the membranes lining the sinuses (cavities inside the bones of the skull surrounding the nasal cavity). Such swelling usually occurs because of sinus infections or allergies. Eyestrain is another common cause of headaches, as is the dilation of cerebral blood vessels, which may be associated with high blood pressure or excessive alcohol consumption.

Not all headaches are created equal though. In fact, very serious headaches may result from increased intracranial pressure. This, in turn, may result from a brain tumor or intracranial bleeding. Inflammation caused by an infection of the meninges (meningitis) or the brain itself (encephalitis), although rare, also produce intense headaches that require immediate attention.

Less threatening, but still extraordinary, are migraines. A migraine headache is a recurrent, rather severe headache. The pain often occurs on one side of the head, and is described as throbbing. Lasting from 4 to 72 hours, migraines are aggravated by movement or physical activity and are typically accompanied by nausea, vomiting, and sensitivity to light and sound.

air, sunshine, or exercise—all of which can counteract depression.

When individuals become aware of their condition, often upon the advice of friends, family, or family physicians, most can pinpoint an event or several events that are responsible for their depression. Most stimuli seem to have one of three features in common: the loss of self-determination (the ability to make choices); the loss of empowerment (feeling you have power to make choices that make a difference); and the loss of self-confidence. In some instances, however, depression appears to have no link to a person's situation. The supposedly spontaneous changes in brain chemistry apparently occur without stimulus—or at least none that can be currently identified.

Although depression can be treated very effectively, many people slip into this state without even realizing it, and sink deeper and deeper in depression unaware that they are spiraling downward and are in need of help. Friends, relatives, and family physicians can help individuals realize that they are depressed.

Interestingly, in most instances, the chemical changes in the brain seem to self-correct—but usually after one to three years without medical treatment. For those who don't want to wait that long to get over depression, there's great hope. Psychological therapy, which addresses the root causes, can be helpful for long-term recovery. Prescription medicines (antidepressants) can also help immensely. Many antidepressants such as Paxil, Luvox, Prozac, and Remeron, are currently available, and they are very effective. In fact, two-thirds of those people treated by any one medication respond favorably. Those who fail to respond to one medication have a great chance of responding to another one.

Antidepressants work by elevating levels of neurotransmitters in the brain, which, for reasons unknown, seems to relieve depression. Antidepressants are not "happy" pills. They don't make one euphoric. They simply lift the feeling of depression.

Antidepressants take a while to work—usually two to three weeks,

but sometimes up to two months—and have some annoying side-effects. Two of the most commonly used antidepressants, Prozac and Paxil, for instance, decrease sexual interest or cause difficulty in achieving an orgasm in about 30% of the patients. Both cause nausea in about 20% of the cases and insomnia in about 15% of the patients. They often cause dry mouth, too

There are no safeguards against depression. But living well—eating right, getting plenty of exercise, balancing work with pleasure, and having a healthy psychological framework—can all help us reduce the likelihood of this sometimes trying condition. For those who contract it, there is hope, and the sooner the problem is recognized, the sooner the cure will take place.

Visit *Human Biology's* Internet site for links to web sites offering more information on this topic.

Migraines afflict an estimated 26 million Americans, about one in ten people, and are often hereditary. They can strike anyone at any age, but are most common in young adult women. Although a cure is not known, there are treatments. Numerous therapies and medications can be used. Some drugs lessen or eliminate the symptoms; others reduce the frequency or duration of a migraine attack.

Like many other neurological disorders, the causes of migraines are not known. Many researchers believe that sudden changes in your body or environment may trigger migraines in individuals who are more sensitive than others. Changes in brain activity result in inflamed blood vessels and nerves around the brain. Relief from medications is due to a quieting of the sensitive nerve pathways or reductions in inflammation.

Section 11-5

The Autonomic Nervous System

As noted earlier, the nervous system consists of two parts: the peripheral nervous system and the central nervous system. The PNS consists of a somatic division and an autonomic division. Each division contains motor and sensory neurons (**FIGURE 11-3**).

The **somatic division** are the nerves or parts of nerves that receive sensory information from the skin, muscles, and joints. This information is transmitted to the CNS. Motor impulses from the CNS, in turn, are sent to skeletal muscles via motor neurons. In contrast, the **autonomic division** is that part of the peripheral nervous system that transmits sensory information from body organs to the CNS. It then delivers motor impulses to smooth muscle, cardiac muscle, and glands. Together,

FIGURE 11-25 Electroencephalogram   Several sample tracings of brain waves during different activities and stages of sleep.

they form the **autonomic nervous system (ANS)**. The ANS functions automatically, usually at a subconscious level. It helps to control internal organs through controls on smooth muscle, cardiac muscle, and glands.

The autonomic nervous system has two subdivisions: the sympathetic and the parasympathetic. The **sympathetic division** of the ANS functions in emergencies and is largely responsible for the **fight-or-flight response.** This response occurs when an individual is startled or faced with danger. A sudden scare results in sympathetic nerve impulses that bring about a whole host of responses, preparing us to fight or flee the scene. One result is a rapid increase in heart rate. The fight-or-flight response also results in pupil dilation and an increase in breathing rate. Dilation of the pupils lets more light in, and presumably helps us see better. Increased breathing delivers more oxygen to the blood. Finally, the fight-or-flight response results in a decrease in blood flow to the intestines, diverting blood from digestion, and an increase in blood flow to the skeletal muscles needed for fighting off danger or making a rapid retreat.

In contrast, the **parasympathetic division** of the ANS brings about internal responses associated with the relaxed state. It therefore reduces heart rate, contracts the pupils, and promotes digestion.

Most organs are supplied with both parasympathetic and sympathetic fibers. As a general rule, these fibers have antagonistic (or opposite) effects. One stimulates activity, and the other reduces activity. This provides the body with a means of fine-tuning organ function.

Section 11-6

Learning and Memory

Few questions intrigue humans more than how the brain functions in learning and memory. **Learning** is a process in which an individual acquires and retains knowledge and skills. Learning usually results from experience, instruction, or some combination of the two, and it depends on one's ability to store information in the brain, a phenomenon called **memory.**

Newly acquired knowledge is first stored in short-term memory. **Short-term memory** holds information for periods of seconds to hours. The phone number you just looked up or the name of a new acquaintance are stashed in short-term memory. If you don't do something to "fix" these memories, they soon vanish. Cramming for tests places a lot of information into short-term memory. Unfortunately, soon after the test is over, the information fades into oblivion. The reason people often cannot recall the details of a traumatic accident is because their short-term memory has been wiped out.

Long-term memory holds information for much longer periods—from days to years—and has a much greater storage capacity than short-term memory "banks."

Transferring information from short-term to long-term memory is called **consolidation.** In the Study Skills section at the front of this book, I described several ways to consolidate information, including repetition, mnemonics, and rhymes.

The process of recalling information stored in either short- or long-term memory is called **remembering.** Short-term memory recall is generally faster than long-term memory recall unless the long-term memory you are retrieving is one that is thoroughly ingrained (for example, your place of birth). By the same token, information lost from short-term memory is generally gone forever. Information you cannot recall from long-term memory is often still there; it just takes time or some special stimulus to extract it.

Memory Is Stored in Multiple Regions of the Brain

Neurons involved in storing memories are widely distributed in the cerebral cortex, especially the temporal lobe. Other regions also hold memories, including the cerebellum and the limbic system. The temporal lobes and a part of the limbic system known as the **hippocampus** (hip-poe-CAMP-us) appear essential for transferring short-term memories into long-term memory.

Short-Term and Long-Term Memory Appear to Involve Structural and Functional Changes of the Neurons

How are memories stored? Although no one knows the precise mechanism for this, evidence points toward certain anatomical and physiological changes in the neuronal circuitry. However, short- and long-term memories probably involve different mechanisms. Studies on slugs and snails suggest that short-term memory may involve transient modifications in the function of existing synapses. Whether this mechanism holds true for humans and other animals remains to be seen.

In contrast, long-term memory appears to involve relatively permanent structural and functional changes in the neurons of the brain. Studies that compared the brains of experimental animals reared in a sensory-deprived environment with those reared in a sensory-rich environment revealed marked differences in the microscopic structures of their brains. The brains of animals exposed to a sensory-rich environment displayed greater branching and elongation of dendrites in regions of the brain thought to serve as memory storage.

Some studies suggest that protein synthesis may be involved in long-term memory because drugs that block protein synthesis interfere with long-term memory. What proteins are involved remains unknown.

New Evidence Suggests that Brain Function Can Be Retained in Old Age.

For years, scientists have thought that thinking and memory faded with age as brain cells died off. But there's startling new evidence that suggests the most unthinkable—that the brain can actually generate new cells, even in elderly individuals. Scientists have also found evidence to suggest that the connections among brain cells strengthen over time if individuals remain intellectually challenged. Because of this, most healthy people can retain their brain power until the end of their lives. Although processing speed—how fast our brains store and retrieve information—does tend to fall

off with in our latter years, we can still learn and remember. We just need a little more time as we grow older. Keeping a mentally active life is all that's needed.

Scientists have also found that regular aerobic exercise such as walking helps eldering people perform certain mental functions, such as switching from one mental task to another. Combined with a lifetime of mental challenges, such as stimulating jobs or hobbies, exercise can ensure good cognitive functions. Although the research is still preliminary, many doctors tell their elderly patients to remain as active as possible.

The loss of mental function is, as you just saw, not a natural consequence of aging. Losses of memory and confusion, however, do occur. Such instances are often a signal of an underlying disease, such as low thyroid hormone production, poor nutrition, or depression. Certain medications can have the same effect, for example drugs for ulcers, high blood pressure, and Parkinson's disease. In some cases, loss of memory and confusion are due to a serious disease known as Alzheimer's disease.

Section 11-7

Diseases of the Brain

The brain, like other important organs, is subject to a wide assortment of diseases, many of which have dire consequences. This section reviews three: Alzheimer's disease, Parkinson's disease, and brain tumors.

Loss of Memory and Confusion in Older Individuals Is Often the Result of Underlying Disease Such as Alzheimer's Disease.

Alzheimer's disease is a progressive loss of mental function, which usually begins later in life. Alzheimer's afflicts an estimated 4 million Americans, mostly people over the age of 65. In fact, it is estimated that about one of ten people over the age of 65 has this terrible disease. Alzheimer's is not life-threatening, but it does result in dramatic changes. Symptoms start out slowly. Forgetfulness is often one of the most common complaints. Irritability and lack of initiative also occur early on. As mental functions decline, patients lose the ability to remember recent events. Over time, losses may be so great that a parent may be unable to recognize his or her own children.

Scientists do not know the cause of Alzheimer's, although there is some evidence to suggest that previous severe brain injuries could be the cause in some instances. Scientists do know that a brain of a person with the disease contains deposits of a material called plaque and fibrous tangles. The plaque consists of a protein known as beta-amyloid. The fibrous clumps are protein from degenerated nerve cells. New research suggests that beta-amyloid binds to nerve cells in the brains, and then causes cell death. This leads to the loss of memory and other symptoms. The tangles of fibers are believed to be remnants of the cells' proteins. They're formed when beta-amyloid binds to the nerve cells.

Experiments with mice suggest that antibodies to beta-amyloid could prevent or slow the development of Alzheimer's disease. When mice who had the disease were given antibodies, beta-amyloid accumulation in the brain was prevented. Existing deposits were removed. Tests will soon begin on people to see if the antibodies work similarly. If they do, this could be great news for those who suffer from this disease or who will develop it as they age. Researchers hope that such treatments may be useful in other brain disorders such as Parkinson's disease and Huntington's disease.

Parkinson's Disease is a Neurological Disorder Caused by a Lack of Dopamine in Certain Regions of the Brain

Another important nervous system disorder is Parkinson's disease. Discussed in Chapter 3, in relation to environmental pollution, Parkinson's disease is caused by a progressive detioration of certain brain centers, those that control movement, especially semiautomatic movements such as swinging the arms when walking. It afflicts about 1 million Americans, most over the age of 60. In fact, approximately one in 100 Americans in this age group has the disease.

Parkinson's disease is characterized by tremors. In many people with the disease, the hands or the head (sometimes both) shake involuntarily. Tremors disappear or decrease, however, when one moves the afflicted part of the body intentionally—for example, when one reaches for an object. If the disease worsens, symptoms worsen and it becomes difficult to write or walk. Speaking may deteriorate too as it becomes difficult to move one's mouth and tongue. Falls become more frequent. It may be difficult to get out of a chair. In later stages of the disease, memory and thinking may deteiorate.

Like Alzheimer's, the cause or causes of Parkinson's are unknown. Chemical pollutants may contribute to the disease. Amalgam fillings in teeth and chemicals used in wood stains may play a role in the onset of the disease. Very likely, there are many causes.

One thing is known, Parkinson's is characterized by a lack of a chemical substance in the brain called *dopamine*. Because of this, patients can be treated with

a drug known as *levodopa*. However, its benefits may diminish over years of use. Some patients suffer severe side effects, including severe nausea and vomiting. Several other drugs are also used.

Recent studies show that fetal cell transplants into the affected brain area may eliminate the symptoms of the disease. A year after receiving a fetal cell transplant, 13 of 19 people showed elevated levels dopamine production. Surgeons can also ablate (destroy) a small region of the brain that appears to be hyperactive in Parkinson's patients. This improves a patient's score on standardized movement tests, although several patients had serious side effects including facial paralysis. Electrodes can also be implanted in the brain to stop uncontrollable movements. Patients are equipped with tiny electronic stimulators, much like pacemakers, which can be switched on or off as needed.

Brain Tumors

Two types of tumors develop in the brain tissue, benign and malignant. Benign tumors are cellular growths in the brain that do not grow rapaciously and do not spread to other parts of the body like malignant tumors. Even as such, benign tumors can cause problems. They may, for instance, place pressure on areas of the brain resulting in definite problems. Benign tumors have distinct borders and can be removed surgically; unlike malignant tumors, they do not recur.

Malignant tumors grow rapidly, especially late in the disease. They are likely to place pressure on neighboring structures and may invade into the tissue around them or to other parts of the body.

Brain tumors occur at any age, although the most common groups are children in the 3- to 12-year-old age bracket and adults in the 40- to 70-year-old bracket. Although researchers still do not know what causes brain tumors, there are some risk factors that increase one's likelihood for developing a cancerous tumor. Workers in certain industries, for example, oil refining, rubber manufacturing, and drug manufacturing, are at a higher risk of developing a brain tumor. Chemists and embalmers have a higher incidence of brain tumors as well. Some researchers believe that exposure to certain viruses may be responsible for brain tumors. And some brain tumors seem to run in families, so there may be a genetic cause that is passed from parents to offspring. In most cases, however, patients with brain tumors have no clear risk factors, so researchers believe that the disease is probably the result of several factors acting together.

There's a great deal of concern these days over the potential of cell phones to cause brain cancer. Although several recent studies show no link, cell phone use is a recent phenomenon. Most cancers take 5 to 30 years to develop. One thing to keep in mind is that cell phones emit radiowaves. Unlike ionizing radiation, for example, from nuclear power plants, radiowaves do not impart much energy in body tissues and may have little, if any, effect on cells of the body. Only time will tell.

Health, Homeostasis, and the Environment

The Violent Brain

The nervous system is one of the body's two control systems (the other being the endocrine system). Receptors perceive changes in the internal and external environment and send signals to the brain and spinal cord, which then respond with corrective actions. This helps maintain physical and chemical conditions essential to life.

Like other organ systems, the nervous system can be damaged by a wide variety of factors. The following case study illustrates an extreme example of what happens when the nervous system comes under attack from poisonous chemicals in the work environment.

Perhaps one of the most disturbing stories of the impacts of hazardous chemicals on the brain is that of David Garabedian, a man described by his family and friends as mild-mannered, passive, even docile. Garabedian worked for a lawn-care company in Massachusetts. On March 29, 1983, he arrived at the home of Eileen Muldoon to estimate the cost of treating her lawn with insecticides. He knocked on the door but found no one at home. Garabedian decided to make an estimate and leave it for her.

After he had completed his work, he experienced a sudden urge to urinate. He went to the backyard and urinated near the house. Just then, Mrs. Muldoon appeared, yelling angrily at him. Garabedian became confused, apologized, and tried to explain his plight. According to his testimony, she turned away from him, refusing to listen. Garabedian tapped her on the shoulder to say he was sorry, but the woman turned on him and clawed his face with her fingernails. Garabedian exploded, grabbing the woman by the neck and strangling her. As she lay motionless on the ground, he hurled large rocks at her head, smashing her skull.

A month before the murder, Garabedian had undergone a remarkable personality change. Usually amicable, he angered easily and was abusive toward his family. He complained of tension, nervousness, impatience, and terrible nightmares. He also complained of numerous physical symptoms such as nausea, diarrhea, headaches, and frequent urination. These symptoms suggested to some that the young man was suffering from pesticide poisoning.

Dr. Peter Spencer, a toxicologist at the Albert Einstein College of Medicine in New York, testified at the trial that "David Garabedian was involuntarily intoxicated with a chemical in the lawn products that he was exposed to on a daily basis." He not only sprayed chemicals on lawns and trees, but also mixed them, pouring large amounts into trucks each night in preparation for the next day's spraying.

One chemical, in particular, has been singled out as the possible culprit. It is carbaryl, a powerful inhibitor of acetylcholinesterase. Physicians believe that the carbaryl, and possibly other pesticides that Garabedian routinely handled, inhibited acetylcholinesterase in his brain. Acetylcholine then accumulated in the synaptic clefts in neurons in his limbic system, triggering uncontrollable rage.

A psychiatrist who testified at the trial said, "In my view, David did not have the capacity to control his behavior because his brain was poisoned." Despite this testimony, Garabedian was found guilty of first-degree murder and is currently serving a life sentence. Drugs, alcohol, pesticides, and industrial chemicals routinely enter our bodies. In small amounts, they may be harmless, but in higher concentrations or in combination, they can disrupt chemical balance and cellular structure, upsetting homeostasis with a wide range of consequences.

Damage in crucial areas of the brain, no matter how slight, can upset its normal operation, resulting in erratic behavior or violent rages. Dr. Richard Restak, a neurologist and author of numerous popular books on the brain, notes that the ingestion of alcohol and other drugs can dismantle (at least temporarily) the brain's intricate system of checks and balances and elicit unusual, and even violent, behavior. "It is humbling and frightening," says Restak, "to consider that our rationality is dependent on the normal function of tissue within our skulls." It is even more frightening to realize that the balance can be so easily upset. "We have the capacity, if everything is operating correctly within our brains, of composing a Bill of Rights or the Constitution," says Restak. "But in the presence of a barely measurable electrical impulse within the limbic system, our much vaunted rationality can be replaced by savage attacks and seemingly inexplicable violence."

Summary

An Overview of the Nervous System

1. The *nervous system* controls a wide range of functions and plays a key role in ensuring homeostasis. The human nervous system also performs many other functions, such as ideation, planning for the future, learning, and remembering.

2. The nervous system consists of two anatomical subdivisions: the *central nervous system (CNS)*, made up of the *brain* and *spinal cord,* and the *peripheral nervous system (PNS)*, which consists of the *spinal* and *cranial nerves.*

3. Receptors in the skin, skeletal muscles, joints, and organs, transmit sensory input to the CNS via *sensory neurons.* The CNS integrates all sensory input and generates appropriate responses. Motor output leaves the CNS in *motor neurons.*

4. The PNS has two functional divisions. The *autonomic division* controls involuntary actions such as heart rate. The *somatic division* largely controls voluntary actions such as skeletal muscle contractions. It also provides the neural connections needed for many reflex arcs.

Structure and Function of the Neuron

5. The fundamental unit of the nervous system is the *neuron.* This highly specialized cell generates and transmits bioelectric impulses from one part of the body to another.

6. Three types of neurons are found in the body: *sensory neurons, interneurons,* and *motor neurons.*

7. All neurons have more or less spherical *cell bodies.* Extending from the cell body are two types of processes: *dendrites,* which conduct impulses to the cell body, and *axons,* which conduct impulses away from the cell body.

8. Many axons are covered by a layer of myelin, which increases the rate of impulse transmission. In the PNS, myelin is laid down by *Schwann cells* during embryonic development. In the CNS, myelin is produced by *oligodendrocytes.*

9. The terminal ends of axons branch profusely, forming numerous fibers that end in small knobs called *terminal boutons.*

10. During cellular differentiation, nerve cells lose their ability to divide. Because of this, neurons that die cannot be replaced by existing cells. Axons often regenerate in the PNS, but only rarely in the CNS.

11. Nerve cells have exceptionally high metabolic rates and require a constant supply of oxygen. Because nerve cells rely exclusively on glucose for energy, decreases in blood glucose levels can have extremely deleterious effects on the nervous system.

12. The small electrical potential across the membrane of nerve cells is known as the *membrane potential* or *resting potential.*

13. When a nerve cell is stimulated, its plasma membrane increases its permeability to sodium ions. Sodium ions rush in, causing *depolarization,* which spreads down the membrane.

14. Depolarization is followed by *repolarization,* a recovery of the resting potential stemming largely from the efflux of potassium ions. The depolarization and repolarization of the neuron's plasma membrane constitute a *bioelectric impulse* or *action potential.*

15. Nerve impulses travel along the plasma membranes of dendrites and unmyelinated axons, but in myelinated axons, impulses "jump" from node to node.

16. When a bioelectric impulse reaches the terminal bouton, it stimulates the release of *neurotransmitters* contained in membrane-bound vesicles.

17. Released into *synaptic clefts,* neurotransmitters diffuse across the cleft, where they bind to receptors in the *postsynaptic membrane.* Neurotransmitters may excite or inhibit the postsynaptic membrane. Whether a neuron fires depends on the sum of excitatory and inhibitory impulses it receives.

18. After stimulating the postsynaptic membrane, neurotransmitters may diffuse out of the synaptic cleft, be reabsorbed by the terminal bouton, or be removed by enzymes.

19. Some insecticides inhibit the activity of the enzymes that deactivate neuro-

transmitters, creating a wide range of nervous system effects.

The Spinal Cord and Nerves

20. The *spinal cord* descends from the brain through the *vertebral canal* to the lower back. It carries information to and from the brain, and its neurons participate in many reflexes.

21. Two types of nerves emanate from the CNS: spinal and cranial. *Spinal nerves* arise from the spinal cord and may be sensory, motor, or mixed. *Cranial nerves* attach to the brain and supply the structures of the head and several key body parts.

22. Spinal nerves are attached to the spinal cord via two roots, a *dorsal root,* which brings sensory information into the cord, and a *ventral root,* which carries motor information out.

23. Sensory fibers entering the cord often end on *interneurons,* which frequently end on motor neurons in the spinal cord, forming *reflex arcs.* Interneurons can also send axons to the brain.

The Brain

24. The brain is housed in the skull. The *cerebrum* with its two *cerebral hemispheres* is the largest part of the brain.

25. The outer layer of each hemisphere is the *cortex.* It contains *gray matter,* which houses nerve cell bodies, and underlying *white matter,* which contains myelinated nerve fibers that transmit nerve impulses to and from the gray matter.

26. The cerebral cortex consists of many discrete functional regions, including motor, sensory, and association areas.

27. Consciousness resides in the cerebral cortex, but a great many functions occur at the unconscious level in parts of the brain beneath the cortex.

28. The *cerebellum* coordinates muscle movement and controls posture. The *hypothalamus* regulates many homeostatic functions. The *limbic system* houses instincts and emotions. The *brain stem,* like the hypothalamus, regulates basic body functions.

29. A watery fluid surrounds the brain and spinal cord. Known as *cerebrospinal fluid (CSF),* it serves as a cushion that protects the brain and spinal cord from traumatic injury. It also fills the central canal of the spinal cord and cavities within the brain, the *ventricles.*

30. Electrodes applied to different parts of the scalp detect electrical activity in the brain and produce a tracing known as an *electroencephalogram (EEG).* The type of brain wave recorded depends on one's level of cortical activity. EEGs are used to diagnose some brain dysfunctions.

31. *Headaches* are the most common form of pain and generally result from tension, swelling of the membranes lining the sinuses, eyestrain, or dilation of the cerebral blood vessels.

32. Very serious headaches may result from increased intracranial pressure caused by a brain tumor, intracranial bleeding, or inflammation caused by an infection of the meninges (meningitis) or the brain itself (encephalitis).

33. Less threatening, but still extraordinary, are migraines, a form of severe, recurrent headache. The pain often occurs on one side of the head, may last 4 to 72 hours, and is aggravated by movement or physical activity. It is typically accompanied by nausea, vomiting, and sensitivity to light and sound.

The Autonomic Nervous System

34. The *autonomic nervous system* or *ANS* is a division of the PNS and transmits motor impulses to smooth muscle, cardiac muscle, and glands.

35. The ANS innervates all internal organs and has two subdivisions: the sympathetic and the parasympathetic.

36. The *sympathetic division* of the ANS functions in emergencies and is responsible in large part for the *fight-or-flight response,* accelerating heart rate and breathing, dilating the pupils, and shunting blood to the skeletal muscles, which provides additional oxygen and nutrients needed to combat an adversary or to escape.

37. The *parasympathetic division* of the ANS reduces heart rate, contracts the pupils, and promotes digestion—responses associated with the relaxed state.

Learning and Memory

38. *Learning* is a process in which an individual acquires knowledge and skills from experience, instruction, or some combination of the two. Learning depends on one's ability to store information in the brain—that is, *memory.*

39. Newly acquired knowledge is first stored in *short-term memory,* which retains information for periods of seconds to hours. Short-term memories may be transferred to *long-term memory,* which holds information for periods of days to years.

40. Memory is stored in multiple regions of the brain.

41. Short- and long-term memory appear to involve structural and functional changes of the neurons.

Diseases of the Brain

42. Alzheimer's disease is a progressive loss of mental function, which usually begins later in life. Symptoms include forgetfulness, irritability, and lack of initiative followed by loss of memory.

43. Scientists do not know the cause of Alzheimer's, although there is some evidence to suggest that previous severe brain injuries could be the cause in some instances.

44. Experiments with mice suggest that antibodies to beta-amyloid, a material found in the brains of Alzheimer's patients, could prevent or slow the development of the disease.

45. Parkinson's disease is a neurological disorder caused by a progressive deterioration of certain brain centers, those that control movement, especially semiautomatic movements such as swinging the arms when walking. It is characterized by tremors that typically worsen as one ages.

46. Like Alzheimer's the cause or causes of Parkinson's are unknown. Chemical pollutants may contribute to the disease. Amalgam fillings in teeth and chemicals used in wood stains may play a role in the onset of the disease. Very likely, there are many causes.

47. Recent studies show that fetal cell transplants into the affected brain area may eliminate the symptoms of the disease. Surgeon can also destroy a small region of the brain that appears to be hyperactive in Parkinson's patients.

48. Electrodes can also be implanted in the brain to stop uncontrollable movements. Patients are equipped with tiny electronic stimulators, much like pacemakers, which can be switched on or off as needed.

49. Two types of tumors develop in the brain tissue, benign and malignant. Benign tumors are growths that do not grow uncontrollably or metastasize like malignant tumors. Benign tumors can cause problems by placing pressure on areas of the brain.

50. Malignant tumors grow rapidly, especially late in the disease. They often place pressure on neighboring structures and may invade the tissue around them or may spread to other parts of the body.

51. Brain tumors occur at any age, although the most common groups are children in the 3- to 12 year old age bracket and adults in the 40- to 70 year-old bracket.

52. Researchers do not know what causes brain tumors, but there are some risk factors that increase one's likelihood for developing a malignant tumor including exposure to chemicals in certain industries, including oil refining, rubber manufacturing, and drug manufacturing, as well as exposure to certain viruses. Some brain tumors seem to run in families, so there may be a genetic cause in some cases. In most cases, however, patients with brain tumors have no clear risk factors, so researchers believe that the disease is probably the result of several factors acting together.

Health, Homeostasis, and the Environment: The Violent Brain

53. Abnormal brain activity can result in bizarre behavior in humans. Brain damage may result from harmful chemicals such as pesticides and drugs.

Critical Thinking

Thinking Critically—Analysis

This Analysis corresponds to the Thinking Critically scenario that was presented at the beginning of this chapter.

The researchers hypothesized that the left prefrontal cortex of the brain may process negative thoughts. Since they found that this cortex is hyperactive in severely depressed subjects, they hypothesized that the hyperactivity results in symptoms of depression. The scientists also conjectured that chemical messengers in the brain that normally dampen the activity of this region are released in abnormally high amounts, causing the brain to malfunction.

To confirm their findings, the researchers compared another group of seven individuals with severe depression to a control group—and found similar results. Although this is encouraging, it is important to note that the sample sizes are rather small. Before one can accept these findings, it's essential that they be repeated by other researchers studying larger sample sizes.

Test of Concepts

1. The nervous system performs a great many functions. Describe them. What functions do you think are unique to humans?

2. Describe how the resting and action potentials are generated. Describe how the plasma membrane of a neuron is repolarized.

3. Draw a typical multipolar neuron, and label its parts. Show the direction in which an action potential travels.

4. Draw a typical synapse, label the parts, and explain how a nerve impulse is transmitted from one nerve cell to another.

5. Describe how each of the following substances affects synaptic transmission: caffeine, cocaine, and malathion (a pesticide).

6. In general, how do anesthetics function?

7. Name and describe the various divisions of the nervous system.

8. Draw a cross section through the spinal cord showing the spinal nerves. Label the parts, and explain a reflex arc and how nerve impulses entering a spinal nerve also travel to the brain.

9. A physician can stimulate various parts of the brain and get different responses. What effects would you expect if the electrodes were placed in the premotor area? The primary motor cortex? The sensory motor cortex?

10. The brain is a delicate organ, and slight shifts in electrical activity can create bizarre behavior. Do you agree with this statement? Give examples.

www.jbpub.com/humanbiology

Connect to this book's web site: www.jbpub.com/humanbiology
The site features eLearning, an online review area that provides quizzes, chapter outlines, and other
tools to help you study for your class. You can also follow useful links for in-depth information,
research the differing views in the Point/Counterpoints, or keep up on the latest environmental
and health news.

The Senses

Organ of Corti.

Thinking **Critically**

Imagine that you suffer from chronic pain. At times the pain in your abdomen becomes unbearable. It wakes you when you sleep. It makes it impossible to sit still and enjoy a movie with your loved ones. It makes you irritable and short-tempered. Yet doctors can't find any cause for it.

Then, one day, your local newspaper runs a story about an experimental procedure pioneered by some researchers at the medical school in your state. This procedure involves the injection of chemical substances into the fluid surrounding the spinal cord. These substances, the researchers believe, bind to nerve cells that carry pain signals to your brain. They've successfully used the procedure on laboratory mice and now are looking for volunteers to test the effectiveness of this procedure on humans.

Would you consider becoming a human guinea pig? If so, what questions would you want answered before you submit to the procedure? ■

ebra Cartwright noticed something strange one day while she was eating dinner. For no apparent reason, she had lost her senses of smell and taste. Doctors were puzzled at first by the finding, for the young lady seemed to be in fine health. She was not suffering from a cold, sinus infection, or even any allergies that might have blocked her nasal passages and impaired her senses of smell or taste. A blood test, however, revealed the cause of her problem: low blood levels of the micronutrient zinc. Her physician prescribed a zinc supplement, and in a few days her senses of smell and taste returned.

This story illustrates the importance of a nutritionally balanced diet and the impact of a dietary deficiency on two important body functions—the senses of taste and smell.[1] It is just one of many examples presented in this book that illustrates how body functions can be altered by external factors such as stress, pollution, and diet.

This chapter examines the senses, dividing the discussion into two broad categories: the general senses and the special senses.

Section 12-1

The General and Special Senses

Staying aware of one's environment and responding to changes in that environment require a system of surveillance not unlike that found at high-security government facilities, where both inside and outside activities are routinely monitored to detect intruders. The surveillance system of the human body, like that of many other animals, consists of numerous receptors, which detect internal and external conditions. In humans, receptors are strategically located in the skin, internal organs, bones, joints, and muscles. They detect stimuli that give rise to the **general senses:** pain, temperature, light touch, pressure, and a sense of body and limb position (**TABLE 12-1**).

The human body is also endowed with five additional senses, known as the **special senses.** They are taste, smell, vision, hearing, and balance. They are generally made possible by highly sophisticated sensory organs—for example, the eye. These marvelously "engineered" detectors increase our ability to perceive stimuli

[1]Zinc deficiencies are quite rare, and dietary supplements containing zinc are generally not needed if you are eating a well-balanced diet. Furthermore, dietary supplements can be dangerous. Just a few times the recommended daily allowance of zinc can cause serious problems.

TABLE 12-1

Summary of General and Special Senses

Sense	Stimulus	Receptor
General senses	Pain	Naked nerve endings
	Light touch	Merkel's discs; naked nerve endings around hair follicles; Meissner's corpuscles; Ruffini's corpuscles; Krause's end-bulbs
	Pressure	Pacinian corpuscles
	Temperature	Naked nerve endings
	Proprioception	Golgi tendon organs; muscle spindles; receptors similar to Meissner's corpuscles in joints
Special senses	Taste	Taste buds
	Smell	Olfactory epithelium
	Sight	Retina
	Hearing	Organ of Corti
	Balance	Crista ampularis in the semicircular canals; maculae in utricle and saccule

in the environment and are one of the most remarkable developments in the evolution of complex multicellular organisms.

Receptors in humans involved in the general and special senses fall into five functional categories: (1) mechanoreceptors, (2) chemoreceptors, (3) thermoreceptors, (4) photoreceptors, and (4) nociceptors (pain receptors). **Mechanoreceptors** are those activated by mechanical stimulation—for example, touch or pressure. **Chemoreceptors** are activated by chemicals in the food we eat, the air we breathe, or in our blood. **Thermoreceptors** are activated by heat and cold, and **photoreceptors** are sensitive to light. **Nociceptors** (no-see-SEP-tors) are pain receptors are stimulated by pinching, tearing, or burning.

Section 12-2

The General Senses

Sit back in your chair for a moment, close your eyes, and concentrate on what you feel. You may detect the pressure of the chair on your buttocks and warmth emanating from a nearby reading lamp. You may feel your cat brushing against the hairs on your arm. You may detect a slight pain from a bruise or gas pressure in your intestines from the burritos you ate for dinner last night. Now move your arm. Even though your eyes are closed, you can feel it moving.

Epithelial cells of epidermis

Pacinian corpuscle (pressure receptor)

Connective tissue cells

Dendrites of sensory neuron

Dendrite of sensory neuron

(a)

(b)

FIGURE 12-1 Receptors General sense receptors are either (a) naked nerve endings or (b) encapsulated nerve endings.

The various sensations you have just experienced fall into the group of general senses. Receptors for the general senses detect internal and external stimuli and relay messages to the spinal cord and brain via sensory nerves (Chapter 11). Sensory input to the central nervous system may elicit a conscious response—for example, the touch of a cat may cause you to reach down and pet your furry friend. Some stimuli will cause unconscious responses—for example, heat may cause you to perspire, or cold may cause you to shiver. Others may simply be registered in the cerebral cortex, making you aware of the stimulus. Still other stimuli may be blocked so they elicit no response at all.

Receptors for the general body senses come in many shapes and sizes, but they generally fit into two groups based on structure: naked nerve endings and encapsulated receptors (**FIGURE 12-1**). As you shall soon see, the naked nerve endings and encapsulated receptors in the body serve very specific roles.

Naked Nerve Endings in Body Tissues Detect Pain, Temperature, and Light Touch

Located in the skin, bones, and internal organs and in and around joints, **naked nerve endings** are the terminal ends of the dendrites of sensory neurons. They are responsible for at least three sensations: pain, light touch, and temperature.

Pain. Physiologists recognize two basic types of pain: somatic and visceral. **Somatic pain** results from injuries in the skin, joints, muscles, and tendons, which stimulates receptors in these areas. Pain receptors are part of a protective mechanism of considerable adaptive value in the evolution of complex multicellular organisms. They signal that something is awry and alert the brain so that appropriate action can be taken.

Somatic pain receptors respond to several types of stimuli. Some respond to cutting, crushing, and pinch-

ing. Others respond to temperature extremes—hot or cold. Still others respond to irritating chemicals released from injured tissues.

Visceral pain results from the stimulation of naked nerve endings in body organs (the viscera). In some body organs, pain receptors are stimulated by distension. In others, they're stimulated by **anoxia** (ah-NOCKS-see-ah), a lack of oxygen. For example, the intestinal pain you feel when you have gas results from the stretching of naked nerve fibers in the wall of the intestine. These nerve endings are mechanoreceptors. In contrast, the pain felt during a heart attack results from a lack of oxygen in the heart muscle.

Visceral pain and somatic pain result from quite different stimuli and are perceived very differently as well. Somatic pain is easily pinpointed. Visceral pain, however, is vague and difficult to localize. Moreover, it is generally felt on the body surface at a site some distance from its origin. For example, pain caused by a lack of oxygen to the heart muscle appears in the chest and along the inside of the left arm (**FIGURE 12-2**).

Visceral pain that appears on the body surface away from the location of the pain is called **referred pain.** Physiologists do not know the cause of this phenomenon, but most think that it results from the fact that pain fibers from internal organs enter the spinal cord at the same location that the sensory fibers from the skin enter. The brain, they hypothesize, interprets the impulses from pain fibers supplying the organs as pain from a somatic source. (Health Note 12-1 describes techniques that relieve pain.)

Light Touch. Light touch is perceived by two anatomically distinct mechanoreceptors. The first receptor is located at the base of the hairs in our skin. As shown in **FIGURE 12-3**, naked nerve endings (dendrites) wrap around the base of the hair follicles. When a hair is moved—for example, by a gentle touch—these nerve fibers are stimulated.

The second light-touch mechanoreceptor is the **Merkel's disc** (MUR-killz). Shown in **FIGURE 12-3**, Merkel's discs consist of small cup-shaped cells on which naked nerve endings terminate. These receptors, located in the outer layer of the epidermis of the skin, are activated by gentle pressure applied to the skin.

Temperature. Naked nerve endings in the skin detect heat and cold. Heat receptors respond to temperatures from 25°C (77°F) to 45°C (113°F). If the temperature of the skin rises above this range, pain receptors are activated, creating a burning sensation. In contrast, cold receptors respond to temperatures from 10°C (50°F) to 20°C (68°F). If the temperature drops below 10°C, pain receptors respond.

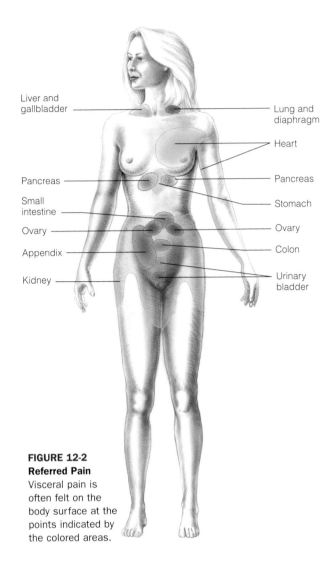

Liver and gallbladder
Lung and diaphragm
Heart
Pancreas
Pancreas
Stomach
Small intestine
Ovary
Ovary
Appendix
Colon
Kidney
Urinary bladder

FIGURE 12-2
Referred Pain
Visceral pain is often felt on the body surface at the points indicated by the colored areas.

Encapsulated Receptors Consist of Naked Nerve Endings Surrounded by One or More Layers of Cells

Shown in **FIGURE 12-3**, the largest encapsulated nerve ending is the **Pacinian corpuscle** (pah-SIN-ee-an CORE-puss-'l). It consists of a naked nerve ending surrounded by numerous concentric cell layers. The Pacinian corpuscle resembles a small onion pierced by a thin wire. Located in the deeper layers of the skin, in the loose connective tissue of the body, and elsewhere, Pacinian corpuscles are stimulated by pressure such as the pressure you feel sitting in your chair.

Another common encapsulated sensory receptor is the **Meissner's corpuscle** (MEIZ-ners). Smaller than Pacinian corpuscles, these oval receptors contain two or three spiraling dendritic ends surrounded by a thin cellular capsule (**FIGURE 12-3**). Like the naked nerve endings surrounding the base of the hair follicle and Merkel's discs, Meissner's corpuscles are thought to respond to light touch. Located just beneath the epithelium in the outermost layer of the dermis, Meissner's

corpuscles are most abundant in the sensitive parts of the body, such as the lips and the tips of the fingers.

Two additional encapsulated receptors are Krause's end-bulbs and Ruffini's corpuscles (**FIGURE 12-3**). Most scientists believe that these receptors are structural variations of the Meissner's corpuscle and are stimulated by light touch.

Proprioception (PRO-pree-oh-CEP-shun; the sense of position) is provided by special encapsulated receptors located in the joints of the body. Resembling Meissner's corpuscles, these receptors inform us of the position of our limbs and alert us to movements of the body.

Proprioception is also served by the muscle spindle and the Golgi tendon organ. **Muscle spindles,** or **neu-**

Epidermis
Meisner's corpuscle

Free dendrite nerve ending (pain)
Merkel's discs (light touch)
Meissner's corpuscle (touch, light pressure)
Ruffini's corpuscle (light touch)
Dendrites (hair movement)
Pacinian corpuscle (deep pressure)

Krause's end-bulb (light touch)
Epidermis
Dermis
Sensory nerve
Subcutaneous fat

Pacinian corpuscle

FIGURE 12-3 General Sense Receptors   The skin houses many of the receptors for general senses. Receptors fall into two categories: naked nerve endings and encapsulated receptors. The Pacinian corpuscle, often located in the dermis of the skin, detects pressure. Meissner's corpuscle, found just beneath the epidermis, detects light touch.

Health Note 12-1

Old and New Treatments for Pain

Millions of people suffer from chronic or persistent pain. In the United States, for example, an estimated 70 to 80 million people are tormented by back pain. Another 26 million suffer from migraine headaches.

Despite its prevalence, pain is one of the least understood medical problems in the world. The study of pain, in fact, is so poorly funded and so widely ignored by the medical community that some have called it an orphan science. Making matters worse, physicians are often poorly trained in dealing with pain.

Minor aches and pains can be treated with aspirin, acetaminophen, and ibuprofen. These pain killers (analgesics) also help reduce fever, and ibuprofen helps reduce inflammation. More intense pain is treated with stronger painkillers, such as codeine and morphine. Codeine is often mixed with ibuprofen and acetaminophen. Although codeine and morphine are both used today, their addictive nature led the medical community to look for other techniques. One promising option is acupuncture, a technique used by the Chinese for thousands of years. Acupuncture relies on thread-thin needles inserted in the skin near nerves (**FIGURE 1**).

No one knows how acupuncture works. The Chinese thought that it interrupted the flow of energy through various pathways in the body, called *meridians*. These meridians, the Chinese contend, are rivers of energy that flow through the body to irrigate and nourish the tissues. They contend that blood and nervous impulses also follow these meridians. Any obstruction in the movement of these energy rivers results in deficiencies of energy, blood, and nerve impulses that may lead to disease. The acupuncture needles, they contend, unblock obstructions and reestablish normal flow.

Neurologists are not certain how acupuncture works, but many think that it blocks pain by overloading the neuronal circuitry. They note that two types of nerve fibers transmit sensory information from the body to the central nervous system: small- and large-diameter fibers. Small-diameter fibers carry pain messages. Large-diameter fibers carry many other forms of sensory information from receptors in the skin—for example, pressure and light touch. The dendrites of both small- and large-diameter sensory nerve cells often terminate in the same location in the spinal cord. From here they send impulses to the brain, signaling pain or some other sense.

Neurobiologists believe that acupuncture needles stimulate the large-diameter nerve fibers. This stimulation blocks nerve impulses carried by the smaller nerve fibers, thus blocking pain messages to the brain. Research on the mechanism of action of acupuncture points to several other possibilities as well. Acupuncture needles, for instance, may stimulate the release of **endorphins**, the body's natural pain killers. Endorphins are produced in the brain. Many U.S. physicians trained to use drugs and surgery to solve most pain remain skeptical about the usefulness of acupuncture. Over the past 20 years, however, a small but steady stream of research has confirmed the painkilling effect of this treatment. Most insurance companies will pay the cost of acupuncture to relieve pain caused, for example, by a car crash.

Joseph Helms, a physician with the American Academy of Acupuncture in Berkeley, California, performed acupuncture on 40 women with menstrual pain. Some women received real acupuncture treatment. Others received placebo treatments (shallow needle treatments that did not reach the acupuncture points). In the group of women receiving acupuncture, 10 out of 11 showed a marked decrease in pain. Patients reported an approximately 50% decrease in pain. In the placebo group, only 4 out of 11 reported a lessening of pain. Only 1 of 10 people given no treatment showed improvement. Acupuncture also reduced the need for painkilling drugs during treatment by over half. Remember, however, that the Critical Thinking section in Chapter 1 suggested that experiments using small numbers of subjects are themselves subject to question. Further studies are needed to confirm these results.

While acupuncture is slowly earning a respected place in the treatment of pain, some health care practitioners are using a procedure called *transcutaneous electrical nerve stimulation,* or TENS. Patients are fitted with electrodes attached to the skin above the nerves that transmit pain signals to the central nervous system. A small battery supplies energy

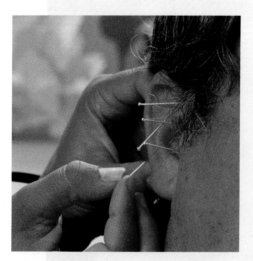

FIGURE 1 Patient Undergoing Acupuncture Acupuncture is generally used to alleviate pain, but it has other applications as well.

that stimulates the electrodes. When the pain begins, patients press a button on the battery pack that sends a tiny current to the electrode. The current is conducted through the skin and blocks the pain impulses. How it blocks pain is currently subject to debate. It may block pain by inhibiting abnormally firing or damaged nerves or blocking pain impulses at the spinal cord. Or, it may stimulate a region of the brain that in turn blocks pain. Finally, it may stimulate the release of endorphins, the body's own pain-killing chemicals.

TENS can be used to reduce pain after surgery. One study showed that this technique reduced the amount of painkillers that doctors had to administer by two-thirds and cut hospital stays by 1 or 2 days. Some day, TENS may be used to reduce the pain of childbirth or pain that athletes often endure.

TENS works like acupuncture, although part of its success may be psychological. In a study of 93 patients with chronic pain, researchers found that over one-third (36%) of them reported no pain or greatly reduced pain when they thought they were being stimulated but really were not. How effective was it when the battery really worked? About half of the patients reported no pain or greatly reduced pain. The slight difference suggests to some physicians that TENS may be overrated. To those suffering from chronic pain, it can be a godsend.

Severe pain can also be treated by surgery. Doctors may cut nerves, sever nerve tracks in the spinal cord that carry pain, or even destroy small parts of the brain to rid a patient of chronic pain. Nerves can also be destroyed by applying certain chemical substances.

Although all of these methods are effective, there are dangers in these procedures. Cutting nerve tracks in the spinal cord, a structure that's approximately the size of your little finger, can be risky. One slip and a surgeon could destroy motor neurons. Nerves carrying pain signals also transmit sensory information. Some doctors think that patients should not risk loss of other senses or motor functions for pain relief. In addition, pain recurs in 9 of 10 patients who have undergone pain-relieving surgery, usually within a year or so.

Recurring pain results from the partial regrowth of axons. Even after another operation, the pain frequently returns, often with much greater intensity. Consequently, physicians are now looking for alternative measures to eliminate chronic pain.

One promising measure is deep brain stimulation. Electrodes can be implanted in parts of the brain and stimulated to block pain impulses before they reach the sensory cortex, where pain is perceived. The electrodes are connected to a portable battery worn on the belt or implanted under the skin. When the pain begins, the patient turns on the current, blocking the pain impulses.

Research shows that deep brain stimulation is an effective blocker of even the most powerful pain stimuli. Yet it does not upset other brain functions. Unfortunately, this technique requires surgery, and implanting electrodes may cause hemorrhaging in some patients, which can result in permanent paralysis or a loss of feeling in parts of the body. Infections may also develop where the electrodes enter the skull. The 75% success rate and the reduced suffering make most patients more than willing to accept the risks.

Another promising approach is molecular neurosurgery. This technique involves the use of toxic chemicals to destroy pain-carrying nerves. Toxic substances are chemically bonded to antibodies that selectively attack sensory nerve fibers. In experiments with laboratory animals, antibody-coupled toxin is injected into the fluid around the spinal cord. In two weeks time, researchers found significant reduction in pain-transmitting neurons.

Antibody-bound toxins are large chemical complexes and do not spread readily through the spinal cord. They are also hard to make. Because of these factors, researchers are also testing the effectiveness of smaller molecules. Nerve cells that respond to tissue damage, for instance, produce a chemical substance simply called P. This peptide consists of 11 amino acids. Scientists speculate that P is a neurotransmitter released by nocicepetor cells that terminate in the spinal cord. It stimulates cells in the spinal cord that transmit the nerve impulses to the brain. When P is released by nociceptor cells, it binds to receptors on the nerve cells in the spinal cord. When substance P is linked to a nerve toxin and injected into the spinal cord fluids of rats, it binds to nerve cells that transmit pain signals to the brain, killing them and relieving chronic pain. Rat studies show that the pain relief lasted a long time and did not affect mild pain, only more intense chronic pain. Although clinical trials are a long way in the future, this too could become an important tool in the medical community's arsenal of pain-relieving treatments.

Visit *Human Biology's* Internet site for links to web sites offering more information on this topic.

romuscular spindles, are located in skeletal muscles. Muscle spindles consist of several modified muscle fibers with sensory nerve endings wrapped around them.

Spindle fibers are stimulated when muscles are stretched. Nerve impulses generated by the spindle are then transmitted to the spinal cord, where they may ascend to the cerebral cortex, helping us remain aware of body position. Others may stimulate motor neurons in the spinal cord, eliciting a reflex contraction of the muscle being stretched. This is what happens when you fall asleep sitting upright in a chair when your head falls forward and quickly snaps back.

Golgi tendon organs (GOAL-jee) are mechanoreceptors named after the Italian cytologist who discovered them. Functionally similar to the muscle spindle, these receptors are located in **tendons**—the structures that connect muscles to bones. Golgi tendon organs are composed of connective tissue fibers surrounded by dendrites and encased in a capsule. When a muscle contracts, the tendon stretches and stimulates the receptor. Like the muscle spindle, this receptor alerts the brain to movement and body position. Impulses from the Golgi tendon organ can also stimulate reflex contraction of muscles. The knee-jerk reflex described in Chapter 11 is a good example.

Many Receptors Stop Generating Impulses After Exposure to a Stimulus for Some Length of Time

Pain, temperature, and pressure receptors are all subject to a phenomenon known as **adaptation.**[2] This occurs when sensory receptors stop generating impulses even though the stimulus is still present. You have probably experienced the phenomenon many times. Recall, for example, the first time you wore a ring or contact lenses. At first, the sensation may have nearly driven you mad, but after a few days or perhaps a few hours, the stimulus seemed to have disappeared. What happened was that pressure receptors that were originally alerting the brain stopped generating impulses, relieving you of what would have otherwise been unrelenting discomfort.

Not all receptors adapt. Muscle stretch receptors and joint proprioceptors are two examples. Because the central nervous system must be continuously apprised of muscle length and joint position to maintain posture, adaptation in these receptors would be counterproductive, even dangerous.

Receptors Play an Important Role in Homeostasis

Many general sense receptors play an important role in homeostasis. Mechanoreceptors that detect changes in blood pressure and chemoreceptors that respond to the ionic concentration of the blood, for example, help maintain blood pressure and proper water balance through mechanisms involving the kidney. Chemoreceptors that detect levels of carbon dioxide and hydrogen ions in the blood and cerebrospinal fluid help to regulate respiration. Chapter 14 describes additional chemoreceptors that detect levels of various hormones, nutrients, and ions in the blood and body fluids. These detectors may stimulate hormonal responses that correct potentially disruptive chemical imbalances.

Section 12-3

Taste and Smell: The Chemical Senses

The special senses are taste, smell, vision, hearing, and balance.

Taste Buds Are the Receptors for Taste and Respond to Chemicals Dissolved in Food

In humans and other mammals, the tongue contains receptors for taste. Known as the **taste buds,** these microscopic, onion-shaped structures are located in the surface epithelium of the tongue and on small protrusions, **papillae** (pah-PILL-ee), on the upper surface of the tongue (**FIGURE 12-4A**). Taste buds are also found on the roof of the oral cavity, the pharynx, and the larynx, but in smaller numbers.

Taste buds are chemoreceptors and are stimulated by chemicals in the food we eat. These substances dissolve in the saliva and enter the **taste pores,** small openings that lead to the interior of the taste bud (**FIGURE 12-4C**). Taste buds contain receptor cells, the ends of which possess large microvilli, known as **taste hairs.** Taste hairs project into the taste pore. The plasma membranes of taste hairs contain clusters of protein molecules that serve as receptors. These receptors bind to food molecules dissolved in water. This, in turn, stimulates the receptor cells, which then stimulate the dendrites of the sensory nerves that are wrapped around the receptor cells.[3] Impulses from the taste buds are then transmitted to the taste centers in the cerebral cortex.

---

[2]Not to be confused with the adaptation occurring in evolution.

[3]Unlike the receptors in the previous section, the receptor cells of taste buds are not part of nerve cells but are independent cells.

FIGURE 12-4 Taste Receptors *(a)* Taste buds are located on the upper surface of the tongue and are concentrated on the *(b)* papillae. *(c)* The structure of the taste bud. *(d)* Taste pore.

In the opening paragraph of this chapter, you were introduced to an unfortunate student who lost her sense of taste because of a dietary zinc deficiency. Research has shown that zinc, which is normally found in low concentrations in the saliva, stimulates division of the cells in taste buds. Because cells of the taste buds are lost from normal wear and tear, a zinc deficiency reduces cellular replacement, and the taste buds eventually cease operation.

The Taste Buds Respond to All Five Primary Flavors But Are Generally Preferentially Responsive to One. Humans can discriminate among thousands of taste sensations. The taste sensations are a combination of five basic flavors: sweet, sour, bitter, salty, and umami. Sweet flavors result from sugars and some amino acids. Sour flavors result from acidic substances. Salty tastes result from metal ions (like sodium in table salt). Bitter flavors result from chemical substances belonging to a group called **alkaloids,** among them caffeine, but also some nonalkaloid substances such as aspirin. Umami is the meaty taste associated with the flavorant MSG (monosodium glutamate) commonly added to Chinese food. All taste buds respond, in varying degree, to all five taste sensations, but they respond preferentially to one taste.

Taste buds are distributed unevenly on the surface of the tongue. A simple experiment in which drops of various substances are placed on the tongue shows that the tip of the tongue is most sensitive to sweet flavors for it contains a higher proportion of taste buds that respond preferentially to sweet flavors. The sides of the tongue are most sensitive to sour flavors, and the back of the tongue is most sensitive to bitter flavors. Salty taste is more evenly distributed, with slightly increased sensitivity on the sides of the tongue near the front. Food contains many different flavors. What we taste, therefore, depends on the relative proportion of the five basic flavors.

The Olfactory Epithelium Is a Patch of Receptor Cells That Detects Odors

Smell, like taste, is a chemical sense. The receptors for smell are located in the roof of each nasal cavity in a patch of cells called the **olfactory epithelium,** or **membrane** (ole-FACK-tore-ee) (**FIGURE 12-5**). Odors are perceived by **receptor cells,** neurons whose dendrites extend to the surface of the olfactory membrane. (**FIGURE 12-5**). In humans, there are an estimated 50 million olfactory receptor cells in the olfactory membrane. These cells terminate in six to eight long projections, **olfactory hairs,** or **olfac-**

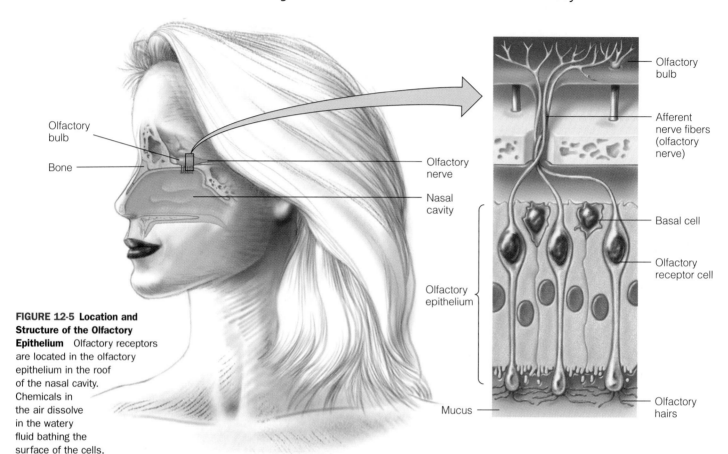

FIGURE 12-5 Location and Structure of the Olfactory Epithelium Olfactory receptors are located in the olfactory epithelium in the roof of the nasal cavity. Chemicals in the air dissolve in the watery fluid bathing the surface of the cells, then bind to receptors on the plasma membranes of the olfactory hairs. The olfactory receptors terminate in the olfactory bulb. From here, nerve fibers travel to the brain.

tory cilia. The olfactory hairs contain protein receptors for molecules. When airborne molecules are trapped on the thin, watery layer on the surface of the cell, they bind to the receptors in the membranes of olfactory hairs. This activates the neurons, causing them to generate impulses that are sent to the **olfactory bulb**, a complex neural structure whose neurons synapse with the dendrites of the receptor cells. Axons of the neurons in the olfactory bulb cells then travel to the brain via the **olfactory nerve.**

Humans can distinguish tens of thousands of odors, many at very low levels. The olfactory receptors are so sensitive, in fact, that even a single molecule binding to the olfactory hairs can produce a bioelectric impulse. But the sense of smell in humans is not as sensitive as that of other animals such as dogs, wolves, and coyotes. A dog's keen sense of smell is due to an olfactory membrane that's about 20 times larger than ours. Humans put the dog's excellent smell to good use. Dogs are used to sniff out drugs at airports and border crossings and to track criminals. Some research suggests that dogs can even detect the odor of skin cancers.

Like taste, odor discrimination is thought to depend on combinations of primary odors. Unfortunately, neuroscientists do not agree on what the primary odors are. One system of classification recognizes seven primary odors ranging from pepperminty to floral to putrid. It is thought that molecules that produce a similar odor are similarly shaped and that specific receptor sites on the olfactory hairs bind to molecules with a common shape. Various combinations of the primary odors give rise to the many odors we perceive. Some researchers hypothesize that there may be thousands of kinds of smell receptors providing odor discrimination. Research shows that there are at least 1000 different protein receptor molecules. New studies suggest that these molecules may be combined in different ways to provide the wide range of odor detection.

Even Though the Olfactory Receptors Are Sensitive and Able to Discriminate Many Odors, They Quickly Become Adapted. Receptors for smell adapt within a short period—about a minute. If you have ever visited a dairy farm or lived near one, you understand (and are grateful for) olfactory adaptation.

Smell Influences Our Sense of Taste, and Vice Versa. Hold a piece of hot apple pie to your nose and take a deep breath. It smells so good you can almost taste it. In fact, you *are* tasting it. Molecules given off by the pie enter the nose, reach the mouth through the pharynx, and dissolve in the saliva, where they stimulate taste receptors. Just as odors stimulate taste receptors, food in our mouths also stimulates olfactory receptors. Molecules released by food enter the nasal cavities, dissolving in the water on the surface of the olfactory membrane and stimulating the receptor cells.

The complementary nature of taste and smell is abundantly evident when a person suffers from nasal congestion. Cold sufferers often complain that they cannot taste their food. This phenomenon results from the buildup of mucus in the nasal cavities, which blocks the flow of air. Mucus may also block the olfactory hairs. Therefore, food loses its "taste" when you have a stuffy nose because your sense of smell is impaired. (You can test this by holding your nose while you eat.)

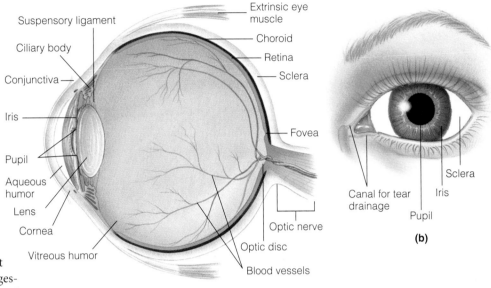

(a)

FIGURE 12-6 Anatomy of the Human Eye

TABLE 12-2

Structures and Functions of the Eye

Structure		Function
Wall		
Outer layer	Sclera	Provides insertion for extrinsic eye muscles
	Cornea	Allows light to enter; bends incoming light
Middle layer	Choroid	Absorbs stray light; provides nutrients to eye structures
	Ciliary body	Regulates lens, allowing it to focus images
	Iris	Regulates amount of light entering the eye
Inner layer	Retina	Responds to light, converting light to nerve impulses
Accessory structures and components		
	Lens	Focuses images on the retina
	Vitreous humor	Holds retina and lens in place
	Aqueous humor	Supplies nutrients to structures in contact with the anterior cavity of the eye
	Optic nerve	Transmits impulses from the retina to the brain

Section 12-4

The Visual Sense: The Eye

The human eye is one of the most extraordinary products of evolution. It contains a patch of photoreceptors that permits us to perceive the remarkably diverse and colorful environment we live in.

The Human Eye Consists of Three Distinct Layers

Human eyes are roughly spherical organs located in the **eye sockets,** or **orbits,** cavities formed by the bones of the skull. The eye is attached to the orbit by six muscles, the **extrinsic eye muscles,** which control eye movement. Small tendons connect these muscles to the outermost layer of the eye.

The Sclera and Cornea. As **FIGURE 12-6** shows, the wall of the human eye consists of three layers (**TABLE 12-2**). The outermost is a durable fibrous layer, which consists of the **sclera,** the white of the eye, and the **cornea,** the clear part in front, which lets light into the interior of the eye (**FIGURE 12-6**). Tendons of the extrinsic eye muscles attach to the sclera.

The Choroid, Ciliary Body, and Iris. As **FIGURE 12-6** shows, the middle layer consists of three parts: the choroid, the ciliary body, and the iris. The **choroid** is the largest portion of the middle layer. It contains a large amount of **melanin** (MELL-ah-nin), a pigment that absorbs stray light the way the black interior of a camera does. The blood vessels of the choroid supply nutrients to the eye. Anteriorly, the choroid forms the ciliary body. The **ciliary body** contains smooth muscle fibers, which control the shape of the lens, permitting us to focus incoming light. The **iris** is the colored portion of the eye visible through the cornea. Looking in a mirror, you can see a dark opening in the iris called the **pupil.** The pupil allows light to penetrate the eye. The blackness you see through the pupil is the choroid layer and the pigmented section of the retina, discussed below. Like the ciliary body, the iris contains smooth muscle cells. The smooth muscle of the iris regulates the diameter of the pupil. Opening the pupil lets more light in, and narrowing it reduces the amount of light that can enter. The pupils open and close reflexively in response to light intensity. This reflex is an adaptation that protects the light-sensitive inner layer, the retina.

The Retina. The innermost layer of the eye is the **retina.** The retina consists of an outer, pigmented layer and an inner layer consisting of photoreceptors (modified nerve cells that detect light) and associated nerve cells. The retina is weakly attached to the choroid and can become separated from it as a result of trauma to the head. A detached retina can lead to blindness if not repaired by surgery. Today, eye surgeons usually repair detached retinas with lasers.

The **photoreceptors** of the retina are highly modified nerve cells. Two types of photoreceptors are present in the retina: rods and cones (**TABLE 12-3**). The **rods,** so named because of their shape, are sensitive to low light (**FIGURES 12-7B** and **12-7C**). Rods function at night and produce grayish, somewhat vague black-and-white images. The **cones,** also named because of their shape, operate only in brighter light. They are responsible for visual acuity—sharp vision—and color vision.

As **FIGURE 12-7B** shows, the rods and cones synapse with the bipolar neurons. These, in turn, synapse with ganglion cells in the retina. The axons of the ganglion cells unite at the back of the eye to form the **optic nerve.** The optic nerve leaves at the **optic disc.** The optic disc is also known as the **blind spot,** because it contains no photoreceptors and is therefore insensitive to light. The blood vessels that enter and leave the eye do so with the optic nerve. These blood vessels and their branches can readily be seen by an ophthalmologist by shining a light through the pupil onto the posterior wall of the eye (**FIGURE 12-8**, page 284).

Rods and cones are found throughout the retina, but the cones are most abundant in a tiny region of each eye lateral to the optic disc. This spot is called the **macula lutea** (MACK-you-lah LEW-tee-ah), literally "yellow spot." In the center of the macula is a minute depression, about the size of the head of a pin, known as the **fovea centralis** (FOE-vee-ah sen-TRAL-iss; meaning central depression). The fovea contains only cones. The sharpest vision occurs at the fovea because it contains the highest concentration of cones and because the bipolar neurons and ganglion cells do not cover the cones in this region as they do throughout the rest of the retina. The number of cones in the retina decreases progressively from the fovea outward, whereas the number of rods increases. Thus, the greatest concentration of rods is found in the periphery of the retina.

Images from our visual field are cast onto the retina, and impulses are transmitted to the visual cortex of the brain's occipital lobe, where they are interpreted. When we focus on an object, the image is projected upside down onto the fovea. Even though the image is upside down, the brain processes the information and gives us a right-side-up image; that is, it allows us to perceive objects in their true position.

The Lens. Light is focused on the retina by the lens. The **lens** is a transparent, flexible structure that lies behind the iris (**FIGURE 12-9**, page 284). The lens is attached to the ciliary body by thin fibers of the **suspensory ligament.** This connection allows the smooth muscle of the ciliary body to alter the shape of the lens, an action necessary for focusing the eye.

In older individuals, the lens sometimes develops cloudy spots, or **cataracts.** The loss of transparency is especially prevalent in people who have been exposed to excessive sunlight or excessive ultraviolet light at work or elsewhere. Patients with this disease complain of cloudy vision. Looking out on the world to them is a little like looking through frosted glass. Interestingly, cataract risk may increase as the Earth's ozone layer, which blocks dangerous ultraviolet radiation from the

TABLE 12-3			
Summary of Rods and Cones			
Photoreceptor	Day or Night	Color Vision	Location
Rods	Night vision	No	Highest concentration in the periphery of the retina
Cones	Day vision	Yes	Highest concentration in the macula and fovea

FIGURE 12-7 The Retina
(a) Cross section through the wall of the eye, showing (b) the arrangement of the cellular components of the retina. (c) The structure of the rods and cones.

subjects had more cataracts than did blue-, gray-, and green-eyed patients. Researchers suggest that melanin in the irises of dark-eyed people may absorb solar radiation, causing more damage to the nearby lens. To lower your risk of cataracts, many eye doctors suggest wearing sunglasses with a coating that reduces ultraviolet penetration. But beware, there is evidence that some manufacturers' claims about ultraviolet protection may be overblown. Regular sunglasses may protect your eyes just fine.

Eye doctors once treated cataracts surgically by removing the afflicted lens. Patients were fitted with a thick pair of glasses or a pair of contact lenses, which compensated for the missing lens. Today, however, the afflicted lenses are routinely replaced by artificial plastic lenses that provide nearly normal vision.

The lens separates the interior of the eye into two cavities of unequal sizes. Everything in front of the lens is the **anterior cavity;** everything behind it is the **posterior cavity.**

The posterior cavity is filled with a clear, gelatinous material, the **vitreous humor** (VEH-tree-ous HUE-mur; "glassy liquid"). Formed during embryonic devel-

sun, is eroded by chlorofluorocarbons from refrigerators, air-conditioning units, and other sources, as discussed in Chapter 24.

Research suggests that the color of one's eyes affects one's risk of developing cataracts. Dark-eyed people run the highest risk of cataracts. Brown- and hazel-eyed

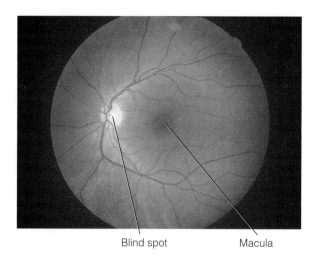

Blind spot   Macula

FIGURE 12-8 View of the Retina This photograph shows the inside back wall of the eye as seen through an ophthalmoscope. The optic disc (blind spot) and macula (site of the fovea centralis) are both indicated.

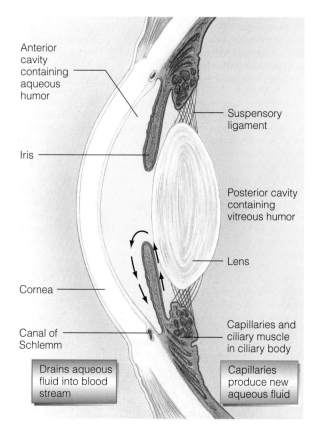

Anterior cavity containing aqueous humor

Iris

Cornea

Canal of Schlemm

Drains aqueous fluid into blood stream

Suspensory ligament

Posterior cavity containing vitreous humor

Lens

Capillaries and ciliary muscle in ciliary body

Capillaries produce new aqueous fluid

FIGURE 12-9 Detailed Cross Section of the Anterior Cavity Arrows show the flow of aqueous humor.

opment, the vitreous humor remains throughout life, holding the lens and retina in place.

The anterior cavity contains a thin liquid, chemically similar to blood plasma, called the **aqueous humor** ("watery fluid"). Unlike the vitreous humor, the aqueous humor is constantly replaced. New fluid is produced by capillaries in the ciliary body and drains into a cavity located at the junction of the sclera and cornea. From here, the plasmalike fluid flows into the bloodstream.

The aqueous humor provides nutrients to the cornea and lens and carries away cellular wastes. In normal, healthy individuals, aqueous humor production is balanced by absorption. If the outflow is blocked, however, the aqueous humor builds up inside the anterior chamber, creating internal pressure. This disease, called **glaucoma** (glaw-COE-mah), progresses gradually and imperceptibly. If untreated, the pressure inside the eye can damage the retina and optic nerve, causing blindness. Because the incidence of glaucoma increases after age 40, doctors recommend an annual eye examination for people over 40. If diagnosed early, glaucoma can be treated with eye drops that increase the rate of drainage. In severe cases, surgery may be required to increase the outflow.

The Lens Focuses Light on the Retina

To understand how the lens operates, you must first understand a little bit about light.

Refraction. First of all, visible light travels in waves. Light waves travel at a constant rate in any given medium such as air or water. When light passes from

one medium to another, however, its velocity changes. For example, when light passes from air to a denser medium such as the cornea of the eye, it slows down. Any time light changes speed in passing from one substance to another, it bends. The bending of light is called **refraction** (ree-FRACK-shun) (**FIGURE 12-10**).

Focusing the Image. The lens of the eye bends incoming light rays, focusing images on the photoreceptors of the retina. Lying in front of the lens is the cornea; it also bends incoming light rays (**FIGURE 12-11**). Although we usually think of the lens as the structure that allows us to focus, most of the bending of incoming rays takes place in the cornea. However, the cornea is a fixed structure. Like the lens on a fixed-focus camera, the cornea cannot be adjusted to focus on nearby objects. Without the adjustable lens, the eye would be unable to focus on objects close at hand.

The lens is a flexible structure whose shape is controlled by the muscles in the ciliary body that are attached via the suspensory ligament. When the muscles of the ciliary body are relaxed, the suspensory ligament is taut, and the lens is somewhat flattened. As **FIGURE 12-11A** shows, light from distant objects comes to the eye as nearly parallel rays. The fixed refractive power of the cornea and the refractive power of the lens in its relaxed state are sufficient to bend these beams to bring them into focus on the retina.

As **FIGURE 12-11B** shows, light rays from nearby objects are divergent. To focus on nearby objects, the lens must become more curved. When the eye focuses on nearby objects, the ciliary smooth muscle contracts, causing the suspensory ligament to relax (**FIGURE 12-12B**). The lens thickens and shortens, becoming more curved, in much the same way that a rubber ball flattened between your hands will return to normal when you reduce the

FIGURE 12-10 Refraction   The pencil in the glass of water appears to bend. Actually, the light rays coming to our eyes are bent as they pass through the water and glass, making the pencil appear bent.

pressure on it. This automatic adjustment in the curvature of the lens as it focuses on a nearby object is called **accommodation** (**FIGURE 12-12**). Accommodation increases the refractive (bending) power of the lens.

Accommodation Is Enhanced by Pupillary Constriction.   As the eyes focus on a nearby object, the pupils constrict. Pupillary constriction is a reflex that eliminates divergent rays of light that would otherwise strike the periphery of the lens. Without pupillary constriction, images of nearby objects would be quite blurred, for the lens would be unable to bend these rays sufficiently to bring them into focus on the retina.

Synchronized Eye Movement and Convergence.   Six muscles located outside the eye, the **extrinsic eye muscles**, are responsible for eye movement (**FIGURE 12-13**). As noted earlier, these muscles attach to the orbit (the bony eye socket) and to the sclera (the white of the eye).

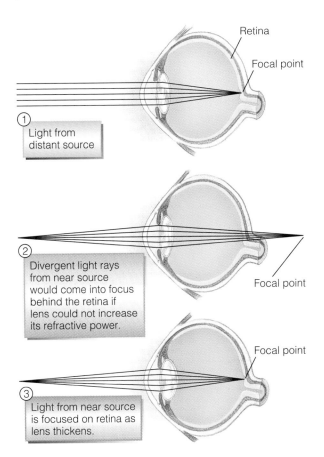

Retina

Focal point

① Light from distant source

② Divergent light rays from near source would come into focus behind the retina if lens could not increase its refractive power.

Focal point

③ Light from near source is focused on retina as lens thickens.

Focal point

FIGURE 12-11 Refraction of Light by the Cornea and Lens
(1) Light rays from distant objects are parallel when they strike the eye. The refractive power of the cornea and resting lens are sufficient to bring them into focus on the retina. (2) Light rays from nearby objects are divergent. The cornea has a fixed refractive power and cannot change. The rays would focus behind the retina if the lens could not alter its refractive power. (3) To focus the image, the ciliary muscles contract. This lessens pressure on the suspensory ligaments, which allows the lens to thicken and shorten, becoming more curved and more refractive.

Relaxed ciliary muscle

Contracted ciliary muscle

Iris

Cornea

Flattened lens

Rounded lens

Taut suspensory ligament

Slackened suspensory ligament

Distant objects in focus
(a)

Close objects in focus
(b)

FIGURE 12-12 Accommodation   (a) The lens is flattened when the ciliary muscles are relaxed. (b) When the ciliary muscles contract, tension on the suspensory ligaments is reduced and the lens shortens and thickens.

FIGURE 12-13 Extrinsic Eye Muscles These muscles move the eye in all directions. They attach to the bony orbit and the sclera.

Eyelid muscle

Optic nerve

Place an index finger gently over the closed lid. Then hold the other hand in front of your face and move it back and forth, then up and down, following it with your opened eye. You should feel your closed eye moving in sync.

When a nearby object is viewed, the eyes turn inward—that is, they converge. **Convergence** ensures that near images are focused on each fovea. Because convergence occurs during all near-point work—reading, writing, sewing, knitting—it tends to strain the extrinsic eye muscles, creating eyestrain.

Alterations in the Shape of the Lens and Eyeball Cause the Most Common Visual Problems

In a relaxed eye with perfect vision, objects farther than 6 meters (20 feet) away fall into perfect focus on the retina (**FIGURE 12-14A**). Many individuals, however, have imperfectly shaped eyeballs or defective lenses. These imperfections result in three visual problems: nearsightedness, farsightedness, and astigmatism.

The eyes generally move in unison like a pair of synchronized swimmers. Synchronized movement is an evolutionary adaptation that ensures that images are focused on the foveas of both eyes at the same time. To test the synchronized movement, close one of your eyes.

FIGURE 12-14 Common Visual Problems

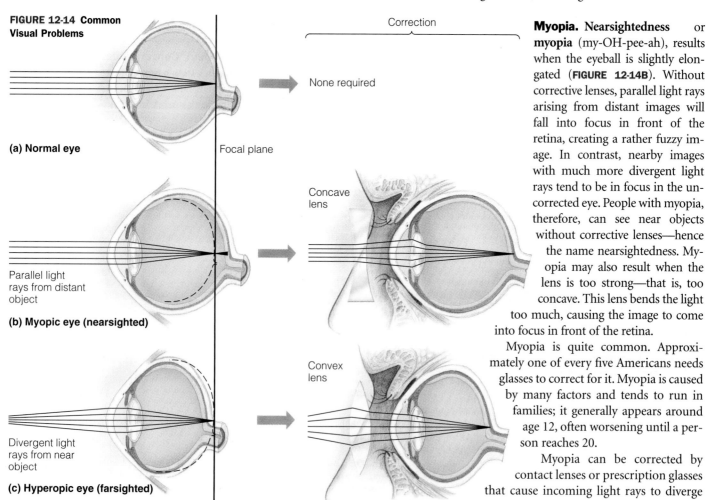

Correction

None required

(a) Normal eye

Focal plane

Concave lens

Parallel light rays from distant object

(b) Myopic eye (nearsighted)

Convex lens

Divergent light rays from near object

(c) Hyperopic eye (farsighted)

Myopia. Nearsightedness or **myopia** (my-OH-pee-ah), results when the eyeball is slightly elongated (**FIGURE 12-14B**). Without corrective lenses, parallel light rays arising from distant images will fall into focus in front of the retina, creating a rather fuzzy image. In contrast, nearby images with much more divergent light rays tend to be in focus in the uncorrected eye. People with myopia, therefore, can see near objects without corrective lenses—hence the name nearsightedness. Myopia may also result when the lens is too strong—that is, too concave. This lens bends the light too much, causing the image to come into focus in front of the retina.

Myopia is quite common. Approximately one of every five Americans needs glasses to correct for it. Myopia is caused by many factors and tends to run in families; it generally appears around age 12, often worsening until a person reaches 20.

Myopia can be corrected by contact lenses or prescription glasses that cause incoming light rays to diverge

(**FIGURE 12-14B**). Contact lenses fit on the surface of the cornea and bend the incoming light rays outward, thereby compensating for the shape of the eye or a defective lens.

Although they're useful in correcting vision, contact lenses can result in serious problems. The largest study of their use in the United States suggests that extended-wear contact lenses, those worn overnight and for up to a week at a time, carry a far greater risk of serious complications than daily-wear lenses. This study of over 22,000 lens wearers showed that sight-threatening complications, such as corneal abrasion, growth of blood vessels into the cornea, corneal ulcers, and severe corneal scarring, were two to four times more prevalent in users of extended-wear contacts than in those using daily-wear lenses. Researchers found that 1 in 2000 daily-wear lens users developed corneal ulcers; and 1 in 300 suffered from other serious complications. In extended-wear users, however, 1 in 500 suffered from corneal ulcers, and 1 in 100 had other serious reactions, suggesting that you should think carefully before choosing extended-wear contacts.

Hyperopia. **Hyperopia** (HIGH-per-OPE-ee-ah), or **farsightedness,** is the opposite of myopia. It results when the eyeballs are too short or the lens is too weak (too convex). In the eyes of farsighted individuals, parallel light rays from distant objects usually fall into focus on the retina, but divergent rays from nearby objects cannot be focused sufficiently. Without corrective lenses, farsighted individuals see distant objects well, but nearby objects are fuzzy. Glasses or contact lenses that bend the light inward bring near objects into sharp focus on the retina (**FIGURE 12-14C**).

Hyperopia is generally present from birth and is usually diagnosed during childhood. Like myopia, it tends to run in families.

Astigmatism. The cornea and lens have uniformly curved surfaces, but either of these surfaces can be slightly disfigured. The surface of the cornea, for example, can have a slightly different curvature in the vertical plane than it does in the horizontal plane. This unequal curvature is called an **astigmatism** (a-STIG-mah-tiz-em). An eye doctor explained it to me as follows. He said that the cornea of a normal eye is round like a basketball. In an astigmatic eye, the cornea is shaped more like the surface of a football.

Astigmatism creates fuzzy images because light rays are bent differently by the different parts of the cornea. Astigmatism is usually present from birth and does not grow worse with age. It can also be corrected with glasses or contact lenses.

Radial Keratotomy and Laser Surgery. Surgeons have also developed a method to correct nearsightedness, called **radial keratotomy (RK)** (RAY-dee-al CARE-ah-TOT-oh-mee). To correct myopia, numerous small, superficial incisions are made in the cornea with a highly precise diamond blade set to a specific depth. Cuts radiate from the center like the spokes of a bicycle wheel. The number of cuts depends on the degree of myopia. This procedure flattens the cornea and reduces its refractive power, causing the rays to diverge and come into focus on the back of the retina.

To correct astigmatism, surgeons make curved or straight incisions in the cornea that help create a round cornea. A round cornea eliminates the blurring caused by distortions in the cornea, as described earlier. Radial keratotomy patients generally recover quickly and suffer minimal discomfort. In studies of the effectiveness of RK, researchers have found that 85 to 99 percent of all RK patients achieve a visual acuity of 20/40 or better. However, the deep incisions required for RK weaken the structural integrity of the eye and make the eye susceptible to traumatic injury. Other problems have also been reported.

Surgeons in the United States and other countries have turned to an even better approach: using lasers to correct myopia. Lasers reshape the surface of the cornea and reduce the amount of refractive error. Two types of laser surgery are widely available in the United States and Canada: PRK and LASIK. Unlike radial keratotomy, in which incisions are made deep into the cornea, laser surgery shaves off microscopic amounts of the cornea, ensuring better structural integrity of the eye.

PRK stands for **photorefractive keratectomy.** In PRK, the surface of the eye is mapped with a sophisticated computer. After mapping, the computer calculates the precise amount of tissue that must be removed to correct vision. It then controls the laser impulses that are used shave off the corneal cells to change the curvature of the lens.

LASIK stands for the tongue twisting scientific description of the process, **lasir in situ keratomileusis** (Care-ah-toe-mill-E-ew-siss). In this procedure, the computer is used to map the eye and calculate the amount of tissue that needs to be removed, as in PRK. However, in LASIK surgery a thin flap of cornea is peeled off using a device known as a microkeratome. The extremely sharp blade shaves off a layer, creating a partial flap, as shown in **FIGURE 12-15A**. The laser is then used to remove tissue and reshape the cornea (**FIGURE 12-15B**). The flap is then folded back into its original position (**FIGURE 12-15C**). It heals shortly.

Laser eye surgery is quick, accurate, but costly. You can pay anywhere from $500 to $2000 per eye, depend-

(a)   **(b)**   **(c)**

FIGURE 12-15 LASIK Surgery   *(a)* Microkeratome slices off a thin layer of corneal tissue *(b)* Laser burns away corneal tissue to correct eyesight. *(c)* Flap is restored, as is vision.

ing on the level of correction and the surgeon. In addition, the procedure appears to be more successful than radial keratotomy as well, with 95 percent of patients achieving 20/40 visual acuity or better. Worldwide, hundreds of thousands of patients have been successfully treated with this procedure. Problems arise in under one percent of the cases.

Eyestrain.   For most of human evolution, people have used their eyes principally for viewing objects at a distance—for example, watching their children play or wild animals roam. Near-point vision probably occupied little of their time. It should come as no surprise, then, to learn that the human eye is best suited for distance vision. Today, however, near-point work is becoming commonplace. This strains the eyes and can cause a progressive deterioration of eyesight. Those who read a lot or spend long periods staring at computer monitors (like textbook authors) often become more nearsighted as they become older. No one knows why, but research suggests that the eye may elongate as a result of constant near-point use.

To reduce eyestrain and the deterioration of eyesight, eye doctors advise that computer operators look away from their screens and that readers look up from their materials regularly, letting their eyes focus on distant objects. This action relaxes the ciliary muscles, reducing eyestrain. (Try it and see if you can feel a difference.) Some ophthalmologists suggest that computer users "blink at every period and look up after every paragraph."

Presbyopia.   The aging process brings with it many joys, among them hair loss, hearing loss, and arthritis. Aging

also results in a decline in the resiliency of the lens. Thus, when the ciliary muscles contract to allow one to focus on a nearby object, the lens responds slowly or only partially, making it difficult to focus. This condition, known as **presbyopia** (PREZ-bee-OPE-ee-a), usually begins around the age of 40 and can be corrected by glasses worn for near-point work such as reading.[4] Presbyopia cannot be corrected by laser eye surgery, because the problem is with the lens, not the cornea.

Color Blindness.   About 5 percent of the human population suffers from color blindness. **Color blindness** is a hereditary disorder, more prevalent in men than women. Characterized by a deficiency in color perception, color blindness ranges from an inability to distinguish certain shades to a complete inability to perceive color. The most common form of this disorder is red-green color blindness.

In individuals with red-green color blindness, the red or green cones may either be missing altogether or be present in reduced number. If the red cones are missing, red objects appear green. If the green cones are missing, however, green objects appear red. Color blindness can be detected by simple tests (**FIGURE 12-16**).

Many color-blind people are unaware of their condition or untroubled by it. They rely on a variety of visual cues such as differences in intensity to distinguish red and green objects. They also rely on position cues. In vertical traffic lights, for example, the red light is always at the top of the signal; green is on the bottom. Al-

---

[4]You may have seen your parents or grandparents holding a phone book at arm's length to read it. They probably argued that their eyes weren't going bad, their arms were just too short!

though the colors may appear more or less the same, the position of the light helps color-blind drivers determine whether to hit the brakes or step on the gas.

Overlapping Visual Fields Give Us Depth Perception

Human eyes are located in the front of the skull, looking forward, much like those of other predatory animals. Each eye has a visual field of about 170 degrees, but the visual fields overlap considerably (**FIGURE 12-17**). This overlapping gives us the ability to judge the relative position of objects in our visual field—that is, it gives us **depth perception,** or **stereoscopic vision.**

Hearing and Balance: The Cochlea and Middle Ear

The human ear is an organ of special sense. It serves two functions: it detects sound, and it detects body position, enabling us to maintain balance (**TABLE 12-4**).

The Ear Consists of Three Anatomically Separate Portions: The Outer, Middle, and Inner Ears

The Outer Ear. The **outer ear** consists of an irregularly shaped piece of cartilage covered by skin, the **auricle**

FIGURE 12-16 Color-Blindness Chart People with red-green color blindness cannot detect the number 29 in this chart.

(OR-eh-kul), and the ear-lobe, a flap of skin that hangs down from the auricle (**FIGURE 12-18**). The outer ear also consists of a short tube, the **external auditory canal,** which transmits airborne sound waves to the middle ear (**FIGURE 12-18A**). The external auditory canal is lined by skin containing modified sweat glands that produce earwax. Earwax traps foreign particles, such as bacteria, and contains a natural antibiotic substance that may reduce ear infections. Earwax may build up in the external auditory canal and, in severe cases, must be flushed out by a doctor or nurse.

The Middle Ear. The **middle ear** lies entirely within the temporal bone of the skull (**FIGURE 12-18B**). The **eardrum,** or **tympanic membrane** (tim-PAN-ick), separates the middle ear cavity from the external auditory canal. The tympanic membrane vibrates when struck by sound waves in much the same way that a guitar string

TABLE 12-4

Structures and Functions of the Ear

Part	Structure	Function
Outer ear	Auricle	Funnels sound waves into external auditory canal
	Ear lobe	
	External auditory canal	Directs sound waves to the eardrum
Middle ear	Tympanic membrane, or eardrum	Vibrates when struck by sound waves
	Ossicles	Transmit sound to the cochlea in the inner ear
Inner ear	Cochlea	Converts fluid waves to nerve impulses
	Semicircular canals	Detect head movement
	Saccule and utricle	Detect head movement and linear acceleration

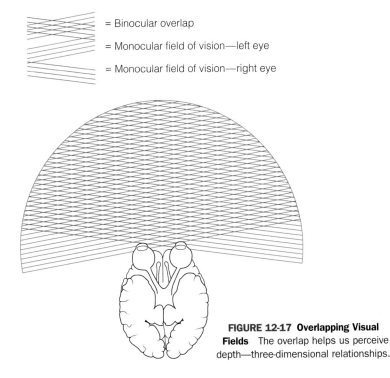

= Binocular overlap

= Monocular field of vision—left eye

= Monocular field of vision—right eye

FIGURE 12-17 Overlapping Visual Fields The overlap helps us perceive depth—three-dimensional relationships.

FIGURE 12-18 The Structures of the Ear   *(a)* Cross section showing the structures of the outer, middle, and inner ears. *(b)* The receptors for balance and sound are located in the inner ear.

vibrates when a note is sounded by another nearby instrument.

Inside the middle ear are three minuscule bones, the **ossicles** (OSS-eh-kuls). Starting from the outside, they are the **malleus** (pronounced MAL-ee-us; hammer), **incus** (IN-cuss; anvil), and **stapes** (STAY-pees; stirrup). As illustrated in **FIGURE 12-18B**, the hammer-shaped malleus abuts the tympanic membrane. When the membrane is struck by sound waves, it vibrates. This causes the malleus to rock back and forth. The malleus, in turn, causes the incus to vibrate, which causes the stapes, the stirrup-shaped bone, to move in and out against the **oval window,** an opening to the inner ear covered with a membrane like the skin on a drum. Thus, vibrations created in the eardrum are amplified as they are transmitted to the inner ear, where the sound receptors are located.

As **FIGURE 12-18** illustrates, the middle ear cavity opens to the pharynx via the **auditory,** or **eustachian, tube** (you-STAY-shun). The eustachian tube serves as a pressure valve. Normally, the eustachian tube is closed. Yawning and swallowing, however, cause it to open, allowing air to flow into or out of the middle ear cavity. This equalizes the internal and external pressure on the eardrum, as you will notice when taking off in an airplane.

Scuba divers and swimmers can sustain considerable damage to an eardrum as they ascend or descend. As a diver descends, for instance, pressure from the water builds, pushing the eardrum inward. To prevent the eardrum from tearing, air must be forced into the middle ear cavity. This can be done by holding one's nose, clamping one's mouth shut, and gently blowing. Air is

forced through the eustachian tube into the middle ear cavity. When a diver ascends, just the opposite happens: Air pressure increases inside the middle ear cavity. The diver must release the pressure or else suffer a broken eardrum. This release usually occurs quite naturally, but it can be facilitated by yawning.

The Inner Ear. The inner ear occupies a large cavity in the temporal bone and contains two sensory organs, the cochlea and the vestibular apparatus. The **cochlea** (COE-klee-ah) is shaped like a snail shell and houses the receptors for hearing.

The **vestibular apparatus** consists of two parts: the semicircular canals and the vestibule (**FIGURE 12-18B**). The **semicircular canals** are three ringlike structures set at right angles to one another. They house receptors for body position and movement. The **vestibule** is a bony chamber lying between the cochlea and semicircular canals. It also houses receptors that respond to body position and movement.

Hearing Requires the Participation of Several Structures

As noted previously, sound waves enter the external auditory canal, where they strike the tympanic membrane, or eardrum. The eardrum vibrates back and forth, causing the ossicles of the middle ear cavity to vibrate. The ossicles, in turn, transmit sound waves to the cochlea, which houses the receptor for sound.

Structure and Function of the Cochlea. The cochlea is a hollow, bony spiral. A cross section through this remarkable structure reveals three fluid-filled canals (**FIGURE 12-19A**). Separating the middle canal from the lowermost one is a flexible membrane called the **basilar membrane** (BAZ-eh-ler). It supports the **organ of Corti,** the receptor organ for sound.

The organ of Corti contains receptor cells, the **hair cells** (**FIGURE 12-19B**). Cellular projections from the hair cells contact the overlying **tectorial membrane** (teck-TORE-ee-al). When sound waves are transmitted from the middle ear to the inner ear, they create pressure waves in the fluid in the uppermost canal of the cochlea, the **vestibular canal.** As shown in **FIGURE 12-20A**, in which the cochlea is unwound, the stirrup transmits vibrations to the drumlike **oval window,** the opening in

the cochlea. Fluid pressure waves created in the vestibular canal then travel through the vestibular membrane into the middle canal, the **cochlear duct** (**canal**). From here, the pressure waves pass through the basilar membrane into the lowermost canal, the **tympanic canal.** Pressure is relieved by the outward bulging of the **round window,** an opening in the bony cochlea, which, like the oval window, is spanned by a flexible membrane.

In their course through the cochlea, the pressure waves cause the basilar membrane to vibrate. This vibration stimulates the hair cells. The hair cells respond by releasing a neurotransmitter, which stimulates the dendrites wrapped around their bases. The nerve impulses travel to the auditory cortex via the **vestibulocochlear nerve** (vess-TIB-you-low-COE-klee-er), one of the 12 cranial nerves.

Distinguishing Pitch and Intensity. A pitch pipe helps a singer find the note to begin a song. It has a range of notes from high to low. The ear can distinguish between these various pitches, or frequencies, in large part because of the structure of the basilar membrane. The basilar membrane underlying the organ of Corti is stiff and narrow at the oval window, where fluid pressure waves are first established inside the cochlea (**FIGURE 12-20B**). As the basilar membrane proceeds to the apex of the spiral, however, it becomes wider and more flexible. The change in width and stiffness results in marked differences in its ability to vibrate. The narrow, stiff end, for example, vibrates maximally when pressure waves from high-frequency sounds ("high

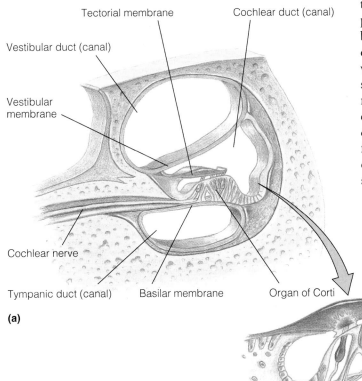

Tectorial membrane

Cochlear duct (canal)

Vestibular duct (canal)

Vestibular membrane

Cochlear nerve

Tympanic duct (canal)   Basilar membrane   Organ of Corti

(a)

FIGURE 12-19 Cross Section Through the Cochlea *(a)* Notice the three fluid-filled canals and the central position of the organ of Corti. *(b)* Hair cells of the organ of Corti are embedded in the overlying tectorial membrane. When the basilar membrane vibrates, the hair cells are stimulated.

Tectorial membrane moves, stimulating the hair cells

Hair cells

(b)

Deflection of basilar membrane, because of fluid movements in the cochlea, stimulates the new cells

FIGURE 12-20 The Transmission of Sound Waves Through the Cochlea   The cochlea is unwound here to simplify matters. *(a)* Vibrations are transmitted from the stirrup (stapes) to the oval window. Fluid pressure waves are established in the vestibular canal and pass to the tympanic canal, causing the basilar membrane to vibrate. *(b)* A representation of the basilar membrane, showing the points along its length where the various wavelengths of sound are perceived. Notice that the basilar membrane is narrowest at the base of the cochlea at the oval window end and widest at the apex. *(c)* High-frequency sounds set the basilar membrane near the base of the cochlea into motion. Hair cells send impulses to the brain, which interprets the signals as a high-pitch sound. Low-frequency sounds stimulate the basilar membrane where it is widest and most flexible.

The numbers indicate the frequencies with which different regions of the basilar membrane maximally vibrate.

notes") are present (**FIGURE 12-20C**). The far end of the membrane vibrates maximally with low-frequency sounds ("low notes"). In between, the membrane responds to a wide range of intermediate frequencies.

Pressure waves caused by any given sound stimulate one specific region of the organ of Corti. The hair cells stimulated in that region send impulses to the brain, which it interprets as a specific pitch. Each region of the organ of Corti sends impulses to a specific region of the auditory cortex in the temporal lobe of the brain. Thus, the auditory cortex can be mapped according to tone in much the same way the motor and sensory cortex can be mapped (Chapter 11).

The intensity of a sound, or its loudness, depends on the amplitude of the vibration in the basilar mem-

brane. The louder the sound, the more vigorous the vibration of the eardrum. The more vigorous the vibration of the eardrum, the greater the deflection of the basilar membrane in the area of peak responsiveness. The greater the deflection of the basilar membrane, the more hair cells are stimulated. Loud rock music or sirens, however, cause extreme vibrations in the basilar membrane, destroying hair cells over time and causing partial deafness.

Hearing Loss. As people grow older, many lose their hearing, but hearing loss usually occurs so slowly that most people are unaware of it. In some cases, though, people lose their hearing suddenly. A loud explosion, for example, can damage the hair cells or even break the ossicles.

Hearing losses may be temporary or permanent, partial or complete. Hearing loss falls into one of two categories, depending on the part of the system that is affected. The first is **conduction deafness,** which occurs when the conduction of sound waves to the inner ear is impaired. Conduction deafness may result from excessive earwax in the auditory canal or a rupture of the eardrum. Damage to the ossicles and rupture of the oval window are additional causes.

Conduction deafness most often results from infections in the middle ear. Bacterial infections may result in the buildup of scar tissue that causes the ossicles to fuse and lose their ability to transmit sound. Infections of the middle ear usually enter through the eustachian tube. Thus, a sore throat or a cold can easily spread to the ear, where it requires prompt treatment. Ear infections are especially common in babies and young children. If undetected, middle ear infections can slow down the development of speech. If untreated, such infections can lead to permanent deafness.

Conduction deafness is treated by hearing aids. A **hearing aid** usually fits in the ear or just behind it (**FIGURE 12-21**). These devices bypass the defective sound-conduction system by transmitting sound waves through the bone of the skull to the inner ear. These cause fluid pressure waves to form in the cochlea and stimulate the basilar membrane.

The second type of hearing loss is neurological and is called **nerve,** or **sensineural, deafness.** Sensineural deafness results from physical damage to the hair cells, the vestibulocochlear nerve, or the auditory cortex. Explosions, extremely loud noises, and some antibiotics can all damage the hair cells in the organ of Corti, creating partial to complete deafness. The auditory nerve, which conducts impulses from the organ of Corti to the cortex, may degenerate, thus ending the flow of information to the cortex. Tumors in the brain or strokes can destroy the cells of the auditory cortex.

Although the ear is vulnerable to loud noise and other problems, it contains a mechanism to protect itself from damage. This mechanism consists of two tiny skeletal muscles (the smallest in the body) located in the middle ear cavity. One of these muscles inserts on the malleus, and the other attaches to the stapes. As noted earlier, the malleus attaches to the eardrum, and the stapes attaches to the oval window. Loud noises stimulate a reflex contraction of the middle ear muscles, pulling them away from their membrane contacts. Whenever an individual is exposed to loud noise, this reflex reduces the conduction of the noise to the inner ear. Unfortunately, the reflex requires about 40 milliseconds, so it cannot protect the ear from explosions.

Correcting Profound Deafness. More than 2 million Americans are profoundly deaf. Until recently, this condition was considered virtually untreatable.

Children who are born deaf or are deafened before they begin to speak often fail to mature emotionally. Even reading comprehension can be impaired. Some profoundly deaf children, in fact, never advance beyond third- or fourth-grade reading levels.

Hearing aids usually cannot help individuals who are born deaf or those who suffer from nerve damage. Researchers, however, have developed a device, called a **cochlear implant**, which simulates the function of the inner ear remarkably (**FIGURE 12-22**). This device picks

FIGURE 12-21 Hearing Aids Worn by people with conduction deafness, hearing aids send sound impulses through the bone of the skull to the cochlea.

FIGURE 12-22 Cochlear Implant The cochlear implant can correct for nerve deafness. Electrodes convey electrical impulses from a small microphone mounted in the ear to the auditory nerve.

up sound and transmits it to a receiver implanted inside the skull. The signal then travels to an electrode implanted in the vestibulocochlear nerve. Electrical impulses in the electrode stimulate the nerve, creating impulses that travel to the auditory cortex.

Today, hundreds of adults and children are equipped with cochlear implants, which detect and transmit a wider range of sounds. Recipients of the new models can perceive many distinct words. Some individuals equipped with these devices have apparently developed a remarkable ability to perceive sounds. Cochlear implants also help the deaf monitor and regulate their voices and make lip reading easier.

The Vestibular Apparatus Houses Receptors That Detect Body Position and Movement

The cochlea lies next to the **vestibular apparatus.** As noted earlier, it consists of the two parts, the semicircular canals and the vestibule. The vestibule is a bony chamber between the cochlea and semicircular canals. The vestibular apparatus houses receptors that detect body position and movement (**FIGURE 12-23**).

The Semicircular Canals. The three semicircular canals are arranged at right angles to one another. Each canal is filled with a fluid called **endolymph.** As **FIGURE 12-23A** shows, the base of each semicircular canal expands to form the **ampulla** (AM-pew-lah). On the inside wall of each ampulla is a small ridge of tissue, or **crista** (CHRIS-tah). Each crista consists of a patch of receptor cells. Each receptor cell contains numerous microvilli and a single cilium embedded in a cap of gelatinous material, the **cupula** (CUE-pew-lah), shown in **FIGURE 12-23B**. Dendrites of sensory nerves wrap around the base of the receptor cells, and the cupula extends into the cavity of the ampulla, where it is bathed in endolymph.

Rotation of the head causes the endolymph in the semicircular canals to move. The movement of the fluid deflects the cupula, which stimulates the hair cells to release a neurotransmitter. This excites the sensory neurons, which send impulses to the brain, alerting it to the rotational movement of the head and body.

Because the semicircular canals are set in all three planes of space, movement in any direction can be detected. By alerting the brain to rotation and movement, the semicircular canals contribute to our sense of balance. They are therefore important to **dynamic balance**— helping us stay balanced when in movement.

The Utricle and Saccule. Two additional receptors play a role in balance and the detection of movement, the **utricle** (YOU-treh-kul) and **saccule** (SACK-yule) (**FIGURE 12-23**). These membranous compartments inside the

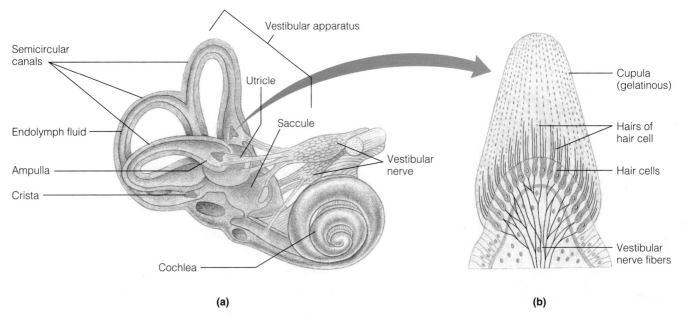

(a)   (b)

FIGURE 12-23 Vestibular Apparatus and Semicircular Canals
(a) This illustration shows the location of the cristae in the ampullae of the semicircular canals. The semicircular canals are filled with endolymph. *(b)* When the head spins, the endolymph is set into motion, deflecting the gelatinous cupula of the crista, thus stimulating the receptor cells.

vestibule provide input under two distinctly different conditions: at rest and during acceleration in a straight line. As a result, these receptors contribute dynamic balance and **static balance**—helping us stay balanced when we are not moving.

The utricle and saccule contain small receptor organs akin to the cristae of the semicircular canals. The nerve impulses generated by the receptors in the semicircular canals and the utricle and saccule are sent to a cluster of nerve cell bodies in the brain stem. Here all of the information the receptors generate on position and movement is integrated with input from the eyes and from receptors in the skin, joints, and muscles (earlier in this chapter). From this center, information flows in many directions. One major pathway leads to the cerebral cortex. This path makes us conscious of our position and movement. Another path leads to the muscles of the limbs and torso. Signals to the muscles maintain our balance and, if necessary, correct body position.

In some people, activation of the vestibular apparatus results in motion sickness, characterized by dizziness and nausea. The exact cause of motion sickness is not known.

Health, Homeostasis, and the Environment

Noise Pollution

The nervous system is essential to homeostasis because it regulates many activities aimed at maintaining a stable internal environment. This, in turn, depends on receptors that provide input essential for homeostasis. While it is fairly obvious that the general senses are involved in regulating key physiological functions essential to homeostasis, what about the special senses?

The special senses help us—and other animals—acquire food, defend ourselves against danger, and affect other behavioral responses that are essential to homeostasis. Damage to these senses may therefore have profound effects. Consider noise.

Noise is one of the most widespread environmental pollutants in modern industrial societies. It may be turning industrial nations into countries of the hearing-impaired. Traffic noise, airport noise, loud music, crowd noise, and other loud sounds so common in modern society may be slowly destroying our hearing. By the time many New York City residents reach the age of 20, their hearing has been so impaired that they hear only as well as a 70-year-old African Bushman who has lived a life free of city noises.

For many years, scientists attributed the decline in hearing to middle ear infections, certain antibiotics, and the natural deterioration of the hair cells. New research, however, suggests that noise is probably the principal cause of hearing loss in modern societies.

Like that of any other pollutant, the damage caused by noise is related to two factors: exposure level (how loud a noise is) and the duration of exposure (how long one is exposed to it). In general, the louder the noise, the more damaging it is. In addition, the longer you are exposed to a damaging level of noise, the more hearing loss you will suffer.

The noise to which people are exposed in factories and at construction sites is sufficient to cause gradual hearing loss. A worker may notice a dulled sense of hearing after working in a noisy environment; this is called a **temporary threshold shift.** Over time, the continued assault leads to a **permanent threshold shift,** complete hearing loss in certain frequencies. In most cases, hearing loss occurs so gradually that workers do not notice it until it is too late.

The intensity of sound is measured in **decibels** (DESS-seh-bells) or **dB. TABLE 12-5** lists the dB level of some common sounds. Surprising new research shows that continuous exposure to sounds over 55 decibels can result in hearing loss. Light traffic and an air conditioner operating 6 meters (18 feet) from you are 60-decibel sounds.

Besides deafening us to the important sounds of modern life, noise disturbs communications, rest, and sleep. The latter two are particularly important to homeostasis and health. Noise also raises our level of stress, which, in turn, shortens our lives. When hearing is impaired, communication falters, and tensions often rise. People who are losing their hearing complain that they feel inadequate in social situations.

Hearing loss is not inevitable. You can take steps to protect your hearing. Keep your stereo at a reasonable level. Avoid noisy events. Cover your ears when an ambulance or fire engine approaches. Wear ear plugs or ear guards when operating firearms or noisy equipment such as vacuum cleaners, chain saws, or construction equipment. Get treatment if you develop an ear infection. Prevention is the best medicine, because once you lose your hearing, it is gone forever.

Recognizing the importance of hearing, a nonprofit organization called Hearing Education Awareness for Rockers (HEAR) works with radio stations in the United States and Canada to protect audiences from loud rock music. In 1996, they gave out over 60,000 earplugs to concert attendees. Even some rock bands, like Motley Crue, now sell ear protectors at concerts.

TABLE 12-5

The Decibel Scale

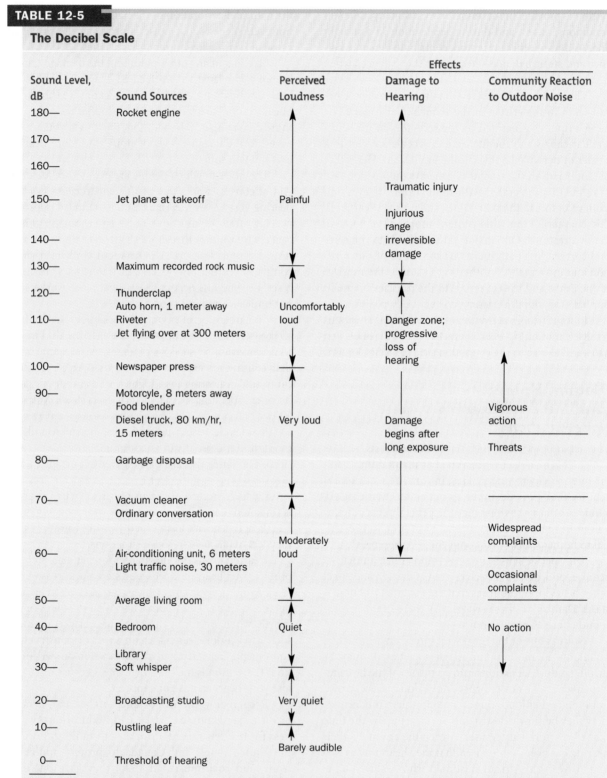

Sound Level, dB	Sound Sources	Effects		
		Perceived Loudness	Damage to Hearing	Community Reaction to Outdoor Noise
180—	Rocket engine			
170—				
160—				
150—	Jet plane at takeoff	Painful	Traumatic injury	
140—			Injurious range irreversible damage	
130—	Maximum recorded rock music			
120—	Thunderclap	Uncomfortably loud		
110—	Auto horn, 1 meter away / Riveter / Jet flying over at 300 meters		Danger zone; progressive loss of hearing	
100—	Newspaper press			
90—	Motorcyle, 8 meters away / Food blender / Diesel truck, 80 km/hr, 15 meters	Very loud	Damage begins after long exposure	Vigorous action
80—	Garbage disposal			Threats
70—	Vacuum cleaner / Ordinary conversation			
60—	Air-conditioning unit, 6 meters / Light traffic noise, 30 meters	Moderately loud		Widespread complaints / Occasional complaints
50—	Average living room			
40—	Bedroom	Quiet		No action
30—	Library / Soft whisper			
20—	Broadcasting studio	Very quiet		
10—	Rustling leaf			
		Barely audible		
0—	Threshold of hearing			

SOURCE: Table from *Environmental Science*, 3rd ed., by Jonathan Turk and Amos Turk. Copyright © 1984 by Saunders College Publishing. Reproduced by permission of the publisher.

Summary

The General and Special Senses

1. The body contains two types of receptors—those that provide general senses and those that provide special senses.

The General Senses

2. The *general senses* are pain, light touch, pressure, temperature, and position sense. Receptors for these senses may be naked or encapsulated nerve endings.

3. Receptors fit into five functional categories: (a) *mechanoreceptors,* (b) *thermoreceptors,* (c) *photoreceptors,* (d) *chemoreceptors,* and (e) *pain receptors (nociceptors).*

4. Sensory stimuli may be internal or external. Some stimuli cause reflex actions. Still others may stimulate physiological changes.

5. The *naked nerve ending receptors* in the body include those stimulated by pain, light touch, and temperature. The *encapsulated receptors* include those that detect pressure *(Pacinian corpuscles),* light touch *(Meissner's corpuscles,* Krause's end-bulbs, and Ruffini's corpuscles), and muscle extension *(muscle spindles* and *Golgi tendon organs).*

6. Many sensory receptors cease responding to prolonged stimuli, a phenomenon called *sensory adaptation.* Pain, temperature, pressure, and olfactory receptors all adapt.

Taste and Smell: The Chemical Senses

7. The *special senses* include taste, smell, vision, hearing, and balance, which are made possible by more elaborate receptor organs.

8. Taste receptors called *taste buds* are located principally on the upper surface of the tongue. Taste buds contain receptor cells. Food molecules dissolve in the saliva and bind to the membranes of the microvilli of the receptor cells.

9. Taste buds respond to five flavors: salty, bitter, sweet, sour, and umami.

10. The receptors for smell are located in the *olfactory membrane* in the roof of the nasal cavities. The receptor cells in the olfactory membrane respond to thousands of different molecules, which bind to membrane receptors on the olfactory hairs, stimulating nerve impulses that are transmitted to the brain via the olfactory nerve.

The Visual Sense: The Eye

11. The *eye* is the receptor for visual stimuli and is located in the orbit, a bony socket.

12. The wall of the human eye consists of three layers. The outermost layer consists of the *sclera* (the white of the eye) and the *cornea* (the clear anterior structure that lets light shine in).

13. The middle layer consists of the *choroid* (the pigmented and vascularized region), the *ciliary body* (whose muscles control the lens), and the *iris* (which controls the amount of light entering the eye).

14. The innermost layer is the *retina,* the light-sensitive layer, which contains two types of photoreceptors: rods and cones. *Rods* function in dim light and provide black-and-white vision, and *cones* operate in bright light and provide color vision. Cones are also responsible for visual acuity. The highest concentration of cones is found in the *fovea centralis.*

15. Light is focused on the retina by the cornea and *lens.* The cornea has a fixed refractive power, but the lens can be adjusted to bend light according to need. The muscles of the ciliary body play an important role in this process. Focusing on near objects is aided by pupillary constriction.

16. The lens may become cloudy with old age or because of exposure to excess ultraviolet radiation. This condition, called *cataracts,* can be corrected by surgically removing the lens and replacing it with a plastic one.

17. The eye is divided into two cavities. The *posterior cavity* lies behind the lens and is filled with a gelatinous material, the *vitreous humor.* The *anterior cavity* is filled with a plasmalike fluid called the *aqueous humor,* which nourishes the lens and other eye structures in the vicinity. If the rate of absorption of aqueous humor decreases, however, pressure can build inside the anterior cavity, resulting in *glaucoma.*

18. As people age, the lens becomes less resilient and less able to focus on nearby objects, a condition called *presbyopia.*

19. *Myopia,* or nearsightedness, results from a lens that is too strong (too concave) or from an elongated eyeball. In the uncorrected eye, the image from distant objects comes in focus in front of the retina.

20. *Hyperopia* results from a weak lens (too convex) or from a shortened eyeball. In the uncorrected eye, light rays from an image nearby would come into focus behind the retina.

21. *Astigmatism* is an irregularly curved lens or cornea that creates fuzzy images.

22. Three types of cones are present in the eye: red, green, and blue. Each type responds maximally to one specific color of light. Intermediate colors activate two or more types of cones.

23. *Color blindness* is a genetic disorder, more common in men than women. It results from a deficiency or an absence of one or more types of cones. Red-green color blindness is the most common type.

Hearing and Balance: The Cochlea and Middle Ear

24. The human ear consists of three portions: the outer, middle, and inner ears.

25. The *outer ear* consists of the *auricle* and *external auditory canal,* both of which direct sound to the *eardrum.*

26. The *middle ear* consists of the eardrum and three small bones, the ossicles, which transmit vibrations to the inner ear.

27. The *auditory tube* equilibrates the pressure inside the middle ear cavity.

28. The *inner ear* contains the cochlea where the receptors for sound are located. The inner ear also houses receptors for movement and head position: the semicircular canals, *utricle,* and *saccule.*

29. The *cochlea* is a spiral-shaped, bony structure that contains three fluid-filled canals. Separating the middle canal from the lower one is the flexible *basilar membrane* which supports the *organ of Corti.* Hair cells in the organ of Corti are embedded in the relatively rigid *tectorial membrane.*

30. Sound waves create vibrations in the eardrum and ossicles, which are transmitted to fluid in the cochlea. Pressure waves in the cochlea cause the basilar membrane to vibrate, which stimulates the hair cells.

31. Pressure waves resulting from any given sound cause one part of the membrane to vibrate maximally. The hair cells stimulated in that region send signals to the brain, which it interprets as a specific frequency.

32. Hearing loss may occur as a result of damage or blockage to the conducting system: the external auditory canal, the eardrum, and the ossicles. Damage to the hair cells, the auditory nerve, or the auditory cortex are forms of *nerve deafness.*

33. The *semicircular canals* are three hollow rings filled with a fluid called *en-*

dolymph. The receptors for head movement are located in an enlarged portion at the base of each canal, the *ampulla.*

34. Fluid movement inside the semicircular canals deflects the gelatinous cap *(cupula)* lying over the receptor cells, stimulating them and alerting the brain to head movements.

35. The semicircular canals are set in all three planes of space so that movement in any direction can be detected.

36. Two membranous sacs in the *vestibule,* the *utricle* and *saccule,* contain receptors that respond to linear acceleration and tilting of the head.

Health, Homeostasis, and the Environment: Noise Pollution

37. Receptors that provide for the general and special senses are extremely important to homeostasis.

38. Noise damages the ears. Extremely loud noises can rupture the eardrum or break the ossicles. Less intense noises, however, generally destroy hearing gradually by damaging hair cells. In most people, hearing loss occurs so gradually as to be undetected.

39. Besides deafening us and cutting us off from the important sounds of modern life, noise disturbs communications, rest, and sleep—the last two of which are particularly important to homeostasis and health. Noise also raises our level of stress, which, in turn, shortens our lives.

Critical Thinking

Thinking Critically—Analysis

This Analysis corresponds to the Thinking Critically scenario that was presented at the beginning of this chapter.

If I were in this predicament, I would want to learn more about the researchers' experiments. Were they conducted properly? Did they have an adequate number of animals? Have others repeated the experiments with the same results? Did the chemical toxins affect other cells of the ner-

vous system? What were the side effects? Did the procedure result in a lasting cure or was it just transient? How long did they follow the rats they used to determine the long-term effectiveness and side effects of the treatment? Has this procedure or any similar procedures ever been tried on people before? What were the results? What kind of care will be provided if you suffer any side effects? Will the procedure render you insensitive to pain medications?

Clearly, there's a lot to be learned before you subject yourself to this potentially beneficial procedure. While the promise of pain relief may be overwhelming, the stakes are high.

Test of Concepts

1. Define the terms *general senses* and *special senses.*

2. Using your knowledge of the senses and of other organ systems gained from previous chapters, describe the role that sensory receptors play in homeostasis. Give specific examples to illustrate your main points.

3. Make a list of both the encapsulated and the nonencapsulated general sense receptors. Note where each is located and what it does.

4. Define the term *adaptation.* What advantages does it confer? Can you think of any disadvantages?

5. Describe the receptors for taste, explaining where they are located, what they look like, and how they operate.

6. Taste buds detect five basic flavors. What are they? How do you account for the thousands of different flavors that you can detect?

7. Describe the olfactory membrane and the structure of the receptor cells. How do these cells operate? In what ways are taste receptors and olfactory receptors similar? In what ways are they different?

8. Explain the following statement: taste and smell are complementary.

9. Draw a cross section of the human eye and label its parts.

10. Define the following terms: retina, rods, cones, fovea centralis, optic disc, ganglion cells, bipolar neurons, and optic nerve.

11. Compare and contrast rods and cones.

12. When focusing on a nearby object, your eyes go through several changes. Describe those changes and what they accomplish.

13. Define the following terms: myopia, hyperopia, presbyopia, and astigmatism.

14. You walk into a dark movie theater and find that you can barely make out the aisle. After a while, your vision recovers. Explain both phenomena.

15. What is color blindness? What is the most common type? Explain what your world would look like if you were afflicted by red-green color blindness.

16. What is a cataract, and how is it treated?

17. Describe the disease known as glaucoma. What causes it, and how is it treated?

18. Describe the anatomy of the ear and the role of the outer, middle, and inner ears in hearing.

19. How do the semicircular canals operate? How do the utricle and saccule operate?

20. Describe the different types of deafness and how they are treated.

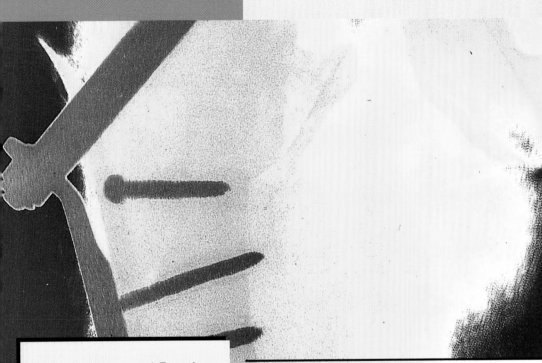

CHAPTER 13

The Skeleton and Muscles

X ray of hip socket and femur showing steel rods used to repair the broken bone.

Thinking **Critically**

A study on osteoporosis in Australian women involving 120 nonsmokers, ranging in age from 50 to 60, concluded that the best prevention against bone fractures is estrogen-replacement therapy. During the 2-year study, the researchers examined the density of bone in the forearms of the women at 3-month intervals. Initial measurements showed very low levels of calcium, which indicates a high risk of fractures.

The women were then divided into three groups. The first group received a placebo, the second group received 1 gram of calcium per day, and the third group received daily doses of estrogen and progesterone (sex steroid hormones). All the women were encouraged to take two brisk 30-minute walks every day and engage in one low-impact aerobics class each week.

The study showed that bone loss continued in the control group (group 1, exercise only) at a rate of 2.5% per year. Bone loss also continued in group 2, which received a daily dose of calcium, but was slower than in group 1 (0.5%–1.3% per year). In group 3, whose participants exercised and received hormone therapy, bone density increased from 0.8% to 2.7% per year.

Given the potential side effects of hormone therapy, the researchers recommended that only women with lowest bone densities receive hormone therapy and that others should exercise and take calcium to reduce their risk of osteoporosis.

Can you pinpoint any potential flaws in the experiment's design or execution? How could they be corrected? ■

Thomas Powers is a 40-year-old college professor. Like many of his friends, he likes to downhill ski. But lately, his skiing has been curtailed by chronic knee pain from an old skiing injury. After visiting his doctor, he found that years ago a spill on the slopes tore some cartilage in his knee. Although it never really healed, the tear caused few problems until he recently took up mountain biking. The additional strain combined with some degeneration of the knee joint itself conspired to create an intolerable situation.

This chapter discusses the human skeleton, including the joints, like those troubling Professor Powers. It also examines the skeletal muscles. Together, the bones, joints, and muscles constitute the **musculoskeletal system**. In adults, bones and muscles make up a remarkable 50%–60% of the body weight.

Section 13-1

Structure and Function of the Human Skeleton

The word **skeleton** is derived from a Greek word that means "dried-up body." Your first impression of bone might not be much different (**FIGURE 13-1**). Bone, after all, appears to be a dry, dead structure. But appearances can be deceiving. The truth be known, bone is a is living, metabolically active tissue. Bone tissue contains numerous cells, known as **osteocytes** (OSS-tee-oh-SITES). These cells are embedded in an extracellular material, known as the **matrix** (MAY-tricks). The matrix consists of calcium phosphate crystals, which impart hardness and strength. It is deposited on an organic component, **collagen fibers** (COLL-ah-gin), made of protein. The collagen imparts flexibility.

FIGURE 13-1 Bone When most people think about bones, they picture a dried-out, lifeless structure. In reality, bones are living tissues that perform many functions essential to homeostasis.

Bones Serve Many Functions and Play an Important Role in Homeostasis

The human skeleton consists of 206 bones, discrete structures made of bone tissue (**FIGURE 13-2**). Bones provide internal structural support, giving shape to our bodies and enabling us to maintain an upright posture. Some bones protect internal organs. The rib cage, for instance, protects the lungs and heart, and the skull forms a protective shell for the brain. Bones serve as the site of attachment for the tendons of many skeletal muscles whose contraction results in purposeful movements. Bones are home to cells that give rise to red blood cells, white blood cells, and platelets. Bones are a storage depot for fat, needed for cellular energy production at work and at rest. Finally, bones are a reservoir of calcium and other minerals. Bones release and absorb calcium as needed, which helps maintain normal blood levels. That's important because calcium is required for muscle contraction. Disturbances in blood calcium levels can impair muscle contraction.

The Human Skeleton Consists of Two Parts

The human skeleton consists of the axial and appendicular skeletons (**FIGURE 13-2**). The **axial skeleton** (AXE-ee-al) forms the long axis of the body. It consists of the skull, the vertebral column, and the rib cage. The **appendicular skeleton** (ah-pen-DICK-you-lar) consists of the bones of the arms and legs as well as the bones of the shoulders and pelvis, to which the upper and lower extremities are attached.

All Bones Have a Hard, Dense Outer Layer That Surrounds a Less Compact Central Region

Take a moment to study the skeleton in **FIGURE 13-2**. As you examine it, you may notice that bones come in a variety of shapes and sizes. Some are long, some are short, and some are flat and irregularly shaped. Nevertheless, all bones share some characteristics. Consider one of the long bones of the body, the **humerus** (HUGH-mer-us), which is located in the upper arm.

FIGURE 13-3 illustrates the anatomy of the humerus. As shown, this bone, like other long bones of the body, consists of a long, narrow shaft, the **diaphysis** (die-AF-eh-siss), and two expanded ends, the **epiphyses** (ee-PIF-eh-seas). The ends of the epiphyses are covered with a thin layer of hyaline cartilage (Chapter 4), which reduces friction in joints.

Like other bones, the humerus consists of an outer shell of dense material called **compact bone.** Inside the humerus is a mass of **spongy bone,** so named because of its spongy appearance. Spongy bone forms an interlacing

Buffer = 5.5

10mL

HA $\longrightarrow$ pka = 5

5mL   5mL $\longrightarrow$ HA + OH$^-$ $\longrightarrow$ A$^-$
HA
              5mL A$^-$

$pH = pka + log \dfrac{A^-}{[HA]}$ $\dfrac{m}{m}$ $\dfrac{mol}{\dfrac{V}{mol}}$

pH
5 = 5

$0.4 = log \dfrac{[A^-]}{[AA]}$

$10^{0.4} = \dfrac{A^-}{[AA]}$

epiphysis

dra

Skull
- Frontal
- Parietal
- Temporal
- Zygomatic
- Maxilla
- Mandible

Pectoral girdle
- Clavicle
- Scapula

Thorax
- Sternum
- Ribs

Vertebral column

Upper limb
- Humerus
- Radius
- Ulna
- Carpals
- Metacarpals
- Phalanges

Pelvic girdle
- Ilium
- Sacrum
- Coccyx
- Ischium
- Pubis

Lower limb
- Femur
- Patella
- Tibia
- Fibula
- Tarsals
- Metatarsals
- Phalanges

Anterior view

FIGURE 13-2 The Human Skeleton Over 200 bones of all shapes and sizes make up the human skeleton. The cartilage is shaded blue.

network and is less dense than compact bone. Spongy bone contains numerous small, adjoining cavities.

On the outer surface of the compact bone is a layer of connective tissue, the **periosteum** (PEAR-ee-oss-TEA-um; "around the bone"). The periosteum serves as the site of attachment for skeletal muscles. It also contains osteogenic (OSS-tea-oh-GEN-ick; "bone-forming") cells

that participate in the production of new bone during remodeling or repair.

The periosteum is richly supplied with blood vessels, which enter the bone at numerous locations. Blood vessels travel through small canals in the compact bone and course through the inner spongy bone, providing nutrients and oxygen and carrying off cellular wastes such as carbon dioxide. The periosteum is also richly supplied with nerve fibers. The majority of the pain felt after a person bruises or fractures a bone results from stimulation of the pain fibers in the periosteum.

Inside the shaft of long bones is a large cavity, the **marrow cavity** (MARE-row). The marrow cavities in most of the bones of the fetus and newborn contain red marrow, so named because of its color. **Red marrow** is tissue that serves as a blood-cell factory, producing red blood cells, white blood cells, and platelets to replace those

- Hyaline cartilage
- Epiphysis
- Spongy bone
- Compact bone
- Marrow cavity
- Red marrow
- Diaphysis
- Periosteum
- Nutrient vessel
- Epiphysis

(a)   (b)

FIGURE 13-3 Anatomy of Long Bones (a) Drawing of the humerus. Notice the long shaft and dilated ends. (b) Longitudinal section of the humerus showing compact bone, spongy bone, and marrow.

FIGURE 13-4 Two Immovable Joints
(a) Many of the bones of the skull are held in place by joints called *sutures*. The bones are linked by fibrous tissue, and the joints are immovable. *(b)* The pubic symphysis is another immovable joint. During childbirth it softens and expands to permit delivery.

routinely lost each day. As an individual ages, most red marrow is slowly "retired" and becomes filled with fat, becoming **yellow marrow**. Yellow marrow begins to form during adolescence and, by adulthood, is present in all but a few bones. Red blood cell formation, however, continues in the bodies of the vertebrae, the hip bones, and a few others. Yellow marrow can be reactivated to produce blood cells under certain circumstances—for example, after an injury.

The Joints Permit Varying Degrees of Mobility

A gymnast races across the mat and leaps into space, twirling effortlessly before landing on her feet. As soon as she lands, she takes off again across the mat in a series of elegant and energetic handsprings. These delightful movements are the result of long hours of practice and exercise and are made possible by joints.

Joints are the structures that connect the bones of the skeleton. They can be classified quite simply by the degree of movement they permit. Those that allow little movement are *slightly moveable*. Those that permit no movement are *immovable joints*, and those that allow free movement are **movable joints**. Consider some examples.

The bones of the skull shown in **FIGURE 13-4A**. As illustrated, these bones interlock to form immovable joints, known as *sutures*. Fibrous connective tissue spans the space between the interlocking bones, holding them together. Another immovable joint is the pubic symphysis (PEW-bick SIM-fa-siss), which is formed by the

two pubic bones (**FIGURE 13-4B**). These bones are held in place by fibrocartilage. Near the end of pregnancy, however, hormones loosen the fibrocartilage of the pubic symphysis, allowing the pelvic outlet to widen enough to permit a baby to pass through—an adaptation of enormous value to our species!

The bodies of the vertebrae are united by slightly movable joints (**FIGURE 13-5**). Each vertebra is separated from its nearest neighbors by an **intervertebral disc**. The inner portion of the disc acts as a cushion, softening the impact of walking and running. The outer, fibrous portion holds the disc in place and joins one vertebra to its nearest neighbor. The joints between the vertebrae offer some degree of movement, resulting in a fair amount of flexibility. If they did not, we would be unable to bend over to tie our shoes or to curl up on the couch for an afternoon snooze.

The most common type of joint is the freely movable, or **synovial joint** (sin-OH-vee-al). The synovial joints are more complex than other types and permit varying degrees of movement. Although synovial joints differ con-

FIGURE 13-5 A Slightly Movable Joint The intervertebral discs allow for some movement, giving the vertebral column flexibility.

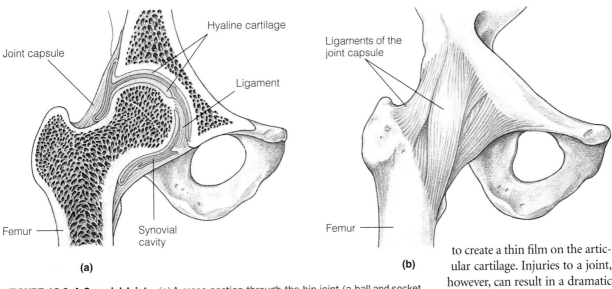

FIGURE 13-6 A Synovial Joint *(a)* A cross section through the hip joint (a ball-and-socket joint) showing the structures of the synovial joint. *(b)* Ligaments in the outer portion of the joint capsule help support the joint.

siderably in architecture, they share several features. The first commonality is the hyaline cartilage located on the articular (joint) surfaces of the bones (**FIGURE 13-6A**). This thin cap of hyaline cartilage reduces friction and facilitates movement. The second commonality is the **joint capsule,** a structure that joins one bone to another (**FIGURE 13-6A**). The outer layer of the joint capsule consists of dense connective tissue that attaches to the periosteum of adjoining bones. In many joints, parallel bundles of dense connective tissue fibers in the outer layer of the capsule form distinct **ligaments.** A ligament is a structure that joins bones to bones together in joints. They provide additional support to the joint.

As a rule, ligaments are fairly inflexible. However, some individuals have remarkably flexible ligaments. Their **tendons,** the connective tissue that joins muscles to bones at their points of origin and insertion, may also be flexible. Because of this, some people exhibit extraordinary flexibility. For example, they may be able to extend their thumbs well beyond the 90 degrees possible for most of us. And some can extend their fingers so much that they can touch the back of their hand. These people are said to be "double-jointed," a misnomer that suggests the flexibility is permitted by the joint when in fact it is due to the tendons and ligaments.

The inner layer of the joint capsule is the **synovial membrane.** It produces a fairly thick, slippery substance called **synovial fluid.** Synovial fluid provides nutrients to the articular cartilage (the hyaline cartilage on the articular surfaces of the bone) and also acts as a lubricant. Normally, the synovial membrane produces only enough fluid

to create a thin film on the articular cartilage. Injuries to a joint, however, can result in a dramatic increase in synovial fluid production, causing swelling and pain in joints.

Tendons and muscles provide additional support in some joints and are commonly associated with synovial joints. In the shoulder, for example, muscles help hold the head of the humerus in the socket (formed by the scapula). Muscles in the hip help hold the head of the femur in place. Because muscles strengthen joints, individuals who are in poor physical shape are much more likely to suffer a dislocation on a ski trip or during exercise than someone who is in good shape. **Dislocation** is an injury in which a bone is displaced from its proper position in a joint due to a fall or some other unusual body movement. In some cases, bones slip out of place, then back in without assistance. In others, the bone can be put back in place only by a trained health care worker.

Synovial joints come in many shapes and sizes and are classified on the basis of structure. Two of the most common are the hinge joint and the ball-and-socket joint. The knee joint is a **hinge joint,** as are the joints in the fingers. Hinge joints open and close like hinges on a door. Such joints provide for movement in only one plane. The hip and shoulder joints are **ball-and-socket joints.** They allow a wider range of motion. (Compare the movements permitted by the shoulder and hip joints to those permitted by the knee joint.)

Arthroscopy Is a Procedure That Permits Surgeons to Repair Injured Joints with a Minimum of Trauma. Joint injuries are common among athletes and other physically active people (**TABLE 13-1**). A hard blow to the knee of a football player, for instance, can tear the

TABLE 13-1

Common Injuries of the Joints

Injury	Description	Common Site
Sprain	Partially or completely torn ligament; heals slowly; must be repaired surgically if the ligament is completely torn.	Ankle, knee, lower back, and finger joints
Dislocation	Occurs when bones are forced out of a joint; often accompanied by sprains, inflammation, and joint immobilization. Bones must be returned to normal positions.	Shoulder, knee, and finger joints
Cartilage tears	Cartilage may tear when joints are twisted or when pressure is applied to them. Torn cartilage does not repair well because of poor vascularization. It is generally removed surgically; this operation sometimes makes the joint less stable.	Knee joint

ligaments inside the knee joint or in the joint capsule. A rough fall can dislocate a skier's shoulder. Improperly lifting an object can strain the ligaments that join the vertebrae of the back.

Torn ligaments, tendons, and cartilage in joints heal very slowly because they have few blood vessels to bring nutrients needed for repair.[1] For years, joint repair required major surgery that was so traumatic it put patients out of commission for several months. Today, however, new surgical techniques allow physicians to repair joints with a minimum of trauma (**FIGURE 13-7**). Through small incisions in the skin over the joint, surgeons insert a device called an **arthroscope** (ARE-

---

[1]Because most cartilage is avascular, it may not heal at all.

throw-scope). It allows them to view the damage inside the joint and to insert instruments that remove damaged cartilage. The surgeon can thus repair damaged cartilage without opening the joint. The damage caused by large incisions is eliminated, and athletes are usually back on their feet and on the playing field in a matter of weeks. New surgical techniques can rebuild torn ligaments and return joints to nearly their original state.

Osteoarthritis Is a Degenerative Bone Disease Caused by Wear and Tear on the Articular Cartilages. Virtually every time you move, you use one or more of your joints. Because of this, problems in joints, which often cause pain, are therefore often quite noticeable. One of the most common problems is called **degenerative joint disease** or **osteoarthritis**. Degenerative joint disease probably results from wear and tear on a joint. Over time, excess wear may cause the articular cartilage on the ends of bones to flake and crack. As the cartilage degenerates, the bones come in contact and may grind against each other during movement. This causes considerable swelling, pain, and discomfort.

Osteoarthritis occurs most often in the weight-bearing joints: the knee, hip, and spine—regions subject to the most wear over time. Osteoarthritis may also develop in the finger joints.

Osteoarthritis is extremely common. X-ray studies of people over 40 years of age show that most people have some degree of degeneration in one or more joints. Fortunately, many people do not even notice the problem, and the disease rarely becomes a serious medical problem.

(b)

(a)

FIGURE 13-7 Arthroscopic Surgery   (a) A physician performing arthroscopic surgery. (b) Inside view of the knee joint through an arthroscope.

FIGURE 13-8 Hand Disfigured by Rheumatoid Arthritis Degeneration of the finger joints causes mild to extreme disfiguration.

Wear and tear on joints is worsened by obesity. The extra pressure wears the cartilage away more quickly. For individuals with a joint problem, weight control can reduce the rate of degeneration and ease the pain.[2] Painkillers such as aspirin and other anti-inflammatory drugs are used to treat the pain and swelling. Injections of steroids may help reduce inflammation, although repeated injections often damage the joint.

Rheumatoid Arthritis Is an Autoimmune Disease.

Another common disorder of the synovial joint is rheumatoid arthritis. **Rheumatoid arthritis** (RUE-mah-toid) is the most painful and crippling form of arthritis. It is caused by an inflammation of the synovial membrane. The inflammation often spreads to the articular cartilages. If the condition persists, rheumatoid arthritis can wear through the cartilage and cause degeneration of the underlying bone. In such cases, the thickening of the synovial membrane and degeneration of the bone often disfigure the joints, reduce mobility, and cause considerable pain (**FIGURE 13-8**). Afflicted joints can be completely immobilized. In severe cases, the bones become dislocated, causing the joints to collapse.

Rheumatoid arthritis generally occurs in the joints of the wrist, fingers, and feet. It can also affect the hips, knees, ankles, and neck.

Research suggests that rheumatoid arthritis results from an **autoimmune reaction**—that is, an immune response to the cells of one's own synovial membrane (Chapter 8). Rheumatoid arthritis occurs in people of all ages, but most commonly appears in individuals between the ages of 20 and 40. Rheumatoid arthritis is usually a permanent condition, although the degree of severity varies widely. Patients suffering from it can be treated with physical therapy, painkillers, anti-inflammatory drugs, and surgery.

Diseased joints can also be replaced by **prostheses** (pross-THEE-seas), artificial

joints that restore mobility and reduce pain. Plastic joints are used to replace the finger joints, greatly improving the appearance of the hands by eliminating the gnarled, swollen joints. Moreover, patients regain the use of previously crippled fingers. Day-to-day chores (buttoning a shirt) that often required assistance become noticeably easier. Once impossible tasks—such as opening screw-top jars—are again feasible. Severely damaged knee and hip joints are replaced with special steel or Teflon substitutes, which, if fitted properly, may last 10–15 years (**FIGURE 13-9**).

In knee-replacement surgery, the ends of the bones are actually sawed off and the artificial joints are glued in place. In a hip replacement, the end of the leg bone, the femur, is sawed off and replaced with an metal substitute. The socket the head of the femur once fit into is replaced with a teflon-coated device into which the new, artificial femur head fits.

Most of the Bones of the Human Skeleton Start Out as Hyaline Cartilage

During embryonic development, hyaline cartilage forms in the arms, legs, head, and torso where bone will eventually be (**FIGURE 13-10**). In short order, the cartilage is converted to bone. This process is known as **endochondral ossification** (en-doh-CON-drall).

Bones Are Constantly Remodeled in Adults to Meet Changing Stresses Placed on Them

Bones are dynamic structures that undergo considerable remodeling in response to changes in our lives. This process begins

FIGURE 13-9 Artificial Joints
An artificial knee joint (a) and hip joint (b).

(a)   (b)

---

[2]Weight control is also a preventive measure that helps people avoid the problem in the first place.

FIGURE 13-10 Human Fetus Eighteen-week-old human fetus showing forming bones. The fetus is six to nine inches in length.

early in life. In a newborn baby, for example, the bones of the leg (the tibia and fibula) are quite bowed. Cramped inside the mother's uterus, the baby's bones do not grow very straight. During the first 2 years of life, however, as the child begins to walk and run, the leg bones generally straighten (**FIGURE 13-11**). The bones are remodeled to meet the markedly different stresses placed on them by upright posture.

Remodeling occurs throughout adult life as well. During sedentary periods, for example, compact bone decreases in thickness. Increasing one's level of activity, however, causes compact bone to thicken, thus helping the bone withstand stresses placed on it by walk-

Tibia

Fibula

Birth

20 months

FIGURE 13-11 Remodeling of a Baby's Leg Bones Notice how dramatically the bones change to meet the changing needs of the toddler.

ing, running, or standing. Spongy bone also undergoes considerable remodeling. Thus, even the internal architecture of a bone changes to meet new stresses.

Two cells are responsible for bone remodeling: osteoclasts and osteoblasts. **Osteoclasts** (OSS-tea-oh-KLASTS) are akin to the wrecking crew that comes into a house to tear out walls before a remodeling job. **Osteoblasts** (OSS-tea-oh-BLASTS) lay down new bone during the remodeling phase like the drywallers and carpenters who rebuild walls after they have been torn down. When an osteoblast becomes surrounded by calcified extracellular material, it is referred to as an osteocyte.

Bone Is a Homeostatic Organ That Helps Maintain Proper Levels of Calcium in the Body

In addition to their role in remodeling bone, osteoblasts and osteoclasts help control blood calcium levels and are therefore part of a homeostatic mechanism. They are controlled by two hormones: parathormone and calcitonin.

When blood calcium levels fall, the **parathyroid glands** (small glands embedded in the thyroid glands in the neck) release a hormone known as **parathormone** (PAIR-ah-THOR-moan) or **PTH** into the bloodstream. PTH travels throughout the body. When it reaches the bone, it stimulates the osteoclasts, causing them to digest bone in their vicinity. The calcium released by the activity of the osteoclasts replenishes blood calcium levels.

When calcium levels rise—for example, after a meal—the thyroid releases **calcitonin** (CAL-seh-TONE-in). This hormone inhibits osteoclasts, stopping bone destruction. It also stimulates osteoblasts, causing them to deposit new bone. The inhibition of osteoclasts and the formation of new bone help lower blood calcium levels, returning them to normal.

Bone Fractures Are Repaired by Fibroblasts and Osteoblasts

If you're like most people, chances are that sometime in your life you'll break a bone. Bone fractures can vary considerably in their severity. Some only involve hairline cracks, which mend fairly quickly. Others involve considerably more damage—a complete break, for instance—that takes much longer to repair. In some instances, the broken ends must be realigned. A plaster cast is then applied to hold the limb in position and keep the ends together to optimize healing. Severe fractures may require surgeons to insert steel pins to hold the bones together.

Bones, like other tissues, are capable of self-repair. As **FIGURE 13-12** illustrates, after a fracture, blood from

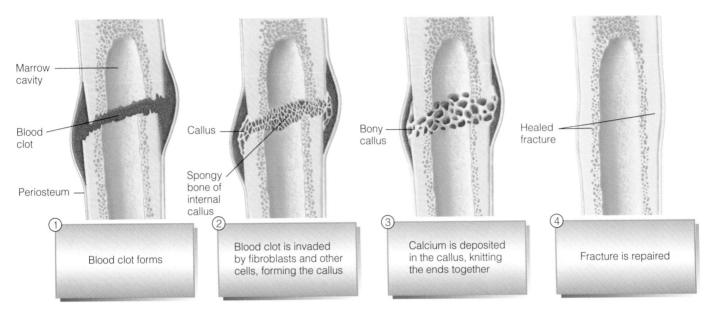

Marrow cavity

Blood clot

Periosteum

Callus

Spongy bone of internal callus

Bony callus

Healed fracture

① Blood clot forms

② Blood clot is invaded by fibroblasts and other cells, forming the callus

③ Calcium is deposited in the callus, knitting the ends together

④ Fracture is repaired

FIGURE 13-12 Stages in Fracture Repair

broken blood vessels in the periosteum and marrow cavity pours into the fracture and forms a blood clot. Within a few days, the clot is invaded by fibroblasts, connective tissue cells from the periosteum. Fibroblasts secrete collagen fibers, thus forming a mass of cells and fibers, the **callus** (CAL-us), which bridges the broken ends internally and externally.

The callus is next invaded by osteoblasts from the periosteum. Osteoblasts slowly convert the callus to bone, thus "knitting" the broken ends together. As **FIGURE 13-12** shows, the callus is initially much larger than the bone itself. But the excess bone is gradually removed

by osteoclasts, leaving little, if any, evidence that a break has occurred.

Osteoporosis Involves a Loss of Calcium, Which Results in Brittle, Easy-to-Break Bones

One of the most common problems adults face is **osteoporosis** (OSS-tea-oh-puh-ROE-siss; "porous bone"), a condition characterized by a progressive loss of bone calcium (**FIGURE 13-13**). In some individuals, calcium loss is so severe that bones become extremely brittle— so much so that even normal activities such as getting

(a)   (b)   (c)   (d)

FIGURE 13-13 Osteoporosis The loss of estrogen or prolonged immobilization weakens bone. In these situations, bone is dissolved and becomes brittle and easily breakable. (a) A section of the body of a lumbar vertebra from a 29-year-old woman. (b) Some thinning is evident in a vertebra of a 40-year-old woman. (c) Bone loss is severe in an 84-year-old woman. (d) Bone loss is most severe in a 92-year-old woman. Osteoporosis is not inevitable and can be prevented by exercise, calcium supplements, estrogen supplements, and other measures.

Health Note 13-1

Preventing Osteoporosis: A Prescription for Healthy Bones

Twenty million Americans, mostly women, suffer from a painful, debilitating disease called osteoporosis (**FIGURE 1**). Caused by a gradual deterioration of the bone, osteoporosis results in nagging pain and discomfort. In more severe cases, bones fracture easily.

If current trends continue, one of every two American women will develop postmenopausal osteoporosis. Each year, nearly 60,000 Americans—most of them women—will die from complications resulting from this common malady. The three most common are hemorrhage; fat embolisms (globules), sometimes released from the yellow marrow of broken bones; and shock. Unfortunately, most women do not realize they have the disease until it has progressed quite far.

FIGURE 1 Bone Deterioration An elderly woman suffering from osteoporosis. Notice the hunched back due to the collapse of vertebrae.

Recent research shows that osteoporosis begins much earlier than researchers once thought—by the time a woman reaches her mid-20s. Bone demineralization occurs very rapidly. In fact, by age 30, many women have lost one-third of their bone calcium! Between the ages of 30 and 50, many women's bones continue to deteriorate, becoming extremely brittle.

Calcium loss begins so early in American women because many weight-conscious women in their mid-20s abstain from fatty foods such as whole milk, cheese, and ice cream to control their weight. Although these foods are fatty, they are also a major source of calcium. Milk products are also shunned by many adults who develop an intolerance to lactose (a sugar) in milk and other dairy products. Lactose intolerance results from a sharp reduction in the production and secretion of the intestinal enzyme lactase as one ages, which makes it difficult to digest lactose. Because of

out of bed in the morning or doing housework cause fractures.

Osteoporosis occurs most often in postmenopausal women. **Menopause** (MEN-oh-pause) usually occurs between 45 and 55 years of age. It results from the loss of estrogen production by a woman's ovaries. Although estrogen is primarily a reproductive hormone, it also helps to maintain bone.

Osteoporosis also occurs in people who are immobilized for long periods. Hospital patients who are restricted to bed for 2 or 3 months, for example, show signs of osteoporosis.

Osteoporosis may also result from environmental factors. In the 1960s, women living along the Jintsu River in Japan developed a painful bone disease known as itai-itai (which literally means "ouch, ouch"). The women lived downstream from zinc and lead mines that released large amounts of the heavy metal cadmium into the river. They used river water for drinking and for irrigat-

ing rice paddies. Even though men, young women, and children were exposed to cadmium, 95% of the cases occurred in postmenopausal women.

Researchers hypothesized that the accelerated bone loss in the postmenopausal Japanese women was due to cadmium and tested this hypothesis by feeding mice diets containing various levels of cadmium chloride. The group receiving the highest dose showed significant reductions in bone calcium when their ovaries had been removed.

These findings may also explain why older women who smoke are more likely to develop osteoporosis and why they experience more bone fractures and tooth loss than nonsmokers. Cadmium is one of several harmful substances present in cigarette smoke. Smoking, however, may also act by decreasing estrogen levels, making it doubly dangerous to a woman's health. For a discussion of ways to prevent osteoporosis, see Health Note 13-1.

these and other factors, adult women often consume only about one-half of the 1000–1500 milligrams of calcium they need every day.

Osteoporosis may be prevented and even reversed by eating calcium-rich foods, such as spinach, milk, cheese, shrimp, oysters, and tofu (soybean curd). Calcium supplements can also help retard or even stop bone deterioration and restore calcium levels. Because vitamin D increases the absorption of calcium in the intestines vitamin supplements can help. (A word of caution, however: excessive vitamin D—five times the RDA—can be toxic.)

Studies also suggest that osteoporosis can be prevented by exercise. Aerobics, jogging, walking, and tennis in conjunction with the dietary changes all help prevent the disease.

Osteoporosis can be *reversed* by exercise even after the disease has reached the dangerous stage. Forty-five minutes of moderate exercise

(walking) 3 days a week, for example, greatly decreases the rate of calcium loss in older individuals. In addition, this exercise regime stimulates the rebuilding process, replacing calcium lost in previous years. Continued exercise increases bone calcium levels and decreases the rate of bone fractures and fatal complications.

Another effective treatment for postmenopausal women is estrogen. Low doses of estrogen halt bone demineralization and promote bone formation. Because women who are given estrogen suffer an increased risk of cancer of the uterine lining, physicians often prescribe a mixed dose of estrogen and progesterone, which reduces the likelihood of this type of cancer.

Studies have also shown that high doses of calcium fluoride stimulate bone development. Calcium fluoride treatment increases bone mass approximately 3%–6% per year and decreases bone fractures. The aver-

age patient in one study experienced one fracture every 8 months before treatment. After treatment, that figure dropped to one fracture every 4.5 years.

Unfortunately, large doses of fluoride may erode the stomach lining, causing internal bleeding. They may also stimulate abnormal bone development and cause pain and swelling in joints. To offset these problems, researchers have developed a pill that releases the fluoride gradually.

For millions of young women, early detection and sound preventive measures, including exercise, vitamin D, dietary improvements, and fluoride treatments, can prevent this unnecessary disease.

Visit *Human Biology's* Internet site for links to web sites offering more information on this topic.

The Skeletal Muscles

Purposeful movement is one of the most distinctive features of animal life. As noted in the introduction to this chapter, in humans, skeletal muscles acting on bones result in movement. Most skeletal muscles are under the control of the nervous system.[3]

FIGURE 13-14 shows some of the skeletal muscles of the body. As illustrated, most skeletal muscles cross one or more joints. When they contract, they produce movement.

As a rule, muscles generally work in groups to bring about various body movements. Groups of muscles are often arranged in such a way that one set produces one movement and another set on the opposite side of the

joint causes an opposing movement. For example, the biceps (BUY-seps) is a muscle in the front of the upper arm. When it and other members of its group contract, they cause the arm to bend, a movement called *flexion* (FLECK-shun). On the back side of the upper arm is another muscle, the triceps (TRY-seps). When it contracts, it causes the arm to straighten, or extend. Such opposing muscles are called **antagonists.** When one muscle contracts to produce a movement, the antagonistic muscles relax.

Not all skeletal muscles make bones move. Some muscles simply steady joints, allowing other muscles to act. These stabilizing muscles are called **synergists** (SIN-er-gists). These muscles help to maintain our posture, permitting us to stand or sit upright despite the constant pull of gravity.

Another group of muscles that don't move bones are the muscles of the face. Anchored to the bones of the skull and to the skin of the face, these muscles allow us to wrinkle our skin, open and close our eyes, and move our lips.

---

[3]Chapter 4 discussed three types of muscle: skeletal, cardiac, and smooth.

FIGURE 13-14 The Skeletal Muscles

Facial
- Temporalis
- Masseter

Platysma

Shoulder
- Trapezius
- Deltoid

Arm
- Triceps brachii
- Biceps brachii

External oblique

Forearm
- Brachioradialis
- Flexor carpi radialis

Pelvis/thigh
- Iliopsoas
- Pectineus

Thigh
- Rectus femoris
- Vastus lateralis
- Vastus medialis

Leg
- Peroneus longus
- Extensor digitorum longus
- Tibialis anterior

Facial
- Frontalis
- Obicularis oculi
- Obicularis oris

Neck
- Sternocleidomastoid

Thorax
- Pectoralis minor
- Pectoralis major
- Intercostals

Abdomen
- Rectus abdominis
- Internal oblique
- Transversus abdominis

Thigh
- Sartorius
- Adductor longus
- Gracilis

Leg
- Tibia
- Gastrocnemius
- Soleus

Nucleus

FIGURE 13-15 Light Micrograph of Skeletal Muscle
Notice the banding pattern on these muscle fibers.

Muscles also produce enormous amounts of heat as a by-product of metabolism. Working muscles produce even more heat—so much, in fact, that you can cross-country ski in freezing weather wearing only a light sweater.

Skeletal Muscle Cells Are Known as Muscle Fibers and Are Both Excitable and Contractile

Skeletal muscles consist of long, unbranched **muscle fibers.** Each fiber contains many nuclei derived from individual cells that fuse during embryonic development to form a fiber. Viewed with the light microscope, skeletal muscle fibers appear striated (STRY-a-tid) or striped (**FIGURE 13-15**).

Like nerve cells, the muscle fiber is an excitable cell. A small potential difference (about –70 millivolts) exists across the plasma membrane of skeletal muscle fibers, as in neurons. Muscle fibers are stimulated by nerve impulses arriving at the terminal boutons of motor nerves. They stimulate the release of a neurotransmitter substance that stimulates a bioelectric impulse in the muscle fiber itself. This new impulse travels along the membrane of the muscle fiber in the same way a nerve impulse travels along an unmyelinated axon or dendrite—like a wave in water.

Muscle fibers are also contractile. When stimulated, the contractile proteins inside the fibers cause the cells to shorten. Muscle fibers are also elastic and therefore capable of returning to normal length after a contraction has ended.

Muscle Fibers Contain Many Small Bundles of Contractile Filaments Known as Myofibrils

Understanding how a muscle contracts first requires an understanding of its structure. To begin, imagine that you could tease a single skeletal muscle fiber (cell) free from a skeletal muscle (**FIGURE 13-16A**). Under the microscope, you would find that each muscle fiber is a long cylinder encased by plasma membrane and containing many nuclei. Each muscle fiber is further characterized by a series of dark and light bands—hence its striated appearance (**FIGURE 13-16B**).

Take the tissue to an electron microscope, and you will find that inside each muscle fiber are lots of threadlike filaments. They exist in tiny bundles called **myofibrils** (MY-oh-FIE-brills) (**FIGURE 13-16B**). Myofibrils contain contractile filaments and, as **FIGURE 13-16C** illustrates, are striated (banded).

The light and dark bands of the myofibril are arranged in a uniform pattern that gives the myofibril and muscle fiber its striated appearance. The details are shown in **FIGURE 13-16C**.

FIGURE 13-16D shows that the myofibrils contain thick and thin filaments. The thick filaments consist of the protein **myosin** (MY-oh-

sin). The thin filaments are composed primarily of the protein **actin** (ACK-tin).

During Muscle Contraction, the Actin Filaments Slide Inward, Causing the Sarcomeres to Shorten

When a muscle contracts, it shortens. This is achieved by the sliding of actin filaments over the myosin filaments. In actuality, the actin filaments do not passively slide to the middle; they are pulled inward by the myosin molecules. How is this accomplished?

FIGURE 13-16 Structure of the Skeletal Muscle Fiber, Myofibril, and Sarcomere *(a)* A single muscle fiber teased out of the muscle. *(b)* Each muscle fiber consists of many myofibrils. *(c)* Note the banded pattern of the myofibril. *(d)* Sarcomeres consist of thick and thin filaments, as shown here. *(e)* Molecular structure of the thick (myosin) and thin (actin) filaments.

FIGURE 13-17 Structure of Myosin Filaments Myosin molecules join to form a myosin filament. Note the presence and orientation of the heads of the myosin molecules.

The contraction of muscle has to rank as one of the most fascinating biological processes. As **FIGURE 13-17** shows, each myosin filament actually consists of numerous golf-club-shaped myosin molecules arranged with their "club ends," or heads, projecting toward the actin filaments. During muscle contraction, the heads of the myosin molecules attach to actin filaments, forming **cross bridges,** which tug the filaments inward.

The attachment of the myosin molecules to the actin molecules is stimulated by the release of calcium inside muscle cells. Calcium is stored in the smooth endoplasmic reticulum, which forms a rather extensive network inside the muscle cells. The release of calcium, in turn, is stimulated by electrical impulses from the nerves. These impulses reach the muscle cell via motor nerves, which form synapses with the muscle cells. Neurotransmitters released from the terminal boutons of the motor nerves cause impulses to be generated in muscle cells. These impulses travel along the membrane of muscle cells and enter the interior via small infoldings of the plasma membrane. These infoldings come in close contact with the smooth endoplasmic reticulum. When an impulse penetrates into the interior, it stimulates calcium release. This causes the heads of the myosin molecules to attach to the actin filaments. ATP in the muscle provides the energy needed to pull the actin filaments inward.

Muscle Cells Use Enormous Quantities of ATP Daily, Which Come From Several Sources. ATP is in relatively short supply in cells, and must be recycled over and over again in rapid succession to meet cellular demands. In muscles, some of the ATP is regenerated by a substance called **creatine phosphate** (CREE-ah-teh-NEEN). This molecule contains a high-energy bond, indicated by the squiggly line (below). Stored in muscle in high concentrations, creatine phosphate reacts with ADP as follows:

$$\text{creatine} \sim \text{P} + \text{ADP} \rightarrow \text{ATP} + \text{creatine}$$

Creatine phosphate replenishes ATP used during muscle contraction.

ATP is also generated by glycolysis, the citric acid cycle, and the electron transport system (Chapter 3). The electron transport system is the main source of ATP. But this process requires oxygen. During vigorous muscle contraction, oxygen supplies inside muscle cells can fall precipitously. If the circulatory system cannot replace oxygen used as quickly as it is being used, the citric acid cycle and electron transport system shut down.

To generate ATP, the cell must resort to fermentation—the metabolic breakdown of glucose in the absence of oxygen. Besides being inefficient, this process results in the buildup of lactic acid. Exercise also depletes the muscle of glycogen, which you may recall is a long-chain molecule in muscle (and liver). It is used to store glucose. The shortage of ATP, the build up of lactic acid, and depletion of muscle glycogen that occurs during vigorous exercise result in muscle fatigue. Oxygen levels are also depleted during exercise, creating an **oxygen debt.**

The shortages of glycogen and oxygen must be replaced in order to continue to function, just as gasoline in your car must be added to continue its functioning. Glycogen is replaced during rest by glucose from the bloodstream. Oxygen is replenished by the diffusion of oxygen from blood capillaries, but this process occurs rather quickly, often right after you exercise, which explains why you keep breathing hard for a while after you stop exercising.

Individual Skeletal Muscle Fibers Contract After Being Stimulated by an Action Potential

The Strength of Muscle Contraction Can Be Increased by Stimulating (Recruiting) Additional Muscle Fibers to Contract. Individual skeletal muscle fibers contract when activated by an action potential. A single contraction, followed by relaxation, is called a **twitch.**

Generating the force needed to move arms and legs or eyelids requires the action of many muscle cells. The engagement of additional muscle fibers during muscle contraction is called **recruitment.**

To understand how recruitment occurs in muscle, we first take a look at **FIGURE 13-18**. The drawing shows that the axons of motor neurons form many branches upon reaching the muscles they supply. A single motor neuron, in fact, may end on dozens of individual muscle fibers in a skeletal muscle. A motor neuron and the muscle fibers it supplies constitute a **motor unit.** When the neuron supplying a motor unit is activated, all of the muscle fibers in the unit are stimulated.

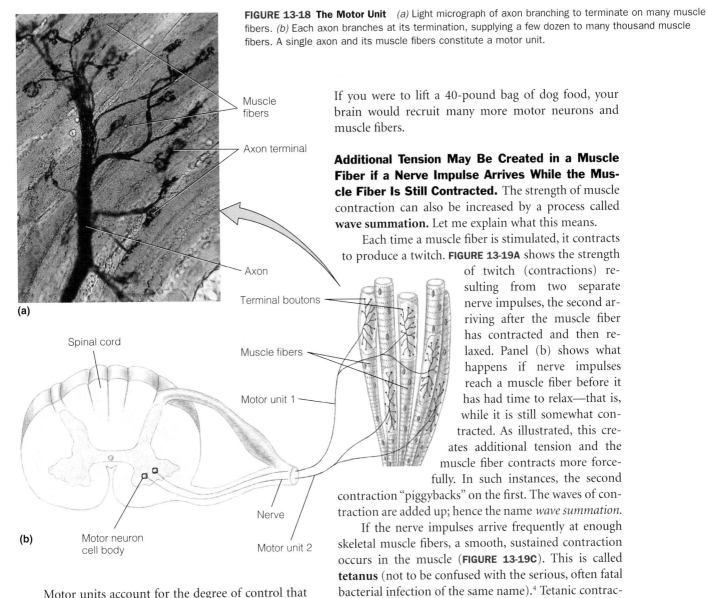

FIGURE 13-18 The Motor Unit *(a)* Light micrograph of axon branching to terminate on many muscle fibers. *(b)* Each axon branches at its termination, supplying a few dozen to many thousand muscle fibers. A single axon and its muscle fibers constitute a motor unit.

(a)

Muscle fibers

Axon terminal

Axon

Terminal boutons

Spinal cord

Muscle fibers

Motor unit 1

(b)

Motor neuron cell body

Nerve

Motor unit 2

If you were to lift a 40-pound bag of dog food, your brain would recruit many more motor neurons and muscle fibers.

Additional Tension May Be Created in a Muscle Fiber if a Nerve Impulse Arrives While the Muscle Fiber Is Still Contracted. The strength of muscle contraction can also be increased by a process called **wave summation.** Let me explain what this means.

Each time a muscle fiber is stimulated, it contracts to produce a twitch. **FIGURE 13-19A** shows the strength of twitch (contractions) resulting from two separate nerve impulses, the second arriving after the muscle fiber has contracted and then relaxed. Panel (b) shows what happens if nerve impulses reach a muscle fiber before it has had time to relax—that is, while it is still somewhat contracted. As illustrated, this creates additional tension and the muscle fiber contracts more forcefully. In such instances, the second contraction "piggybacks" on the first. The waves of contraction are added up; hence the name *wave summation.*

If the nerve impulses arrive frequently at enough skeletal muscle fibers, a smooth, sustained contraction occurs in the muscle (**FIGURE 13-19C**). This is called **tetanus** (not to be confused with the serious, often fatal bacterial infection of the same name).[4] Tetanic contractions occur in your arm muscles when you carry a bag of groceries. In such instances, the muscles contract to support the weight and remain contracted throughout the activity. Tetanic contractions eventually cause muscle fatigue and muscles stop contracting, even though the neural stimuli may continue.

Muscle Tone Results from the Contraction of a Small Number of Muscle Fibers That Keep Muscles Slightly Tense

Touch one of your muscles. Even if you are not in peak physical condition, you will notice that the muscle is rel-

Motor units account for the degree of control that various muscles exert. The fewer muscle fibers in a motor unit, the finer the control. Such is the case in the muscles of the fingers, which are capable of very fine movements. In contrast, the more muscle fibers in a motor unit, the cruder the control. Thus, the neurons that supply the muscles of the leg, which produce a crude but strong propulsive force, may end on as many as 2000 muscle fibers. Each time an impulse is delivered to the motor unit, it stimulates all 2000 muscle fibers.

How does this process relate to recruitment? To increase the force of contraction in a skeletal muscle, more motor neurons are stimulated and therefore more muscle fibers are called into action. Therefore, if you were to lift a piece of Styrofoam, only a small fraction of the motor neurons going to the arm muscle would be used.

---

[4]The bacterial infection is called *tetanus* because the toxins from the bacterial infection cause the muscle to lock.

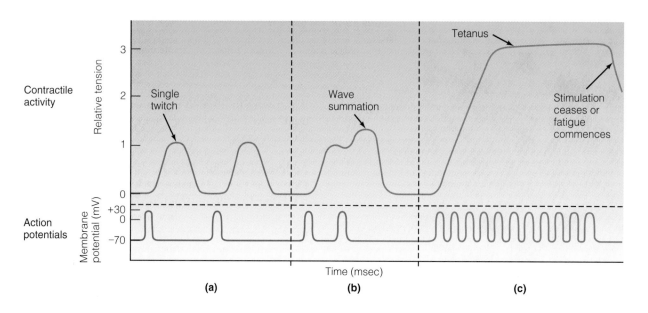

The duration of the action potentials is not drawn to scale, but is exaggerated.

FIGURE 13-19 Graph of Muscle Contraction *(a)* The force generated by two separate stimuli (action potentials from motor neuron). *(b)* The force generated by two closely timed stimuli. *(c)* The force generated by many closely spaced stimuli.

atively firm. This firmness is called **muscle tone.** Muscle tone is essential for maintaining posture. Without it, you would fall into a heap on the floor. Muscle tone also generates heat in warm-blooded animals like us.

Muscle tone results from the contraction of muscle fibers during periods of inactivity. But not all fibers contract—just enough of them to keep the muscles slightly tense. Muscle tone is maintained, in part, by the muscle spindle, a receptor that monitors muscle stretching (Chapter 12). The spindle "alerts" the brain and spinal cord to the degree of stretching. When muscles relax, signals travel to the spinal cord, and then back out to motor axons, which stimulate a low level of muscle contraction, maintaining muscle tone.

Two Types of Muscle Fibers Are Found in Skeletal Muscle, Slow- and Fast-Twitch

Physiological studies have revealed the presence of two types of skeletal muscle fibers: fast-twitch and slow-twitch fibers.[5] **Slow-twitch muscle fibers** contract relatively slowly but have incredible endurance. It is not surprising, then, that the muscles of endurance athletes (for example, long-distance runners) contain a high proportion of slow-twitch muscle fibers (**FIGURE 13-20**).

[5]In truth, there are three types—one kind of slow-twitch and two types of fast-twitch. One type of fast-twitch fiber fatigues rather easily, whereas the other type is fatigue resistant.

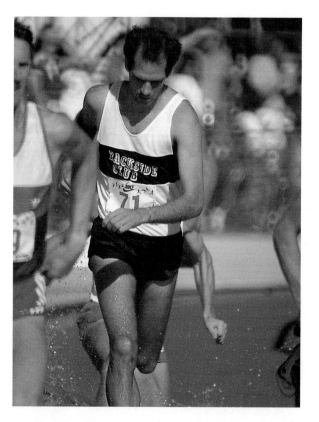

FIGURE 13-20 Built to Last An abundance of slow-twitch fibers gives the Olympic long-distance runner endurance.

These permit such athletes to perform for long periods without tiring. The flight muscles of birds, which can travel long distances without stopping, are similarly made.

Fast-twitch muscle fibers contract swiftly. The muscles of sprinters and other athletes whose performance depends on quick bursts of activity contain a high proportion of fast-twitch fibers.

Skeletal muscles generally contain a mixture of slow- and fast-twitch fibers, giving each muscle a wide range of performance abilities. However, a muscle that performs one type of function more often than another tends to have a disproportionately higher number of fibers corresponding to the type of activity it performs. The muscles of the back, for example, contain a larger number of slow-twitch fibers. These muscles operate throughout the waking hours to maintain posture. They do not need to contract quickly, but they must be resistant to fatigue. In contrast, the muscles of the arm are used for many quick actions—waving, playing tennis, or grasping falling objects. Fast-twitch fibers are more common in the muscles of the arm.

Genetic Differences May Account for Differences in Athletic Performance.

New research suggests that one of the reasons some people excel in certain sports may lie in the relative proportion of fast- and slow-twitch fibers in their muscles. In fact, a study of the skeletal muscles of world-class long-distance runners suggests that their physical endurance is primarily due to a high proportion of slow-twitch fibers, a trait that may be genetically determined. Biochemical studies also show that the muscle cells in endurance athletes have a higher level of ATP, both at rest and during exercise, thus providing more energy for muscle contraction. Endurance athletes start out with a larger storehouse of energy and maintain a larger supply throughout exercise.

Exercise Builds Muscles and Increases Endurance

Milo of Croton was a champion wrestler in ancient Greece who stumbled across a revolutionary way to build muscle. His method was simple. Milo borrowed a newborn calf, then proceeded to carry the animal around every day. Day after day, he faithfully followed this routine so that by the time the calf had become a bull, so had he. Milo's program worked, for he went on to win six Olympic championships in wrestling.

The Greek wrestler discovered a principle of muscle physiology familiar to weight lifters today: When muscles are made to work hard, they respond by becoming larger and stronger. The increase in size and strength results from an increase in the amount of contractile protein inside muscle cells.

Unfortunately, muscle protein is quickly made and quickly destroyed. In fact, about half of the muscle you gain in a weight-lifting program is broken down 2 weeks after you stop exercising. In order to build muscle, then, the rate of formation must exceed the rate of destruction. If you don't keep up with your exercise program, your newly developed biceps will disappear quickly.

High-intensity exercise, such as weight lifting, builds muscle, and it takes surprisingly little exercise to have an effect. Working out every other day for only a few minutes will result in noticeable changes in muscle mass. According to some sources, 18 contractions of a muscle (in three sets of six contractions each) are enough to increase muscle mass, if the contractions force your muscles to exert over 75% of their maximum capacity.

Low-intensity exercise, such as aerobics and swimming, tends to burn calories but not build muscle bulk. Aerobic exercise therefore helps increase endurance—that is, it increases one's ability to sustain muscular effort. Stamina or endurance results from numerous physiological changes. One of the most important changes occurs in the heart. The heart responds to exercise like any other muscle—it grows stronger and enlarges. A well-exercised heart beats more slowly but pumps more blood with each beat, as explained in Chapter 6. The net result, then, is that the heart works more efficiently, delivering more oxygen to skeletal muscles.

Increased endurance also results from improvements in the function of the respiratory system. For example, exercise increases the strength of the muscles involved in breathing. These muscles become stronger and can operate longer without tiring. Breathing during exercise becomes more efficient.

Increased endurance may also be attributed to an increase in the amount of blood that occurs as a result of exercise. An increase in blood volume, in turn, results in an increase in the number of RBCs, which increases the amount of oxygen available to cells. This improvement, combined with others, allows an individual to work out longer without growing tired.

When you set out on an exercise program, it is important to establish your goals first. If you are interested in increasing your endurance, you should pursue an exercise regime that works the heart and muscles at a lower intensity over longer periods such as riding a stationary bicycle. If you are after bulk, the answer lies in high-intensity exercises such as weight lifting that result in increased muscle mass.

Many health clubs and university gyms offer advice and exercise programs to help you achieve your goals. And many offer a variety of machines to help you build muscles or simply tone them up. Most of the exercise machines work one particular muscle group—for example, the muscles of the upper arm or the muscles of the chest. In most gyms, a half-dozen or more machines are usually placed in a line so you can go down the line, working one set of muscles after another until you have exercised your entire body.

Exercise machines are popular because they are safer than free weights (barbells and dumbbells). Progressive resistance machines eliminate the chances of your dropping a weight on your toes—or someone else's! Moreover, it is almost impossible to strain your back if you make a mistake using one. In contrast, lifting free weights requires care and training as well as brawn.

These machines also reduce the amount of time a person needs to exercise by about half because they've been designed to require work when a joint is both flexed and extended. The biceps machine, for example, requires you to pull the weights up, then return them slowly. Your muscles are being forced to work in both directions.

Such machines also permit individuals to lift heavier weights. The reason for this is simple. With free weights, you can only lift a weight that can safely be moved through the part of the exercise where your muscle is the weakest. Any more, and you can tear a muscle or drop a weight. One previously popular brand of progressive-resistance machine, Nautilus, alters the resistance automatically as you perform an exercise. In the weakest phase of the exercise, the machine reduces the resistance to prevent damage. Throughout the rest of the exercise, however, the resistance is full.

Health, Homeostasis, and the Environment
Athletes and Steroids

The skeleton and muscles provide many obvious benefits, the most evident one being mobility. These two systems also contribute to homeostasis. The skeleton, for instance, serves as a calcium reservoir, essential for controlling blood levels of calcium, which are crucial for normal muscle function. Muscle helps provide the heat necessary for the normal operation of cells.

This section is a departure from previous Health, Homeostasis, and the Environment sections, which have shown how health is affected by environmental pollution or adverse environmental conditions that up-set homeostatic workings of cells and various organ systems. Here we will discuss how an intentional action (taking anabolic steroids) to improve a body system (the muscles) can upset other systems.

Anabolic steroids are synthetic hormones that resemble the male sex hormone, testosterone. When taken in large doses, anabolic steroids stimulate muscle formation. They increase muscle size and strength by stimulating protein synthesis in muscle cells. High doses may also reduce the inflammation that frequently results from heavy exercise, allowing athletes to work out harder and longer.

When it comes to building muscle, steroids and exercise are an unbeatable combination. Some users claim that steroids even increase aggression, which may be helpful to competitive athletes such as football players.

Despite the benefits of steroids, most physicians view them as a dangerous proposition. For example, steroids can result in psychiatric (mental) and behavioral problems. One set of researchers interviewed 41 athletes who used steroids in doses 10–100 times greater than those used in medical treatment. The athletes also reported using as many as five or six steroids simultaneously in cycles lasting 4–12 weeks, a practice known as "stacking." In this study, researchers found that one-third of the athletes developed severe psychiatric complications.

Athletes in the study reported episodes of severe depression during and after steroid use. Some reported feelings of invincibility. One man, in fact, deliberately drove a car into a tree at 40 miles per hour while a friend videotaped him. Some subjects reported psychotic symptoms in association with steroid use, including auditory hallucinations (hearing voices). Withdrawal from steroids resulted not only in depression, but also in suicidal tendencies.

Other studies have shown that steroids used in excess may damage the heart and kidneys and reduce testicular size in men. In women, steroids deepen the voice and may cause enlargement of the clitoris. Steroids also cause severe acne and liver cancer. Unfortunately, there are no scientific studies on the long-term health effects of steroids.

Despite the fact that anabolic steroids are banned by the National Football League, the International Olympic Committee, and college athletic programs, athletes continue to use them. Although periodic drug tests are often made, these steroids escape detection, along with a host of other performance-enhancing drugs, including stimulants and even a substance known as EPO (short for erythropoeitin) which increases the production of red blood cells.

U.S. athletes are subjected to numerous unannounced drug tests. Other countries are far more lenient. Most steroids used in the United States are imported illegally from Mexico and Europe. Because of a federal crackdown on the importation of steroids, some experts believe that the inflow may be slowing. Others are not so optimistic, contending that the $100-million-a-year black market will not be easily deterred.

A recent survey of 46 public and private high schools across the United States involving over 3000 teenagers suggests that steroid use is especially prevalent in high school seniors. About 1 of every 15 senior boys reported taking anabolic steroids. The study also showed that the use of anabolic steroids begins in ju-nior high school. Two-thirds of the students surveyed said that they had used steroids by age 16. Nearly half the users said they took the drugs to boost athletic performance, and 27% said their primary motive was to improve their appearance. Researchers say that adolescents who use steroids may be putting themselves at risk of stunted growth, infertility, and psychological problems.

Steroid use in the United States illustrates our dependence on quick fixes. It is a tragic result of the almost obsessive focus on performance and achievement in our highly competitive society, a social environment that may be endangering the health of our children and our athletes.

Summary

Structure and Function of the Human Skeleton

1. *Bones* serve many functions. They provide internal support, allow for movement, and help protect internal body parts. They also produce blood cells and platelets, store fat, and help regulate blood calcium levels.

2. Most bones have an outer layer of *compact bone* and an inner layer of *spongy bone*. Inside the bone is the *marrow cavity,* filled with either fat cells *(yellow marrow)* or blood cells and blood-producing cells *(red marrow)* or with combinations of the two.

3. The *joints* unite bones. Three types of joints are found: immovable, slightly movable, and freely movable. The movable joints allow for flexion, extension, and other important movements.

4. Joints are vulnerable to injury and disease. Torn ligaments and ripped cartilage are common injuries among athletes. Wear and tear on some joints can cause the articular cartilage to crack and flake off, resulting in degenerative joint disease, or *osteoarthritis. Rheumatoid arthritis* results from an autoimmune reaction that produces a painful inflammation and thickening of the *synovial membrane,* disfiguring and stiffening joints.

5. Most of the bones form from hyaline cartilage in a process called *endochondral ossification.*

6. Bone is constantly remodeled after birth to accommodate changing stresses. During bone remodeling, *osteoclasts* destroy bone. *Osteoclasts* are stimulated by *parathormone,* produced by the parathyroid glands.

7. Osteoclasts also participate in the homeostatic control of blood calcium levels. When activated, these cells free calcium from the bone, raising blood calcium levels.

8. *Osteoblasts* are bone-forming cells stimulated by *calcitonin* from the thyroid gland. Calcitonin secretion decreases blood calcium levels and increases the amount of calcium in bones.

9. *Osteoporosis* is a disease of the bone caused by progressive decalcification. The bones become brittle and easily broken. Osteoporosis is most common in postmenopausal women and results from the loss of the ovarian hormone estrogen. It also occurs in people who are immobilized for long periods.

10. Osteoporosis can be prevented and reversed by exercise, calcium supplements, calcium-rich foods, vitamin D, and estrogen therapy.

The Skeletal Muscles

11. *Skeletal muscles* are involved in body movements; they help maintain our posture and produce body heat both at rest and while we are working or exercising.

12. Each skeletal muscle consists of many long, unbranched, multinucleated cells known as *muscle fibers.* Muscle fibers are both excitable and contractile.

13. Inside each muscle fiber are numerous *myofibrils,* bundles of the contractile filaments *actin* and *myosin.*

14. Contraction occurs when the heads of the myosin filaments attach to binding sites on the actin filaments, then pull the actin filaments inward.

15. Muscle contraction is stimulated by nerve impulses from motor neurons that cause the release of acetylcholine.

16. The energy for muscle contraction comes from ATP. ATP is replenished by creatine phosphate, glycolysis, and cellular respiration.

17. Individual muscle fibers contract when stimulated by an action potential, producing a *twitch.* Contractions of varying strength (graded contractions) can be generated in whole muscles by recruitment and by wave summation.

18. *Recruitment* results from the engagement of many motor units. A *motor unit* is a motor axon and all of the muscle cells it innervates.

19. *Wave summation* is a piggybacking of muscle fiber contractions that occurs when stimuli arrive before the fiber relaxes.

20. *Muscle tone* is the rigidity of resting muscle caused by low-level contraction of some muscle fibers.
21. The body contains two types of skeletal muscle fibers: *slow-twitch* and *fast-twitch fibers*. Skeletal muscles generally contain a mixture of the two types, but fast-twitch fibers are found in greatest number in muscles that perform rapid movement. Slow-twitch fibers are found in muscles such as those of the back that perform slower motions or are involved in maintaining posture.
22. Muscle mass can be increased by certain forms of exercise, such as weight lifting. An increase in muscle mass results from an increase in the amount of contractile protein (actin and myosin) in muscle fibers.
23. Endurance can be increased by other forms of exercise such as aerobics.
24. Endurance is a function of at least three factors: the condition of the heart, the condition of the muscles of inspiration, and the blood volume. Improvement in all three factors increases the efficiency of oxygen delivery to muscles.

Health, Homeostasis, and the Environment: Athletes and Steroids

25. Many athletes are using synthetic anabolic steroids to improve performance and build muscle.
26. Unfortunately, massive doses of steroids have many harmful effects. They can increase aggression, cause psychiatric imbalance such as severe depression and result in damage to the heart and kidneys.

Critical Thinking

Thinking Critically— Analysis

This Analysis corresponds to the Thinking Critically scenario that was presented at the beginning of this chapter.

If you noted that no mention was made of dietary calcium intake by the various groups, you're correct. Unfortunately, the diets of the women in this study were not monitored to determine how much calcium was being ingested through food and beverages. Second, this study focused on the bones of the forearm, not the load-bearing bones that are at greatest risk of fractures. Walking would probably influence the bones of the legs, hips, and back. To accurately assess the effects of the exercise regime prescribed in this study, the researchers probably should have looked at bone density in all three sites, not the arms. Given these inadequacies, do you think this study's conclusions are reliable?

Exercising Your Critical Thinking Skills

A friend is selling an all-natural supplement guaranteed to give you more energy and help you sleep better at night. She cites a number of examples of users who feel energized and are sleeping better. She also notes that the developer of the product has a Ph.D. in nutrition. She wants you to try the product, which costs $40 a bottle. Using the critical thinking rules you learned in Chapter 1, describe what you might do in this situation. How would you evaluate the evidence your friend has given supporting the use of this supplement? What additional information would you want?

Test of Concepts

1. Describe the functions of bone. In what ways does bone participate in homeostasis?

2. The synovial joints move relatively freely. What structures support the joint, helping keep the bones in place?

3. A young patient comes to your office with swollen joints and complains about pain and stiffness in the joints. Friends have suggested that the boy has arthritis, but his parents argue that he is too young. Only old people get arthritis, they say. How would you answer them?

4. Describe the process of bone formation. Be sure to define the following terms: primary and secondary centers of ossification, osteoclasts, perichondrium, osteoblasts, and osteocytes.

5. Bone is constantly remodeled, from infancy through adulthood. Explain when bone remodeling occurs and what cells and hormones participate in the process.

6. Using what you know about bone, explain why an office worker who exercises very little is more likely to break a bone on a skiing trip than a counterpart who works out every night after work.

7. Describe how a bone heals after being fractured.

8. A 30-year-old friend of yours who smokes, exercises very little, and avoids milk products because of her diet says: "Why should I worry about osteoporosis? That's a disease of old women." Based on what you know about bone, how would you respond to her?

9. Describe the major functions of skeletal muscle.

10. Describe the detailed structure of a skeletal muscle fiber.

11. Describe the molecular events involved in muscle contraction.

12. Define the term *graded contraction*, and describe how they are achieved.

13. Describe the two types of skeletal muscle fibers, and explain how they differ.

14. A friend comes to you complaining that he can't seem to lose weight. He works out on barbells three times a week for an hour or so each time. His diet hasn't changed much, but with the increase in exercise, he thinks he should be losing weight, rather than staying even. Why do you think he isn't losing weight?

15. A friend is thinking about using anabolic steroids to improve his performance in gymnastics. He argues that he is young and will be taking the drug only for a year or so. He points out that other young men are using steroids and they really help build muscle and endurance. What advice would you give him?

www.jbpub.com/humanbiology

Connect to this book's web site: www.jbpub.com/humanbiology
The site features eLearning, an online review area that provides quizzes, chapter outlines, and other tools to help you study for your class. You can also follow useful links for in-depth information, research the differing views in the Point/Counterpoints, or keep up on the latest environmental and health news.

CHAPTER 14

The Endocrine System

Thinking Critically

One of the hormones you'll learn about in this chapter is growth hormone. As its name implies, it stimulates growth. Some individuals' bodies produce inadequate amounts, resulting in mild to severe stunted growth.

With the advent of genetic engineering, growth hormone is now commercially available. As a result, physicians can now treat patients whose bodies produce inadequate amounts, permitting them to grow more or less normally. Some parents and doctors are treating children who might be normally small. Should growth hormone be given to these "normal" children to enhance their growth—for example, to make them better basketball players? ■

Special image of the human thyroid gland.

One day while on his morning jog, president George Bush (the elder) began to feel weak. His heartbeat became irregular. He felt breathless. Fearing a heart attack, his security entourage rushed the president to the hospital where a blood test revealed elevated levels of a hormone called *thyroxine*. Thyroxine is a hormone produced by a gland in the neck known as the thyroid gland (THIGH-roid). This substance accelerates cellular energy production and affects a number of mental as well as physical processes. Elevated levels are indicative of a condition known as **hyperthyroidism** (HIGH-per-THIGH-roid-izm), or **Grave's disease** (after its discoverer, not the final outcome). This rare disease can occur at any age. It is just one of many diseases caused by a hormonal imbalance. This chapter discusses hormones of the endocrine system and presents some interesting examples of homeostatic imbalance caused by endocrine disorders.

Principles of Endocrinology

The human **endocrine system** consists of numerous small glands scattered throughout the body (**FIGURE 14-1**). These highly vascularized glands produce and secrete chemical substances known as **hormones** (HOAR-moans). (The word *hormone* comes from the Greek *hormon*, which means "to stimulate" or "excite.") A hormone is a chemical produced and released by cells or groups of cells that constitute the endocrine (ductless) glands.

All hormones are transported in the bloodstream to distant sites where they exert some effect. The hormone insulin, for example, is produced by the pancreas and travels in the blood to skeletal muscle and other body cells, where it stimulates glucose uptake and glycogen synthesis. The cells affected by a hormone are called its **target cells**. For a discussion of some of the early research that contributed to our understanding of hormones, see Scientific Discoveries 14-1.

Hormones function in five areas: (1) homeostasis; (2) growth and development; (3) reproduction; (4) energy production, storage, and use; and (5) behavior. At any one moment, the blood carries dozens of hormones. The cells of the body are therefore exposed to many different chemical stimuli. How does a cell keep from responding to all of these signals?

Target Cells Contain Receptors for Specific Hormones

Despite the fact that they're literally flooded with hormonal signals, target cells respond only to specific ones. Selectivity is conferred by protein **receptors**. In some target cells, the hormone receptors are embedded in the plasma

FIGURE 14-1 **The Human Endocrine System** The endocrine system consists of a scattered group of glands that produce hormones, chemicals that regulate growth and development, homeostasis, reproduction, energy metabolism, and behavior.

Scientific Discoveries that Changed the World 14-1

Pancreatic Function: Is It Controlled by Nerves or Hormones?
Featuring the Work of Bayliss and Starling

The concept of chemical control of body functions, like many other important biological ideas, is rooted in numerous experiments.

Of the many experiments crucial to our understanding of endocrinology, one by two British physiologists, W. M. Bayliss and E. H. Starling, stands out. Published in 1902, this experiment set to rest a debate about the mechanism controlling the release of pancreatic secretions.

Several experiments before the publication of this work suggested that hydrochloric acid in chyme (produced in the stomach) stimulated nerve endings in the small intestine. This, in turn, triggered a reflex that caused the release of pancreatic juices containing sodium bicarbonate, which neutralizes the acid. In these studies, researchers injected substances into the small intestine of anesthetized dogs to see what stimulated the release of pancreatic secretions. To determine the nature of the reflex, the researchers cut the nerves supplying the small intestine. Even though severing the nerves did not halt the pancreas, these researchers still argued that a nervous system reflex was involved. They hypothesized that clumps of nerve cells (ganglia) and their network of interconnected fibers in the wall of the intestine participated in local reflex arcs.

Bayliss and Starling repeated these experiments but were careful to sever all nerve connections to the small intestine. They then tied off a piece of the small intestine and injected small amounts of hydrochloric acid into it. This treatment resulted in the produc-

---

membrane; in others, they're located in the cytoplasm. (More on this later.) Each cell contains receptors for the hormones it's genetically programmed to respond to.

Hormones Stimulate the Synthesis and Release of Other Hormones or Activate Cellular Processes

Hormones fall into two broad categories. The first are the trophic or more commonly today, tropic hormones (TROW-pick; "to nourish"). **Tropic hormones** stimulate the production and secretion of hormones by other endocrine glands. An example is **thyroid-stimulating hormone** (**TSH**). Produced by the pituitary gland, TSH travels in the blood to the thyroid gland located in the neck on either side of the larynx. In the thyroid, TSH stimulates the release of a hormone, thyroxine (thigh-ROX-in).

Thyroxine, in turn, circulates in the blood and stimulates metabolism in many types of body cells. Thyrox-

ine is a **nontropic hormone**. Nontropic hormones stimulate cellular growth, metabolism, or other functions.

Hormones can also be classified into three groups according to their chemical composition: (1) steroids, (2) proteins and polypeptides, and (3) amines.

Steroid hormones are derivatives of cholesterol. **FIGURE 14-2** illustrates two common steroid hormones. Only minor differences in the chemical structure of these molecules exist, but they produce profound functional differences. **Protein** and **polypeptide hormones** are the largest group of hormones. As you may recall from Chapter 3, proteins and polypeptides are polymers of amino acids. Growth hormone and insulin are two examples. **Amine hormones** are much smaller mole-

(a) Thyroxine

(b) Epinephrine

FIGURE 14-3 Representative Amine Hormones *(a)* Thyroxine from the thyroid and *(b)* adrenalin (epinephrine) from the adrenal medulla.

Testosterone,
a masculinizing
hormone

(a)

Estradiol,
a feminizing
hormone

(b)

FIGURE 14-2 Two Common Steroids

tion of pancreatic juices. Because it was previously known that acid introduced into the bloodstream had no effect on the release of pancreatic secretions, the researchers concluded that "the effect was produced by some chemical substance finding its way into the veins of the loop of jejunum in question. . . ." This substance, they wrote, was "carried in the bloodstream to the pancreatic cells."

To verify their hypothesis, the researchers tried another experiment. In this one, they scraped off the cells lining the section of the small intestine, exposed them to acid, ground them up, and then extracted the fluid, which they injected into the bloodstream. After a brief latent period, the pancreas began secreting, a clear indication that these cells were producing a chemical substance that stimulated the pancreas.

Bayliss and Starling referred to the mystery substance as "secretin," because it stimulated pancreatic secretion. This name remains in use today.

Besides settling the debate over the control of pancreatic function, Bayliss and Starling helped clarify our understanding of endocrinology, furnishing definitions for some of the most important terms in the field. One good example is the term *endocrine gland*, which they defined as an organ that secretes specific substances into the blood that affect some other organ or process located at a distance from the gland.

cules derived from the amino acid tyrosine (TIE-row-seen). **FIGURE 14-3** shows the structure of two of the four amine hormones produced in the body.

Hormone Secretion Is Often Controlled by Negative Feedback Mechanisms

Hormones help to control many homeostatic mechanisms. Not surprisingly, their production and release are generally controlled by **negative feedback loops**, described in Chapter 4. In negative feedback loops in humans and other living things, the end product of some biochemical process inhibits its production. Consider the hormone glucagon (GLUE-ka-gone).

Glucagon is secreted (seh-CREET-ed) by cells in the pancreas when glucose concentrations fall—for example, between meals. After being released into the bloodstream, glucagon circulates throughout the body. In the liver, it stimulates the breakdown of glycogen stored inside liver cells. Glucose released from this process diffuses into the bloodstream, restoring normal levels. When normal glucose levels are achieved, the glucagon-producing cells in the pancreas cease secretion.

Not all feedback loops are as simple as this one. Some involve intermediary compounds. Nevertheless, all operate on the same basic principle.

Positive feedback loops are also encountered in the endocrine system, but only rarely. A **positive feedback loop** results when the hormonal product of a cell or organ stimulates the production of another hormone. This, in turn, causes more secretion and so on and so on. (The noise in a restaurant is a good example of a positive feedback. As the noise level increases, people talk louder. This increases the overall noise, forcing people to talk even louder.)

Positive feedback loops perform specialized functions. Ovulation (OV-you-LAY-shun), the release of the ovum from the ovary, for example, is stimulated by a positive feedback loop discussed in Chapter 19. Fortunately, each positive feedback loop has a built-in mechanism that ends the escalating cycle, preventing the response from getting out of hand.

Most Hormones Undergo Periodic Fluctuations in Their Release

The fact that hormones are controlled by negative feedback loops does not mean that hormone concentrations in the blood are constant 24 hours a day, 365 days a year. In fact, virtually all hormones undergo periodic

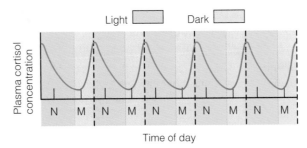

N is noon; M is midnight.

FIGURE 14-4 Cortisol Secretion Cortisol secretion follows a diurnal (daily) rhythm with highest levels occurring in the night just before waking. N = noon and M = midnight. Adapted with permission from George A. Hedge, Howard D. Colby, and Robert L. Goodman, *Clinical Endocrine Physiology* (Philadelphia: W. B. Saunders Company, 1987), Figure 4-4, p. 80.

fluctuations in their release, causing many body functions to also fluctuate. These natural fluctuations in body function are called **biological cycles**, or **biorhythms**, and were described in Chapter 4.

Biological cycles vary in length. Some hormones are released in hourly pulses, or cycles. Others are released in daily cycles. Cortisol (CORE-te-zol) is a steroid hormone produced by the adrenal cortex in a 24-hour, or **circadian rhythm** (sir-KAY-dee-an) (**FIGURE 14-4**). Cortisol has many functions, one of which is to increase levels of blood glucose. Its secretion increases during the night, reaching a peak just before one awakens, then falls sharply during the day.

Other hormones are released in monthly cycles. For example, the ovarian hormones estrogen and progesterone are released in a 28-day menstrual cycle. Still other hormones are released in seasonal cycles. In humans, thyroid hormone is released in greater amounts during the winter than during the summer. Thyroid hormone stimulates metabolism, which raises body temperature—a great adaptation for those of us who live in colder climates.

Most hormonal cycles are controlled by biological clocks, those regions of the brain that regulate biological cycles (Chapter 4). The biological clock is generally controlled by environmental conditions, primarily day length. Seasonal cycles are also typically controlled by environmental conditions—for example, temperature or photoperiod (day length). Such an interplay permits an organism to function in sync with its environment.

The Chemical Nature of a Hormone Determines How It Is Transported in the Blood and How It Acts on Cells

Protein and polypeptide hormones are water-soluble and, therefore, readily dissolve in the plasma of the blood. In contrast, steroid hormones are lipids and do not dissolve in water. To be transported, they must be bound to much larger plasma proteins like albumin.

When they arrive at their target cells, protein and polypeptide hormones bind to receptors in the plasma membrane. This binding of hormone to receptor stimulates a series of metabolic changes that activate the target cell. Steroid hormones, being lipid-soluble, pass through the plasma membrane of target cells into the cytoplasm where they bind to their receptors. This, in turn, results in numerous internal changes.

The Endocrine System and the Nervous System Are Both Control Systems, But They Operate in Markedly Different Ways

In the last two chapters, you studied the nervous system and the ways it controls basic body functions. The endocrine system also plays an important role in controlling the body's many functions. In fact, these two systems operate quite similarly. Both systems, for instance, send signals to distant sites that initiate a variety of important changes. But that's where the similarities end. A careful analysis reveals many profound differences. Perhaps the most important is that the nervous system typically elicits a rapid, short-lived response (for example, a muscle contraction). Although there are a few notable exceptions to this rule, the endocrine system generally brings about much slower, longer lasting responses (such as a change in body temperature).

The differences between the nervous and endocrine system can be attributed in part to the type of signal found in each system. For example, in the nervous system messages are conveyed by bioelectric impulses that travel very rapidly along the nerves of the body. In the endocrine system, messages are chemical in nature and are transmitted much more slowly through the bloodstream.

Despite these differences, the endocrine and nervous systems both promote homeostasis. As you will soon see, these systems sometimes work in concert.

With these basic facts in mind, let's begin to study the various endocrine glands and the hormones they produce. We'll start with the master gland, the pituitary, and the hypothalamus.

The Pituitary and Hypothalamus

Attached to the underside of the brain by a thin stalk is the **pituitary gland** (peh-TWO-eh-TARE-ee) (**FIGURE 14-5**). About the size of a pea, the pituitary lies in a depression in the base of the skull.

The pituitary gland is one of the most complex of all the endocrine organs. It is divided into two major parts: the anterior pituitary and the posterior pituitary. Together, they secrete a large number and variety of hormones, affecting a great many of the body's functions. Let's begin with the anterior pituitary.

The anterior pituitary produces seven protein and polypeptide hormones, six of which are discussed in this chapter (**TABLE 14-1**). One of the first things you discover when studying this fascinating little gland and the hormones it produces, however, is that the anterior pituitary does not work alone. It is controlled by a region of the brain known as the **hypothalamus.**

Lying just above the pituitary gland, the hypothalamus contains receptors that monitor blood levels of hormones, nutrients, and ions. When activated, the receptors stimulate specialized nerve cells within the hy-

FIGURE 14-5 The Pituitary Gland (a) A cross section of the brain showing the location of the pituitary and hypothalamus. (b) The structure of the pituitary gland. (c) Releasing and inhibiting hormones travel via the portal system from the hypothalamus to the anterior pituitary, where they affect hormone secretion.

pothalamus. These cells are a special brand of neurons called **neurosecretory neurons**—so named because they synthesize and secrete hormones. The hormones they produce control the production and release of hormones by its near neighbor, the anterior pituitary (**FIGURE 14-5**).

The hypothalamus produces two types of hormones—those that stimulate the release of anterior pituitary hormones, which are called **releasing hormones,** designated **RH,** and those that inhibit the release of hormones from the anterior pituitary. They're

called **inhibiting hormones,** designated **IH.** How do these hormones travel to the pituitary?

The releasing and inhibiting hormones are produced in the cell bodies of the neurosecretory neurons. They travel down the axons of the neurosecretory cells, which terminate in the lower part of the hypothalamus, just above the pituitary gland. The hormones are stored in the axon terminals until needed.

When released, the hormones diffuse into nearby capillaries. As shown in **FIGURE 14-5**, these capillaries drain into a series of veins in the stalk of the pituitary.

TABLE 14-1

Hormones Secreted by the Pituitary Gland

Hormone	Function
Anterior pituitary	
Growth hormone (GH)	Stimulates cell growth. Primary targets are muscle and bone, where GH stimulates amino acid uptake and protein synthesis. It also stimulates fat breakdown in the body.
	Stimulates release of thyroxine and triiodothyronine.
Thyroid-stimulating hormone (TSH)	Stimulates secretion of hormones by the adrenal cortex, especially glucocorticoids.
Adrenocorticotropic hormone (ACTH)	Stimulate gamete production and hormone production by the gonads.
Gonadotropins (FSH and LH)	Stimulates milk production by the breast.
Prolactin	Function in humans is unknown.
Melanocyte-stimulating hormone (MSH)	
Posterior pituitary	
Antidiuretic hormone (ADH)	Stimulates water reabsorption by nephrons of the kidney.
Oxytocin	Stimulates ejection of milk from breasts and uterine contractions during birth.

ng/ml = nanograms per mililiter

FIGURE 14-6 Growth Hormone Secretion in an Adult Growth hormone stimulates muscle and bone growth and is released during exercise and at night.

These veins drain into a capillary network located in the anterior pituitary. From here, the hormones diffuse into the anterior pituitary. They then bind to their target cells, causing them to release hormones.

This unusual arrangement of blood vessels where a capillary bed drains to a vein, which then drains into another capillary bed, is called a **portal system.**[1]

The Anterior Pituitary Secretes Seven Hormones with Widely Different Functions

The pituitary produces a number of hormones that profoundly influence our bodies. We will now discuss the major ones produced by the anterior pituitary gland.

---

[1]Another portal system is associated with the liver and digestive tract.

Growth Hormone Stimulates Cell Growth, Primarily Targeting Muscle and Bone.

It never fails to amaze me how much people differ. One of the most noticeable differences is in height and body build. What causes such variation?

These differences are largely attributable to **growth hormone (GH)** a protein hormone produced by the anterior pituitary. As its name implies, growth hormone stimulates growth in the body. It does so by promoting cellular enlargement (hypertrophy; HIGH-per-TROW-fee) and an increase in the number of cells through division (hyperplasia; HIGH-per-PLAY-za).

Although growth hormone affects virtually all body cells, it acts primarily on bone and muscle. In muscle, it stimulates the uptake of amino acids and protein synthesis. In bone, growth hormone stimulates cell division and protein synthesis in bone cells, resulting in an increase in both the length and width of bone.

Recent evidence shows that growth hormone actually operates via intermediaries—several polypeptide hormones produced largely by the liver. Known as **somatomedins** (so-MAT-oh-ME-dins), these hormones directly stimulate bone and cartilage cells. Their production in and release from the liver, however, are stimulated by GH.

As a rule, the more growth hormone produced during the growth phase of an individual's life cycle, the taller and heftier he or she will be.[2] In men, body growth is also stimulated by testosterone, an anabolic steroid produced by the testes, which stimulates bone and muscle growth, explaining why men are generally taller and more massive than women.

Growth hormone secretion undergoes a diurnal (daily) cycle. As **FIGURE 14-6** shows, the highest blood levels are present during sleep and during strenuous exercise. It is no wonder that sleep is so important to a growing child. Growth hormone secretion declines gradually as we age.

The secretion of growth hormone is controlled by a releasing hormone (GH-RH) produced by the hypothalamus. Growth hormone participates in a classic negative feedback loop. When levels are low, GH-RH is released from the hypothalamus, causing the anterior pituitary to produce and release more GH.

---

[2]Growth hormone production levels are ultimately determined by the genes.

(a)

FIGURE 14-7 Disorders of Growth Hormone Secretion
(a) Pituitary dwarves. *(b)* Pituitary giant.

(b)

(a)

(b)

(c)

(d)

FIGURE 14-8 Acromegaly Hypersecretion of growth hormone in adults results in a gradual thickening of the bone, which is especially noticeable in the face, hands, and feet. There is no sign of the disorder at age 9 *(a)* or age 16 *(b)*. Symptoms are evident at age 33 *(c)* and age 52 *(d)*.

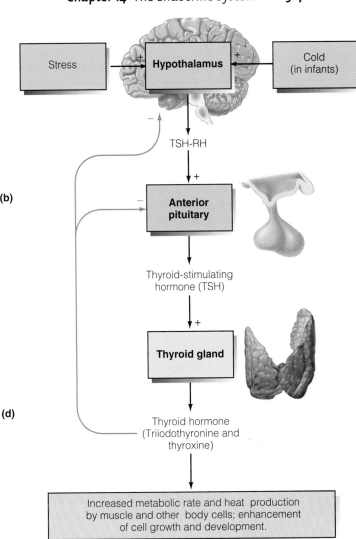

FIGURE 14-9 Negative Feedback Control of TSH Secretion Triiodothyronine (T₃) and thyroxine levels are detected by receptors in the hypothalamus. They also feedback on the anterior pituitary. When levels of T₃ and thyroxine are low, the hypothalamus releases TSH-RH, which stimulates the pituitary to release TSH. TSH, in turn, stimulates the thyroid gland to secrete T₃ and thyroxine. Other factors such as stress and cold influence the release of TSH via the hypothalamus. (A + denotes stimulation; a − denotes inhibition.)

Growth homone release is also stimulated directly through the nervous system. Studies show that stress and exercise both stimulate the hypothalamus via neural pathways to release GH-RH.

Deficiencies in growth hormone can result in dramatic changes in body shape and size, depending on when the deficiency occurs. Undersecretion, or **hyposecretion** (HIGH-poe-seh-KREE-shun), occurring during the growth phase of a child is one cause of stunted growth (dwarfism) (**FIGURE 14-7A**). Oversecretion, or **hypersecretion** (HIGH-per-seh-KREE-shun), results in **giantism** (GIE-an-tizm) if the excess occurs during the growth phase (**FIGURE 14-7B**). If the pituitary begins producing excess growth hormone after growth is complete, the result is a relatively rare disease called **acromegaly** (AH-crow-MEG-al-ee). Facial features become coarse, and hands and feet continue to grow throughout adulthood (**FIGURE 14-8**). Growth of the vertebrae results in a hunched back. The tongue, kidneys, and liver often become quite enlarged in patients with acromegaly.

Thyroid-Stimulating Hormone Stimulates the Thyroid Gland to Produce Thyroxine. Thyroid-Stimulating Hormone (TSH) is a protein hormone produced by the anterior pituitary and is controlled by **TSH-RH** (**TSH-releasing hormone**) from the hypothalamus. Day-to-day levels are primarily regulated by the level of thyroxine in the blood in a classical negative feedback loop relying on receptors in the hypothalamus that detect the level of circulating thyroxine. When circulating levels are low, these receptors signal the hypothalamus to release TSH-RH. When the level of thyroxine increases, TSH-RH secretion declines (**FIGURE 14-9**). TSH-RH secretion, however, is also stimulated by cold and stress. When you're under a lot of stress, TSH-RH secretion will be higher than when you are calm.

TSH-RH travels to the anterior pituitary, where it stimulates the production and release of TSH. TSH then travels in the blood to the thyroid gland, located in the neck (**FIGURE 14-1**). TSH stimulates the production and release of two thyroid hormones, thyroxine (thigh-ROX-in) and triiodothyronine (try-eye-OH-doe-THIGH-row-neen). These hormones circulate in the bloodstream and influence many body cells. One of

their chief functions is to stimulate the breakdown of glucose by body cells. Because this process produces energy and heat, increased levels of these hormones also raise body temperature—in the same way that adding wood to a fire increases its heat output.

ACTH Stimulates the Release of Hormones from the Adrenal Cortex. Another important hormone is **ACTH**, also known as **adrenocorticotropic hormone** (ad-REE-no-core-tick-oh-TRO-pick). ACTH is produced by the anterior pituitary. Its target organ is a layer of hormone-producing cells located in the outer regions of the adrenal gland. This portion of the adrenal gland is known as the **adrenal cortex**.

As shown in **FIGURE 14-10**, ACTH stimulates the production and release of a group of steroid hormones known as the **glucocorticoids** (GLUE-co-CORE-teh-KOIDS). Glucocorticoids like the hormone cortisol are steroids. Their main function is to increase blood glucose levels, thus helping maintain homeostasis.

As in other anterior pituitary hormones, ACTH secretion is controlled by the hypothalamus. As shown in **FIGURE 14-10**, the hypothalamus releases a small peptide known as ACTH-RH. Like other releasing hormones, it travels to the pituitary in the portal system.

ACTH-RH plays a pivotal role in the release of adrenal hormones via ACTH. But ACTH secretion is controlled by several other factors, two of which are discussed here. The first is the level of circulating glucocorticoids. These hormones are produced by the adrenal cortex and participate in a classical negative feedback loop (**FIGURE 14-10**). ACTH-RH secretion is also controlled by stress, acting through the nervous system. When we're under stress, ACTH-RH secretions increase, which causes an increase in ACTH release. This stimulates an increase in the release of glucocorticoids by the adrenal cortex. Glucocorticoids increase blood glucose levels, which ensures that we have the additional energy we need to operate body systems, especially muscles, when we are under stress.

The Gonadotropins Are Hormones That Stimulate the Ovaries and Testes. Reproduction in both males and females is under the control of the anterior pituitary. It produces two hormones that affect the gonads, appropriately known as **gonadotropins** (go-NAD-oh-TROW-pins). Because these hormones are discussed in detail in the next chapter, a few words will suffice for now.

The pituitary's gonadotropins are follicle-stimulating hormone and luteinizing hormone. **Follicle-stimulating hormone (FSH)** pro-

FIGURE 14-10 Feedback Control of ACTH Cortisol regulates hypothalamic and pituitary activity, but stress and the biological clock also influence the release of ACTH-RH.

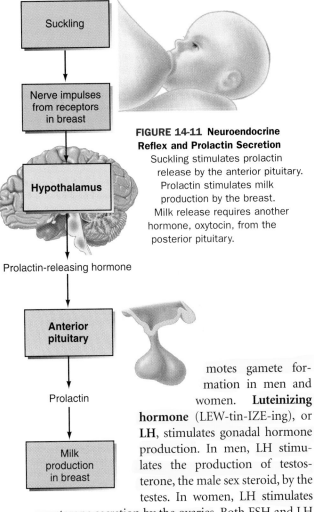

FIGURE 14-11 Neuroendocrine Reflex and Prolactin Secretion Suckling stimulates prolactin release by the anterior pituitary. Prolactin stimulates milk production by the breast. Milk release requires another hormone, oxytocin, from the posterior pituitary.

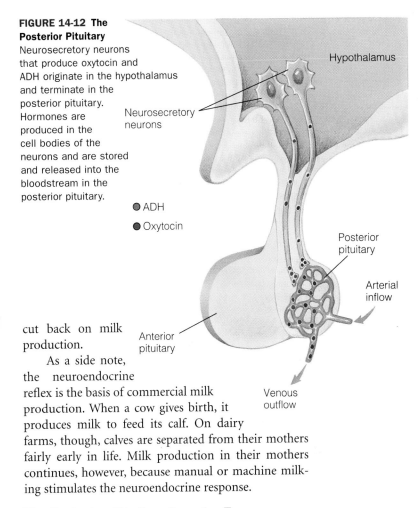

FIGURE 14-12 The Posterior Pituitary Neurosecretory neurons that produce oxytocin and ADH originate in the hypothalamus and terminate in the posterior pituitary. Hormones are produced in the cell bodies of the neurons and are stored and released into the bloodstream in the posterior pituitary.

● ADH
● Oxytocin

motes gamete formation in men and women. **Luteinizing hormone** (LEW-tin-IZE-ing), or **LH**, stimulates gonadal hormone production. In men, LH stimulates the production of testosterone, the male sex steroid, by the testes. In women, LH stimulates progesterone secretion by the ovaries. Both FSH and LH are under the control of **gonadotropin releasing hormone**, produced and secreted by the hypothalamus.

Prolactin Stimulates Milk Production in the Breasts of Women.

Prolactin (pro-LACK-tin) is a protein hormone produced by the anterior pituitary. In women, prolactin is secreted at the end of pregnancy and acts on the mammary glands (breasts), stimulating milk production.

Prolactin secretion is controlled by a **neuroendocrine reflex,** a reflex involving both the nervous and endocrine systems. As **FIGURE 14-11** shows, suckling stimulates sensory fibers in the breast. Nerve impulses travel to the hypothalamus via sensory neurons. In the hypothalamus, these impulses stimulate the release of prolactin releasing hormone (PRH). This hormone, in turn, travels to the anterior pituitary in the bloodstream, where it stimulates the secretion of prolactin. As long as suckling continues, prolactin secretion will continue. Prolactin production continues for many months as long as suckling continues. As babies begin to eat solid food, they reduce their dependence on their mother's milk. Reduced suckling shuts down prolactin secretion and the breasts

cut back on milk production.

As a side note, the neuroendocrine reflex is the basis of commercial milk production. When a cow gives birth, it produces milk to feed its calf. On dairy farms, though, calves are separated from their mothers fairly early in life. Milk production in their mothers continues, however, because manual or machine milking stimulates the neuroendocrine response.

The Posterior Pituitary Secretes Two Hormones

Have you ever wondered why alcoholic beverages make a person urinate so much or what actually causes milk to flow from a woman's breast? Have you ever wondered why a woman's uterus contracts when she delivers a baby?

These phenomena can be attributed to two hormones from the posterior pituitary. Like the hypothalamus, the **posterior pituitary** is a neuroendocrine gland—that is, a gland made of neural tissue that produces hormones. Derived from brain tissue during embryonic development, the posterior pituitary remains connected to the brain throughout life.

The posterior pituitary secretes two hormones: **oxytocin** (OX-ee-TOE-sin) and **antidiuretic hormone** (an-tie-DIE-yur-ET-ick) (ADH). Both hormones consist of nine amino acids. As shown in **FIGURE 14-12**, ADH and oxytocin are produced in the cell bodies of the neurosecretory cells located in the hypothalamus. They then travel down the axons into the posterior

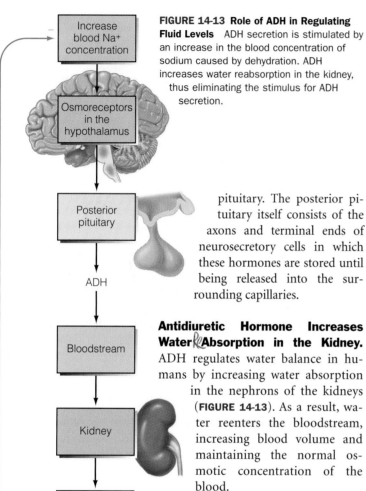

FIGURE 14-13 Role of ADH in Regulating Fluid Levels ADH secretion is stimulated by an increase in the blood concentration of sodium caused by dehydration. ADH increases water reabsorption in the kidney, thus eliminating the stimulus for ADH secretion.

pituitary. The posterior pituitary itself consists of the axons and terminal ends of neurosecretory cells in which these hormones are stored until being released into the surrounding capillaries.

Antidiuretic Hormone Increases Water Absorption in the Kidney. ADH regulates water balance in humans by increasing water absorption in the nephrons of the kidneys (**FIGURE 14-13**). As a result, water reenters the bloodstream, increasing blood volume and maintaining the normal osmotic concentration of the blood.

ADH secretion is controlled by a negative feedback loop (**FIGURE 14-13**). Receptors in the hypothalamus monitor the concentration of dissolved substances (especially sodium ions) in the blood. When the concentration exceeds the normal level—for example, during dehydration—ADH is released into the bloodstream. ADH stimulates the reabsorption of water by the nephrons, thus diluting the blood. When the osmotic concentration of the blood approaches homeostatic levels, ADH secretion ceases.

As Chapter 10 notes, ADH is inhibited by ethanol in alcoholic beverages. The reduction in ADH decreases water reabsorption in the kidneys and increases urine output. This, in turn, can lead to dehydration—the dry mouth and intense thirst a person may experience as part of a hangover.

ADH secretion may also decline as a result of traumatic head injuries that damage the hypothalamus. Such injuries can cause a sharp decline in ADH output. In the absence of ADH, the kidneys produce several gal-

lons of urine a day. To keep up with the water loss and to prevent dehydration, an individual must drink enormous quantities of water. This condition is known as **diabetes insipidus** (Chapter 10).

Because of its ability to increase arterial blood pressure, ADH is sometimes referred to as **vasopressin** (VEY-zoh-PRESS-in). Under most conditions, however, it is doubtful that enough ADH is secreted to increase blood pressure. ADH secretion in levels sufficient to exert a vasopressive effect occurs when an individual suffers an extreme loss of blood. When released in massive quantities, ADH constricts the walls of severed arteries, reducing blood loss. Clotting factors in the blood also help seal damaged vessel walls. ADH causes vasoconstriction throughout the cardiovascular system, which helps maintain blood pressure. This process is important because a large decrease in blood pressure can reduce the flow of blood to body cells, resulting in death.

Oxytocin Facilitates Birth and Stimulates Milk Let-Down. Prolactin from the anterior pituitary stimulates milk production in the breasts. But it's oxytocin from the posterior pituitary that actually "pumps" the milk from the glands by stimulating the contraction of the smooth-muscle-like cells around the glands in the breast.

Oxytocin release is stimulated by suckling. Sensory fibers in the breast conduct nerve impulses to the hypothalamus, triggering the release of oxytocin. The hormone travels in the blood to the breast, where it stimulates **milk let-down**—the ejection of milk from the glands soon after suckling begins.

Oxytocin also plays a role in the birth of a child. At the end of pregnancy, in the hours prior to delivery, the walls of the uterus and cervix stretch. Impulses from the stretch receptors in the uterus travel to a region of the neurosecretory cells in the hypothalamus that produce oxytocin. Impulses from the stretch receptors cause the neurosecretory cells to release the hormone. Oxytocin travels in the blood to the uterus, where it stimulates smooth muscle contraction, aiding in the expulsion of the baby.

Section 14-3

The Thyroid Gland

On a 50° day in the fall, you bundle up in a sweater to feel warm. However, 50° in the spring feels warm. You may not even need a sweater. Why the difference?

The answer lies in the thyroid gland and two of its hormones. The **thyroid gland** is a U- or H-shaped gland (it varies from one person to the next) located in

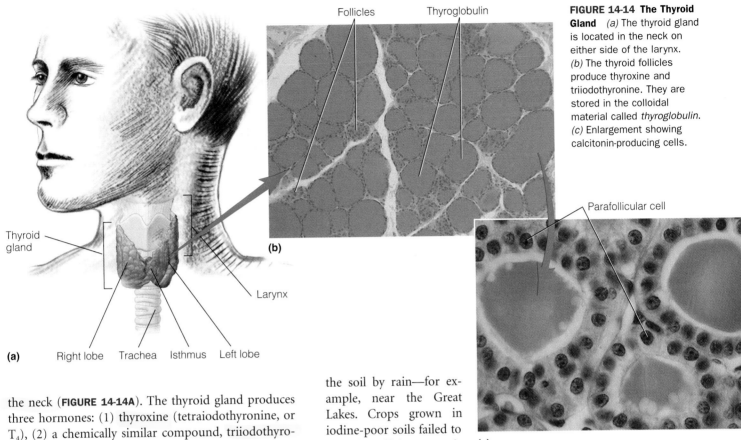

Follicles   Thyroglobulin

(b)

Thyroid gland

Larynx

(a) Right lobe   Trachea   Isthmus   Left lobe

Parafollicular cell

(c)

FIGURE 14-14 The Thyroid Gland *(a)* The thyroid gland is located in the neck on either side of the larynx. *(b)* The thyroid follicles produce thyroxine and triiodothyronine. They are stored in the colloidal material called *thyroglobulin*. *(c)* Enlargement showing calcitonin-producing cells.

the neck (**FIGURE 14-14A**). The thyroid gland produces three hormones: (1) thyroxine (tetraiodothyronine, or T_4), (2) a chemically similar compound, triiodothyronine (T_3), and (3) calcitonin. The first two are involved in controlling metabolism and heat production; the last helps regulate blood levels of calcium.

As **FIGURE 14-14B** shows, the thyroid gland consists of large, spherical structures known as **follicles** (FOLL-ick-als). Each follicle consists of a central region containing a gel-like glycoprotein called **thyroglobulin** and a surrounding layer of cuboidal follicle cells that produce thyroglobulin. **Thyroxine** and **triiodothyronine** are relatively small molecules (amines) derived from much larger thyroglobulin molecules in each follicle.

To make T_3 and T_4, the thyroid requires large quantities of iodide, I^-, which is actively transported into the cell. A shortage of iodide in the diet results in a decline in the levels of thyroxine and triiodothyronine in the blood. The hypothalamus responds by producing more TSH. TSH causes the thyroid to increase thyroglobulin production. Without sufficient iodide, however, the thyroid gland cannot produce thyroxine and triiodothyronine. As a result, the thyroid gland continues to produce thyroglobulin. This causes the gland to enlarge, sometimes forming softball-sized enlargements on the neck. This condition is known as **goiter** (GOY-ter) (**FIGURE 14-15**).

Goiter was once common in areas of Europe and the United States where iodine had been leached out of

the soil by rain—for example, near the Great Lakes. Crops grown in iodine-poor soils failed to provide sufficient quantities. To counteract this deficiency, iodine was added to table salt. Today, few people in industrialized nations develop goiter because they eat iodized salt or ingest sufficient quantities of iodine in their food or through mineral supplements.

FIGURE 14-15 Goiter An enlargement of the thyroid gland most often results from a lack of iodine in the diet.

Thyroxine and Triiodothyronine Accelerate the Breakdown of Glucose and Stimulate Growth and Development

Thyroxine and triiodothyronine are virtually identical and, as a result, have nearly identical functions. Both hormones, for example, accelerate the rate of glucose breakdown in most body cells. Thyroid hormones also stimulate cellular growth and development. Bones and muscles are especially dependent on them during the growth phase. Even normal reproduction requires these hormones. A deficiency of T_3 and T_4, for example, delays sexual maturation in both sexes. In children, depressed thyroid output stunts mental as well as physical growth. If the deficiency is not detected and treated, the effects are irreversible.

In adults, reduced thyroid activity, or **hypothyroidism**, is less severe. Hypothyroidism decreases the metabolic rate, making a person feel cold much of the time. People suffering from hypothyroidism also feel tired and worn out. Even simple mental tasks become difficult. Their heart rate may slow to 50 beats per minute. Hypothyroidism is treated by pills containing artificially produced thyroid hormone.

Excess thyroid activity, **hyperthyroidism**, in adults results in elevated metabolism, excessive sweating (due to overheating), and weight loss, despite increased food intake. The increase in thyroid hormone levels results in increased mental activity, resulting in nervousness and anxiety. People suffering from hyperthyroidism often find it difficult to sleep. Their heart rate may accelerate, as in the case of former President Bush, and they may lose their sensitivity to cold. Some people suffering from hyperthyroidism exhibit a condition called **exophthalmos** (EX-oh-THAL-mus), or bulging eyes. It is brought about by a swelling of the soft tissues of the orbit, or eye socket, which causes the eyes to bulge forward. In such individuals, the eyes may protrude so much that the eyelids cannot close completely. Exophthalmos can cause double vision or blurred vision.

Hyperthyroidism is treated in a number of ways. Patients may be given antithyroid medications, drugs that block the effects of thyroid hormones. Surgery may be required to remove part or all of the gland if it has become cancerous. The most common treatment for hyperthyroidism, however, is radioactive iodine. Iodine is concentrated in the thyroid gland. Radioactive iodine therefore accumulates in the cells of the thyroid follicle, damaging them and reducing their output of thyroid hormones. This procedure, while effective, may lead to other problems (notably cancer) later in life.

Calcitonin Decreases Blood Levels of Calcium

Large, round cells in the perimeter of the thyroid follicles produce **calcitonin**, or **thyrocalcitonin**, a polypeptide hormone (**FIGURE 14-14C**). Calcitonin lowers the blood calcium level in one of three ways: (1) by inhibiting osteoclasts, bone-resorbing cells, thus reducing the release of calcium from bone. (2) by stimulating bone-forming cells, osteoblasts, causing calcium to be deposited in bone. (3) by increasing the excretion of calcium (and phosphate) ions by the kidneys.

Calcitonin is involved in a simple negative feedback loop with calcium ions in the blood. When the calcium-ion concentration increases, calcitonin secretion increases. As calcium concentrations fall, calcitonin secretion falls.

Section 14-4

The Parathyroid Glands

The **parathyroid glands** are four small nodules of tissue embedded in the back side of the thyroid gland. These glands, once mistaken by anatomists for undeveloped thyroid tissue, are actually independent endocrine glands. They produce a polypeptide hormone known as parathyroid hormone, or **parathormone** (**PTH**).

Parathyroid hormone increases blood calcium levels. Its secretion is stimulated when calcium levels in the blood drop. PTH restores blood calcium levels by (1) increasing intestinal absorption of calcium, (2) stimulating bone destruction by osteoclasts, and (3) increasing calcium reabsorption in the kidney.

Calcium homeostasis is also influenced by vitamin D, available in some of the foods we eat, such as milk. Vitamin D is also produced in the skin under the influence of sunlight. Vitamin D increases calcium absorption in the intestine. It also increases the responsiveness of bone to parathyroid hormone.

As in other glands, the parathyroid may malfunction. **Hyperparathyroidism**, excess secretion of parathyroid hormone, is the most common condition. It may result from tumors in the parathyroid glands, which cause the secretion of excess PTH. Excess PTH results in a loss of calcium from the bones and teeth. Excess PTH also upsets several metabolic processes, resulting in indigestion and depression. Because bones contain enormous amounts of calcium, most symptoms of hyperparathyroidism (except high blood calcium) do not appear until 2–3 years after the onset of the disease. Therefore, by the time the disease is discovered, kidney stones may already

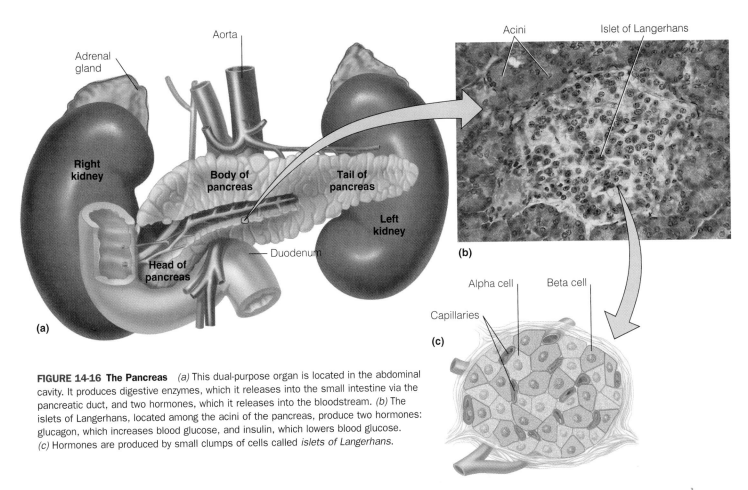

FIGURE 14-16 The Pancreas *(a)* This dual-purpose organ is located in the abdominal cavity. It produces digestive enzymes, which it releases into the small intestine via the pancreatic duct, and two hormones, which it releases into the bloodstream. *(b)* The islets of Langerhans, located among the acini of the pancreas, produce two hormones: glucagon, which increases blood glucose, and insulin, which lowers blood glucose. *(c)* Hormones are produced by small clumps of cells called *islets of Langerhans.*

have formed from calcium, cholesterol, and other substances, and bones may have become more fragile and susceptible to breakage. To prevent further complications, parathyroid tumors must be removed.

Section 14-5

The Pancreas

A young girl's parents complain to the daughter's doctor of frequent urination, bladder infections, fatigue, and weakness. Tests show that she is suffering from **diabetes mellitus,** a disorder of the pancreas. Diabetes mellitus has several causes, but in young people it is generally caused by a lack of insulin production.

Insulin is a hormone produced by the pancreas. It has many functions, but one of the most important is that it stimulates the uptake of glucose by body cells. It also stimulates the synthesis of glycogen in liver and muscle cells. As noted in Chapter 5, glycogen is a polysaccharide containing many glucose molecules. It's the way the body stores glucose for use between meals.

In healthy individuals, the amount of glycogen in the liver increases immediately after meals, then begins to decline in the period between feedings as the body uses up its storage depots to supply body cells with glucose. Muscle glycogen also increases after eating, then declines as the muscles break it down to produce glucose needed to provide energy.

Insulin is produced by the **pancreas** (PAN-kree-us), a dual-purpose organ located in the abdominal cavity and described in Chapter 5 (**FIGURE 14-16A**). The head of the pancreas lies in the curve of the duodenum, and its tail stretches to the left kidney. Most of the pancreas consists of tiny clumps of cells called **acini** (A-sin-eye). These cells produce digestive enzymes and sodium bicarbonate. Scattered throughout these enzyme-producing cells, however, are small islands of hormone-producing cells, known as the **islets of Langerhans** after the cytologist who first described them (EYE-lits of LANG-er-hahns). **FIGURE 14-16B** shows the acini and islets.

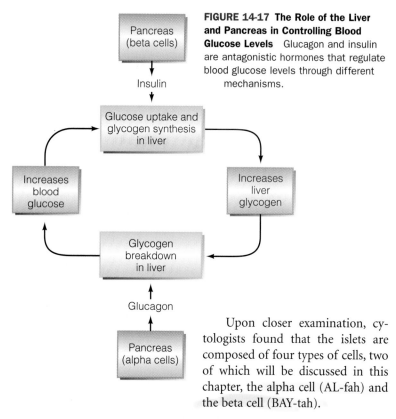

FIGURE 14-17 The Role of the Liver and Pancreas in Controlling Blood Glucose Levels Glucagon and insulin are antagonistic hormones that regulate blood glucose levels through different mechanisms.

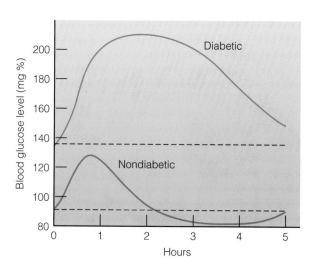

FIGURE 14-18 Glucose Tolerance Test In a diabetic (pink line), blood glucose levels increase rapidly and remain high after ingestion of glucose. In a normal person (blue line), blood glucose levels rise but are quickly reduced by insulin.

Upon closer examination, cytologists found that the islets are composed of four types of cells, two of which will be discussed in this chapter, the alpha cell (AL-fah) and the beta cell (BAY-tah).

Insulin Is a Glucose-Storage Hormone and Is Produced by the Beta Cells

The **beta cells** produce insulin, a protein hormone released within minutes after glucose levels in the blood begin to rise. Insulin affects a number of cellular processes and a number of different cells (**FIGURE 14-17**). Its principal targets, however, are skeletal muscle cells, liver cells, and fat cells. In this chapter we examine a few of its major functions, beginning with skeletal muscles.

Skeletal muscle cells are virtually impermeable to glucose in the absence of insulin. When insulin is present, however, the glucose transport into muscle cells increases dramatically. Glucose uptake rises because insulin stimulates facilitated diffusion. Insulin also increases glycogen synthesis in skeletal muscle cells. This not only helps store glucose for later use, it also lowers intracellular concentrations, thus accelerating diffusion (by maintaining a concentration gradient). Insulin also increases the uptake of amino acids by muscle cells and stimulates protein synthesis in them, thus promoting muscle formation.

In contrast, the plasma membrane of liver cells is quite permeable to glucose, so glucose enters with great ease whether or not insulin is present. Nevertheless, insulin still increases the uptake of glucose by liver cells by stimulating the addition of phosphate groups to glucose

molecules that have entered the cytoplasm. Because phosphorylated glucose cannot diffuse through the plasma membrane, glucose is trapped in the liver cell. Insulin also increases glycogen formation, creating glucose stores for times of need (**FIGURE 14-17**). Phosphorylation and glycogen synthesis decrease the cytoplasmic concentrations of glucose, thus maintaining the concentration gradient between the blood and the cytoplasm, which ensures a steady influx of glucose into the liver cell.

In fat cells, insulin increases glucose uptake and also stimulates lipid synthesis, creating food stores for times of need.

Glucagon Increases Blood Levels of Glucose, Thus Opposing the Actions of Insulin

A successful homeostatic mechanism often requires antagonistic—or opposing—controls. (In a car, we have an accelerator and brakes to control speed. In Congress, we have Democrats and Republicans.) In glucose homeostasis, the antagonistic control is provided by **glucagon**.

Produced by the **alpha cells** of the islets of Langerhans, glucagon is a polypeptide hormone that increases blood levels of glucose by stimulating the breakdown of glycogen in liver cells (**FIGURE 14-17**). This process, called **glycogenolysis** (GLY-co-jeh-NOL-i-sis), helps maintain proper glucose levels in the blood between meals. One molecule of glucagon causes 100 million molecules of glucose to be released.

TABLE 14-2

Type I and Type II Diabetes

Characteristic	Type I Diabetes	Type II Diabetes
Level of insulin secretion	None or almost none	May be normal or exceed normal
Typical age of onset	Childhood	Adulthood
Percent of diabetics	10%–20%	80%–90%
Basic defect	Destruction of beta cells	Reduced sensitivity of insulin's target cells
Associated with obesity?	No	Usually
Genetic and environmental factors important in precipitating overt disease?	Yes	Yes
Speed of development of symptoms	Rapid	Slow
Development of ketosis	Common if untreated	Rare
Treatment	Insulin injections; dietary management	Dietary control and weight reduction; occasionally oral hypoglycemic drugs

Glucagon also elevates blood glucose levels by stimulating the synthesis of glucose from amino acids and glycerol molecules derived from the breakdown of triglycerides. This process is called **gluconeogenesis** (GLUE-coe-KNEE-oh-GEN-eh-siss). Gluconeogeneis occurs in the liver.

Glucagon secretion, like that of insulin, is regulated by a negative feedback mechanism stimulated by glucose concentrations in the blood. When glucose levels fall, the alpha cells release the hormone into the bloodstream. When glucose levels rise, glucagon secretion declines. Glucagon release is also stimulated by an increase in the concentration of amino acids in the blood. Because glucagon stimulates gluconeogenesis, this process ensures that excess amino acids in high-protein meals are used to produce glucose.

Diabetes Mellitus Is a Disease Resulting from an Insulin Deficiency or a Decrease in Tissue Sensitivity to Insulin

FIGURE 14-18 shows a graph of blood glucose levels in nondiabetic and diabetic people obtained during a **glucose tolerance test**. During this test, physicians give their patients an oral dose of glucose, then check blood levels at regular intervals. The blue line on the graph in **FIGURE 14-18** represents the blood glucose levels in a normal person with a healthy pancreas. As illustrated, glucose levels increase slightly after the administration of glucose at time zero. However, within 2 hours, glucose levels have decreased to normal, thanks to insulin secretion.

The pink line illustrates the response in a diabetic person, who produces insufficient amounts of insulin or whose cells have become unresponsive to insulin. Glucose levels rise considerably in these people after they've been given an oral dose of glucose and they remain elevated for 4–5 hours. A similar response is seen in untreated diabetics after they have eaten a meal. In both instances, blood glucose levels remain high for such a long period because there are few places for the glucose to go. Virtually no glucose can enter skeletal muscle cells. Liver uptake is also greatly reduced, as is glycogen synthesis in liver and muscle cells.

Glucose levels eventually decline as this nutrient is used by brain cells, red blood cells, and others. The kidneys also excrete excess glucose. Unfortunately, this wastes a valuable nutrient and causes the kidneys to lose large quantities of water. Excess urination and constant thirst are the chief symptoms of untreated diabetes. Diabetics may have to urinate every hour, day and night.

Diabetes Is Really Two Diseases with Similar Symptoms But Different Causes. Physicians recognize two types of diabetes (**TABLE 14-2**). **Type I diabetes** occurs mainly in young people and results from a deficiency in insulin production. Also called **juvenile diabetes** or **early-onset diabetes,** Type I diabetes is believed to be caused by damage to the insulin-producing cells of the pancreas. A leading hypothesis suggests that it is the result of an autoimmune reaction. In some cases, however, there is no evidence of an autoimmune reaction. In such instances, individuals develop the disease very rapidly, which leads researchers to speculate that Type I diabetes is caused by a viral infection or an environmental pollutant that damages the cells that produce insulin.

Insulin production varies in patients with Type I diabetes. In some, it is only slightly reduced; in others, it is completely suppressed. In the latter, the absence of insulin starves body cells for glucose. Energy must be provided by the breakdown of fats.

Type II diabetes usually occurs in people over 40 and is also called **late-onset diabetes** (**TABLE 14-2**). In this disease, the beta cells produce normal or above-normal levels of insulin. However, because of a decline in the number of insulin receptors in target cells, cells are unresponsive to insulin.

Type II diabetes is commonly associated with obesity, a problem growing rapidly in more developed nations like the United States where people dine on high-fat, high-calorie diets. In the United States, for example, more than half (54%) of all adults are overweight. Not surprisingly, diabetes has increased 76% from 1990 to 1998 in individuals in their thirties. The increase is almost entirely due to a rise in Type II diabetes. But the increase in Type II diabetes is not just in older individuals. Physicians in the United States and Canada are also reporting a dramatic rise of Type II diabetes in overweight children. Lack of exercise and high-fat diets are the main culprits. Researchers predict that Type II diabetes will increase and that we will pay a high price for it. Disability, death, and medical expenses are all bound to escalate.

Heredity may also be an important contributor, as it is in Type I diabetes. In fact, studies show that about one-third of the patients with Type II diabetes have a family history of the disease. Critical thinking rules in Chapter 1 suggest the need to look for other explanations. Perhaps it may be the obesity that is inherited, rather than the tendency to develop diabetes.

Although Type I and Type II diabetes have different causes, both forms of this disease exhibit similar symptoms. Excess urination and thirst are generally the first signs of trouble. Patients often feel tired, weak, and apathetic. Weight loss and blurred vision are also common. Excess glucose in the urine may result in frequent bacterial infections in the bladder.

Although Symptoms Are Similar, Treatments for Type I and Type II Diabetes Are Quite Different.

Early-onset diabetes (Type I) is treated with insulin in-

jections and therefore is often called **insulin-dependent diabetes.** Patients receive regular injections of insulin—usually two to three times per day. Patients are also required to eat meals and snacks at regular intervals to maintain constant glucose levels in the blood and to ensure that regular insulin injections always act on approximately the same amount of blood glucose.

Insulin injections are tailored to an individual's lifestyle and body demands. To mimic the body's natural release, medical researchers have developed a device called an **insulin pump**. This device delivers predetermined amounts of insulin. Because the pump cannot actually measure blood glucose levels, it may deliver inappropriate amounts at certain times. Medical researchers are also experimenting with ways to transplant healthy beta cells into the pancreas of a diabetic.

Others are working on a nasal spray to dispense insulin, and so far clinical trials are proving to be quite promising. A two-year study in Israel showed that inhalants were as effective as injections at controlling blood sugar levels in people with Type I diabetes. Although diabetics may never be free from their needles, researchers believe that inhalants could reduce the number of injections they require to stay healthy.

Researchers are also working on ways to monitor blood glucose in diabetics. Currently, diabetics must prick their skin three or more times a day to gather a drop of blood which allows them to test blood glucose levels. A new experimental device is now being tested by a company based in California. This device measures glucose from moisture absorbed through the skin. The device, called GlucoWatch, resembles a wrist watch. It has an absorbent pad that sops up moisture and a measuring device that monitors glucose continuously. Studies on patients indicate a high degree of accuracy and the company is currently applying to the Food and Drug Administration for approval of their device.

In a recent study, researchers from the University of Florida reported findings that may help prevent Type I diabetes. The scientists withdrew blood from 5000 young children who showed no symptoms of early-onset diabetes. Next, they analyzed the blood for antibodies produced by an autoimmune reaction and followed the children's health status over time to determine which ones developed diabetes. During the study, 12 of the subjects developed early-onset diabetes. Blood samples from these individuals all contained an antibody that attacks a protein on the surface of the beta cells of the pancreas. The antibody was found in blood samples taken as many as 7 years before the onset of diabetes.

The antibody to the surface protein of the beta cell may provide a biochemical marker, an advance notice of the disease. Eventually, researchers hope to find ways to attach chemicals to the surface proteins of the beta cells that would neutralize or destroy the antibodies that bind to them, thus preventing the disease from developing. If this research proves fruitful, regular blood tests could be used to screen children. When the antibodies are found, special treatment could be used to annihilate them before they have time to attack the islet cells. This could free millions of people from a lifetime of insulin injections and the risk of blindness and other serious medical problems later in life.

Type II diabetes is also called **insulin-independent diabetes** because insulin injections are useless, given the fact that the disease very likely stems from a lack of insulin receptors in target cells. In many patients, Type II diabetes can be eliminated by weight loss. In others, the disease can be controlled by diet and exercise. For example, physicians restrict carbohydrate intake of their patients and instruct them to eat small meals at regular intervals during the day. Candy, sugar, cakes, and pies are strictly off-limits. Glucose must be supplied by complex carbohydrates, such as starches.

The treatments described above have dramatically changed the prognosis for diabetics. At one time the disease was fatal. Today, patients can live fairly normal lives. However, risks are still present. Type I diabetics, for example, may suffer from diabetic comas, or unconsciousness, when they receive insufficient amounts of insulin or if they go without an insulin injection for a prolonged period. Without insulin, the body cells become starved for glucose (even though blood levels are high) and begin breaking down fat. Excessive fat catabolism releases toxic chemicals (called *ketones*) that cause the patient to lose consciousness.

Diabetics may also suffer from **insulin shock** caused by an overdose of insulin. This reduces blood glucose levels, creating hypoglycemia. In mild cases, symptoms include tremor, fatigue, sleepiness, and the inability to concentrate. These symptoms result from a lack of glucose in the brain. In severe cases, unconsciousness and death may occur.

Early- and late-onset diabetics may also suffer from loss of vision, nerve damage, and kidney failure 20–30 years after the onset of the disease, even if they are being treated. Damage to the circulatory system can cause gangrene (GANG-green), requiring amputation of limbs, especially the lower extremities. These serious complications result from the inevitable elevations in blood glucose levels that occur periodically over the years. Elevated levels of glucose can damage nerve cells and blood vessels.

The Adrenal Glands

You stand on the banks of a raging river. Your raft is tied to a tree and floating in the calm water of an eddy above the tumultuous white water. As you watch kayakers and rafters head into the rapids, your heart starts to race, and your intestines churn in excitement (and fear).

This natural response results from the secretion of two of the many hormones produced by the **adrenal glands** (ah-DREE-nal). As **FIGURE 14-19** shows, the adrenal glands perch atop the kidneys, and each consists of two zones. The central region, or **adrenal medulla**, produces the hormones that increase the heart rate and accelerate breathing when a person is excited or frightened. The outer zone, the **adrenal cortex**, produces a number of steroid hormones discussed in more detail shortly.

The Adrenal Medulla Produces Stress Hormones

The adrenal medulla produces two hormones: **adrenalin** (epinephrine) and **noradrenalin** (norepinephrine). In humans, about 80% of the adrenal medulla's output is adrenalin. Helping us meet the stresses of life, adrenalin and noradrenalin are instrumental in the **fight-or-flight response**—the physiological reactions that take place when an animal is threatened. It enhances our ability to fight or flee. Adrenalin and noradrenalin are secreted under all kinds of stress—for example, when a careless driver cuts in front of you in heavy traffic or as you wait outside a lecture hall, anticipating an exam. Nerve impulses traveling from the brain to the adrenal medulla trigger the release of adrenalin and noradrenalin. The response is part of the autonomic nervous system (Chapter 11).

The physiological changes these hormones cause are many. For example, adrenalin and noradrenalin elevate blood glucose levels, making more energy available to cells, particularly skeletal muscle cells. They also increase breathing rate, which provides additional oxygen to skeletal muscles and brain cells. These hormones cause heart rate to accelerate as well. This increases circulation and ensures adequate glucose and oxygen for cells that might be called into action. In addition, adrenalin and noradrenalin cause the bronchioles in the lungs to dilate, permitting greater movement of air in and out of them. Furthermore, these hormones cause blood vessels in the intestinal tract to constrict, putting digestion on temporary hold, while the blood vessels in skeletal muscles dilate, increasing flow through them. Mental alertness increases as a result of increased blood flow and hormonal stimulation. You are ready to fight or flee.

The Adrenal Cortex Produces Three Types of Hormones with Markedly Different Functions

Surrounding the medulla is the adrenal cortex (**FIGURE 14-19**). The adrenal cortex produces three types of steroid hormones, each of which has a different function. The first group, the **glucocorticoids**, affect glucose metabolism and maintain blood glucose levels. The second group, the **mineralocorticoids** (MIN-er-al-oh-CORE-teh-KOIDS), regulate the ionic concentration of the blood and tissue fluids. The final group, the **sex steroids**, are identical to the hormones produced by the ovaries and testes. In healthy adults, the secretion of adrenal sex steroids is insignificant compared to the amounts produced by the gonads.

Glucocorticoids. The prefix *gluco* reflects the fact that these steroid hormones affect carbohydrate metabolism. (Glucose, of course, is one of many carbohydrates in living things.) The secretion of glucocorticoid is governed by ACTH from the anterior pituitary, as noted earlier. Several chemically distinct glucocorticoids are secreted, the most important being **cortisol**. Cortisol increases blood glucose by stimulating gluconeogenesis (the synthesis of glucose from amino acids and glycerol). This makes more glucose available for energy production in times of stress. Cortisol also stimulates the breakdown of proteins in muscle and bone, freeing amino acids that can then be chemically converted to glucose in the liver.

In pharmacological doses (levels beyond those seen in the body), cortisol inhibits inflammation, the body's response to tissue damage. Pharmacological doses of glucocorticoids also depress the allergic reaction. Cortisol brings about its effects by inhibiting the movement of white blood cells across capillary walls, thus impeding their migration

into damaged tissue. Cortisol also reduces the number of circulating lymphocytes by destroying them at their site of formation.

Because they reduce inflammation, cortisol and other glucocorticoids (particularly cortisone, a synthetic glucocorticoid-like hormone) can be used to treat inflammation resulting from diseases such as rheumatoid arthritis or physical injuries. However, the benefits must be weighed carefully against the damage that can be caused by upsetting homeostasis.

Mineralocorticoids. The mineralocorticoids are involved in electrolyte or mineral salt balance. The most important mineralocorticoid is **aldosterone**. It is the most potent mineralocorticoid and constitutes 95% of the adrenal cortex's hormonal output.

Although mineralocorticoids regulate the level of several ions, their main function is to control sodium- and potassium ion concentrations, and their chief target is the kidney. As noted in Chapter 10, aldosterone increases the movement of sodium ions out of the nephron and into the blood, a process called *tubular reabsorption*. Aldosterone also stimulates sodium ion reabsorption in sweat glands and saliva and potassium excretion by the kidney. When sodium is shunted back into the blood in the kidney and the skin, water follows. Aldosterone therefore helps conserve body water.

Aldosterone secretion is controlled by the sodium ion concentration in a negative feedback loop. As sodium levels fall, aldosterone secretion increases. As sodium levels are restored, aldosterone secretion declines. As you might expect, aldosterone secretion is also stimulated when potassium levels climb and when blood volume and blood pressure decline.

Diseases of the Adrenal Cortex. **Cushing's syndrome** generally results from pharmacological doses of cortisone. Cortisone is a synthetic glucocorticoid used to treat rheumatoid arthritis or asthma. In a few instances, the disease may be caused by a pituitary tumor that produces excess ACTH or a tumor of the adrenal cortex that secretes excess glucocorticoid.

Patients with Cushing's disease often suffer persistent **hyperglycemia**—high blood sugar levels—because of the presence of high levels of glucocorticoid. Bone and muscle protein may also decline sharply, because glucocorticoids stimulate the breakdown of protein. Individuals complain of weakness and fatigue. Loss of bone protein increases the ease with which bones fracture.

Water and salt retention are also common in Cushing's patients, resulting in tissue edema (swelling). Because of this, Cushing's patients typically have a rounded "moon face." Swelling occurs because gluco-

Adrenal gland

Adrenal cortex
Adrenal medulla

Kidney

FIGURE 14-19 Adrenal Gland   The adrenal glands sit atop the kidney and consist of an outer zone of cells, the adrenal cortex, which produces a variety of steroid hormones, and an inner zone, the adrenal medulla. The adrenal medulla produces adrenalin and noradrenalin, the secretion of which is controlled by the autonomic nervous system.

TABLE 14-3

Summary of Some Endocrine Disorders

Disease	Cause	Symptoms
Giantism	Hypersecretion of GH starting in infancy or early life	Excessive growth of long bones
Dwarfism	Hyposecretion of GH in infancy or early life	Failure to grow
Acromegaly	Hypersecretion of GH after bone growth has stopped	Facial features become coarse; hands and feet enlarge; skin and tongue thicken.
Hyperthyroidism	Overactivity of the thyroid gland	Nervousness; inability to relax; weight loss; excess body heat and sweating; palpitations of the heart
Hypothyroidism	Underactivity of the thyroid gland	Fatigue, reduced heart rate; constipation; weight gain; feel cold; dry skin
Hyperparathyroidism	Excess parathyroid hormone secretion, usually resulting from a benign tumor in the parathyroid gland	Kidney stones; indigestion; depression; loss of calcium from bones
Hypoparathyroidism	Hyposecretion of the parathyroid glands	Spasms in muscles; numbness in hands and feet; dry skin
Diabetes insipidus	Hyposecretion of ADH	Excessive drinking and urination; constipation
Diabetes mellitus	Insufficient insulin production or inability of target cells to respond to insulin	Excessive urination and thirst; poor wound healing; urinary tract infections; excess glucose in urine; fatigue and apathy
Cushing's syndrome	Hypersecretion of hormones from adrenal cortex or, more commonly, from cortisone treatment	Face and body become fatter; loss of muscle mass; weakness; fatigue; osteoporosis
Addison's disease	Gradual decrease in production of hormones from adrenal gland; most common cause is autoimmune reaction.	Loss of appetite and weight; fatigue and weakness; complete adrenal failure

corticoids, in high concentrations, have mineralocorticoid effects.

Because most cases of Cushing's syndrome result from steroids taken for health reasons, treatment is a simple matter: by gradually reducing the glucocorticoid dose. Tumors in the pituitary and the adrenal cortex may be treated with radiation or surgically removed.

Another disease of the adrenal cortex is **Addison's disease**. Most cases of Addison's disease are thought to be autoimmune reactions in which the cells of the adrenal cortex are recognized as foreign and are then destroyed by the body's own immune system. Addison's disease is characterized by a variety of symptoms caused by the loss of hormones from the adrenal cortex. These include loss of appetite, weight loss, fatigue, and weakness. Although insulin and glucagon are still present, the absence of cortisol upsets the body's homeostatic mechanism for controlling glucose. The body's reaction to stress is also impaired. The lack of aldosterone results in electrolyte imbalance. Because aldosterone maintains sodium levels and blood pressure, patients with Addison's disease have low blood sodium levels and low blood pressure. Addison's disease can be treated with steroid tablets that replace the missing hormones. Treatment allows patients to lead fairly normal, healthy lives.

Health, Homeostasis, and the Environment

Herbicides and Hormones

Hormones orchestrate an incredible number of body functions, and help to create a dynamic balance that is vital for good health. Hormones influence homeostasis primarily by controlling the rate of various metabolic reactions and by regulating ionic balance. When this balance is altered, human health suffers (**TABLE 14-3**). The endocrine system, like other systems, is sensitive to outside factors. Stress, for example, can lead to an imbalance in adrenal hormones, resulting in high blood pressure and other complications. High blood pressure, in turn, puts strain on the heart.

Hormonal balance can also be upset by toxic pollutants. One example is dioxin (die-OX-in), a contaminant found in some herbicides and in paper products. Infamous for its presumed carcinogenic properties, dioxin was found in the chemical known as Agent Orange, which was used in the Vietnam War to kill vegetation to reduce hiding spots for enemy soldiers. Oil spread on dirt roads in Times Beach, Missouri, also contained dioxin, deliberately added to the oil by a less-than-honest waste disposer. In 1983, after considerable public debate, the U.S. government bought up the town for $35 million, moved the residents out, and fenced it off.

New evidence suggests, however, that dioxin may be carcinogenic primarily at high levels—those in the workplace and those associated with chemical spills. The low levels found in Times Beach, in fact, may have little effect on human cancer.

Before you write your congressional representative to complain about the costly buyout, consider recent studies that suggest that at low levels dioxin may suppress immune functions. Scientists believe that it binds to plasma membranes and cytoplasmic receptors to which hormones normally attach, upsetting body functions. Thus, some researchers are calling dioxin an "environmental hormone." One form of dioxin, TCDD, suppresses the immune system in mice at least 100 times more effectively than corticosterone, one of the body's glucocorticoids.

TCDD also causes a variety of other direct biological effects. In some cells, it causes rapid cell growth. In others, it may alter cellular differentiation. Nonetheless, its effect on the immune system may be far more important than its impact on cancer.

Dioxin is not the only dangerous chemical in the environment. Studies suggest that a number of common herbicides (the thiocarbamates) may upset the thyroid's function and result in the formation of thyroid tumors. These herbicides are chemically similar to thyroid hormone and therefore block the secretion of TSH, resulting in goiter. At higher levels, they may cause thyroid cancer.

The overall impact on human health of toxic chemicals released into the environment is probably small, especially compared with the impact of tobacco smoke. However, not everyone agrees. The Point/Counterpoint in Chapter 17 debates this subject, which is an issue worth thinking about. This is an important debate, and it will be around for years.

Summary

Principles of Endocrinology

1. The *endocrine system* consists of a widely dispersed set of highly vascularized ductless glands that produce *hormones*.

2. Hormones affect five vital aspects of our lives: (a) homeostasis; (b) growth and development; (c) reproduction; (d) energy production, storage, and catabolism; and (e) behavior.

3. Hormones act on specific cells. Specificity results from the presence of hormone receptors on target cells. Steroid hormone receptors are generally located in the cytoplasm, and protein and polypeptide hormone receptors are located in the plasma membrane.

4. Three types of hormones are produced in the body: (a) steroids, (b) proteins and polypeptides, and (c) amines.

5. Hormone secretion is controlled principally by negative feedback loops, many of which involve the hypothalamus.

6. The endocrine and nervous systems are similar in several respects. They both send signals that regulate cell structure and function. Both help coordinate body functions.

7. The endocrine and nervous systems differ in several key respects. The nervous system elicits rapid, generally short-lived responses. The endocrine system elicits slower, longer-lasting responses.

The Pituitary and Hypothalamus

8. The *pituitary* is a pea-sized gland suspended from the *hypothalamus* by a thin stalk. It consists of two parts: the anterior pituitary and the posterior pituitary.

9. The *anterior pituitary* produces seven protein and polypeptide hormones. Their release is controlled by *releasing* and *inhibiting hormones* produced by the hypothalamus, which are transported to the anterior pituitary via a portal system.

10. The hypothalamic hormones are produced by *neurosecretory neurons*. Their release is controlled by chemical stimuli and nerve impulses.

11. The hormones of the anterior pituitary and their functions are summarized in **TABLE 14-1**.

12. The *posterior pituitary* is derived from brain tissue during embryonic development and consists of axons and terminal ends of neurosecretory cells whose cell bodies are located in the hypothalamus. Hormones are produced in the cell bodies and transported down the axons to the posterior pituitary, where they are stored in the axon terminals until released.

13. The posterior pituitary produces two hormones, *antidiuretic hormone* (*ADH*) and *oxytocin*, whose functions are also summarized in **TABLE 14-1**.

The Thyroid Gland

14. The *thyroid gland* is located in the neck, on either side of the trachea near its junction with the larynx. The thyroid produces three hormones: thyroxine (T_4), triiodothyronine (T_3), and calcitonin.

15. *Thyroxine* and *triiodothyronine* accelerate the rate of glucose breakdown in most cells, increasing body heat. These hormones also stimulate cellular growth and development.

16. Thyroxine and triiodothyronine both require iodine for their synthesis. A deficiency of this element in the diet results in *goiter*, an enlargement of the thyroid gland.

17. *Calcitonin* lowers blood calcium levels by inhibiting osteoclasts, thus reducing bone destruction and the release of calcium from bone. Calcitonin also increases formation of bone by osteoblasts and increases the excretion of calcium in the kidneys.

The Parathyroid Glands

18. The *parathyroid glands* are located on the back of the thyroid gland and produce a polypeptide hormone called *parathyroid hormone* (*PTH*), or *parathormone*.

19. PTH is released when calcium levels in the blood drop. This hormone increases

blood calcium levels by stimulating bone reabsorption by osteoclasts, increasing intestinal absorption, and increasing renal reabsorption of calcium.

The Pancreas

20. The *pancreas* produces two hormones, insulin and glucagon, from the *islets of Langerhans.*

21. *Insulin* is the glucose-storage hormone. It stimulates the uptake of glucose by many body cells and stimulates the synthesis of glycogen in muscle and liver cells. Insulin also increases the uptake of amino acids and stimulates protein synthesis in muscle cells.

22. *Glucagon* is an antagonist to insulin. It raises glucose levels in the blood between meals by stimulating glycogen breakdown and the synthesis of glucose from amino acids and fats (gluconeogenesis).

23. *Diabetes mellitus* is a disease involving insulin and blood glucose. It has two principal forms: Type I and Type II. *Type I*, also called *early-onset diabetes*, occurs early in life and may be caused by an autoimmune reaction that destroys the beta cells of the pancreas. It can be treated by insulin injections.

24. New methods of measuring blood glucose and administering insulin are under development and could help diabetics manage their blood glucose levels much better.

25. Type II, or late-onset, diabetes, results from a reduction in the number of insulin receptors on target cells. It is caused by obesity and genetic factors and can often be treated successfully by dietary management. Because of rising levels of obesity in the U.S. population, the incidence of Type II diabetes has begun to rise dramatically.

The Adrenal Glands

26. The *adrenal glands* lie atop the kidneys and consist of two separate portions: the adrenal medulla, at the center, and the adrenal cortex, a surrounding band of tissue.

27. The *adrenal medulla* produces two hormones under stress: adrenalin and noradrenalin. These hormones stimulate heart rate and breathing, elevate blood glucose levels, constrict blood vessels in the intestine, and dilate blood vessels in the muscles.

28. The *adrenal cortex* produces three classes of hormones: glucocorticoids, mineralocorticoids, and sex steroids.

29. The *glucocorticoids* affect carbohydrate metabolism and tend to raise blood glucose levels. The principal glucocorticoid is cortisol.

30. In pharmacological doses, cortisol inhibits the immune system and allergic reactions and is used to treat allergies or inflammation caused by injury and infections. High doses, however, have many adverse impacts on the body.

31. The chief *mineralocorticoid* is *aldosterone*. It acts on the kidneys, sweat glands, and salivary glands, causing sodium and water retention and potassium excretion.

Health, Homeostasis, and the Environment: Herbicides and Hormones

32. Hormones influence an incredible number of body functions, fostering homeostasis, a dynamic balance necessary for good health. When homeostasis is altered, our health suffers.

33. The endocrine system, like others, is sensitive to upset from stress and environmental factors such as pollutants.

34. Dioxin, a contaminant in some herbicides and paper products, may exert most of its effects through the endocrine system.

35. A number of common herbicides (the thiocarbamates) upset the thyroid's function and may even cause thyroid tumors.

Critical Thinking

Thinking Critically— Analysis

This Analysis corresponds to the Thinking Critically scenario that was presented at the beginning of this chapter.

This ethical dilemma hinges on several key questions—for example, should people be tinkering with nature? It is also a medical dilemma. For example, will growth hormone injections over a long period have any adverse effects?

As it turns out, no one knows the answers to the medical questions, but some studies suggest that prolonged usage may result in diabetes or high blood pressure. A recent study showed that growth hormone therapy in normal children, while greatly increasing height and muscle mass, dramatically reduced body fat. Children appeared gangly and raw-boned (emaciated). What effects these might have in the long term, no one knows. Some scientists believe that subtle abnormalities may develop in the cells, tissues, and organs of these individuals.

Clearly, the jury is still out on the long-term effects of growth hormone therapy in children. Parents who are subjecting their children to such treatment may be essentially creating a generation of human guinea pigs.

Test of Concepts

1. Define the following terms: endocrine system, hormone, and target cell.

2. Hormones function in five principal areas. What are they? Give some examples of each.

3. Describe the concept of specificity. How is it created in the nervous system? How is it created in the endocrine system?

4. Compare and contrast the functions of the nervous and endocrine systems.

5. The endocrine system elicits slower, longer-lasting responses than the nervous system. Do you agree or disagree? Explain your reasons.

6. Define the terms *tropic* and *nontropic hormones*, and give several examples of each.

7. Give two examples of negative feedback loops in the endocrine system, a simple feedback mechanism and a more complex one that operates through the nervous system.

8. Define the term *neuroendocrine reflex*, and give some examples.

9. Give several biological reasons for the following observations: (a) the endocrine response tends to be delayed; (b) the endocrine response tends to be prolonged; (c) some hormones perform several different functions.

10. List the hormone(s) involved in each of the following functions: blood glucose levels, growth, milk production, milk let-down, calcium levels, and metabolic rate.

11. Describe the role of the hypothalamus in controlling anterior pituitary hormone secretion.

12. Describe the ways in which the posterior pituitary differs from the anterior pituitary.

13. Explain the hormonal reasons for each of the following: acromegaly, dwarfism, and giantism. Acromegaly and giantism are both caused by the same problem. Why are these conditions so different?

14. ACTH is controlled by levels of glucocorticoid and by a biological clock. How are the controls different?

15. Describe the neuroendocrine reflex involved in prolactin secretion.

16. Offer some possible explanations for the following experimental observation: Milk production occurs late in pregnancy and is thought to be stimulated by the hormone prolactin. A nonpregnant rat is injected with prolactin but does not produce milk.

17. Where is ADH produced? Where is it released? Describe how ADH secretion is controlled. What effects does this hormone have?

18. Where is oxytocin produced? Where is it released? Describe how oxytocin secretion is controlled. What effects does this hormone have?

19. A patient comes into your office. She is thin and wasted and complains of excessive sweating and nervousness. What tests would you run?

20. A patient comes into your office. He is suffering from indigestion, depression, and bone pain. An X-ray of his bone shows some signs of osteoporosis. You think that the disorder might be the result of an endocrine problem. What test would you order?

21. How are the two basic types of diabetes mellitus different? How are they similar? How are they treated, and why are these treatments chosen?

22. Describe the physiological changes that occur under stress. What hormones are responsible for them?

23. What is gluconeogenesis? What hormones stimulate the process?

24. Cortisone depresses the allergic response. A patient comes to your office and asks that you treat her allergies with cortisone. What would you tell her?

25. Aldosterone is a mineralocorticoid. Describe its chief functions. How does it help retain body fluid? Under what conditions is aldosterone secreted?

www.jbpub.com/humanbiology

Connect to this book's web site: www.jbpub.com/humanbiology
The site features eLearning, an online review area that provides quizzes, chapter outlines, and other tools to help you study for your class. You can also follow useful links for in-depth information, research the differing views in the Point/Counterpoints, or keep up on the latest environmental and health news.

Chromosomes, Cell Division, and Cancer

Thinking Critically

Since the 1970s, environmentalists have been warning people of the increasing danger of a global calamity caused by the release of a class of chemicals called chlorofluorocarbons or CFCs for short. Used in refrigerators, freezers, and many other products, CFCs drift into the upper atmosphere where sunlight causes them to dissociate, producing a chemical that many scientists believe could seriously deplete the ozone layer, which protects us and many other species from dangerous ultraviolet radiation. Ultraviolet radiation, of course, can cause skin cancer, cataracts, and other problems. As the ozone layer thins, skin cancer rates and mortality from skin cancer could skyrocket.

Against this gloom and doom, a loud dissenting voice was raised on the airways of America, led in large part by radio and television celebrity Rush Limbaugh. He called the ozone threat a "scam." He said scientists were behind it, in part, because they viewed it as a way to enhance their funding. He and others alleged that claims by environmentalists and scientists were wrong.

Environmentalists countered that Limbaugh and others like him were spreading misinformation—or more bluntly, falsehoods. How would you go about analyzing this debate? ■

Human cell arrested in cell division.

Electricity flowing through wires produces a magnetic field. Since the discovery of this phenomenon, scientists have been interested in it mostly as a matter of curiosity. In 1979, though, two researchers from the University of Colorado discovered a potential dark side to this natural phenomenon. They reported the health effects of extremely low frequency (ELF) magnetic waves generated by high-voltage power lines. Their studies suggested that these magnetic fields may increase the incidence of leukemia (a cancer of the white blood cells) in children who live near high-voltage power lines. The cancer death rates in these children were twice what would have been expected in the general public. In November 1986, researchers from the University of North Carolina published reports showing a fivefold increase in childhood cancer (particularly leukemia) in families living 25–50 feet from wires transporting electricity from power substations to neighborhood transformers (**FIGURE 15-1**).

Studies of human health, such as these, are part of the science of **epidemiology** (EP-uh-DEEM-ee-OL-uh-ge), literally, "the study of epidemics." Epidemiological studies depend primarily on statistical analysis to examine potential correlations between cause and effect. Today, they're used to study the impacts of a wide range of substances and physical agents such as mag-

netic fields on human health. One epidemiological study by itself rarely proves a point. But when several studies report the same correlation, as in the ELF case, the results are more reliable.

Experimental work in the laboratory also lends support to epidemiological studies. In the ELF controversy, additional evidence in favor of the hypothesis came from a researcher who found that ELF fields increased the growth rate of cancer cells in tissue culture. They also rendered the cells 60%–70% more resistant to the immune system's naturally occurring killer cells, which attack cancer cells.

Some studies showed that numerous household items, such as water bed heaters and electric blankets, produce magnetic fields and that these devices increased the likelihood of miscarriage (spontaneous abortion of an embryo or fetus). In October, 1996, however, a panel of scientists convened by the prestigious National Research Council concluded that electromagnetic fields associated with power lines, appliances, and other sources *do not* pose a health risk to humans. Their conclusion was based on an exhaustive analysis of over 500 studies on the subject performed over a 17-year period. Although some studies do show an effect, the bulk of the evidence shows no credible link, they concluded. In those studies that demonstrated a link, scientists suggested that other unmeasured factors may have been responsible.

This chapter provides basic information about chromosomes and cell division that will help you understand this debate as well as the information on cancer, the other main topic of this chapter.

Section 15-1

The Cell Cycle

As noted in Chapter 1, all cells arise from preexisting cells via cell division. This process is the basis of reproduction and growth and is therefore essential to all forms of life. In humans and other multicellular organisms, cell division also plays an important role in the repair of damaged tissues and organs. Without it, we'd be in grave trouble.

Cell division is a well-orchestrated process, occurring during a distinct part of the life cycle of a cell, commonly referred to as the **cell cycle** (**FIGURE 15-2**). As illustrated, the cell cycle is divided into two parts: cell division and interphase. During **cell division**, the nucleus and the cytoplasm divide, splitting the cell more or less equally, thus forming two new cells. **Interphase** is the period between cell divisions.

FIGURE 15-1 Too Close for Comfort?   Some studies suggest that extremely low frequency radiation from power lines may increase the incidence of cancer, especially childhood leukemia, in nearby residents. A recent analysis of the research, however, indicates that this link between cancer and electrical lines is *not* real.

Interphase Is Divided into Three Parts

Once thought to be a resting period, interphase is now known to be a time of intense metabolic activity. During interphase, for example, cells replicate their DNA. They also replicate many cytoplasmic components, including organelles, a process that prepares cells for division. Thus, when cells divide, their offspring, or daughter cells, receive an adequate supply of the organelles and molecules needed to function normally.

Interphase is divided into three phases: G_1, S, and G_2 (**FIGURE 15-2** and **TABLE 15-1**). G_1 (**gap 1**) begins immediately after a cell divides. During G_1, the nuclear DNA orchestrates the cell's synthesis of RNA, proteins, and other molecules vital for proper cellular function and growth. These molecules also serve as a stockpile that ensures each daughter cell an adequate supply of nutrients.

The length of G_1 varies considerably from one cell to another. Some cells in an organism spend only a few minutes or hours in G_1; others spend weeks or even months. Cells such as nerves that never divide remain locked in G_1 for life. In general, mammalian cells in culture spend 8–10 hours in G_1 (**FIGURE 15-2**).

TABLE 15-1

Phases of the Cell Cycle

Phase	Characteristics
Interphase	
G_1 (gap 1)	Stage begins immediately after mitosis.
	RNA, protein, and other molecules are synthesized.
S (synthesis)	DNA is replicated.
	Chromosomes become double stranded.
G_2 (gap 2)	Mitochondria divide; precursors of spindle fibers are synthesized.
Mitosis	
Prophase	Chromosomes condense.
	Nuclear envelope disappears.
	Centrioles divide and migrate to opposite poles of the dividing cell.
	Spindle fibers form and attach to chromosomes.
Metaphase	Chromosomes line up on equatorial plate of the dividing cell.
Anaphase	Chromosomes begin to separate.
Telophase	Chromosomes migrate or are pulled to opposite poles.
	New nuclear envelope forms.
	Chromosomes uncoil.
Cytokinesis	Cleavage furrow forms and deepens.
	Cytoplasm divides.

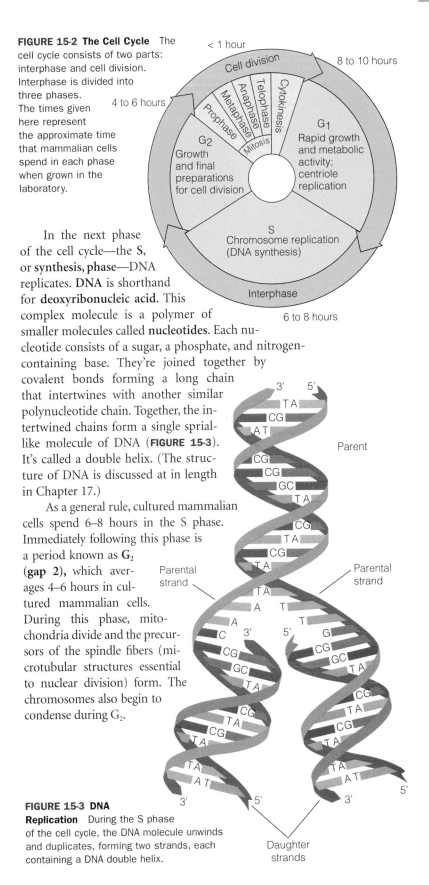

FIGURE 15-2 The Cell Cycle   The cell cycle consists of two parts: interphase and cell division. Interphase is divided into three phases. The times given here represent the approximate time that mammalian cells spend in each phase when grown in the laboratory.

In the next phase of the cell cycle—the **S**, or **synthesis, phase**—DNA replicates. **DNA** is shorthand for **deoxyribonucleic acid**. This complex molecule is a polymer of smaller molecules called **nucleotides**. Each nucleotide consists of a sugar, a phosphate, and nitrogen-containing base. They're joined together by covalent bonds forming a long chain that intertwines with another similar polynucleotide chain. Together, the intertwined chains form a single sprial-like molecule of DNA (**FIGURE 15-3**). It's called a double helix. (The structure of DNA is discussed at in length in Chapter 17.)

As a general rule, cultured mammalian cells spend 6–8 hours in the S phase. Immediately following this phase is a period known as G_2 (**gap 2**), which averages 4–6 hours in cultured mammalian cells. During this phase, mitochondria divide and the precursors of the spindle fibers (microtubular structures essential to nuclear division) form. The chromosomes also begin to condense during G_2.

FIGURE 15-3 DNA Replication   During the S phase of the cell cycle, the DNA molecule unwinds and duplicates, forming two strands, each containing a DNA double helix.

Nuclear and Cytoplasmic Division Occur Separately

Interphase is followed by cell division, a rapid event by cell standards, which lasts only about 1 hour in mammalian cells. During cell division, the nucleus and cytoplasm both divide. However, nuclear division, commonly known as **mitosis** (my-TOE-siss), precedes cytoplasmic division.

Mitosis involves a series of rather dramatic and fascinating structural changes. In order for the replicated chromosomes to divide, they must first condense. During this process, the chromosomes become compact structures that are clearly visible in ordinary light microscopic preparations (**FIGURE 15-4**). Condensation facilitates chromosomal segregation. Without it, cell division would be a nightmare. Dividing the 46 unravelled chromosomes in humans would result in a tangled mass of broken chromosomes. Cell division without chromosome compaction would be like trying to separate a plate of spaghetti into two equal piles without breaking a single strand.

In addition, for mitosis to occur smoothly, the chromosomes must line up in the center of the cell. From this position, the two chromatids of each chromosome can easily be drawn apart and then be divvied up, one-half going to each new daughter cell.

Cytoplasmic division, or **cytokinesis** (literally, "cell movement," pronounced SITE-toe-ki-NEE-siss), occurs independently of mitosis and usually toward the end of it. With this overview of cell division, we now turn our attention to one of the main actors in this exciting cellular drama, the chromosome.

The Chromosome

As you surely know by now, chromosomes contain the genetic information of cells, DNA, which directs most cellular events. (For a discussion of the scientific work that led to the discovery of DNA, see Scientific Discoveries 15-1; for a review of terminol-

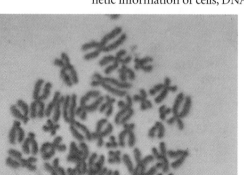

FIGURE 15-4 Metaphase Chromosomes Taken from a human cell during metaphase, these chromosomes are clearly visible under a light microscope.

TABLE 15-2	
Review of Terminology	
Chromatin	General term referring to a strand of DNA and associated histone protein
Chromatin fiber	Strand of chromatin
Chromosome	Structure consisting of one or two chromatin fibers
Chromatid	Generally used to refer to one of the chromatin fibers of a replicated chromosome
Centromere	Region of each chromatid to which a sister chromatid attaches

ogy see **TABLE 15-2**.) All organisms have a set number of chromosomes. All of the cells in your body, for example, contain 46 chromosomes, except for the gametes (or germ cells—the sperm and egg), which contain half that number.

Each type of chromosome contains very specific genetic information and is different from every other type. Chromosomes also differ in several other key respects, such as size, location of the centromere, and banding patterns (**FIGURE 15-5**). By studying these features, **geneticists**, scientists who study chromosomes, genes, and heredity, have found that chromosomes in

FIGURE 15-5 Karyotype Chromosomes from a normal human female arranged in order of decreasing size. Note that there are 46 chromosomes—or 23 pairs—in somatic cells. Each pair is similar in size, banding pattern, and location of the centromere.

FIGURE 15-6 Chromosome Structure
(a) The DNA helix wraps around histone molecules to form a chromatin fiber. During prophase, the chromatin fiber coils tightly, forming the densely packed chromosome. *(b)* Transmission electron micrograph of a metaphase chromosome.

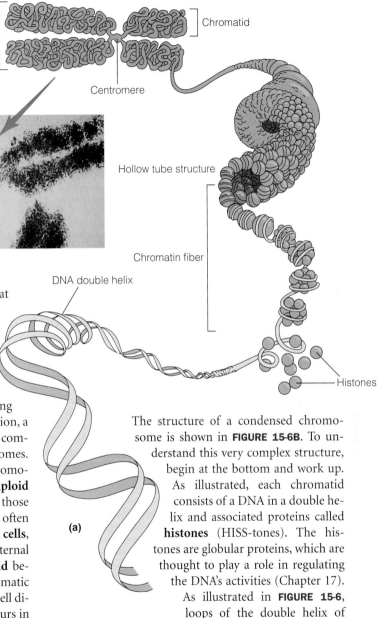

Metaphase chromosome

Chromatid

Centromere

Hollow tube structure

Chromatin fiber

DNA double helix

Histones

(b)

(a)

most of the cells of the body exist in pairs. In humans, for example, geneticists can distinguish 23 structurally similar pairs. As shown in **FIGURE 15-5**, each pair has the same length, banding pattern, and centromere position. Such chromosomes are described as **homologous** (ha-MOLL-ah-GUS).

Homologous chromosomes contain genes that control the same inherited traits. For example, if a gene for hair color is located on one chromosome of a pair, another gene of similar structure will be found at the same location (or **locus**) on the other member of the pair.

The presence of homologous chromosome pairs results from sexual reproduction—the uniting of a sperm and an ovum. During sexual reproduction, a new individual is created when the sperm and egg combine. Both the sperm and egg contain 23 chromosomes.

Cells that contain the full complement of chromosomes—that is, 46 chromosomes—are said to be **diploid** (diploid = twofold). In humans, all body cells, like those of skin and muscle, are diploid. Such cells are often called **somatic cells** to distinguish them from **germ cells**, the sperm and ovum, which carry paternal and maternal chromosomes, respectively. Germ cells are **haploid** because they contain half the chromosomes of somatic cells. Germ cells are produced by a special kind of cell division known as **meiosis** (my-OH-siss), which occurs in the gonads (ovaries and testes). Meiosis is discussed in Chapter 16.

Chromosomes Condense After Replication, Forming Tightly Coiled Structures in the Nucleus

Soon after replication, the chromosomes of the cell begin to coil, compacting in much the same way that a stretched phone cord shortens and compacts when the tension is removed. Unlike a phone cord, which functions just as well when it is stretched or compacted, chromosomes in the condensed state are metabolically inactive—that is, unable to produce either RNA or DNA.

The structure of a condensed chromosome is shown in **FIGURE 15-6B**. To understand this very complex structure, begin at the bottom and work up. As illustrated, each chromatid consists of a DNA in a double helix and associated proteins called **histones** (HISS-tones). The histones are globular proteins, which are thought to play a role in regulating the DNA's activities (Chapter 17).

As illustrated in **FIGURE 15-6**, loops of the double helix of DNA encircle the histones, forming small clusters. The small clusters along the DNA molecule compact to form hollow tubules. These tubules, in turn, form coils like those of a phone cord. When the coils are compacted, they form the body of the chromosomes.

Chromosomal condensation is of great importance to cells, as pointed out earlier. It also has many practical applications. For example, it provides physicians and geneticists an opportunity to search for genetic defects. This is especially useful to expectant parents who are concerned about possible genetic defects in their babies.

In order to acquire fetal cells, physicians extract fluid from the liquid-filled cavity surrounding the grow-

Unraveling the Structure and Function of DNA

Featuring the Work of Miescher, Griffith, Avery, Watson, Crick, Wilkins, and Franklin

In a word-association test, when the tester says "hot," you'd probably answer "cold." If he or she said "DNA," a biologist would probably answer "Watson and Crick." James Watson and Francis Crick, to be exact.

In 1953, Watson and Crick published a brief paper that proposed a model (hypothesis) for the structure of

FIGURE 1 The Double Helix Model for DNA Watson and Crick and their double helix model.

DNA (**FIGURE 1**). They suggested that DNA was a double helix and explained how the nucleotides fit together.

Like many other scientific advances that changed our understanding of the world and, in some cases, our way of life, the discovery of the structure of DNA resulted from the efforts of many scientists over many years. In fact, work on DNA began in the 1860s, when Frederick Miescher launched an inquiry into the chemical composition of white blood cells. In 1868, Miescher separated the nuclei of white blood cells from their cytoplasm. He then began to study the chemical nature of the material he had extracted. Research by other scientists using his techniques revealed the presence of two types of molecules in the nucleus: RNA and DNA.

Over the next 80 years, evidence that DNA played a role in heredity steadily accumulated. In 1920, for example, Frederick Griffith discovered a chemical substance in bacteria he called the "transforming factor." When transmitted from one bacterium to another, this substance caused specific structural changes in

the recipient. In 1944, Oswald Avery and his colleagues identified the transforming factor as DNA. They showed that DNA extracted from one strain of bacteria produced an altered capsule in a recipient strain. Furthermore, this trait was passed to all offspring of the recipient.

To confirm the hypothesis that DNA was the transforming agent, Avery and co-workers treated the extracts from the first bacteria with enzymes that destroy protein and RNA. They found that removing protein and RNA did not affect transformation. To test their hypothesis that DNA was the hereditary molecule, the researchers treated the preparation with an enzyme that destroys DNA. As they had expected, this blocked transformation altogether.

This work led some scientists to conclude that DNA is the genetic material and that it controls the synthesis of specific cellular products. Prior to this time, most scientists believed that proteins were the most likely candidate for hereditary molecules. In fact, this notion persisted until the mid-1940s because many scientists

ing fetus through a long needle inserted through the mother's abdomen (**FIGURE 15-7**, page 350). This process is called **amniocentesis** (AM-knee-oh-cen-TEE-siss).

Fetal skin cells present in the fluid are separated from it, and then grown in culture dishes. There, they proliferate, dividing by mitosis. After the number of cells has increased, the tissue culture is treated with a chemical substance that arrests cell division. The cells are then removed from the culture, placed on a glass slide, and stained. A small piece of glass or plastic is placed over them and compressed, causing the cells to flatten out. The chromosomes are then photographed through a camera mounted on the microscope. Chromosomes are then cut out of the photos, and arranged

in homologous pairs with the largest first, as shown in **FIGURE 15-5**. The resulting display is called a **karyotype** (CARE-ee-oh-TYPE).

Nowadays, computers are usually used to produce karyotypes. A camera mounted on the microscope projects the image onto a computer screen. Technicians then isolate the chromosomes on the screen and assign each one a number; the computer then creates the karyotype.

Lining the chromosomes up like this helps geneticists locate obvious structural defects—for example, extra chromosomes or missing segments. More subtle changes cannot be detected this way. As the next chapter explains, gross defects in chromosomes can have serious consequences. In many cases, chromosomal thought that nucleic acids, which contain only four different nucleotide building blocks, lacked the complexity needed to carry and transmit the vast amount of genetic information required by most species. Proteins, on the other hand, contain as many as 20 different amino acid subunits. As a result, scientists reasoned, proteins probably offered a level of complexity needed to transmit thousands of traits, an assumption that clearly thwarted scientific understanding.

Once it was established that DNA was the molecule responsible for heredity, scientists turned their attention to unraveling its structure. This work began in the mid-1940s and culminated in the publication of Watson and Crick's paper in 1953. Watson and Crick used available information from other researchers. One vital piece came from Rosalind Franklin, who worked in the laboratory of British researcher Maurice Wilkins. Franklin produced X-ray photographs of crystals of highly purified DNA (**FIGURE 2**). Her remarkable photographs suggested that the DNA molecule was helical.

Another vital piece of evidence came from the laboratory of Erwin Chargaff and his colleagues, who had spent years studying the chemical nature of DNA. Chargaff's lab showed that the amount of purine in DNA always equals the amount of pyrimidine and that the ratios between adenine and thymine and between cytosine and guanine are always 1 : 1.

Armed with these and other vital details, Watson and Crick devised an ingenious model that fit the chemical and physical data. They published their results in 1953 in the journal *Nature,* and 2 months later they published a second paper proposing that the complementary strands of their model could explain replication. In addition, Watson and Crick hypothesized that genetic information could be stored in the sequence of bases and that mutations might result from a change in that sequence.

In the ensuing years, numerous scientists have provided hard evidence that supports the model proposed by Watson and Crick. And in 1962, Watson, Crick, and Wilkins

FIGURE 2 Discovering DNA's Helical Shape The famous X-ray diffraction photograph of DNA by Rosalind Franklin.

were awarded the Nobel Prize for their discovery. Interestingly, although much of the X-ray data on which the Watson-Crick model was based had come from Franklin, she was not included in the celebrations. She couldn't be. Unfortunately, Rosalind Franklin died of cancer in 1958, and Nobel Prizes are awarded only to living scientists. Had she been alive, it is likely that she too would have shared in this coveted prize and been a household name as well.

analysis assures parents that their child has no obvious genetic defects, alleviating worry during a period of heightened anxiety. It has the added benefit of helping parents learn the sex of their baby, which, of course, helps them determine the color to paint the baby room, illustrating the importance of science to our daily lives.

Although Somatic Cells Contain a Set Number of Chromosomes, the Number of Chromatids Varies, Depending on the Stage of the Cell Cycle

The study of genetics can be quite confusing at first, in part, because chromosomes may contain one or

two chromatids, depending on the stage of the cell cycle. For example, as noted earlier, during G_1 of interphase, each chromosome consists of a single DNA molecule (a double helix) and associated protein. The 46 unreplicated chromosomes in the human cell are packed loosely in the nucleus in an apparently random fashion. During the S phase, however, the DNA strands replicate (**FIGURE 15-3**). Each chromosome now consists of two identical chromatids held together at the centromere. Each chromatid is a molecule of DNA, arranged in a double helix, with its associated proteins. When a cell divides, these chromosomes are split in half, with one chromatid going to each daughter cell.

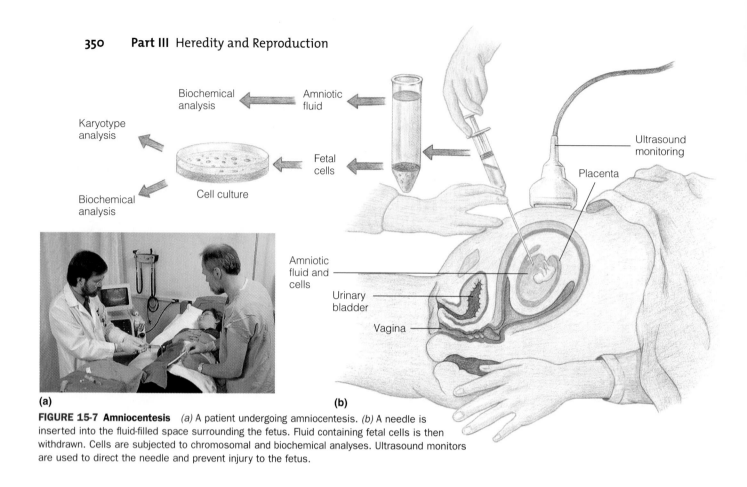

FIGURE 15-7 Amniocentesis *(a)* A patient undergoing amniocentesis. *(b)* A needle is inserted into the fluid-filled space surrounding the fetus. Fluid containing fetal cells is then withdrawn. Cells are subjected to chromosomal and biochemical analyses. Ultrasound monitors are used to direct the needle and prevent injury to the fetus.

FIGURE 15-8 Mitosis

Cell Division:
Mitosis and Cytokinesis

With this background information in mind, let's explore some of the changes occurring during cell division, beginning with mitosis, nuclear division.

Mitosis Is Divided Into Four Stages

The four stages of mitosis are prophase, metaphase, anaphase, and telophase (**FIGURE 4-2**).[1]

Prophase. Prophase begins immediately after interphase, a time during which the chromosomes replicate. During prophase, the replicated chromosomes shorten and thicken considerably, forming compact structures (**FIGURES 15-8A** and **15-8B**). In addition, the nucleoli, regions of active rRNA synthesis, gradually disappear.

Two events of great importance occur in the cytoplasm during prophase. The first is the division of the cell's centrioles. Shown in **FIGURE 15-9**, each **centriole**

consists of two small, cylindrical structures identical to the basal bodies (Chapter 3). Like other organelles, centrioles replicate during interphase. During prophase, the centrioles separate, migrating to opposite ends of the nucleus.

The second cytoplasmic event of importance is the formation of the mitotic spindle. The **mitotic spindle** is an elaborate array of microtubules responsible for subsequent movement of the chromosomes. As biologist Norman Wessels writes, "Just as a dancing puppet is operated by moving strings, the dance of the chromosomes is choreographed and controlled by the action of the spindle fibers."

As shown in **FIGURE 15-10**, two types of fibers are found in the mitotic spindle: **polar fibers**, which extend from the spindle pole inward toward the center of the cell; and **chromosomal fibers**, which also extend from the poles inward, but attach to individual chromosomes via their centromeres. Each fiber is actually a bundle of microtubules composed of tubulin molecules. These molecules are derived from the disassembly of the cell's cytoskeleton during mitosis.

Also associated with the centrioles in animal cells is a star burst of microtubules called the **aster**. Its role in

---

[1]You can use the acronym PMAT to remember these steps.

(d) Metaphase   **(e) Anaphase**   **(f) Telophase and cytokinesis**

FIGURE 15-8 Mitosis—continued

FIGURE 15-9 Centriole *(a)* The centriole, like the basal body, consists of nine sets of microtubules with three in each set. Centrioles are found in the cytoplasm and replicate during interphase. *(b)* They migrate to opposite poles of the nucleus during mitosis.

(a)

(b) Nucleus

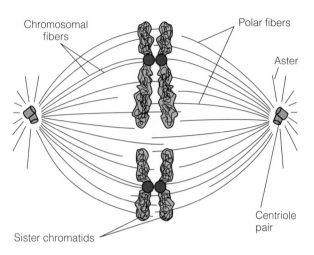

FIGURE 15-10 Mitotic Spindle The mitotic spindle, made of microtubules, forms during prophase in the cytoplasm of the cell. Chromosomal fibers connect to the chromosomes, and polar fibers extend from a pole to the equatorial region of the spindle. In ways not currently understood, the mitotic spindle separates each double-stranded chromosome during mitosis.

cell division remains unclear, although it may anchor the spindle to the plasma membrane.

Late in prophase (**FIGURE 15-8C**), the nuclear envelope begins to disintegrate. This permits the chromosomal fibers of the mitotic spindle to attach to the chromosomes, setting the stage for the next step, metaphase.

Metaphase. Before chromosomes can be divided equally, they are lined up in the center of the cell an equal distance from the two poles of the mitotic spindle with their centromeres located along the equatorial plane (**FIGURE 15-8D**). This alignment occurs during metaphase and greatly facilitates the separation of chromatids.

Anaphase. When the chromatids of each chromosome begin to separate, the cell enters anaphase. The shortest part of mitosis, anaphase lasts only a few minutes (**FIGURE 15-8E**). During anaphase, the chromatids of the homologous chromosomes are drawn toward opposite poles of the mitotic spindle and therefore toward opposite ends of the cell. As shown in **FIGURE 15-8E**, the chromosomes are dragged centromere-first, with their arms trailing behind. All of the chromosomes begin to separate simultaneously.

Telophase. The final stage of nuclear division is telophase (**FIGURE 15-8F**). Telophase begins when the chromosomes complete their migration to the poles, and it involves a series of changes in the nuclei that is essentially the reverse of prophase.

During telophase, nuclear envelopes form around the chromosomes of each daughter cell. New nuclear envelopes are produced by the endoplasmic reticulum. They soon fuse into one. Also during telophase, the spindle fibers disappear, and the chromosomes uncoil, regaining their threadlike appearance. Nucleoli reappear. Telophase ends when the nuclei of the daughter cells appear to be in interphase.

Cytokinesis Is the Division of the Cytoplasm

As **FIGURE 15-8** shows, cytokinesis usually begins late in anaphase or early in telophase. Cytokinesis is brought about by a dense network of contractile fibers, or microfilaments, that lies beneath the plasma membrane. These microfilaments, which are part of the cytoskeleton of the cell, are composed of the same proteins found in muscle cells.

When the time comes for the cytoplasm to divide, the microfilaments along the midline of the cell contract and pull the membrane inward (**FIGURE 15-11**). The membrane furrows as if it were being constricted by a thread tied around the cell, then tightened. As cytokinesis proceeds, the furrow deepens, eventually pinching the cell in two. This results in two daughter cells with more or less equal amounts of cytoplasm. With this equal allocation of cytoplasm to the daughter cells comes a sharing of the cell's organelles.

Control of the Cell Cycle

What stimulates the replication of DNA and the division of organelles? What causes a cell to divide?

Despite years of intensive research, our understanding of the controls of the cell cycle is far from complete. Some experiments suggest that chemical messages from the cytoplasm control the cell cycle. If cytoplasmic signals control the nucleus, the next logical question is, What controls the cytoplasm?

Unfortunately, no one knows for sure. Research shows that certain external signals may exert some control over cytoplasmic events. Studies of **cell cultures**—that is, cells grown in the laboratory under precise conditions—have shown that normal cells migrate and divide until they spread evenly across the bottom surface of culture dishes. At this point, the cells stop dividing, even though nutrients are plentiful. The contact of cells with one another apparently inhibits further growth; this process is called **contact inhibition**. Contact inhibition also occurs in the tissues of the body.

Interestingly, one of the reasons cancer cells grow uncontrollably is that they lose contact inhibition. Thus, in a culture dish, cancer cells proliferate wildly, growing on top of one another and quickly utilizing nutrients in the nutrient bath they're immersed in. In the body, cancer cells grow in a similar way, forming large growths, called **tumors**, that may eventually destroy vital organs and cause death.

Hormones affect the cell cycle as well. During each menstrual cycle, the hormone estrogen released from a woman's ovaries stimulates the growth of breast tissue and the uterine lining in preparation for pregnancy. Several other hormones also stimulate the division of body cells.

Growth-promoting and growth-inhibiting factors likewise play a role in controlling the cell cycle. Skin cells, for example, produce a growth-inhibiting factor that prevents cell division. However, damage to the skin—say, a cut or burn—reduces the number of skin cells and presumably reduces the amount of inhibiting factor at the site of injury. This, in turn, releases cells from inhibition. Cells proliferate and repair the damaged area. When the tissue is repaired, the rate of cell division returns to normal.

Obviously, there is no single answer to the question of what controls the cell cycle. Many factors play a role, depending on the type of cell. In time, other factors are sure to be discovered. These factors may act directly on the cytoplasm but more likely induce changes in the genes in the nucleus that regulate the cell cycle. Activa-

FIGURE 15-11 Cytokinesis *(a)* The cytoplasm of a cell is divided in two by the contraction of a ring of contractile microfilaments. Cytokinesis begins late in anaphase or early in telophase. *(b)* Cell undergoing cytokinesis.

tion of these genes may, for example, lead to the production of chemicals in the cytoplasm that diffuse back into the nucleus, thus causing the nuclear changes of mitosis.

Cancer: Understanding a Deadly Disease

In the early 1970s, Americans were shocked by reports of hazardous wastes seeping into their drinking water, pesticides contaminating the food they ate, and pollution fouling the air they breathed. Many feared that these conditions would lead to an increase in cancer. In fact, some experts estimated that 90% of all cancers were caused by environmental and workplace pollution and by other agents such as X-rays, ultraviolet light, and viruses. That conjecture caused a storm of controversy and a flurry of research into cancer, a disease that kills over 560,000 Americans each year. (**TABLE 15-3** lists the most common human cancers.)

TABLE 15-3

Most Common Cancers

Skin	Uterus	Bladder
Breast	Lymph glands	Rectum
Kidney	Lung	Prostate
Colon	Pancreas	Bone marrow
Ovary		

Are We Facing an Epidemic of Cancer?

America's Epidemic of Chemicals and Cancer

Lewis G. Regenstein

Lewis Regenstein, an Atlanta writer, is author of Cleaning Up America the Poisoned *and is president of the Interfaith Council for the Protection of Animals and Nature.*

America is in the throes of an unprecedented cancer epidemic, caused in part by the pervasive presence in our environment and food chain of deadly, cancer-causing pesticides and industrial chemicals.

Today, significant levels of hundreds of toxic chemicals known to cause cancer, miscarriages, birth defects, immune and central nervous system damage, and other health effects are found regularly in our food, our air, our water—and our own bodies. Accompanying this widespread pollution has been a dramatic and alarming rise in the cancer rate in recent decades (which has only now begun to abate for some cancers, with the restricting of some of the most dangerous chemicals).

Over 4.6 billion pounds of active pesticide ingredients are used in the United States each year—mainly on farms—which amounts to some 18 pounds for every man, woman, and child in the country. Some 75 million pounds of pesticides are used on just lawns and turf. Of the 36 most widely used lawn chemicals, 13 can cause cancer; 14 can cause birth defects, 11 can cause reproductive effects, 15 can damage the liver, and 21 can harm the nervous system.

Indeed, pesticides are used almost everywhere in our society: in homes, schools, restaurants, hospitals, parks, offices, hotels—they are virtually inescapable. One EPA study found 23 pesticides in indoor dust and air, many of which had not been used on the premises; another found that most households had at least five pesticides in indoor air, often at levels ten times higher than outdoors.

So it should not be surprising that by the time restrictions were placed on some of the deadliest compounds, such as DDT, dieldrin, and BHC, these carcinogens were being found in the flesh tissues of literally 99 percent of all Americans tested, including mother's milk.

Numerous studies link exposure to pesticides to incidences of cancer, especially in children. Higher rates of childhood brain cancers, leukemia, and soft tissue sarcomas are found in homes where pesticides are used. Indeed, a child in a household where home and garden pesticides are used has a 6.5 fold increased risk of contracting leukemia.

The U.S. National Research Council and the EPA have estimated that pesticide residues in food may be responsible for 20,000 to 60,000 excess cancer cases in America each year. And the American Academy of Pediatrics has warned that infants and children are at particular risk, since "the government is permitting 100 to 500 times as much chemicals in the food as a health basis number would dictate."

Cigarette smoking is by far the biggest cause of cancer, mainly of the lung; and diet can also be an important risk factor, especially the frequent consumption of meat and other high fat foods. But the constant, unavoidable, lifelong chemical onslaught to which we are subjected, from conception on, also plays a role in this disease, once considered rare, that now strikes 1.2 million Americans a year. (This does not count the rapidly growing number of usually non-fatal skin cancers, now a million cases a year. These are mainly caused by exposure to sunlight and increased ultraviolet radiation resulting from the ongoing depletion of the earth's protective ozone layer, which is also caused by pesticides and other synthetic chemicals.) One American in three can now expect to contract a potentially fatal cancer, which kills some 570,000 of us every year—more Americans than were killed in combat in World War II, Korea, and Vietnam combined.

And cancer has now become a common disease of the young as well as the old, with the actual incidence (and not just detection) of childhood cancers, especially leukemia and brain tumors, mounting sharply in recent years.

The response of the U.S. government, through various administrations, has been largely weak or non-existent enforcement of the nation's health and environmental protection laws. EPA, under pressure from Congress and chemical and agricultural interests, has, with few exceptions, refused to carry out its legal duty to ban or restrict cancer causing pesticides.

Thus, we are even now acting to ensure that the current cancer epidemic will continue long into the future. Only time will tell what will be the effect on this generation of Americans, and future ones—the chemical industry's ultimate guinea pigs.

Sharpening Your Critical Thinking Skills

1. Regenstein asserts that America is in the midst of a cancer epidemic caused in large part by pesticides and industrial chemicals. Eaton argues the opposite. He says that the death rate for all types of cancer except lung cancer is actually declining. Summarize the supporting data of each author.

2. Using the critical thinking skills described in Chapter 1, analyze each argument.

"America's Epidemic of Chemicals and Cancer"— Myth or Fact?

David L. Eaton, Ph.D.

There is no debate that cancer is a devastating and deadly disease. One in three people living in the United States today will contract some form of cancer in his or her lifetime, and one in four will die from it, if current rates continue. Are cancer rates increasing in epidemic proportions? The total number of people and the fraction of all deaths attributable to cancer have increased dramatically in the past 75 years. However, cancer is largely a disease of old age, and thus it is necessary to adjust such statistics for changes in the age distribution of our population. Annual mortality statistics from both the American Cancer Society and the National Cancer Institute indicate that age-adjusted deaths from all causes of cancer have not increased significantly in the past several decades *if lung cancer mortality is excluded*. There is no question that we have experienced an epidemic of lung cancer in the 20th century. The age-adjusted mortality for lung cancer in both males and females has increased over 50-fold since the early 1900s, peaking in the late 1980s in men and late 1990s in women. About 85-90% of all lung cancer is directly attributable to smoking. Per capita consumption of cigarettes increased 5-fold in men from 1900–1960, and with it concomitant increase in lung cancer. This pattern was repeated, 20 years later, in women. Tobacco products also increase the risk of several other types of common cancers (e.g., cancers of the bladder, kidney, esophagus and mouth). In contrast, there was an equally dramatic decline in the incidence of stomach cancer in the US, during the first half of the 20th century. This decline was mostly likely due to changes in dietary habits that came with the widespread use of refrigeration and possibly antioxidant food preservatives (versus the older methods of smoking and salting methods used to preserve foods). Although mortality statistics have not

risen sharply, the incidence (number of cases per 100,000 population) of certain cancers has been increasing in the past several decades. For example, the incidence of childhood leukemia and brain cancers, and adult cases of non-Hodgkin's lymphoma, have increased significantly. While at least part of these increases are likely to be due to better disease surveillance and reporting, the cause(s) of these increases are not known and may be related to as yet unidentified environmental factors. Infectious agents also cause many cancers. For example, nearly all cases of cervical cancer are thought to result from papilloma virus infection that is spread by sexual activity. Likewise, many cases of liver cancer are from hepatitis virus infections, and stomach cancer risk is increased by certain bacterial infections.

Finally, recent advances in the understanding of the biology of cancer suggest that spontaneous or background alterations in DNA may explain much of the cause of cancer. The use of modern techniques in molecular biology has revealed that DNA is inherently unstable and can be altered by normal errors in DNA replication. Within our life span, our cells undergo about 10 trillion cell divisions. Spontaneous errors in this process, which lead to mutations and cancer, accumulate with age. DNA is also subject to extensive oxidative damage from processes associated with normal cellular metabolism that occurs in each cell every day of our lives. Although most of this damage is repaired in the cells, over many years, small amounts of unrepaired damage to DNA accumulates. It is not surprising then that cancer is a frequent outcome of old age. One reason that diet is an important risk factor for many types of cancer is because of the presence of naturally occurring "antioxidants" found in fruits and vegetables. These chemicals help protect against DNA damage from normal cellular metabolism, and may also offer protection against other DNA damaging chemicals found in cigarette smoke, our diet, and other environmental sources of exposure.

The vast majority of cancer researchers throughout the world do not support the view that we are in an overall cancer epidemic caused largely by industrial chemicals. Unfortunately, it will take some time for the political arena, influenced greatly by public fears, to come to grips with the fact that further reduction in exposure of the general public to trace amounts of synthetic chemicals will not have a measurable impact on overall cancer incidence.

David L. Eaton *is Professor of environmental health and Associate Dean for Research in the School of Public Health and Community Medicine at the University of Washington. He has an active research program on the molecular mechanisms by which chemicals cause cancer.*

Hundreds of billions of dollars are spent each year on pollution reduction in the US alone, often under the rubric of reducing cancer risk to the public. I believe that much of these expenditures are justified to enhance the quality of our environment, protect valuable natural resources, and ensure the habitability of our planet for our children and our children's children. But these expenditures for pollution prevention are not going to have a significant impact on cancer incidence and mortality in the US. Certainly we must continue our efforts to identify potentially cancer-causing industrial chemicals and take appropriate actions to minimize occupational and environmental exposures to such chemicals. However, if our society is truly concerned about reducing the human tragedy from cancer, more efforts should be focused on eliminating smoking and alcohol abuse and increased public education about dietary risk factors. More research into the biochemical and molecular events that lead to cancer will ultimately lead to more effective prevention and treatment of cancer.

Visit *Human Biology's* Internet site for links to web sites offering more information on this topic.

More recent studies suggest that the early estimates were probably in error. Today, in fact, many health experts believe that only 20%–40% of all cancers arise from environmental and workplace pollutants. Most of the rest are caused by smoking, diet, and natural causes.

No matter what the cause, cancer is a disease that most of us will have close experience with. According to national statistics, one of every three Americans will contract cancer, and one of every four will die from it. For a debate on whether America is in a cancer epidemic see the Point/Counterpoint discussion.

Fortunately, new drugs have helped boost the survival rate of individuals suffering from certain types of cancer, such as childhood leukemia. Surgery also works effectively for some cancers, notably certain types of skin cancer. Radiation treatment and chemotherapy are successful in still others. Despite an outpouring of cancer treatments, one of the most productive advances in the treatment of cancer is not a drug or radiation; it is early detection. The earlier a cancer is detected, the greater one's chances of survival. The reason for this is that when a cancer is detected early, there's less chance that it will have spread to other parts of the body. Even so, the war on cancer seems to be a losing battle—with only marginal gains in survival rates after years of intensive research.

Although we often think of cancer as a human disease, in actuality, cancer occurs in a wide range of animals and plants (**FIGURE 15-12**). This section looks at cancer in humans. It will familiarize you with terms and concepts that you will encounter throughout your lifetime.

Two Types of Tumors Are Encountered in Humans

As mentioned, **cancer** is a disease in which cells divide uncontrollably, often invading other parts of the body. But not all abnormal cellular proliferation is cancerous. Some cells, in fact, form small masses that reach a certain size, then stop growing. These are called **benign tumors**. As a rule, they pose no significant medical problems unless they put pressure on nerves or block blood vessels.

Of great concern, however, are the **malignant tumors**, which continue to grow and often spread to other parts of the body, where they may destroy vital organs. The term *cancer* is reserved for malignant tumors, of which there are over 100 different types, such as brain cancer, lung cancer, liver cancer, and so on. Even within these general categories are subtypes; for example, there are several different types of skin cancer. Almost every type of cell in the body can become malignant. Notable exceptions include neurons and muscle cells. What is more, each type of cancer has its own unique properties.

Cancer Cells Break Loose From Their Site of Origin and Often Set Up Residence in Other Parts of the Body, with the Lung Being the Most Common Site.

Malignant tumors spread when individual cells or clusters of cells break loose from the original tumor, known as the **primary tumor**. They then can travel through the body in the circulatory system, or blood vessels, and in the lymphatic system, a network of vessels that drains excess fluid from body tissues (Chapter 6). These cells may settle in other sites, most commonly, the lungs and, secondarily, the liver, where they can divide uncontrollably to form **secondary tumors**. The spread of cells from one region of the body to another is called **metastasis** (ma-TASS-tah-SISS).

The ability to metastasize is one of the main reasons cancers are so lethal. Acquiring the ability to metastasize is, therefore, a key event in the development of most cancers. What allows cancer cells to break away from the primary tumor?

Most cells in the body stay in place. They're joined in tissues and organs by molecules on their surfaces, known as **cell-cell adhesion molecules.** In cancer cells, these molecules are lacking or altered, so that the cells are no longer constrained. They are said to have lost their anchorage. Interestingly, experimentally restoring these molecules in cancer cells grown in culture dishes can render cancer cells ineffective when transplanted into mice.

Not all cells that break away from the primary tumor survive to form a secondary tumor. In fact, researchers estimate that only one in 10,000 cancers cells that enter the circulatory system are successful in establishing a secondary tumor.

As noted earlier, most cancerous cells metastasize to the lungs. After leaving the organ in which the primary

FIGURE 15-12 Cancer in Plants Cancers occur in a number of different species, not just humans.

tumor is located, the first vascular bed most cells encounter is in the lung, which you may recall from Chapter 10 has an extensive network of capillaries. Cancer cells quickly attach to the lining of the small blood vessels, where they set up residence. The liver is the second most common site for secondary tumors.

Interestingly, some types of cancer show a preference for certain organs other than the lung and liver. Prostate cancer cells, for instance, tend to settle in the bones. It is believed that molecules on the prostate cancer cells bind specifically to molecules on the cells lining the blood vessels in bone.

Tumors Can be Removed Surgically or Can be Treated with Chemotherapy and Radiation

Primary tumors can often be removed surgically or destroyed by radiation. The removal of the original tumor, however, is fruitless unless secondary tumors are destroyed. Unfortunately, finding secondary tumors is extremely difficult, for there are literally thousands of places where the cells can become established. Cancer cells from the breast, for example, may lodge in the brain or lungs or in **lymph nodes**, organs interspersed along the lymphatic system to filter the fluid coursing through the lymphatic vessels. Physicians can take tissue samples of lymph nodes to assess the spread of the cancer and can remove cancerous nodes.

When a secondary tumor is difficult to remove, physicians generally use radiation or **chemotherapeutic drugs**, highly toxic drugs that attack rapidly dividing cells of tumors. This shotgun approach has many side effects, including nausea, hair loss, and general sickness, but it may be a patient's only hope. Some new developments in cancer treatment are noted in Health Note 15-1.

The Conversion of a Normal Cell to a Cancerous One Involves Two Steps

Few questions interest cell biologists more than what causes a cell to begin dividing uncontrollably. A growing body of research suggests that the production of a malignant tumor (cancer) actually involves two steps that may take place over a long period of time: (1) conversion and (2) development and progression (**FIGURE 15-13**).

The **conversion** of a normal cell to a cancerous one typically begins with a **mutation**, a change in the DNA caused by a chemical, physical, or biological agent (a virus, for example). Those agents that cause the initial transformation are known as **co-carcinogens**. Mutating just any gene won't do, though. In order to produce a mutation that sets the stage for a cancerous growth, the mutation must occur in one of the 50 genes that control the replication of cells.

Two groups of genes are primarily responsible for triggering cancer. These genes are responsible for regulating the cell cycle. One group, called **proto-oncogenes**, plays a role in stimulating cell division. The second group, the **tumor suppressor genes**, inhibit growth in the cell. (They're described more fully in Health Note 15-1.) When mutations occur in these genes, cells may be partially or completely released from the normal growth controls.

Partially released cells often remain dormant for long periods, presumably repressed by chemicals released by nearby cells, often called *tissue factors*. This homeostatic control keeps the cancer cell from dividing and thus provides an important measure of protection. Unfortunately, this safeguard can be overridden. In some instances, for example, certain hormones produced by the body can stimulate the growth of mutated (precancerous) cells. Such cancers are said to be hormone-dependent.

The second stage leading to cancer is called **development** and **progression**. It occurs when a chemical substance stimulates the growth of a mutated cell. Those chemical substances that influence the second stage of carcinogenesis are called **promoters**. Promoters stimulate cells to divide uncontrollably. Once released, cells begin a frenzy of growth that, if unchecked, usually kills the host.

FIGURE 15-13 Stages Leading to Cancer.

Health Note 15-1

Cancer: Ultimately, You May Hold the Key to a Cure

Hardly a year goes by without headlines announcing several promising new treatments for cancer.

ANTICANCER VACCINES

Efforts to treat cancers with a vaccine date back to the beginning of the field of immunology. Early researchers used malignant cells, either from the patient's own turmors or from other patients. The tumor cells were irradiated so they would not continue to divide. They were then injected into the bloodstream. The goal behind this was to stimulate the immune system to make antibodies and T cells that would attack not just the cells being injected, but the tumor itself. Such efforts were never very successful.

In 1998, however, researchers reported preliminary results of a clinical study using a "vaccine" against lung cancer, a disease that annually kills 160,000 Americans. The new vaccine contained antigens taken from the plasma membranes of tumor cells.

The lung cancer vaccine is not really a vaccine in the traditional sense, because it does not prevent the disease. This treatment is actually an immune system boost, which helps fight off an existing disease. In the study, 34 patients with early-stage lung cancer were treated with a plasma membrane protein extracted from lung cancer cells. When given to patients in early stages of lung cancer, the protein appears to stimulate the patient's immune system. The immune system, in turn, mounts an assault on the foreign protein in the blood. But because the protein is also attached to the plasma membrane of lung cancer cells, the immune system attacks and kills the cancer cells, especially those that have spread to other sites.

In clinical studies, this experimental therapy greatly increased the subjects' 5-year survival rates. Normally, only 1 patient in 10 who is diagnosed with lung cancer is alive 5 years after diagnosis and conventional treatment (surgery followed by chemotherapy). Five years after the immune system boost, 5 of 10 patients were still alive. Spurred by this research and others, scientists now have a rapidly growing list of tumor antigens, many of which are being tested in clinical trials.

MICROSPHERES AND MONOCLONAL ANTIBODIES

In recent years, some scientists have expressed their enthusiasm for lipid microspheres (liposomes) containing cancer-killing chemicals, or oncotoxins. Liposomes can be designed to target cancer cells, in the process delivering small doses of the lethal drugs to cancer cells and sparing the rest of the body. Targeting cancer cells is the job of antibodies, special proteins incorporated in the membrane of the liposome. These antibodies bind to proteins in the plasma membrane of cancer cells, allowing the "toxic bullet" to find its target.

Oncotoxins may also be attached directly to monoclonal antibodies, which are synthesized by the immune system of animals that have been injected with human cancer cells. These antibodies can be chemically bonded to **oncotoxins**, either a chemotherapeutic drug or a radioactive compound, and then administered to patients. Inside the body of the patient, the antibody-oncotoxin complex binds to the cell surface of cancer cells.

The poisonous chemotherapuetic agent would destroy the cell. A radioactive compound would have a similar effect by bombarding the cell with radiation. Laboratory and clinical trials have shown some promising results. Interestingly, studies show that anitbodies themselves can also effectively eliminate tumor cells.

ATTACKING A CANCER'S BLOOD SUPPLY

Another promising development in the treatment of cancer involves techniques that attack its blood supply. Early on, cancerous tumors remain fairly small. For example, it may take a tumor a decade to reach the size of a pea. Blood vessels on the periphery of the tumor supply blood, but the tumor cannot grow larger because of a lack of blood to its interior.

But then something happens. New blood vessels begin to form. They invade the tumor, previously held in check by a lack of internal capillaries. The formation of new blood vessels is called **angiogenesis**.

New blood vessels supply the tumor cells with nutrients and growth factors that can cause the mass to expand. In fact, researchers believe that neovascularization (another name for the development of new blood vessels) "is one of the crucial steps in a tumor's transition from a small, rather harmless cluster of mutated cells to a large, malignant growth capable of spreading to other organs throughout the body," says oncologist Judah Folkman. Growth promoting factors may come from a variety of sources: the tumor cells themselves, nearby tissue cells, or perhaps even macrophages.

Interestingly, not all newly vascularized tumors take off. Researchers have found that certain cancer cells produce proteins, some of which stimulate angiogenesis and others that inhibit it. The balance between them may explain why some newly vascularized tumors do not grow. If the cells produce an excess of inhibitory molecules, the spread of new capillaries is thwarted. The tumor's growth is restricted.

Researchers are now testing a variety of antiangiogenic drugs in hopes that they can shrink tumors. Numerous compounds are under study at university and pharmaceutical laboratories around the world. One of the most promising is a protein known as angiostatin. It has been shown to stop angiogenesis in large primary tumors and secondary tumors in laboratory animals. Used in conjunction with chemotherapeutic agents or radiation, angiostatin or other similar drugs could help treat cancer. They may eventually be used for long-term treatment of cancer patients after they've undergone more traditional treatments such as surgery, chemotherapy, or radiation.

ATTACKING CANCER AT THE LEVEL OF THE GENES

Advances in molecular biology have widened our understanding of the genetic changes occurring in human cancer. Researchers have found that key groups of genes are responsible for cell growth and reproduction. Mutations in these genes are largely responsible for the deadly shift from a normal cell to a cancerous one. Knowledge of these mutations, in turn, have enabled researchers to develop new drugs that act on the disrupted gene or the proteins produced under their direction. Their hope is to restore normalcy in malignant cells or to selectively kill malignant cells.

Researchers are targeting three groups of genes: oncogenes, tumor suppressor genes, and a third group that controls the replication and repair of DNA. **Oncogenes** are a mutated version of genes that regulate cell growth, called proto-oncogenes. (You'll learn more about them in Chapter 17.) **Tumor suppressor genes** are naturally occurring genes that normally keep cells from becoming malignant.

Because treatment of cancer at the genetic level would require a chapter to adequately explain, let me choose just one example to give you an idea of the possibilities. We'll look at the most common cancer-causing mutation, which occurs in a gene known as the *ras gene*. The ras gene is a proto-oncogene. It is responsible for the production of a protein that acts as a relay switch in a biochemical pathway that triggers cell division. When external stimuli are present, for example, growth hormones, the gene signals the production of the ras protein. It activates the process of cell division. When no signals are present, the ras protein is inactive.

When the ras gene is mutated, however, the cell acts as if the relay switch is stuck in the *on* position. As a result, the cell and its offspring continue to replicate. Blocking this protein could represent a viable means of stopping cellular proliferation in malignant cells.

When ras protein is first formed, it is in an immature state. In order to become an active relay switch, it must undergo some chemical changes. Researchers are experimenting with ways to interfere with the maturation of the ras protein. Studies of cultured tumor cells have shown that blocking an enzyme in the pathway responsible for making the ras protein functional effectively prevents the formation of new tumors.

By blocking genes involved in cell replication or altering their products, researchers hope to find ways to target cancer cells specifically. Their hope is that such treatments at the genetic level will help them stop cancer dead in its tracks, while reducing toxic side effects seen with other forms of treatment such as chemotherapy.

Some researchers are even studying ways to correct the genetic defects in cancer cells that lead to uncon-

trolled replication. Take the tumor suppressor gene, for example. Tumor suppressor genes code for the production of a suppressor protein that, in normal cells, serves as a brake to DNA replication. Mutations of the gene can render the protein inactive. Cells that are normally held in check are unleashed to proliferate madly. By inserting normal tumor suppressor genes in tumor cells, researchers hope to return them to normalcy. Encouraging results are being produced in laboratory studies.

TREATING CANCER WITH LIGHT

Scientists have found that certain drugs, when activated by laser light, can kill cancer cells. In one therapy, patients with tumors in the lining of the esophagus and the bronchi of the lung are given the drug Photofrin (porfimer sodium). After the drug circulates in the blood and bathes the cancer cells, the researchers insert a small fiberoptic fiber in the affected area. A laser beam is trained on the cancer and, when turned on, activates the chemical, which selectively destroys the cancer cells. This treatment has been approved in the United States for certain forms of advanced esophageal cancer. One of the chief advantages is that photodynamic therapy, as it is called, poses little risk to adjacent tissues and can be repeated several times and combined with other therapies.

EARLY DETECTION

Besides finding ways to kill tumors, researchers are working on ways to detect cancers earlier. New technologies make it possible to detect cancer cells in the blood of patients after they have broken away from the primary tumor, long before any clinical signs of a secondary tumor have appeared. Additional assays permit researchers to identify the origin of

Continued

Health Note 15-1

Cancer: Ultimately, You May Hold the Key to a Cure—cont'd

cells, too. Researchers hope that these techniques will someday help oncologists, physicians who treat cancer, determine whether additional treatment is needed for what appears to be an otherwise self-contained tumor.

PREVENTION

Despite the promising new developments in cancer treatment, many experts stress the importance of prevention. By quitting smoking or not taking it up in the first place, by limiting exposure to X-rays and UV light, and by choosing a safe occupation and dwelling, you can greatly reduce your likelihood of contracting cancer.

As noted in Chapter 5, proper diet may also help prevent cancer. Dietary fiber in grains and vegetables,

for example, may help reduce your chances of contracting colon cancer, a leading killer of men (**FIGURE 1**).

Other substances in food known as phytochemicals may also help reduce the risk of cancer. Many **phytochemicals** are **antioxidants**, as explained in Chapter 5. They remove free radicals that can trigger early changes in the DNA that may eventually lead to cancer.

Recent research suggests that a chemical substance called ellagic acid, which is found in raspberries, blackberries, strawberries, and other fruit and nuts, may destroy carcinogenic molecules in the body, reducing the likelihood of developing cancer. Scientists studying carcinogenic agents found in tobacco smoke, auto exhaust, and foods noted that in lab-

oratory animals, ellagic acid reduced DNA damage caused by one prevalent carcinogen by 45–70%.

Ellagic acid has to be added before or during exposure to a carcinogen, and researchers have not yet identified the mechanism by which this substance works in people. They suspect that it competes for binding sites on the DNA molecule to which carcinogens attach. Studies are currently underway in humans to determine if ellagic acid is an effective anticancer agent.

EMOTIONS AND CANCER

Recent studies indicate that there may be a link between one's emotional state and the likelihood of developing cancer. Researchers at Johns Hopkins University studied

---

Mutations, like those that result in cancer, occur with great frequency. Fortunately, though, cells have evolved an intricate mechanism to repair genetic damage. Thus, if a mutation that transforms a cell into a cancerous one can be repaired before the cell divides, the cancer is eliminated. These mechanisms must also be considered part of the body's homeostatic weaponry. The immune system can also locate and destroy tumor cells.

Unfortunately, not all cancerous mutations are repaired in time or eliminated by the immune system. Given the large number of mutations occurring every day in our bodies and the longer lives we now lead, it is little wonder that one out of every three of us will develop some form of cancer in our lifetime.

Some Carcinogens Exert Their Effect Outside of the DNA

As mentioned above, many chemical carcinogens induce cancer by altering the DNA of cells. These are generally referred to as **DNA-reactive carcinogens**. A growing body of evidence, however, indicates that many chemical substances act outside the DNA—that is, they do not react with DNA. These carcinogens, known as **epigenetic carcinogens**, operate by eliciting other biological effects. For example, some may cause a hormonal imbalance that leads to cellular proliferation.

Others may suppress the immune system, which, in turn, permits cellular proliferation. Still others may cause chronic (persistent) tissue injury. Evidence suggests that some epigenetic carcinogens stimulate changes in the DNA indirectly and may facilitate tumor development from already-converted cells. For example, alpha particles are a form of radiation that can cause direct damage to DNA. However, when alpha particles miss the nucleus, they can cause the formation of **free radicals**, highly reactive chemicals that possess an extra electron. These highly reactive substances can diffuse into the nucleus, where they affect the DNA.

Interestingly, seemingly innocuous chemicals can turn into dangerous substances inside the body. A good example is the nitrites. Nitrites are used as a food preservative, for example, in sandwich meats like bologna and in hot dogs. Although normally harmless, nitrites are converted to carcinogenic nitrosamines inside the human body. (See the Health, Homeostasis, and the Environment section in Chapter 2.) The enzymes responsible for this conversion reside in the smooth endoplasmic reticulum (SER) of liver cells and possibly others. Although the liver's SER is usually an ally in detoxifying chemical substances, in this instance it converts a harmless substance into a potentially lethal one.

medical students subjected to personality tests between 1948 and 1964 and compared the results of the tests with subsequent health records. They found that over a 30-year period students characterized as "loners," who suppressed emotions beneath a bland exterior, were 16 times more likely to develop leukemia and several other cancers than a group that gave vent to emotions and took active measures to relieve anger and frustration. Why this might be so is anyone's guess.

Corroborating these results, a 17-year study of nearly 7000 people in Alameda County, California, showed that two types of social isolation (having few close friends and feeling alone even in the presence of friends)

elevated the risk of certain cancers in women. A study in Yugoslavia also showed that repression and denial of emotions both on a regular basis and in response to stress were related to an increase in cancer and heart disease.

Despite these gains from years of research and billions of dollars spent studying cancer, modern science may actually be losing the war against many types of cancer. For example, long-term survival rates in cancer patients over the past decade or so have increased only 4.2% compared with an overall increase of 5.1% in survival rates for all other diseases. Because of this statistic, many agree that the cheapest and most effective cure is prevention.

FIGURE 1 Reducing Cancer by Eating Right Fruits, vegetables, and grains provide fiber and phytochemicals that help reduce the incidence of colon cancer.

Visit *Human Biology's* Internet site for links to web sites offering more information on this topic.

Cancers Develop Many Years After the Initial Exposure to a Carcinogen

As a rule, mutations do not manifest themselves immediately in cancer. In fact, many tumors form 20 or 30 years after the mutation. A few cancers such as leukemia occur within 5 years. The period between exposure and the emergence of a cancerous tumor is called the **latent period**. Because the latent period is long, it has been extremely difficult for medical researchers to determine the exact causes of many cancers, a fact that has hindered public health research considerably. Studies on cell phone use for periods of up to three years, which are being cited in newspaper articles on the safety of cell phone use in 2001, for example, show no link to brain cancer. Although this may eventually be found to be true, studies of brain cancer that survey usage over a period of three years are of little value.

Several Physical and Biological Agents Are Also Responsible For Producing Cancer

Chemicals are not the only cause of cancer. X-rays that physicians use to diagnose disease, ultraviolet radiation from the sun or a tanning salon, and radon gas given off by soils in some parts of the country can lead to mutations that result in cancer.

Biological agents also cause cancer. In 1911, Peyton Rous discovered that a certain virus produced cancerous growths in chickens. Since that time, researchers have discovered many viruses that cause cancer in a wide variety of animals, including humans. Unlike physical and chemical carcinogens, which alter DNA structure, carcinogenic viruses contain genes that, when inserted into the genetic material of the cells, may cause uncontrollable cell division.

Health, Homeostasis, and the Environment
Depleting the Ozone Layer

Encircling the Earth, 12–30 miles above your head, is a layer of air rich in a naturally occurring substance known as **ozone** (O_3) (**FIGURE 15-14**). Ozone consists of three covalently bonded oxygen molecules. The region of the upper atmosphere is called the **ozone layer**. Although the ozone layer may seem far removed from the discussion at hand, it's not. It is vital to the protection of our genes. As such, it is crucial to maintaining homeostasis and our health.

The ozone layer forms an invisible shield that filters out most (99%) of the **ultraviolet (UV) radiation** emitted from the sun. Ultraviolet radiation is invisible, but

FIGURE 15-14 The Ozone Layer   High above our heads lies the ozone layer of the atmosphere. The ozone layer shields the Earth from most of the ultraviolet radiation in sunlight.

dangerous. It can cause mutations and cancer in animals and may suppress photosynthesis in plants. Consequently, the ozone layer protects all living things—from plants to humans—from damaging UV light. Interestingly, biologists believe that the formation of the ozone layer over 1 billion years ago was probably necessary for the evolution of life on land (Chapter 21). Without it, terrestrial life could probably not exist or would have evolved thick, protective shields.

Today the ozone layer is disappearing. In 1974, two chemists warned that chemical substances used as spray-can propellants and refrigerants, known as the **chlorofluorocarbons (CFCs),** were eroding the ozone layer. Over the next decade and a half, numerous estimates of ozone depletion were presented, but because of conflicting results and because the ozone concentrations in the ozone layer fluctuate naturally from year to year, atmospheric scientists could not tell for certain whether the projections were accurate.

Then, in 1988, a group of 100 scientists, working under the auspices of the National Aeronautics and Space Administration (NASA), gathered to review the data of nearly 20 years of atmospheric monitoring. They found that the computer collecting data from satellites had been programmed to omit low readings. When these were taken into account, it was evident that the protective ozone layer was indeed declining and that levels over the poles had fallen by as much as 10% since 1969. The decline over the heavily populated regions of North America and Europe over the same period was 3%. More recent studies show that an overall decline of 3% over the entire planet, and a 13%–14% decline over the northern hemisphere since the early 1970s.

One area of greatest concern is Antarctica. In 1985, British scientists noted extreme losses of ozone over Antarctica during the winter months. Since then, the region of depletion, called the *ozone hole,* has spread and now covers an area twice the size of the United States. In the spring, the ozone hole breaks up. Ozone-depleted air spreads out over much of the southern hemisphere.

A similar hole has been discovered over the North Pole, too. Although ozone depletion in the Arctic ozone

hole is less, it is still of great concern, because of its proximity to heavily populated countries in the Northern Hemisphere.

Scientists predict that each 1% decrease in the ozone layer will increase the incidence of skin cancer by 2% to 4%. If this prediction proves correct, the 3% decline over North America could increase the skin cancer rate by 6% to 8%.[3] This would result in an additional 20,000–60,000 cases of skin cancer each year in the United States alone. Given that 4% of all skin cancers are fatal, an additional 800–2400 Americans could die each year from skin cancer. A 13% decline would lead to a far greater incidence of skin cancer. Some scientists believe that ozone levels over North America may plummet by as much as 30%.

Scientists are now documenting increased levels of ultraviolet light and are witnessing record high levels of skin cancer in areas where ozone depletion and ultraviolet light penetration are most noticeable, particularly along the northern coast of Australia.

In September 1987, about a year before the NASA report, representatives from 24 nations met in Montreal to work out a treaty to restrict the use of most CFCs and a few related chemicals also thought to destroy the ozone layer. The nations agreed to cut their use to one-half of the 1986 levels by 1999. Given the accumulation of CFCs in the upper atmosphere since the 1950s, many critics warned that this reduction would not save the ozone layer.

Much to the surprise of the critics, Du Pont, a world leader in CFC production, agreed in 1988 that further cuts were necessary and called for a total worldwide ban on CFC production. The company argued that stronger regulations could eliminate CFC production by the end of the century. Two years after the Montreal Treaty, the signatories met in London and agreed to a complete phase-out of CFCs and other ozone-depleting chemicals by 2000.

In 1992, another treaty was signed in Copenhagen, calling for an acceleration of the phaseout of CFCs and other ozone-depleting chemicals. The three treaties have resulted in a dramatic decline in the production and release of ozone-depleting chemicals. While that is cause for celebration, many scientists point out that the ozone layer will continue to deteriorate because massive amounts of ozone-depleting chemicals can still be found in the stratosphere and because these chemicals last for decades. Although no one knows for sure, scientists estimate that it may take 50 to 200 years before the ozone layer is back to normal.

---

[3]More recent estimates suggest that each 1% decline in the ozone layer will result in a 4% increase in skin cancer.

Summary

1. Researchers have found a disturbing correlation between extremely low frequency (ELF) magnetic radiation and leukemia in children. At least one study shows that ELF radiation accelerates the growth of cancer cells and increases their resistance to the body's natural killer cells.

2. ELF magnetic fields are generated by power lines and by electric appliances, water bed heaters, and electric blankets.

3. An analysis of all published studies, however, concludes that there is no correlation between ELF magnetic radiation and cancer.

The Cell Cycle

4. The life cycle of a cell is called the *cell cycle* and consists of two parts: interphase and cell division.

5. *Interphase* is a period of active cellular synthesis and is divided into three phases: G_1, S, and G_2.

6. During G_1, the cell produces RNA, proteins, and other molecules; G_1 is the period during which a cell carries out its normal activities. It is also a period of preparation for division.

7. During the S phase, the DNA replicates. After replication, each chromosome in the nucleus of the cell contains two chromatin fibers, or chromatids.

8. G_2 is a much shorter period and is relatively inactive.

9. During interphase, the cell replicates its organelles and molecules needed by the two daughter cells.

10. *Cell division* follows interphase. It requires two separate but related processes: *mitosis*, or nuclear division, and *cytokinesis*, or cytoplasmic division.

The Chromosome

11. Each organism has a set number of chromosomes. All body cells, except the germ cells, are called *somatic cells*; they contain a full complement of chromosomes and are described as *diploid*.

12. *Germ cells* or *gametes* contain half the number of chromosomes of somatic cells and are referred to as *haploid cells*.

13. Gametes are produced by a special type of cell division known as *meiosis*, which occurs in the gonads (ovaries and testes).

14. The chromosomes are loosely arranged in the nucleus during interphase but condense during prophase. Condensation facilitates chromosome separation.

15. Chromosomal condensation also allows physicians to study the morphology of chromosomes. Chromosomes arranged according to size form a *karyotype*, which allows geneticists to count the chromosomes and to locate gross abnormalities.

Cell Division: Mitosis and Cytokinesis

16. During cellular division, the cell divides its chromosomes equally and distributes its cytoplasm and organelles more or less evenly between the two daughter cells.

17. Cell division is essential to reproduction and growth. It is the basis of tissue repair and provides replacements for cells lost through normal wear and tear.

18. *Mitosis*, nuclear division, is divided into four stages: prophase, metaphase, anaphase, and telophase. **TABLE 15-1** summarizes the major changes in each stage.

19. Successful mitosis depends on the presence of the *mitotic spindle*, an array of microtubules that forms during prophase. Some of the spindle fibers attach to the chromosomes and help pull them apart during anaphase.

20. *Cytokinesis*, the division of the cytoplasm, begins in late anaphase or early telophase. In human cells, cytokinesis results from the contraction of microfilaments lying beneath the plasma membrane.

Control of the Cell Cycle

21. Research suggests that the cell cycle is controlled in part by substances produced in the cytoplasm. These chemicals cause changes in the nucleus of the cell.

22. External controls, such as hormones, growth regulators, cell contact, and others, are also imposed on the cell.

Cancer: Understanding a Deadly Disease

23. Cancer is a disease characterized by uncontrolled cell division. Current estimates suggest that 20%–40% of all cancers arise from environmental and workplace pollutants. The remaining cases are caused by smoking, diet, and natural causes.

24. No matter what the cause, cancer is a disease that most of us will have close experience with. One out of three Americans will contract the disease, and one out of four will die from it.

25. Cells that divide uncontrollably form *tumors*. Tumors that fail to grow and spread are *benign* and rarely cause medical problems.

26. *Malignant tumors* are those that continue to grow, often spreading to other parts of the body and invading vital organs. The term *cancer* is reserved for malignant tumors.

27. Malignant tumor cells spread (*metastasize*) through the body via the circulatory and lymphatic systems, often becoming established in distant sites, where they form *secondary tumors*. The lungs are one of the main sites of metastasis.

28. Tumors can be removed surgically or destroyed with radiation, but successful treatment depends on the location and destruction of secondary tumors.

29. Patients can also be treated with chemotherapeutic agents, chemical substances that attack rapidly dividing cells.

30. The transformation of a normal cell into a cancerous one often results from a mutation, a change in the DNA resulting from a chemical, biological, or physical agent. These agents are called *co-carcinogens*.

31. The initial mutation, caused by a co-carcinogen, may or may not result in a cancerous growth. A second factor, a *promoter*, however, may stimulate the cell to proliferate uncontrollably.

Health, Homeostasis, and the Environment: Depleting the Ozone Layer

32. The ozone layer, found in the upper atmosphere, filters out most of the incoming ultraviolet light, protecting many life-forms from harmful burns and damaging mutations that can lead to cancer.

33. Unfortunately, certain chemicals called *chlorofluorocarbons* (CFCs) are destroying the ozone layer. In industrialized nations, CFCs were used as spray-can propellants, refrigerants, coolants, cleaning agents, and blowing agents for foam.

34. CFCs have caused a 3% decline in ozone levels globally and a 13% decline over North America.

35. CFC production and release have been nearly eliminated thanks to international treaties.

www.jbpub.com/humanbiology

Connect to this book's web site: www.jbpub.com/humanbiology
The site features eLearning, an online review area that provides quizzes, chapter outlines, and other
tools to help you study for your class. You can also follow useful links for in-depth information,
research the differing views in the Point/Counterpoints, or keep up on the latest environmental
and health news.

Critical Thinking

Thinking Critically— Analysis

This Analysis corresponds to the Thinking Critically scenario that was presented at the beginning of this chapter.

First and foremost, one should examine the source of information and look for hidden bias. First, you will find that Rush Limbaugh is not a scientist and has little knowledge of the atmospheric science necessary to understand ozone depletion. Furthermore, Limbaugh is a powerful advocate of free enterprise and takes a dim view of government regulation. In other words, he's not exactly an unbiased observer.

Furthermore, if you read his work, you'll find that he gets most of his facts from the late Dixie Lee Ray, also an avowed anti-environmentalist. According to author Robert Boyle, she, in turn, gets much of her information from Rogelio Maduro, an associate editor of *21st Century*. Maduro coauthored a book entitled *The Holes in the Ozone Scare*. It asserts that efforts to ban CFCs stem in large part from a corporate plot led by Du Pont, the world's leading manufacturer of CFCs. According to Maduro, they are eager to profit from substitutes for CFCs, which they developed.

Unfortunately, this characterization is in error. Du Pont and other chemical companies actually opposed bans on ozone-depleting CFCs for many years. Only when the evidence that CFCs were damaging the ozone layer became irrefutable did Du Pont back down and support a ban.

Articles in *Science* and *Chemical and Engineering News* have systematically refuted the claims made by Limbaugh, Ray, and Maduro. Unfortunately, few people will ever read these journals to explore the scientific treatment of this subject.

This controversy, like others, illustrates the importance of examining the source of information and looking for hidden bias.

Test of Concepts

1. Describe the cell cycle, and explain what happens during each part.
2. Discuss the factors that control the cell cycle. Is it likely that many factors play a role in determining when and how often a cell divides?
3. Draw a diagram of the cell cycle, and note how many chromosomes are found in the cell at each stage and whether they are single- or double-stranded.
4. List the stages of mitosis, and describe the major nuclear changes occurring in each stage. When does cytokinesis occur? What are the major cytoplasmic changes?
5. In what ways are cancer cells different from normal cells? What events lead to a cancer? Why don't more cells become cancerous? What is the difference between a benign and a malignant tumor?
6. The Health, Homeostasis, and the Environment section argues that chemical substances produced by modern society—notably, the chlorofluorocarbons—may be making our environment hazardous to human health. Describe how.
7. Cancer is often considered a disease of aging. Given the fact that cancer is caused by DNA mutation, why is this assertion correct? Can you think of some reasons why the incidence of some cancers has risen in the past 20 years?

Principles of Human Heredity

Scanning electron micrograph of human chromosomes.

Thinking **Critically**

More than a hundred years after his death, President Abraham Lincoln has become the subject of a scientific controversy. The debate among some scientists is not over who killed him or why but, rather, over the possibility that he suffered from a genetic disorder called **Marfan's syndrome.**

Marfan's syndrome is an extremely rare disorder that affects the skeletal system, the eyes, and the cardiovascular system. It is difficult to diagnose and is usually identified only after its victims die. Flo Hyman, the star of the 1984 U.S. women's Olympic volleyball team had Marfan's syndrome. In 1986, Hyman collapsed on the volleyball court and died from a ruptured aorta, the huge blood vessel that carries blood away from the heart to the body.

Marfan's victims typically have exceedingly long arms and legs, which make them excellent volleyball and basketball players. In normal individuals, the arm span (the distance from fingertip to fingertip) is equal to their height. In Marfan's syndrome, however, arm span exceeds height.

Nearsightedness and lens defects are also common among Marfan's patients. The most serious problem, however, is enlargement and weakening of the aortic arch, caused by a degeneration of the connective tissue in the wall of this vessel. If untreated, the aorta can burst, causing instant death.

Evidence suggests that Lincoln had Marfan's syndrome. He was tall and lanky, for example, and he wore glasses. And, his great-great-grandfather had the disease, making it possible that Abe had received the Marfan's gene. What additional evidence might you look for to confirm this hypothesis? What critical thinking rule(s) do(es) this exercise illustrate? ■

For most of us, life is an emotional roller coaster. That is, unless you're numb to the world, your emotions tend to fluctuate with changing circumstances. Some events bring elation, while others evoke anger, fear, or other deep-seated emotions. Such peaks and troughs are quite normal. But for some people, the emotional roller coaster ride is intense—their feelings swing erratically for little or no reason. One minute they are in a state of elated overactivity (mania), the next they fall into a state of depressed inactivity. This condition, known as **manic-depression,** is a psychological disorder characterized by cyclic mood swings that are unrelated to external events.

Manic-depression varies widely from one person to the next. In some, it persists for only a short time. In others, it continues for years. During mania, the animated and highly energetic state, manic-depressives often act irrationally or obnoxiously. Such behavior can ruin relationships and can lead to financial disaster, especially if it interferes with decision making. When in a state of deep depression, victims sometimes threaten suicide, although their lack of energy often prevents them from following through. In some cases, however, the self-destructive yearning persists after the period of depression and results in suicide.

Manic-depression occurs in about 3% of the U.S. population and tends to run in families, a fact that suggests a genetic link. Researchers, in fact, recently located a gene near the tip of chromosome 11 that may predispose its bearers to manic-depression and possibly severe depression.

Genes on chromosomes determine the structure and function of cells and organs. Growing evidence suggests that they also influence behavior, sometimes profoundly. New evidence also strongly suggests that a gene or several genes may influence children's susceptibility to ear infections. Children with this as yet unidentified gene are more prone to ear infections than those without them.

This chapter examines how genes are passed from parent to offspring. In other words, we'll be looking at the inheritance of traits. We begin with an overview of meiosis, a special kind of cell division responsible for gamete formation in humans and other sexually reproducing organisms. We then focus our attention on some basic principles of heredity.

Section 16-1

Meiosis and Gamete Formation

Body cells contain 46 chromosomes. For successful reproduction to occur, we must have some mechanism to produce gametes with half the number of chromosomes of somatic cells. Thus, when the male and female gametes unite, the offspring will have the normal (diploid) number of chromosomes. The mechanism responsible for reducing the number of chromosomes in sex cells is called **meiosis** (my-OH-siss).

Meiosis is a type of nuclear division that occurs in germ cells and yields haploid gametes. Germ cells are formed in the reproductive organs, the ovaries (OH-var-ees) of women and testes (TESS-tees) of men. When germ cells unite, they form a zygote with 46 chromosomes, 23 coming from the mother and 23 coming from the father. The zygote continues to divide and eventually forms an embryo, then a fetus, and after birth, a baby who grows to become an adult. Each of the body or somatic cells in these different forms of human life will contain 46 chromosomes.

As you may recall from Chapter 15, chromosomes occur in pairs, called **homologous pairs,** because they are the same length, have the same appearance, and contain the same genes. In humans there are 22 pairs of autosomes and 1 pair of sex chromosomes. During meiosis, the homologous pairs in the cells that give rise to gametes are split so that each gamete ends up with one chromosome of each pair.

Meiosis Involves Two Cellular Divisions

Meiosis is a rather complicated but fascinating process with many resemblances to mitosis, discussed in Chapter 15. If you haven't read that section or have forgotten some of the details, you may want to reread it now.

Unlike mitosis, meiosis involves two nuclear divisions. The two nuclear divisions are referred to as meiosis I and II. Let's consider the main details of each one, drawing on your knowledge of mitosis.

Meiosis I Is a Reduction Division

Meiosis I is often called a **reduction division. FIGURE 16-1** illustrates the process. Take a moment to look at the figure. One of the first things you will note is that meiosis contains the same four steps as mitosis: prophase, metaphase, anaphase, and telophase.

Just as in mitosis, chromosomes duplicate in interphase, so that each chromosome contains two chromatids. During prophase I, the chromosomes condense, just as they do in mitosis. However, something unusual occurs in prophase I of meiosis; that is, homologous chromosomes "pair up." In other words, chromosome 1 from the mother and chromosome 1 from the father become attached. Chromosome 2 from the mother pairs with chromosome 2 of the father and so on down the line. During metaphase I of meiosis I, the homologous pairs line up along the equatorial plate. During anaphase I, the pairs separate, with one member of each pair going to each daughter cell. As a result, each daugh-

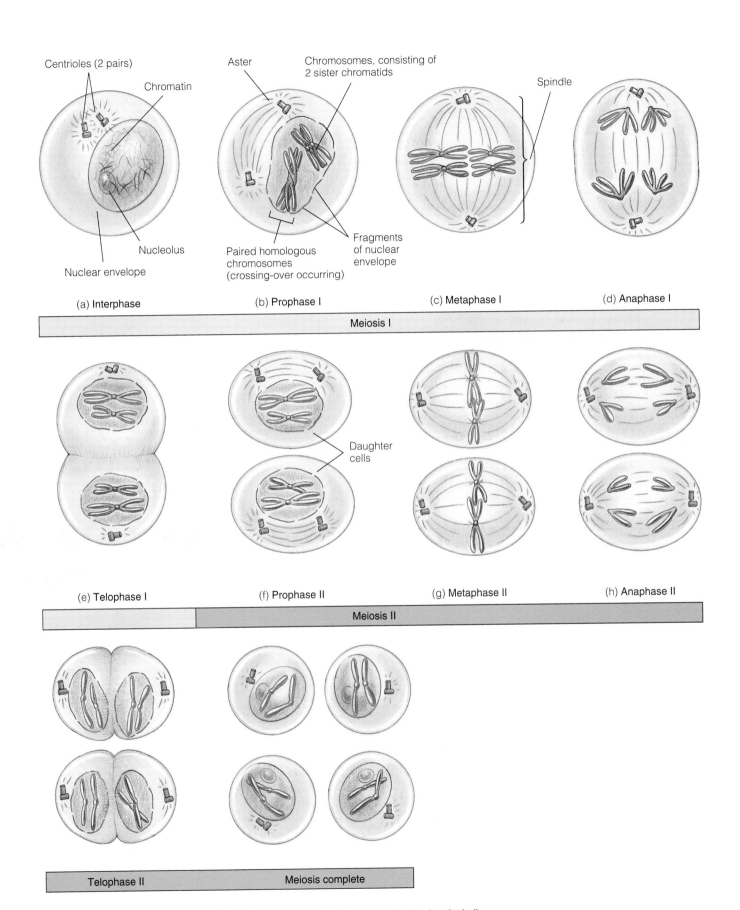

Centrioles (2 pairs)

Chromatin

Nucleolus

Nuclear envelope

(a) Interphase

Aster

Chromosomes, consisting of 2 sister chromatids

Paired homologous chromosomes (crossing-over occurring)

Fragments of nuclear envelope

(b) Prophase I

Spindle

(c) Metaphase I

(d) Anaphase I

Meiosis I

Daughter cells

(e) Telophase I

(f) Prophase II

(g) Metaphase II

(h) Anaphase II

Meiosis II

Telophase II

Meiosis complete

FIGURE 16-1 Meiosis. Note that meiosis is divided into two phases: meiosis I and meiosis II.

ter cell ends up with half the number of chromosomes (23) of the parent cell (46) from which it was formed. Each chromosome contains two chromatids. Because the number of chromosomes decreases by half during this process, meiosis I is called a reduction division. In mitosis, in contrast, duplicated chromosomes simply line up "single file" along the equatorial plate and split down the middle so that each daughter cell contains the same number of chromosomes as the parent cell.

Meiosis II Is Akin to Mitotic Division

The second division, **meiosis II,** also resembles mitosis, except for one difference: The cells start out as haploid.

As illustrated in **FIGURE 16-1**, the chromosomes of the haploid cells condense during prophase II, then line up in single file along the equatorial plate during metaphase II. During anaphase II, the chromatids dissociate, one going to each pole. The result is two cells, each containing a haploid number of single-stranded (unreplicated or one-chromatid) chromosomes. It is these cells give that rise to the haploid gametes.

Although this may sound confusing, take a few minutes to review mitosis. Then go over the steps In meiosis, paying attention primarily to two things: the number of chromosomes and the number of chromatids in each one. Here's a recap of what you'll find: In meiosis I the cells begin with 46 chromosomes—each with two chromatids. During meiosis I, these cells divide. Each daughter cell ends up with 23 chromosomes.

Each chromosome has two chromatids. During meiosis II, the 23 chromosomes split apart, and each daughter cell ends up with 23 chromosomes—each with one chromatid.

In Males, Meiosis Produces Four Gametes; In Females, It Produces Only One

Meiosis differs between males and females. In males, the process is much as I have described above. Thus, a single diploid cell in the gamete-producing **testis** (singular; pronounced TESS-tiss) gives rise to four sperm cells. During this process, the cytoplasm of the original cells that give rise to the sperm is divided equally among the four germ cells. However, during the final stages of sperm development, much of the cytoplasm is discarded to produce a highly streamlined sperm capable of swimming up the female reproductive tract (**FIGURE 16-2**).

In females, the single diploid cell gives rise to only one egg (**FIGURE 16-3**). Thus, all of the cytoplasm is retained in one cell, and the extra chromosomal material is systematically discarded during the two meiotic divisions. This difference reflects the fact that the egg is fairly sedentary. It's the sperm that must do most of the work during fertilization! This early division of labor also ensures that adequate cellular organelles (supplied by the female) are available for the fertilized ovum, or **zygote** (ZYE-goat).

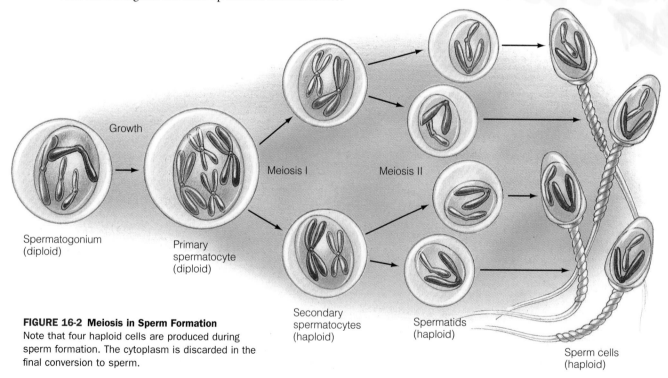

Growth

Meiosis I

Meiosis II

Spermatogonium (diploid)

Primary spermatocyte (diploid)

Secondary spermatocytes (haploid)

Spermatids (haploid)

Sperm cells (haploid)

FIGURE 16-2 Meiosis in Sperm Formation
Note that four haploid cells are produced during sperm formation. The cytoplasm is discarded in the final conversion to sperm.

FIGURE 16-3 Meiosis in Ovum Formation   Note that only one haploid cell is formed, containing all of the cytoplasm. Nuclear material is discarded along the way.

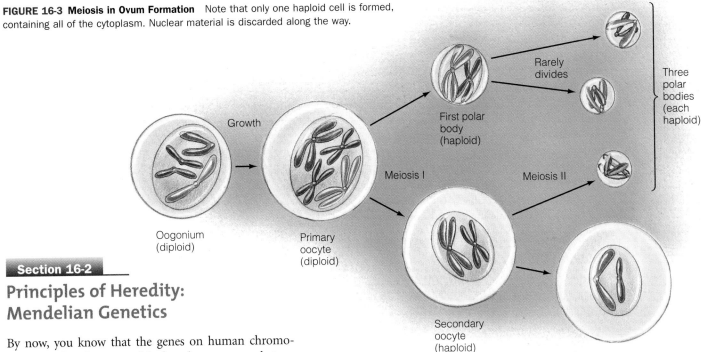

Growth

Oogonium
(diploid)

Primary
oocyte
(diploid)

Meiosis I

First polar
body
(haploid)

Rarely
divides

Meiosis II

Three
polar
bodies
(each
haploid)

Secondary
oocyte
(haploid)

Ovum
(haploid)

Section 16-2

Principles of Heredity: Mendelian Genetics

By now, you know that the genes on human chromosomes are largely responsible for who we are—what we look like and, at least partly, how we behave. The gene-bearing chromosomes are divvied up during meiosis into germ cells. The germ cells combine during fertilization to form a new being. With these basics in mind, we turn our attention to heredity—the transmission of genes from parents to offspring.

Heredity is one aspect of the study of genetics. The formal study of genetics began with a look at heredity at the organismic level carried out by a 19th-century monk, Gregor Mendel, working in his garden (**FIGURE 16-4**).

Born in Eastern Europe in 1821, Mendel entered an Augustinian monastery in Brno, in what is now the Czech Republic, at the age of 21.[1] After completing his studies, Mendel enrolled at the University of Vienna, where he studied botany, mathematics, and other sciences. Returning to the monastery, he began a series of experiments on garden peas—studies that would reveal several fundamental principles of genetics.

During Mendel's time, many scientists believed that the traits of a child's parents were blended in the offspring, producing a child with intermediate characteristics. In addition, because the ova of sexually reproducing organisms are much larger than the sperm, some scientists believed that the female had a greater influence on the characteristics of the offspring than the male.

---

[1]Brno is now the city of Brunn.

(b)

FIGURE 16-4 Mendel and His Garden   (a) Gregor Mendel worked out some of the basic rules of inheritance in the mid-1800s in his research on garden peas. (b) Mendel's garden at the monastery in Czechoslovakia as it appears today.

(a)

Mendel's studies were designed to examine these two assumptions.

Mendel was a careful scientist. He spent 2 years selecting an organism to study and eventually settled on one species of garden pea. Over a 10-year period, he studied inheritance in approximately 28,000 pea plants, thereby avoiding problems that might have arisen from a small sample size. Proper sample size, of course, is a requirement of a good experiment, as noted in the critical thinking section of Chapter 1. Mendel also repeated his experiments, ensuring that his results were reproducible. Finally, he analyzed his results according to principles of probability and was very likely the first scientist in history to use this kind of analysis in biological research.

Mendel Discovered That the Traits He Was Studying Did Not Blend

Mendel's first discovery was that the physical characteristics of the parents did not blend to produce offspring with intermediate traits. When he bred a pea with a white flower to a pea with a purple flower, he did not produce pea plants with intermediate pink flowers as many would have hypothesized, based on existing assumptions. Instead, these crosses produced plants with purple flowers, for reasons that will be discussed later. Experiments that Mendel performed on the inheritance of other traits showed similar results—refuting the prevailing notion that parental traits blended in offspring.

Mendel Discovered That the Parents Contributed Equally to the Characteristics of Their Offspring

Mendel's research led him to conclude that adult plants contain pairs of hereditary factors for each trait (for example, seed color) and that each pair governed the inheritance of a single trait. Today, we refer to Mendel's hereditary factors as the genes, which we know are located in the DNA of the chromosomes.

Mendel reasoned that, because a male gamete and a female gamete combine to form a new organism and an adult contains only two hereditary factors for any given trait, each gamete must contain only one hereditary factor (gene) for each trait. Mendel's studies therefore suggested that the paired hereditary factors of the mother and father must separate during gamete formation so that each gamete contributes one and only one hereditary factor to the zygote. The separation of hereditary factors during gamete formation is known as the **principle of segregation.**

Because the gametes of the parents combine to produce an offspring and because each gamete contains one hereditary factor for each trait, Mendel concluded that the contributions of the parents must be equal. That is, each parent contributes one hereditary factor, or gene, for each trait.

These conclusions may seem unremarkable to us today, especially with our knowledge of meiosis and gamete formation. However, remember that Mendel performed his experiments in the 1850s and 1860s, long before chromosomes had been discovered! In fact, he hypothesized the presence and behavior of genes long before scientists knew even the most basic facts of cell biology and inheritance.

Mendel Also Discovered the Principle of Dominance

Mendel postulated that hereditary factors (genes) are either **dominant** or **recessive** (**TABLE 16-1**). When a dominant factor and a recessive factor are present in a pea, Mendel concluded, the dominant factor is always expressed. A recessive factor is expressed only when the dominant factor is missing.

An alternative form of the same gene is called an **allele** (ah-LEEL). Thus, dominant and recessive factors are known today as dominant and recessive alleles. Dominant alleles are designated by capital letters; recessive alleles are signified by lowercase letters. In Mendel's peas, for instance, the gene for flower color is the P gene. The dominant form is P (purple flowers), and the recessive form is p (white flowers). The P and p genes are both alleles of the flower-color gene.

For genes with two alleles, three combinations are possible during fertilization. The first consists of two dominant genes—for example, PP. This individual is said to be **homozygous dominant** (hoe-moe-ZYE-gus) for that particular trait. The second consists of two recessive alleles—in this example, pp—and the individual

TABLE 16-1

Genetic Traits Studied by Mendel

Structure Studied	Dominant Trait	Recessive Trait
Seeds	Smooth	Wrinkled
	Yellow	Green
Pods	Full	Constricted
	Green	Yellow
Flowers	Axial (along stems)	Terminal (top of stems)
	Purple	White
Stems	Long	Short

is said to be **homozygous recessive** for that trait. The third occurs when dominant and recessive alleles are present (*Pp*), and the individual is **heterozygous.** Take a moment to memorize these terms. They're essential to your understanding of much of the rest of the material in this chapter.

The Genotype of an Organism Is Its Genetic Makeup; the Phenotype Is Its Appearance

As noted earlier, Mendel determined that blending did not occur in the inheritance of traits, such as flower color. Thus, a pea plant with purple flowers (*PP*) bred with a pea plant with white flowers (*pp*) produced offspring with purple flowers and not pink flowers, which would occur if blending took place. Mendel proposed that the purple-flowered offspring of this cross were heterozygous—*Pp*. In such cases, he argued, the recessive hereditary factors (genes) are masked by the dominant hereditary factors (genes). Because of dominance, Mendel noted, the outward appearance of a plant—its **phenotype** (FEEN-oh-type)—does not always reflect its genetic makeup, or **genotype** (JEAN-oh-type). In fact, in this example, two different genotypes lead to the same phenotype (*PP* = purple and *Pp* = purple) (**FIGURE 16-5**). As a general rule, a homozygous dominant individual and a heterozygous individual are indistinguishable on the basis of phenotype.

Genotypes and Phenotypes Can Be Determined by the Punnett Square

To track the genotypes and phenotypes of breeding experiments, such as those that Mendel performed, geneticists use a relatively simple tool known as the **Punnett square** (**FIGURE 16-6**). To illustrate the process, consider one of the traits that Mendel studied—seed-coat texture. The gene for seed-coat texture has two alleles: one that codes for smooth seeds (*S*) and one that codes for wrinkled seeds (*s*). As indicated by the capital *S*, the smooth-seed allele is dominant.

Suppose that you bred a homozygous-dominant plant (*SS*) with a homozygous-recessive plant (*ss*). **FIGURE 16-6** lists the genotypes of each parent and the possible genotypes of the gametes. Determining the genotype is a rather simple affair. If a diploid parent is *SS*, its haploid gametes are all *S*. If a parent is *ss*, the gametes are all *s*.

To determine the outcome of crossing these two plants, all of the possible gametes produced from one plant are listed along the top of the Punnett square, and all of the possible gametes from the other are listed along the side. The gametes are then combined as shown, producing all of the possible genotypes present in the offspring.

Genotype	PP Homozygous dominant	Pp Heterozygous	pp Homozygous recessive
Phenotype	Purple	Purple	White

FIGURE 16-5 Blending Traits Mendel's experiments showed that traits did not blend, as was commonly thought during his time.

As this example illustrates, a cross between a homozygous-dominant (*SS*) individual and a homozygous-recessive (*ss*) individual produces only heterozygous (*Ss*) offspring. Thus, the offspring are phenotypically uniform, and all of them resemble the homozygous-dominant parent—they have a smooth seed coat.

In the language of genetics, when one organism is bred to another to study the transmission of a single trait, the procedure is called a **monohybrid cross** (MON-oh-HYE-brid). In a monohybrid cross, the organisms that are bred initially constitute the P_1 generation (P for parents). The first set of offspring constitutes the F_1 generation (first filial generation; *filialis* is Latin for "of a son or daughter"). In this example, the F_1 offspring could be bred to produce additional offspring, the F_2 generation (second filial generation).

FIGURE 16-6 Mendel's Early Experiments When studying the inheritance of seed conformation, Mendel first crossed homozygous-recessive (*ss*) and homozygous-dominant (*SS*) plants. The offspring were all heterozygotes (*Ss*).

To determine the genotypes and phenotypes of such a cross, the Punnett square can be used once again. As **FIGURE 16-7** shows, the gametes of the F₁ generation are *S* and *s* because all of the parents are heterozygous (*Ss*). All of the possible gametes from the father are placed along the top of the Punnett square, and all of the possible gametes of the mother are placed along the side. The gametes are combined as before in the appropriate boxes.

As shown in **FIGURE 16-7**, this cross produces three different genotypes: *SS, Ss,* and *ss.* The ratio of genotypes, or the genotypic ratio of the F₂ generation, is one *SS* to two *Ss* to one *ss,* or 1 : 2 : 1. Thus, if 100 offspring are produced, you would expect 25 of them to be *SS* (homozygous dominant), 50 to be *Ss* (heterozygous), and 25 to be *ss* (homozygous recessive). Because of dominance, though, this cross yields only two phenotypes: plants with smooth seeds (*SS* and *Ss*) and plants with wrinkled seeds (*ss*). The ratio of phenotypes, or the phenotypic ratio, is three smooth to one wrinkled, or 3 : 1.

Genes on Different Chromosomes Segregate Independently of One Another During Gamete Formation

In his later experiments, Mendel tracked two traits at the same time, a procedure geneticists refer to as a **dihybrid cross** (DIE-HIGH-brid) (**FIGURE 16-8**). This work led to the **principle of independent assortment**—the idea that genes located on different chromosomes segregate independently during meiosis. To understand what this principle means and how Mendel arrived at it, consider another example that examines seed-coat texture and seed color.

As noted above, peas contain a gene for seed-coat texture, the *S* gene. The dominant form is *S* (smooth), and the recessive form is *s* (wrinkled). Peas also contain a gene for seed color; the dominant form (*Y*) yields yellow seeds, and the recessive form (*y*) yields green seeds.

To study the inheritance of these two genes, Mendel crossed homozygous-dominant plants with smooth, yellow seeds (*SSYY*) with homozygous-recessive plants (*ssyy*). As **FIGURE 16-8** shows, the genotype of the F₁ generation was *SsYy.* Con-

sequently, the offspring were phenotypically identical, and all displayed the dominant characteristics (smooth, yellow seeds).

When Mendel crossed two of the F₁ offspring (genotype = *SsYy*), however, he got a mixture of phenotypes (**FIGURE 16-8**). To produce this combination of offspring, Mendel concluded, the hereditary factors *S* and *s* must have segregated independently of *Y* and *y* during gamete formation. Translated into modern terms, this means that the *Y* and *S* genes (and their alleles *y* and *s*) were on different chromosomes and separated independently of each other during gamete formation (meiosis). Because of independent assortment, the *gametes* of the F₁ generation contain all combinations of the alleles in

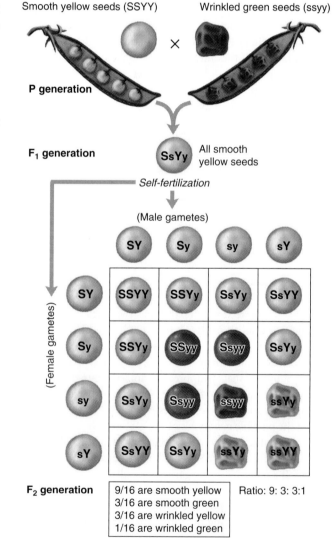

FIGURE 16-8 Dihybrid Cross The dihybrid cross examines the inheritance of two traits. Independent assortment of genes produces a large number of genotypes.

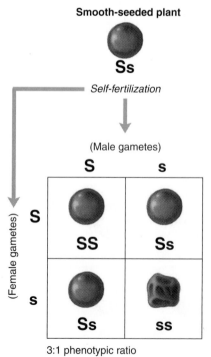

FIGURE 16-7 Monohybrid Cross In Mendel's early work, he crossed offspring from his F₁ generation (*Ss*) and found a variety of genotypes and phenotypes.

equal proportions: *SY, Sy, sY,* and *sy.* Fertilization also occurs at random, giving rise to 16 possible genetic combinations (see F$_2$ genotypes in **FIGURE 16-8.**

This research led Mendel to propose the principle of **independent assortment**, which states that the segregation of the alleles of one gene on one chromosome is independent of the segregation of the alleles of another gene on a second chromosome during gamete formation.

Mendel may have been one of the luckiest scientists in the world—or maybe he was divinely blessed. We'll never know. In either case, he fortuitously chose to study seven traits, listed in **TABLE 16-1,** each of which scientists now believe is on a different chromosome. (This assumption has not yet been proved.) If two genes under study were located on the same chromosome, Mendel might have never discovered his principle of independent assortment because such genes tend to be inherited together. All this is to say, as you'll soon see, that independent assortment is not a universal truth. It holds only for genes located on different chromosomes.

| Section 16-3 |

Mendelian Genetics in Humans

What do studies on garden peas have to do with humans? It's simple. Much of what Mendel discovered in garden peas pertains to human genes and human inheritance. **TABLE 16-2** lists a number of human traits and diseases whose inheritance follows basic Mendelian principles. This section describes the inheritance of those traits, using several common diseases as examples.

Autosomal-Recessive Traits Are Expressed Only When Both Alleles Are Recessive

Human cells contain 23 pairs of chromosomes. They can be divided functionally into one pair of sex chromosomes and 22 pairs of autosomes (AU-toe-zomes).

The **sex chromosomes** are involved in sex determination—that is, determining whether we turn out male or female—as well as a few other functions. Two types of sex chromosomes exist, X and Y. Females have two homologous X chromosomes; their genotype is therefore XX. Males have a nonhomologous pair, consisting of one X chromosome and one Y chromosome. Their genotype is XY.

The remaining 22 pairs of chromosomes are called the **autosomes.** The autosomes contain numerous genes that control a variety of traits. This section examines several **autosomal-recessive traits.** These are traits expressed only when both recessive alleles are present.

Over 600 traits in humans have been identified as autosomal recessive, and another 800 are strongly suspected of being autosomal recessive. Some autosomal-recessive traits are the cause of abnormalities, among them albinism and cystic fibrosis.

Albinism. Albinism is one of the most common genetic defects known to science. It occurs in 1 of every 38,000 Caucasian births and in 1 of every 22,000 African-American births. Among the Hopi and Navajo Indians of the American Southwest, the incidence is 1 in every 200.

Albinism in humans and other animals as well (rabbits and rats, for example) occurs when two

TABLE 16-2		
Traits and Diseases Carried on Human Chromosomes		
Autosomal recessive		
Albinism	Lack of pigment in eyes, skin, and hair	
Cystic fibrosis	Pancreatic failure, mucus buildup in lungs	
Sickle-cell anemia	Abnormal hemoglobin leading to sickle-shaped red blood cells that obstruct vital capillaries	
Tay-Sachs disease	Improper metabolism of a class of chemicals called gangliosides in nerve cells, resulting in early death	
Phenylketonuria	Accumulation of phenylalanine in blood; results in mental retardation	
Attached earlobe	Earlobe attached to skin	
Hyperextendable thumb	Thumb bends past 45° angle	
Autosomal dominant		
Achondroplasia	Dwarfism resulting from a defect in epiphyseal plates of forming long bones	
Marfan's syndrome	Defect manifest in connective tissue, resulting in excessive growth, aortic rupture	
Widow's peak	Hairline coming to a point on forehead	
Huntington's disease	Progressive deterioration of the nervous system beginning in late twenties or early thirties; results in mental deterioration and early death	
Brachydactyly	Disfiguration of hands, shortened fingers	
Freckles	Permanent aggregations of melanin in the skin	

recessive genes are inherited from one's parents. The recessive genes result in a deficiency in the metabolic pathways leading to the production of melanin. **Melanin** is the brown pigment responsible for coloration of the eyes, skin, and hair. Individuals who are homozygous-recessive for albinism have no melanin at all or may have reduced levels (**FIGURE 16-9**). Consequently, the skin of an albino is pale, and the hair is white. The eyes of albino children are pink, because there is no pigment in the iris or retina.

In most of us, melanin in the skin protects against the effects of ultraviolet light. Its absence in albinos makes them highly susceptible to sunburn and skin cancer. Moreover, the lack of pigment in the eyes may result in damage in the light sensitive region, the retina, which is essential to vision. This, in turn, may result in blindness.

Cystic Fibrosis. **Cystic fibrosis** (SISS-tick fie-BRO-siss) is an autosomal-recessive disease that leads to early death. The presence of two recessive alleles for the disease alters the function of sweat glands of the skin, mucous glands in the respiratory system, and the pancreas. Defective sweat glands, for example, release excess amounts of salt, a marker that helps physicians diagnose the disease. The most significant symptoms, however, occur in the pancreas and lungs.

In individuals with cystic fibrosis, the ducts that drain digestive enzymes from the pancreas into the small intestine become clogged. This not only impairs digestion, but also causes a buildup of enzymes in the organ that results in the formation of cysts. Over time,

the pancreas begins to degenerate, and fibrous tissue replaces glandular tissue—hence, the name *cystic fibrosis* (**FIGURE 16-10**).

Despite adequate nutritional intake, victims of cystic fibrosis often show signs of malnutrition. To enhance digestion, patients must eat powdered or granular extracts of animal pancreases containing digestive enzymes. Massive doses of vitamins and nutrients must also be taken.

The respiratory systems of most victims of cystic fibrosis produce copious amounts of mucus. Mucus blocks the passages, making breathing difficult. Thus, patients must be treated several times a day to remove the mucus (**FIGURE 16-11**). Despite antibiotic therapy and other treatments, most cystic fibrosis patients live only into their late teens or early twenties.

Cystic fibrosis is one of the most common genetic diseases known to medical science. Surprisingly, 1 of every 22 Caucasians carries a gene for this disease, and approximately 1 of every 2000 Caucasians born in the United States suffers from it. In the African-American population, only about 1 in 100,000–150,000 individuals is a carrier. New hope may be around the corner, however. Researchers have recently found that the plasma membranes of cells in the lungs and pancreases of mice with the same genetic defect as humans with cystic fibrosis have lower levels of a fatty acid called DHA (docosahexaenoic acid). When they were fed a diet rich in DHA, this corrected the imbalance and erased previous damage. Human trials are currently under way.

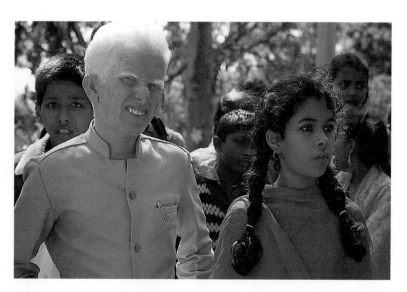

FIGURE 16-9 Albinism Albinism is an autosomal-recessive trait. An albino man with his wife in India.

(a)   (b)

FIGURE 16-10 Comparison of a Pancreas from Patient with Cystic Fibrosis with a Normal Pancreas Cystic fibrosis is a disease caused by an autosomal-recessive gene. *(a)* It results in a blockage of the ducts draining the pancreas, leading to cysts in the pancreatic tissue. The tissue degenerates and is replaced by fibrous connective tissue. *(b)* Normal pancreas.

FIGURE 16-11 Cystic Fibrosis   Inhalants, antibiotics, and physical therapy are used to treat patients with cystic fibrosis. To remove mucus from the lungs, parents or physical therapists must treat the patient two or three times a day. Pounding on the rib cage with a cupped hand (clopping) loosens the mucus.

Autosomal-Dominant Traits Are Expressed in Heterozygous and Homozygous-Dominant Individuals

Many human traits are autosomal dominant; that is, they are carried on the autosomes and are expressed in heterozygous (Aa) and homozygous-dominant (AA) individuals. To date, nearly 1200 human traits have been identified as autosomal dominant, and 1000 others are suspected. The absence of dermal ridges (which give rise to fingerprints), short fingers and toes, freckles, cleft chin, and drooping eyelids are all autosomal-dominant traits. Marfan's syndrome, discussed in the Thinking Critically section in this chapter, is an autosomal-dominant disease. This section discusses two other examples: widow's peak and achondroplasia.

Widow's Peak. Take a moment to examine the hairlines of your friends and classmates. In some individuals, the hairline runs straight across the forehead. In others, it juts forward in the center, forming a "widow's

(a)

(b)

FIGURE 16-12 Widow's Peak   (a) The widow's peak is a dominant trait carried on one of the autosomes. (b) A straight hairline is a recessive trait. Simple Mendelian genetics can be used to determine the genotype of the offspring.

peak" (**FIGURE 16-12**). Widow's peak is determined by an autosomal-dominant gene, indicated by W. Because the W allele is dominant, this phenotype is expressed in homozygous-dominant individuals (WW) and also heterozygotes (Ww). Individuals with the genotype ww have a straight hairline.

Achondroplasia. The boy shown in **FIGURE 16-13** has a genetic disease called **achondroplasia** (a-CON-drow-PLAY-zee-ah), one form of dwarfism. Individuals with this disease have short, stubby legs and arms but a relatively normal-sized trunk. As a rule, they do not grow taller than 4 feet. Surgeons have developed a technique to lengthen the arms and legs of people with this disorder. In this procedure, the leg and arm bones of the person are fractured (under anesthesia), and the patient is fitted with a traction device. Traction is applied to the broken bones, causing them to separate. New bone is formed in the gap, and the bones slowly elongate.

Achondroplasia afflicts about 1 of every 10,000 children born in the United States and results from an autosomal-dominant gene. Most cases are believed to arise from spontaneous mutations, because the majority of children with the condition are born to phenotypically normal parents.

FIGURE 16-13 Achondroplasia   Achondroplasia, one form of dwarfism, is an autosomal-dominant disorder.

Variations in Mendelian Genetics

Mendel presented his work at meetings of the Natural Science Society in Czechoslovakia in 1865 and published his results the following year. Like many ideas ahead of their time, Mendel's conclusions went largely unnoticed. It was not until 1900, 16 years after he died, that Mendel's studies received the attention they deserved. At that time, the publication of three other studies confirmed Mendel's findings. More studies followed, and excitement began to mount. The scientific community realized that Mendel's principles pertained to a great many organisms. Since that time, researchers have uncovered additional modes of inheritance and gene expression.

Incomplete Dominance Results in Intermediate Traits—That Is, a Kind of Blending of Traits

One example of another form of inheritance is a phenomenon called **incomplete**, or **partial**, **dominance**. Incomplete dominance occurs when heterozygous offspring exhibit intermediate phenotypes. In other words, incomplete dominance produces F_1 offspring with phenotypes intermediate to the parental phenotypes. This is the kind of blending that Mendel said didn't exist!

Incomplete dominance occurs in the snapdragon flower. **FIGURE 16-14** shows a cross between a plant with red flowers (*II*) and one with ivory flowers (*ii*). Even though the red color is dominant, this cross produces offspring with pink flowers, an intermediate phenotype (**FIGURE 16-14**). That's because the *I* gene does not exert complete dominance. Interestingly, incomplete dominance also occurs in a number of human disorders, including sickle-cell anemia.

Sickle-Cell Anemia. Sickle-cell anemia affects the blood, and chiefly afflicts African Americans and Caucasians of Mediterranean descent. Sickle-cell anemia is caused by a genetic defect that leads to abnormal hemoglobin (HEME-oh-GLOW-bin) formation. Hemoglobin is a protein found in red blood cells, which carry oxygen to body cells.

Sickle-cell anemia occurs in individuals that are homozygous recessive. The abnormal hemoglobin causes red blood cells to convert to sickle-shaped cells when they encounter low oxygen levels in the blood—for example, when blood cells flow through capillaries (small blood vessels) in metabolically active tissues.

Sickle cells are larger than red blood cells and inflexible. As a result, sickle cells clog capillaries and reduce oxygen flow to brain cells, heart cells, and other organs. In homozygous-recessive individuals, sickle-cell anemia is usually lethal. In fact, most individuals with the disease die by their late twenties.

Individuals who are heterozygous for the trait are referred to as **carriers,** because they can pass the gene on to their children. Carriers generally lead relatively normal lives, but they are subject to occasional problems. Although their red blood cells appear normal,

FIGURE 16-14 Incomplete Dominance Incomplete dominance involves two alleles, neither of which is dominant over the other. The result is an intermediate phenotype as shown here in the snapdragon flower.

they actually contain 50% normal and 50% abnormal hemoglobin. Moderate sickling occurs when these cells are exposed to low oxygen.

Approximately 1 in every 500 African Americans born in the United States is homozygous recessive, and about 1 of every 12 is heterozygous (a carrier) for the sickle-cell trait. Why is this allele so prevalent?

In tropical climates, from which African Americans come, the sickle-cell allele protects carriers and homozygous-recessive individuals from malaria, a deadly disease prevalent in humid, tropical regions. Although homozygous-recessive individuals die earlier, the selective advantage that carriers enjoy has caused the allele to increase in the population.

Malaria is caused by a microscopic parasite called *Plasmodium* (plaz-MOW-dee-um), which is transmitted from one person to the next by certain mosquitoes. Inside the body, the parasites invade and colonize the liver, where they multiply rapidly. New parasites leave the liver and enter the bloodstream, where they attack and destroy red blood cells. Many of the parasites remain in the liver, however, continuing to reproduce and periodically release new offspring. Unless treated, a victim of malaria suffers from repeated attacks of chills followed by fever. Each attack corresponds with the release of a new batch of *Plasmodia* from the liver.

How does the sickle-cell allele protect people? As noted earlier, the hemoglobin in the red blood cells of carriers and individuals who are homozygous recessive is altered by the sickle-cell allele. For reasons not entirely clear, the presence of altered hemoglobin changes the plasma membrane of red blood cells and prevents the parasite from entering. As a result, both homozygous-recessive individuals and carriers (heterozygotes) are relatively immune to the parasite.

Because the sickle-cell allele confers a selective advantage on those who have it and because heterozygotes suffer relatively few problems, in East Africa, where the malaria parasite is quite common, 45% of all blacks are carriers of the trait (heterozygotes). In the United States, where malaria is virtually nonexistent, the frequency of the sickle-cell allele has decreased considerably.

Some Genes Have Multiple Alleles

Mendel studied seven characteristics of peas. Each characteristic is determined by a gene with two alleles—two alternative forms. In human and other species, however, researchers have shown that some genes can have more than two alleles; such a gene is said to have **multiple alleles.**

Consider blood types. One gene that controls blood type is called the *I* **gene** (for isoagglutinin; pronounced EYE-sa-AH-glue-TEH-nin). The *I* gene is located at a

FIGURE 16-15
Codominance
Codominant genes are expressed fully when present in the same cell. In blood type AB, both *A* and *B* genes produce their characteristic glycoproteins. Type A (genotype AO) cells have only type A glycoprotein, and type B (genotype BO) cells have only type B glycoprotein. Type O cells have neither. Note that type A blood may also be in people with the AA genotype and that type B blood may be in people with the BB genotype.

particular site (or locus) on one pair of chromosomes. But unlike the genes Mendel studied, which had only two alleles, the *I* gene exists in one of three distinct forms. The three alleles are I^A, I^B, and I^O. Note, however, that even though there are three possible alleles in human beings, an individual can have only two of the alleles in his or her **genome** (genome refers to all of one's genes), one on each homologous chromosome. It's like having three mittens. You can only wear two at a time.

Four possible blood types exist: A, B, AB, and O. **TABLE 16-3** lists the four blood types and the six different genotypes that give rise to them. Take a moment to study them.

As shown, the A blood type occurs when an individual has two *A* alleles of the *I* gene or an *A* and an *O*. Type B occurs when an individual has two *B* alleles of the *I* gene or a *B* and an *O*. Type AB has both *A* and *B* alleles. Type O occurs when two *O* alleles of the *I* gene are present.

The *I* gene is responsible for the production of glycoproteins (proteins with carbohydrate attached) that project from the surface of red blood cells. Thus, the *A* and *B* alleles of the *I* gene produce A and B glycoproteins, respectively. The *O* allele, on the other hand, pro-

TABLE 16-3

Phenotype and Genotype in ABO system

Phenotype (blood type)	Genotypes
Type A	$I^A I^A$, $I^A I^O$
Type B	$I^B I^B$, $I^B I^O$
Type AB	$I^A I^B$
Type O	$I^O I^O$

(a)

(b)

(c)

(d)

(e)

FIGURE 16-16 Polygenic Inheritance Skin color is probably determined by at least two, perhaps as many as eight, genes, resulting in a wide range of phenotypes: *(a)* black, *(b)* dark, *(c)* mulatto, *(d)* light, and *(e)* white.

duces neither type of cell-surface glycoprotein. If you know this, you can determine the type of glycoproteins in the different phenotypes. For example, AA individuals have only A glycoproteins, and BB individuals have only B glycoproteins. In AO and BO individuals, the red blood cells contain only type A glycoproteins and B glycoproteins, respectively (top, **FIGURE 16-15**). Type AB individuals have both A and B glycoproteins.

Both A and B are dominant genes, and the O allele is recessive. Therefore, the I^A and I^B genes are said to be co-dominant. **Codominant genes** are expressed fully and equally. So not only are blood types an example of multiple genes, they are also an example of codominance, another type of inheritance.

Incomplete dominance (blending), multiple alleles, and codominance are three exceptions to Mendel's principles. But don't be too quick to dismiss Mendel. These examples do not negate his discoveries. They are simply additional modes of gene expression. Moreover, Mendelian principles can be used to predict the genotypic ratios and patterns of inheritance in these alternative forms of inheritance.

Some Traits Are Determined by More Than One Gene Pair

For many years, geneticists believed that each gene controls a single trait. In humans and other animals, however, many

TABLE 16-4

Possible Skin-Color Genotypes and Phenotypes with Two Skin-Color Genes*

Genotype	Phenotype	Number of Recessive Genes
AABB	Black	0
AABb	Dark	1
AaBB	Dark	1
AaBb	Mulatto	2
AAbb	Mulatto	2
aaBB	Mulatto	2
Aabb	Light	3
aaBb	Light	3
aabb	White	4

*Skin color probably involves many more genes.

traits are controlled by a number of genes—from a few to perhaps hundreds. Skin color, for example, is controlled by as many as eight genes. This type of inheritance is called **polygenic inheritance** (polly-JEAN-ick). Polygenic inheritance results in incredible phenotypic variation.

To see how polygenic inheritance leads to such wide phenotypic variation, consider an example using two genes for skin color, designated *A* and *B*. In this example, we will say that the genotype of an African American is *AABB* and the genotype of a Caucasian is *aabb*. **TABLE 16-4** lists all of the possible genotypes in this example with possible phenotypes; **FIGURE 16-16** shows what they look like. Take a moment to study the table and the figure.

Polygenic inheritance is also responsible for height, weight, intelligence, and a number of behavioral traits. But in each instance, the genes are not the only factors controlling these traits. As a rule, the genotype establishes the range in which a phenotype will fall, but environmental factors (for example, diet) determine exactly how much of the potential will be realized for many genes. For example, although genes determine height, this trait is also influenced by one's diet. The better one eats from infancy to adolescence, the taller he or she will be.

Genes Located on the Same Chromosome Are Said To Be Linked

As pointed out earlier, Mendel found that during gamete formation, the seven genes under study in his pea plants were segregated independently. Also noted earlier, independent assortment generally occurs *only* when the genes under study are on different chromosomes. As a rule, if two genes are on the same chromosome, they do not segregate independently.

Humans have an estimated 100,000 genes on their 46 chromosomes. Those genes located on the same chromosome tend to be inherited together and are said to be **linked.**

(a)

(b)

FIGURE 16-17 Linkage *(a)* Hypothetical dihybrid cross with no linkage. *(b)* Hypothetical dihybrid cross with linkage. Linkage reduces the number of genotypes in the offspring.

To illustrate the concept, imagine that you are studying two traits. Designate the dominant form of the first trait *A* and the recessive allele *a*. The dominant form of the second trait is designated *B* and the recessive form is *b*. Suppose we cross a homozygous-dominant individual (*AABB*) with a homozygous-recessive mate (*aabb*). This scenario is shown in **FIGURE 16-17A**. Take a moment to study the top part of the figure.

As shown, if the *A* and *B* genes are *not* linked, this cross produces an F_1 generation that's entirely heterozygous (*AaBb*). Furthermore, F_1 offspring will produce four genetically different gametes: *AB*, *Ab*, *aB*, and *ab*. If an F_1

offspring mates with another F_1 offspring (of the opposite sex of course), the result is an F_2 generation with nine distinct genotypes and four different phenotypes. You can take my word for this, or examine **FIGURE 16-17A** for yourself.

If the *A* and *B* genes are on the same chromosome (they're linked) and the *a* and *b* genes are on the other (also linked), the outcome changes dramatically. First, as **FIGURE 16-17B** shows, only two gametes are produced: *AB* and *ab*. Second, as **FIGURE 16-17B** also shows, all members of the F_1 generation are heterozygous, *AaBb*. This is the same as if the genes were unlinked. However, because the *A* and *B* genes are on the same chromosome, the F_1 generation produces only two types of gametes, *AB* and *ab*. Consequently, only two phenotypes are produced in the F_2 generation.

So can we conclude that independent assortment does not occur when genes are linked? Yes—at least most of the time. When two genes are on the same chromosome, they tend to be inherited together. However, there is one exception—a phenomenon called crossing-over.

Crossing-over occurs during meiosis: when the homologous chromosomes come together, or "pair up," in

FIGURE 16-18 Crossing-Over The crossing-over shown here increases genetic variation in gametes and offspring and occurs during meiosis.

prophase I. During this process, the chromatids of homologous chromosomes fuse at one or more points, as shown in **FIGURE 16-18**. Later, when the chromosomes separate, arms of one chromosome may end up with the other. In this process, then, chromosomes actually exchange segments of their chromatin with chromatids on homologous chromosomes. There's a kind of genetic swapping. When this occurs, genes that were linked are no longer linked and are not necessarily inherited together.

Crossing-over "unlinks" genes and increases genetic variation in gametes; this, in turn, leads to genetic variation in offspring. (Other factors also contribute to genetic variation.) The more variation, the more genotypes and possible phenotypes in a population. As Chapter 21 points out, variation is essential to evolution. Genetic variants may have characteristics that give one organism an advantage over another. In a very general sense, then, crossing-over provides variation that ensures the survival of populations in changing environmental conditions. It's a protective mechanism of sorts.

Crossing-over can occur anywhere along the length of a chromosome. However, the greater the distance between two genes on the same chromosome, the more likely it is that a crossover will occur between them. This fact helped scientists map the human genome.

The Human Genome Project Seeks To Determine the Sequence of Bases in Human DNA and the Location of All of the Genes

In the 1990s scientists the world over embarked on what is conceivably the largest unified biological research project of its kind in human history. It was designed to determine the location of all of the genes on all 46 chromosomes and the precise sequence of bases of the human genes and intervening DNA in the chromosomes. With an estimated 100,000 genes and three billion bases in the human DNA, costs of this monumental task were estimated to be $3 billion dollars. Time to complete the task was estimated to be 15 years or longer.

The **Human Genome Project,** as it is called, began in earnest in 1991. Scientists found that the first part of the project—mapping the location of the 100,000 or so genes—occurred at a much faster pace than anticipated. By November, 1998, geneticists had pinpointed the location of 95% of the human genes. The remaining 5% were mapped out two years later.

Why is it important to know the location of human chromosomes? First, it adds to our overall knowledge of human genetics. Second, it provides scientists a way to isolate and synthesize human genes. For example, a gene that controls the production of useful products (hormones, blood-clotting factors, etc.) could be synthesized in the lab and used to mass produce the product to treat various illnesses. Chapter 18 discusses this process in more detail.

A third practical, but controversial, application of this research is that it could help medical geneticists locate disease-producing genes. This would allow geneticists to screen unborn fetuses to determine if they contain any life-threatening or debilitating disorders. If results show this to be so, parents may choose to abort their offspring. For those for whom abortion is not an option, genetic screening with this kind of power could help prepare parents for the challenges that await them with their specially challenged child.

Fourth, knowing the location of disease genes also leads some scientists to speculate on the possibility of genetic repair—for example, finding ways to splice normal genes in place of defective ones, avoiding problems altogether. A parent, faced with the possibility of having a severely physically impaired child because of a genetic disorder, for example, might opt to have gene replacement therapy on the unborn fetus in hopes of having a healthy child. Although this prospect may be years away from successful completion, some early research seems promising.

Researchers are currently experimenting with ways to replace mutated tumor suppressor genes. As you may recall from Chapter 15, tumor suppressor genes are normal genes that hold cells in check. When mutated, cells can undergo rapid division. By replacing the defective gene in tumor cells with intact tumor suppressor genes, researchers hope someday to tame malignancies, bringing the cells back under control.

The Human Genome Project is not without opposition. Some critics argue that knowledge gained from knowing the human genome intimately could lead to a potentially tricky situation in which a physician can diagnose an illness through genetic means long before cures are available. Some individuals are concerned that insurance companies could access a person's records and, by examining his or her genetic code, would be in a position to deny coverage. Finally, some critics worry about the possibilities the Human Genome Project will present for manipulation of the human genes. Is it opening doors to genetic manipulation that should be better left to evolution? Are we playing God with our own genome?

One upshot of this project has been the mapping of chromosomes in nonhuman species, a step that could help bring important genetic improvements, in the case of livestock, or in the case of disease organisms could help scientists find better tools to combat them.

Section 16-5

Sex-Linked Genes

Earlier, I noted that the sex chromosomes determine an individual's sex. The truth of the matter is that the sex of an individual is determined by the Y chromosome. If the Y chromosome is present, an individual becomes a male. The absence of the Y chromosome results in the development of a female phenotype.

The Y chromosome exerts its effect during embryonic development. Interestingly enough, males and females start out looking alike. That is, early in the embryo's development, the gonads, which develop in the abdominal cavity, are identical. When the Y chromosome is present, however, the embryonic gonad becomes a testis—thanks, at least in part, to the presence of the *t* gene (testis-determining gene). The testis, in turn, produces testosterone and other androgens, which are responsible for the male secondary sex characteristics—hair growth, body shape and size, and so on (Chapter 19). The absence of the Y chromosome results in the development of an ovary with its hormones and the resultant female phenotype.

The X and Y chromosomes also carry genes that determine many other traits. Genes situated on the X and Y chromosome are therefore known as **sex-linked genes.** So far, the majority of the sex-linked genes discovered by geneticists are located on the X chromosome. These are known as **X-linked genes.** The following sections describe the inheritance of some common sex-linked genes.

Recessive X-Linked Genes Are the Best Understood of the Sex-Linked Genes

At least 124 genes have been assigned to the X chromosome. At least 160 more are also thought to be located on it. Color blindness, discussed in detail in Chapter 12, and certain forms of hemophilia are examples of recessive traits carried on the X chromosome.

In order for a female (XX) to display a recessive sex-linked trait, each of her X chromosomes must carry the recessive gene. For males (XY), however, only one recessive allele is required. Why? Because the Y chromosome is not genetically equivalent to the X chromosome.[2] Thus, in males, only one recessive gene is needed to exhibit a recessive X-linked trait.

FIGURE 16-19 shows four possible genetic combinations leading to color blindness. This illustration also introduces you to a genetic-tracking system used to

(a)   (b)

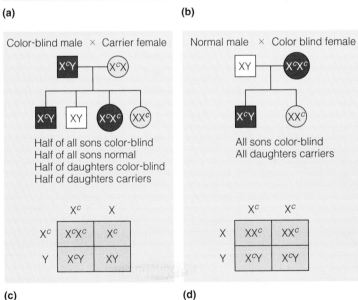

(c)   (d)

FIGURE 16-19 Inheritance of Color Blindness Four possible genetic ways a sex-linked recessive gene such as color blindness can be passed to offspring. Males are indicated by boxes and females by circles. In this scheme, green boxes and circles represent men and women with color blindness. Light blue boxes represent men and women who are carriers. White boxes and circles represent men and women without the color blindness gene. The notation X^c indicates an X chromosome carrying the gene for color blindness.

---

[2]The X and Y chromosomes are believed to share few genes, and only part of the Y chromosome is homologous with the X chromosome.

follow traits in families, known as a **pedigree.** In a pedigree, squares represent men and circles represent women. (We assume the square for males is not social commentary.) The horizontal line linking a square to a circle indicates a mating. Offspring are shown below their parents. When a square is lightly shaded, the individual is a carrier of the gene. He or she does not have the disease, but does carry the recessive gene and can pass it on to his or her offspring. A darkly shaded square or circle indicates the person has the trait.

In **FIGURE 16-19A,** for example, a man and a woman have four children, two boys and two girls. The woman (light blue circle) is a carrier of color blindness. Her cells contain one X chromosome with a recessive allele for color blindness (designated X^c) and another X chromosome with the normal allele. Consequently, half of her ova will contain the recessive allele, and the other half will contain the normal allele. As shown, the woman's husband (white square) is not color-blind. He produces sperm containing either an X or a Y chromosome. When one of his X-bearing sperm unites with one of her ova bearing an X chromosome with the allele for color blindness, the result is a daughter who is a carrier, indicated by a light blue circle. When one of his X-bearing sperm unites with an ovum carrying a normal X chromosome, the result is a daughter who is neither a carrier nor color blind (white circle).

Now what about male children of these parents? Males are produced when a Y-bearing sperm unites with an ovum carrying an X chromosome. If the X chromosome carries the recessive allele for color blindness, the boy is color-blind (green square). If the X chromosome is normal, the boy's color vision is unimpaired (white square). Take a moment to study the other possibilities in **FIGURE 16-19.**

Dominant X-Linked Genes Are Relatively Rare

Recessive X-linked genes are the most common sex-linked trait in humans. However, there are a few noteworthy examples of dominant X-linked genes. One of the best understood is a disorder with a tongue-twisting name of **hypophosphatemia** (high-poe-FOS-fuh-TEEM-ee-uh). This disease is

FIGURE 16-20 Hypophosphatemia
People with hypophosphatemia, a dominant X-linked genetic disorder, resemble this child with rickets, which usually results from inadequate vitamin D intake.

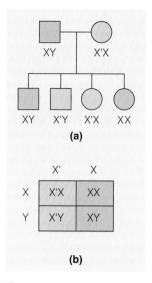

FIGURE 16-21 Inheritance of a Sex-Linked Dominant Gene (*a*) Pedigree. (*b*) Corresponding Punnett square.

characterized by low phosphate levels in the blood and tissues of the body. This, in turn, results in a form of **rickets** (RICK-its), or bowleggedness (**FIGURE 16-20**). Rickets usually results from a dietary deficiency of vitamin D or insufficient exposure to sunlight (Chapter 5). Alleviating the dietary deficiency usually solves the problem. In this genetic disease, however, vitamin D cannot reverse the symptoms.

Hypophosphatemia occurs when either the male (XY) or the female (XX) has one X chromosome containing the dominant gene, indicated as X′ (X prime). **FIGURE 16-21** illustrates the pattern of inheritance when a woman who is heterozygous (X′X) for the trait mates with a man who does not carry the trait (XY). Study the figure and see if you can determine any rules that apply to the inheritance of X-linked dominant genes.

What you should have discovered is that, whenever the dominant gene is present, it is expressed—regardless of the sex of the individual.

Both Dominant and Recessive Y-Linked Genes Are Always Expressed

The genes that control gonadal differentiation, sperm production, and male secondary sex characteristics are thought to be on the Y chromosome. The Y-linked genes have a simple and distinct pattern of inheritance. Because only males have Y chromosomes, Y-linked traits only appear in males. Obviously, Y-linked genes can only be transmitted from fathers to sons. Because the X and Y chromosomes in men are not homologous, each gene on the Y chromosome has only one allele. Thus, both dominant and recessive Y-linked genes are always expressed.

The Action of Some Genes Is Influenced by the Sex of an Individual

In one of the most interesting twists on basic genetics, it turns out that certain autosomal genes behave differently in the two sexes. In one sex, for example, an allele will be dominant; in the other sex, it will be recessive. These genes are known as **sex-influenced genes.**

The best-known example is the gene for pattern baldness. **Pattern baldness** is the loss of hair that often begins in a man's twenties. The name of this condition results from the fact that affected individuals do not go completely bald; they retain a rim of hair on the temples and back of the head.

The gene for pattern baldness is present in men and women, but in men the gene acts as if it is autosomal-dominant. That is, it is expressed in both heterozygous and homozygous-dominant individuals, which means that lots of men end up with pattern baldness. In contrast, in women the allele acts as if it is autosomal-recessive. Only women who are homozygous recessive for the trait exhibit baldness, which means very few end up with this affliction. For more on the causes and cures of baldness, see Health Note 16-1.

What accounts for the different behavior of these genes in men and women? Geneticists believe that the genes are influenced by testosterone, a sex steroid hormone found in far greater concentration in the blood of men than women. In this case, the genotype and hormonal environment interact to determine the expression of the pattern-baldness gene.

Section 16-6

Chromosomal Abnormalities and Genetic Counseling

A young couple wait in their doctor's office for the results of a genetic test on cells of their unborn baby, which were drawn via amniocentesis, described in Chapter 15. They will soon learn that the studies have revealed an abnormal number of chromosomes.

Abnormal Chromosome Numbers Generally Result from a Failure of Chromosomes to Separate During Gamete Formation (Meiosis)

During meiosis I, homologous chromosomes pair, then separate—with one member of each pair going to each daughter cell (**FIGURE 16-22A**). If a homologous pair fails to separate during meiosis, however, one of the new cells will end up with an extra chromosome (**FIGURE 16-22B**). The other cell will be short one chromosome. The failure of homologous chromosomes to separate is called **nondisjunction** (non-diss-JUNK-shun).

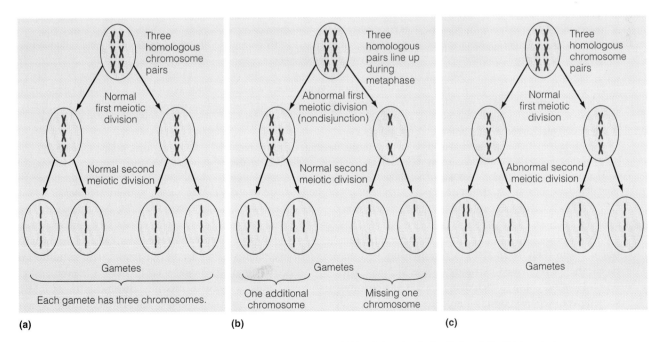

(a)   (b)   (c)

FIGURE 16-22 Meiosis and Abnormal Chromosome Numbers
(a) A simplified version of meiosis. During the first meiotic division, the homologous pairs line up, then separate, producing daughter cells with one-half the number of chromosomes. In the second meiotic division, the chromosomes line up single file and separate, with one chromatid going to each daughter cell.

(b) Nondisjunction in the first meiotic division. A chromosome pair may fail to separate during meiosis I, resulting in abnormal gametes. Half are missing a chromosome, and the other half have an extra chromosome. *(c)* Nondisjunction in second meiotic division, resulting in two normal gametes, one gamete with two chromosomes, and one gamete with four.

Health Note 16-1

Going, Going . . . Gone: The Causes and Cures of Baldness in Men and Women

Americans and others in Western society spend billions of dollars a year on their hair—styling it, coloring it, cutting it, and, yes, preventing its loss. Hair loss, however, is as inevitable as death itself. All of us lose hair as we age, but some people lose a lot more than others—and, for some, hair loss begins early in life, even in childhood.

Doctors recognize three types of hair loss. Partial hair loss involves the loss of small, isolated patches of hair. The second type, pattern baldness, involves the loss of most or all of the hair on the head. Total body hair loss is the complete loss of hair from every part of the body: head, eyelids, eyebrows, arms, legs, and so on.

Hair loss strikes both sexes, all ethnic groups, and all age groups. In fact, two of every three American men will develop some form of balding. An even larger percentage of men and women will lose some hair.

Hair loss is not a life-threatening condition, but can have severe emotional impacts on individuals. Men whose hair begins to thin in their twenties often feel self-conscious and anxious in public. They may feel isolated from their cohorts, for hair loss often makes them look five to ten years older than their peers. Friends may poke fun at them, further adding to their self-conscious feelings. Even in older men, whose friends are balding, hair loss can result in depression, feelings of low self-esteem, and a general sense of inadequacy. In women, hair loss can have even more devastating effects. What causes hair loss?

A surprising number of factors can cause hair to fall out. One of the most widely recognized is chemotherapy—chemical treatments used to fight cancer. These drugs attack rapidly dividing cells in the body such as cancer cells and the cells in hair follicles. High fever, severe infections, and severe cases of the flu also cause hair loss that mysteriously begins four weeks to twelve months after the illness. Many prescription drugs also cause hair loss. Thyroid disease—either an overactive or an underactive thyroid—can cause hair to fall out. Birth control pills, iron deficiencies, and protein-deficient diets can have a similar effect in some patients. Many women report excessive hair loss after pregnancy. But the most common cause of all is genetic.

Hereditary balding (pattern baldness) or thinning, described in the chapter, results from genes that arise from either the mother's or the father's side of the family. In men, this condition results in near total or complete loss of hair. Women, on the other hand, tend to experience excessive thinning, but rarely go completely bald. What can be done to combat balding?

Two lines of attack are possible: medicinal and surgical. Consider the medicinal approach first.

Several medicines, some of which are over the counter, are available. One of the most widely publicized is Rogaine. In a study of 2300 patients with male pattern baldness, Rogaine treatment resulted in moderate to marked hair growth in 39% of the patients, compared to 11% of those in the control group.

For Rogaine to be effective, however, a man must be prepared for a lifetime of work because this drug must be applied twice a day every day of one's life. Stopping treatment causes bald spots to reappear, and reverting to once a day results in continued hair loss. A one-year supply of Rogaine costs $600 to $1000 per year, depending on the size of one's bald spot.

Rogaine also creates some discomfort in the form of itching, headaches (in 40% of the patients), dizzy spells, and an irregular heart-

---

Nondisjunction can also occur in the second meiotic division (**FIGURE 16-22C**). In this division, you may recall, the 23 replicated chromosomes split apart, with one chromatid going to each daughter cell. If a chromosome fails to separate into its two chromatids, the result is the same as nondisjunction in meiosis I—a daughter cell with an extra chromosome and another daughter cell missing one chromosome.

When a gamete with one extra chromosome unites with a normal gamete, the zygote produced will contain 47 chromosomes. The zygote may be able to divide successfully by mitosis, producing an embryo all of whose cells will have an additional chromosome. Thus, instead of the normal 23 chromosome pairs, each cell in the embryo contains 22 pairs and one triplet. This condition is called **trisomy** (TRY-sew-mee; literally, "three bodies").

Gametes with a missing chromosome can also unite with normal gametes. This results in individuals with 45 chromosomes—22 chromosome pairs and a chromosome singlet. This condition is called **monosomy** (MON-oh-SO-me).

Surprisingly, one of every two conceptions contains an abnormal chromosome number. Most of these embryos and fetuses die in utero. This condition is believed to be responsible for 70% of all early embryonic deaths and 30% of all fetal deaths. It is also beat in some patients. Rogaine is recommended for younger men from ages 20 to 30 who have begun to lose hair within the last five years. Men who are completely bald are poor candidates for treatment.

Antiandrogens can be given to women. These drugs inhibit the binding of androgens (male hormones found in women's blood) to the hair follicles. For reasons not well understood, this treatment can result in a complete reversal of hair loss, but only if it is begun within two years of the onset of hair loss. Men can also be treated with antiandrogens, but not without significant problem, for these drugs cause a loss of sex drive and an undesirable elevation of the voice.

For those who do not respond to drugs, surgery is an option. But surgery can be quite expensive, costing as much as $15,000. Despite its potentially high price tag, an estimated 250,000 American males elect to have one of several different types of surgical procedures each year.

One of the most common is hair transplantation (**FIGURE 1**). In this operation, small plugs of hair are taken from the sides and back of the scalp where hair grows thickly. These plugs are placed in the bald spot. De-

pending on the size of the bald spot, up to four sessions may be required. To make the graft look more natural, surgeons often place single-hair follicle or several-hair follicle grafts along the hair line.

Another common procedure is scalp reduction. In this procedure, surgeons remove well-defined bald spots (up to 2 by 7 inches) in the top of the scalp. The edges of the incision are then drawn together, thus reducing the area of baldness. Hair transplants may also be performed in conjunction with this procedure to fill in the remaining area.

Another option is a wig or toupee. Although wigs or toupees have improved dramatically and well-crafted hair pieces made from real or synthetic hair are very difficult to distinguish from the real thing, there are enough bad ones around that this option is often looked upon with disfavor by many men. Hair pieces can even be sutured in place.

Certain cosmetic remedies are also available. For example, cutting one's hair short tends to make baldness less obvious. Dark hair can be lightened so that it is more closely matched in color with the scalp, thus making the contrast between hair and scalp less obvious.

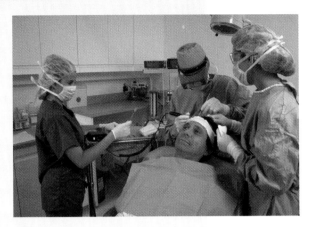

FIGURE 1 Patient undergoing hair transplant surgery.

People who are experiencing baldness should seek medical attention quickly to determine if it is transient, as in the case of post-pregnancy; medicinally induced loss; or heredity. With their doctor's help, they can plot a strategy, if they so desire, to ward off balding. Or, they can simply accept their fate and learn to live with—or even appreciate—it.

Visit *Human Biology's* Internet site for links to web sites offering more information on this topic.

---

associated with an increased miscarriage rate in older mothers.

Down Syndrome Is Trisomy 21. One of the most common trisomies is **Down syndrome,** or **trisomy 21.**[3] Approximately 1 of every 700 babies born in the United States has Down syndrome. Down syndrome children are typically short with round, moonlike faces (**FIGURE 16-23**). Their tongues protrude forward,

forcing their mouths open, and their eyes slant upward at the corners. These children have IQs that are rarely over 70. A significant number of Down syndrome babies die from heart defects and respiratory infections in the first year of infancy. Modern medical care, especially antibiotics, has reduced early death, and many individuals with Down syndrome live to age 20 or beyond.

The incidence of Down syndrome (and many other monosomies and trisomies) increases with maternal age. As **FIGURE 16-24** shows, a woman's chances of having a Down syndrome baby increase dramatically after age 35. For this reason, many couples choose to have their children

---

[3]Contemporary geneticists generally refer to this as Down syndrome, rather than Down's syndrome.

(a)   Female with Down Syndrome (47,XX,+21)

FIGURE 16-23 Down Syndrome *(a)* Karyotype of Down syndrome girl. Note trisomy of chromosome 21. *(b)* Notice the distinguishing characteristics described in the text.

(b)

for the rise in Down syndrome children later in life may be related to the mother's ability to carry such a fetus to term. This study suggests that the number of trisomy 21 conceptions is the same in all women regardless of age. The embryos are simply less likely to be naturally aborted in older women. Why? No one knows.

Nondisjunction of the Sex Chromosomes. Nondisjunction can occur in any chromosome—that is, in both autosomes and sex chromosomes. Nondisjunction of the sex chromosomes can lead to a variety of nonlethal genetic disorders. One of the most common is Klinefelter syndrome.

Klinefelter syndrome occurs when an ovum with an extra X chromosome is fertilized by a Y-bearing sperm, resulting in an XXY genotype (**FIGURE 16-25**). This condition occurs in about 1 of every 700 to 1000 newborn males.[4] Although Klinefelter syndrome patients are males, masculinization is incomplete. The males' external genitalia and testes are unusually small, and about 50% of them develop breasts. Spermatogenesis is abnormal, and Klinefelter patients are generally sterile.

Another common disorder resulting from nondisjunction of the sex chromosomes is **Turner syndrome,** a monosomy. Turner syndrome results when an ovum lacking the X chromosome is fertilized by a X-bearing sperm. It may also result when a genetically normal ovum is fertilized by a sperm lacking an X or Y chromosome (**FIGURE 16-25**). In either case, the result is an offspring with 22 pairs of autosomes and a single, unmatched X chromosome (XO).

Turner syndrome patients are phenotypically female and are characteristically short with wide chests and a prominent fold of skin on their necks (**FIGURE 16-26**). Because their ovaries fail to develop at puberty, Turner syndrome patients are sterile, have low levels of estrogen, and have small breasts.[5] For the most part, they lead fairly normal lives. Mental retardation is not associated with the disorder, although some studies suggest that Turner patients are not as capable at numerical skills and spatial per-

earlier in the woman's child-bearing years. If the woman does get pregnant after age 35, many couples choose to have amniocentesis. If the test shows that the fetus has Down syndrome, a couple may decide to opt for an abortion. Amniocentesis also enables parents for whom abortion is not an option to prepare psychologically and to seek education that will help them care for their child.

Why does the incidence of Down syndrome increase with age? A recent study suggests that the reason

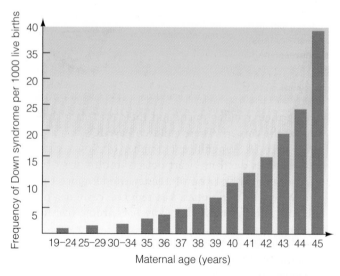

FIGURE 16-24 Incidence of Down Syndrome Babies at Various Maternal Ages The incidence of Down syndrome rises quickly after the maternal age of 35.

---

[4]Nondisjunction can also occur in sperm development, resulting in an XY sperm. The XY sperm can fertilize a normal ovum, resulting in an XXY individual.

[5]Note that some estrogen is released from the adrenal cortex, but not enough to permit breast development.

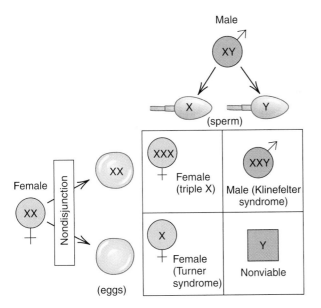

FIGURE 16-25 **Nondisjuction of sex chromosomes can result in two syndromes: Klinefelter Syndrome and Turner syndrome.**

TABLE 16-5

Chromosome Deletions

Syndrome	Phenotype
Wolf-Hirschhorn syndrome	Growth retardation, heart malformation, cleft palate; 30% die within 24 months.
Cri-du-chat syndrome	Infants have catlike cry, some facial anomalies, severe mental retardation.
Wilm's tumor	Kidney tumors, genital and urinary tract abnormalities
Retinoblastoma	Cancer of eye, increased risk of other cancers
Praeder-Willi syndrome	Infants are weak and grow slowly; children and adults are obese and are compulsive eaters.

ception as genetically normal children. Turner syndrome occurs in 1 of every 10,000 female births. The rarity of this condition, compared with Klinefelter's syndrome, is due to the fact that the XO embryo is more likely to be spontaneously aborted.

Genetic Disorders May Also Result from Variations in Chromosome Structure

Another defect in chromosomes involves alterations in chromosome structure, the most common of which are (1) **deletions,** the loss of a piece of chromosome, and (2) **translocations,** breakage followed by reattachment elsewhere.

Deletions. Most deletions are deleterious, and embryos with them are usually eliminated early in pregnancy. Nevertheless, some embryos whose cells contain deletions do survive. **TABLE 16-5** lists a few disorders caused by deletions. One of the more striking is called Praeder-Willi syndrome (PRAY-der Will-ee).

Praeder-Willi syndrome occurs in 1 in 10,000–25,000 births. It is caused by the loss of one of the arms of chromosome 15 during gamete formation and is characterized by slow infant growth, compulsive eating, and obesity. Babies born with the syndrome are weak. They have a poor suckling reflex and do not feed well. By age 5 or 6, however, these children become compulsive eaters. Parents must lock their cupboards and refrigerators. Neighbors must be warned to discourage begging and must keep their garbage cans under lock and key. The urge to eat results in obesity, which often leads to diabetes. If food intake is not restricted, victims can literally eat themselves to death. Researchers believe that the eating disorder may result from an endocrine imbalance caused by the deletion—illustrating how a genetic defect can lead to an upset in homeostasis.

Translocations. Translocations occur when a segment of a chromosome breaks off and reattaches to another site on the same chromosome or to another chromosome. Although this might at first seem innocuous, movement of a segment of a chromosome to another site can upset the delicate balance of gene expression and alter homeostasis. Translocations, for example, may be the cause of certain forms of leukemia.

Genetic Screening Allows Parents to Determine Whether They Will Have a Genetically Normal Baby

Chapter 15 noted that parents can now find out the sex of their child and the presence of certain genetic defects

FIGURE 16-26 **Turner Syndrome** *(a)* In a person with Turner syndrome only one X chromosome is present. *(b)* Characteristic physical features of a Turner syndrome girl.

(a) X   Y

(b)

well before birth via amniocentesis. This procedure permits geneticists to search for abnormal chromosome numbers, as well as deletions and translocations. Biochemical tests can also be run to pinpoint metabolic disease, although only a dozen or so are routinely screened.

Amniocentesis increases the risk of spontaneous abortion by about 1%. It also slightly increases the risk of maternal uterine infection. Therefore, this procedure is usually recommended only if one or more of the following conditions are met: (1) a woman is over 35, (2) she has already delivered a baby with a genetic defect, (3) she is a carrier of an X-linked genetic disorder, or (4) she or the father has a known chromosomal or genetic abnormality.

As a rule, amniocentesis is usually not performed until the sixteenth week of pregnancy.[6] Before this time, there is not enough fluid surrounding the fetus, and the needle could damage the fetus. Analysis of the fetal cells withdrawn from the amnion requires 10–15 additional days. If a serious defect is observed, a couple may elect to have an abortion. However, the risk of an abortion to the mother is slightly greater at this time than it is during the 12- to 16-week period, and some state laws do not permit abortion after 16 weeks.

To permit earlier detection of genetic defects, a new procedure, known as **chorionic villus biopsy** (CORE-ee-on-ick VILL-us BYE-op-see), has been developed. Chorionic villi are composed of embryonic tissue that form the fetal portion of the placenta (plah-SEN-tah), a structure that nourishes the growing fetus. To perform this procedure, physicians first insert a device into the uterus through the vagina. It is used to remove a small sample of a villus. The cells of the villus are then examined for chromosomal abnormalities, much the same way as those removed during amniocentesis.

Because a biopsy can be performed much earlier than amniocentesis, abortions can be performed between 8 and 12 weeks of gestation; these abortions are safer than those performed between 16 and 20 weeks. Although chorionic villus biopsy allows for earlier detection, it poses a slightly higher risk to the mother and her fetus.

DNA Abnormalities May Also Occur in Mitochondria, Resulting in Diseases

Mitochondria contain a tiny fraction (about 0.3%) of a cell's DNA. As noted in Chapter 3, the DNA inside a mitochondrion may be an evolutionary remnant from the time when the mitochondrion was a free-living organism. Until recently, though, the significance of mitochondrial DNA was not well understood.

A few years ago, however, researchers discovered a rare form of blindness in humans linked to a defect in the mitochondrial DNA. This finding confirmed suspicions that defective mitochondrial genes result in defects, and it also suggests an additional mechanism for inheriting genetic diseases.

The defective gene in the mitochondria that leads to blindness codes for a protein required in the first step of ATP production. The absence of this protein in the neurons of the optic nerve results in their death, which, in turn, leads to blindness usually by age 20.

Because mitochondria are passed on by the mother, all of the children of a woman with the defective gene will inherit it. Only a small fraction of the children who inherit the defective gene actually go blind, so it is thought that the mutation only predisposes people to blindness. Other factors may also contribute to blindness.

Several rare genetic diseases may also result from mitochondrial DNA defects. Researchers suggest that even some of the more common diseases may be caused by genetic defects in mitochondrial DNA. Some cases of heart, kidney, and central nervous system failure, whose causes are now unknown, may one day be linked to defective mitochondrial DNA.

Health, Homeostasis, and the Environment
Nature Versus Nurture

Throughout this book, the central theme—the idea that homeostasis and human health are profoundly influenced by our environment—has emerged repeatedly. Put in other words, the environment, which includes our social, psychological, and physical environments, has a profound impact on our internal environment (homeostasis) and our health.

In this section, we examine a controversy that has raged in science for decades over the connection between our genes and our environment. We will look at two basic questions: How do our genes contribute to our personalities? What is the role of our environment in determining our personality and behavior and, perhaps, even our health?

At one time, psychologists viewed the baby as a blank slate. A child's personality, they said, develops through interaction with its environment—its parents, friends, teachers, and so on. However, extensive research now suggests that our personalities are also influenced by our genes. Thus, our genes and our environment probably operate together in determining personality.

Michael Lewis, a researcher at the Robert Wood Johnson Medical School, studies infant response to stress. His research shows that newborn babies differ

---

[6]Improvements in this technique now allow physicians to perform the procedure as early as the fourteenth week, although risks of spontaneous abortion increase somewhat.

markedly in how they respond to the stress of a blood test performed well before their environment could have affected their personality. Lewis found that some children wail when poked with a needle during routine blood tests in the first few days of life; others hardly seem to notice. Of the newborns who cry, some quickly dampen their response. Others seem to go on forever, much to their parents' chagrin.

Lewis notes that a child's reaction to stress at this time is likely to be repeated 3 months later when the child receives an inoculation. He believes that the difference in response to stress is genetically based and that the inherent differences will persist.

Lewis has also found that babies differ in how they react to frustration. He performed a series of experiments to test infant response to a frustrating situation. Most children responded with anger. Some, however, showed no response at all, and others displayed sadness. These innate differences in behavior, occurring too early to stem from differences in upbringing, probably result from genetic differences. They may help account for the profound differences in responses to stress seen in adults.

Psychologist Nathan Fox has performed some intriguing studies on shy and extroverted children. His studies show that shy children cling to their mothers when a clown suddenly appears; extroverted children eagerly engage the clown in play. Fox has found that shy children show greater electrical activity in the right part of the brain; extroverted children show a higher level of activity in the left side. Because the children's personalities differ at birth and because the personality differences are reflected in differences in brain activity, genetics may be playing a powerful role in personality development.

Allison Rosenberg, a researcher at the National Institutes of Health, has also studied shy and outgoing children. Her work shows marked differences between these two groups in heart rate and the release of the hormone cortisol, further supporting the notion that there are inherent physiological differences in children from the outset. These are related to early differences in personality and, very possibly, to differences in genetic makeup. Interestingly, geneticists have recently discovered a gene dubbed the *Prozac gene*. It is not responsible for the production of Prozac, an antidepressant, but rather is believed to be responsible for mild-mannered behavior in those who have it.

Similar findings have been reported in other primates. Infant monkeys, for instance, display a wide range of personality traits early in life. Research shows that timid animals differ physiologically from their braver counterparts. Stephen Soumi, a researcher at the National Institutes of Health, believes that the individual differences seen in personality and in response to stress are so pro-

nounced that they must be genetically based. Furthermore, he and his colleagues have found that shyness and extroversion tend to run in families, further suggesting a link between early behavior and genetics.

Soumi notes, however, that environmental effects, especially events very early in life, can modify genetically programmed behavior. If a shy baby monkey is paired with an exceptionally nurturant mother, he finds, the shy animal develops rapidly and actively explores its environment.

Another example of the genetic basis of behavior and the role of one's environment in modifying genetically predisposed behavioral patterns comes from research on thrill seeking. Psychologists believe that some individuals are naturally born thrill seekers, or type T people (**FIGURE 16-27**). Some researchers believe that thrill seeking may be genetically based. One theory is that risk takers, the type T or "big T" individuals, may be hard to excite and, therefore, may attempt extraordinary feats for excitement. At the opposite end of the spectrum are "small t" people, risk avoiders, who are easily aroused. They seek to avoid stimulation. Presumably, there's a whole spectrum of folks in the middle.

Some researchers believe that type T individuals have an imbalance of a neurotransmitter known as monoamine oxidase (MAO) in the brain. Thrill seeking supposedly increases the MAO levels in the brain, creating a feeling of exhilaration.

Type T behavior can be modified by an individual's upbringing and turned in a negative or positive direction, say some psychologists. A positive direction might lead an individual to play for the Green Bay Packers football team. A negative direction might lead that same individual, under different environmental conditions, into gang fighting and crime in the streets.

Peers, teachers, relatives, ministers, parents, and others make up the environment. Their influence may turn the type T child to healthy, constructive opportunities or unhealthy, destructive ends. Environmental influences, then, may affect health in a roundabout way. Children who respond abnormally to stress, for instance, may be steered toward mechanisms that reduce stress, resulting in a more healthy life-style. Homeostasis is, therefore, broadly affected by the psychological environment.

FIGURE 16-27 Type T Behavior Thrill seeking, or type T behavior, is thought to have a genetic basis.

Summary

Meiosis and Gamete Formation

1. Sexually reproducing organisms halve the number of chromosomes in germ cells through *meiosis,* a type of nuclear division found only in germ-cell production in the gonads of sexually reproducing animals.

2. Meiosis involves two nuclear divisions. During the first division, *meiosis I,* the chromosome number is halved. Thus, a diploid cell produces two haploid cells.

3. The second meiotic division, *meiosis II,* is virtually identical to mitosis, except for the fact that the cells are haploid. When haploid cells divide in meiosis II, they produce two new cells, each containing a haploid number of single-stranded (unreplicated, or one-chromatid) chromosomes.

4. In males, meiosis produces four gametes, but in females it produces only one.

Principles of Heredity: Mendelian Genetics

5. Gregor Mendel, a nineteenth-century monk, derived several important principles of inheritance from his work on garden peas. Mendel determined that, in peas, traits do not blend as was commonly thought at the time. He also postulated that each adult has two hereditary factors for a given trait and that these factors (genes) separate during gamete formation. He called this notion the *principle of segregation.*

6. Mendel also postulated that a hereditary factor might be either dominant or recessive. A *dominant factor* masks a recessive factor. A *recessive factor* is expressed only when the dominant factor is missing. The dominant and recessive genes are alternative forms of the gene, or *alleles.*

7. Three genetic combinations are possible for a given trait: *heterozygous, homozygous dominant,* and *homozygous recessive.*

8. The genetic makeup of an organism is called its *genotype.* The physical appearance, which is determined by the genotype and the environment, is the *phenotype.*

9. From his studies, Mendel concluded that the hereditary factors were separated independently of one another during gamete formation. This is the principle of *independent assortment* and holds true only for nonlinked genes.

Mendelian Genetics in Humans

10. Human cells contain 23 pairs of chromosomes: 22 pairs of *autosomes* and 1 pair of *sex chromosomes.* Chromosomes carry dominant and recessive traits, and inheritance of these traits is consistent with Mendel's principles of inheritance, although additional mechanisms are at work in humans and other organisms.

11. Sickle-cell anemia, cystic fibrosis, and albinism are *autosomal-recessive traits* and are expressed only in homozygous-recessive individuals.

12. Widow's peak, achondroplasia, and Marfan's syndrome are *autosomal-dominant traits* and are expressed in heterozygous and homozygous-dominant genotypes.

Variations in Mendelian Genetics

13. Genetic research since Mendel's time has turned up several additional modes of inheritance. One mode is *incomplete dominance.* It occurs when an allele exerts only partial dominance, producing intermediate phenotypes.

14. Some genes have more than two possible alleles. *Multiple alleles* result in more genotypes and phenotypes in a population. Because chromosomes exist in pairs, individuals can have only two of the possible alleles.

15. *Codominance* occurs in multiple-allele genes. Codominant genes are expressed fully and equally.

16. Some traits are controlled by many genes. This phenomenon is referred to as *polygenic inheritance.*

17. Genes that are found on the same chromosome are said to be *linked.* If crossing-over does not occur, these genes are inherited together.

Sex-Linked Genes

18. The X and Y chromosomes are commonly referred to as the sex chromosomes. However, studies suggest that the real determinant of sex is the Y chromosome. If it is absent, the individual (XX) is a female. If it is present, the individual (XY) is a male.

19. The sex chromosomes also carry genes that determine physical traits. A trait determined by a gene on a sex chromosome is a *sex-linked trait.* Most sex-linked traits occur on the X chromosome. Both dominant and recessive sex-linked traits can be present.

Chromosomal Abnormalities and Genetic Counseling

20. Abnormalities in the human genome arise from mutations (changes in DNA structure), abnormalities in chromosome number (aneuploidy and polyploidy), and alterations in chromosome structure (deletions and translocations).

21. Alterations in the number of chromosomes result chiefly from errors in gamete formation when chromosomes fail to separate during meiosis. This process is called *nondisjunction.*

22. Variations in chromosome structure result from two occurrences: *deletions,* or the loss of a piece of chromosome, and *translocations,* or breakage followed by reattachment elsewhere.

23. Embryos with abnormal chromosome numbers or abnormal chromosome structure are likely to die and be aborted spontaneously.

Health, Homeostasis, and the Environment: Nature Versus Nurture

24. At one time, psychologists thought that a child's personality developed principally through interaction with the environment—parents, friends, and teachers. New research suggests, however, that our personalities are also influenced by our genes.

Critical Thinking

Thinking Critically— Analysis

This Analysis corresponds to the Thinking Critically scenario that was presented at the beginning of this chapter.

To begin, reread the previous material in this exercise and make a list of the symptoms characteristic of Marfan's syndrome.

They are aortic weakening, abnormally long legs and arms, excellence on the basketball and volleyball court, and nearsightedness.

Although you won't be able to find any information about aortic weakening, you could possibly find information on Lincoln's health—perhaps old medical files. In fact, Lincoln's medical records are available, and they show that the former president displayed no signs of cardiovascular disease. That doesn't really prove anything, by itself.

As for the president's skill on the basketball court or volleyball court . . . we'll never know. The sports hadn't even been invented yet. But, more seriously, it just so happens that Lincoln's lanky limbs were within the normal dimensions of tall people. As for the president's eyesight, it turns out that Lincoln was farsighted, not nearsighted.

This evidence strongly suggests that Abe Lincoln did not have this genetic disorder. This exercise illustrates the importance of a close examination of the facts.

Exercising Your Critical Thinking Skills

The sex of a child is determined by the presence or absence of the Y chromosome. As you learned in this chapter, the sex chromosomes in males are XY; in females, they are XX. Thus, the presence of a Y chromosome yields a male; its absence produces a female.

Since 1959, geneticists have been searching for the specific gene on the Y chromosome responsible for male characteristics. In 1983, a group of scientists was studying a rare condition—males with XX chromosomes. This anomaly occurs in approximately 1 of every 20,000 males. When they examined the X chromosomes of these males, the researchers discovered that the X chromosomes (presumably from the father) carried a small fragment from a Y chromosome. Maleness, they concluded, comes from the presence of a gene on that segment exchanged with the X chromosome.

The magazine article in which I read this report noted that the researchers had studied several dozen XX males with these fragments. After examining the fragments, they isolated a specific gene and identified it as the possible sex determiner. This astounding finding was reported with much fanfare by the news media in 1987.

When I went to the original research publication, however, I found that the researchers had not reported how many XX males in their study had the fragment from the Y chromosome. Was it all XX males or just a few? (The editors should have insisted on full disclosure.) Given the conclusions of the study and my faith in scientific publications, I surmised (uneasily) that all of the XX males studied had the Y fragment—that is, that this phenomenon occurred in 100% of the XX males.

A few years later, though, a second report hit the press. In this study, researchers found that three XX males in their study group did not have the much-heralded gene, suggesting that in the earlier research the same phenomenon might have occurred.

The second study clearly illustrates the importance of good follow-up research, which allows scientists to check the results of earlier work and find weaknesses. As pointed out in the Thinking Critically section in Chapter 1, follow-up research is essential to good science! Critical thinkers must demand it.

Continuing the saga, a more recent study uncovered another gene that researchers think may be the sex determiner. Their studies suggest that this gene may be something of a master gene—that is, it may control other genes involved in sexual development. The sex-determining gene controls sexual development by inducing testicular development. Subsequent male sexual differentiation is a consequence of testosterone, a hormonal product of the testis. Interestingly, the sex-determining gene appears to work just prior to the development of male sex organs in the embryo.

If this gene is indeed responsible for sex determination, it would be expected to be found in all mammals. Research shows that an almost identical gene is present in many mammals, including mice, rabbits, chimpanzees, horses, and tigers.

The research team that discovered the "master gene" is hesitant to announce that it has found the sex determiner gene even with all this evidence. Because any announcement would be met with at least some skepticism, the evidence must be concrete before definite conclusions can be made. In other words, more studies are needed.

Using your knowledge of genetics, can you think of any way to test whether this gene is the sex determiner? Pause for a few minutes and jot down your ideas.

Here's what the research team is doing: They are using a procedure that allows them to insert the gene into mouse embryos with two X chromosomes. These embryos would normally develop into females. If the gene is the sex determiner, the researchers assert, the embryos should develop into males.

Test of Concepts

1. Explain the process of meiosis in general terms. Where does it occur? What does it accomplish?

2. Draw a diagram showing the various stages of meiosis I and meiosis II. Make a note of the number of chromosomes at each stage and their condition—that is, whether they have one chromatid or two. Which division is the reduction division?

3. How is mitosis different from meiosis? How is it similar?

4. Mendel's research was designed to answer two basic questions. What were the questions and what were his findings?

5. Define the following terms: principle of segregation, principle of independent assortment, allele, phenotype, genotype, heterozygous, homozygous, monohybrid cross, and dihybrid cross.

6. Freckles are an autosomal-dominant trait. A woman with freckles (*Ff*) marries and has a baby by a man without freckles (*ff*). What are the chances that their children will have freckles?

7. Two freckled adults marry and have children. The first baby has no freckles. What are the genotypes of the parents?

8. Attached earlobes (*A*) are an autosomal-dominant trait. The *A* allele is dominant over the *a* allele, which produces unattached earlobes in homozygous-recessive individuals. A woman with freckles and attached earlobes (*FfAa*) marries a man who has freckles and attached earlobes (*FfAa*). Draw a Punnett square showing the various gametes as well as the genotypes of the offspring. List all possible phenotypes and the genotypes that correspond to them.

9. An albino guinea pig with the genotype *ccBB* is mated to a brown guinea pig with the genotype *CCbb*. Using a Punnett square, determine the genotype and phenotype of the F₁ generation.

10. What is sickle-cell anemia? What causes it? Why can a person be a carrier of the disease but not display outward symptoms?

11. How do incomplete dominance and codominance differ? Give examples of each.

12. Assuming that two genes (A and B) control height, list all of the possible genotypes, and indicate the phenotype associated with each.

13. Describe how crossing-over works. What impact does it have on the genotype of a person's gametes?

14. Color blindness is a recessive, X-linked gene. A color-blind man and his wife have four children, two boys and two girls. One boy and one girl are color-blind, and the other two are normal. What is the genotype of the woman?

15. What is a sex-influenced gene? Give some examples. What criteria would you use to assess whether a trait was sex-influenced?

16. Explain how each of the following genetic defects could arise: trisomy 18, monosomy 10, triploidy, and tetraploidy.

www.jbpub.com/humanbiology

Connect to this book's web site: www.jbpub.com/humanbiology
The site features eLearning, an online review area that provides quizzes, chapter outlines, and other tools to help you study for your class. You can also follow useful links for in-depth information, research the differing views in the Point/Counterpoints, or keep up on the latest environmental and health news.

CHAPTER 17

Molecular Genetics

HOW GENES WORK AND HOW GENES ARE CONTROLLED

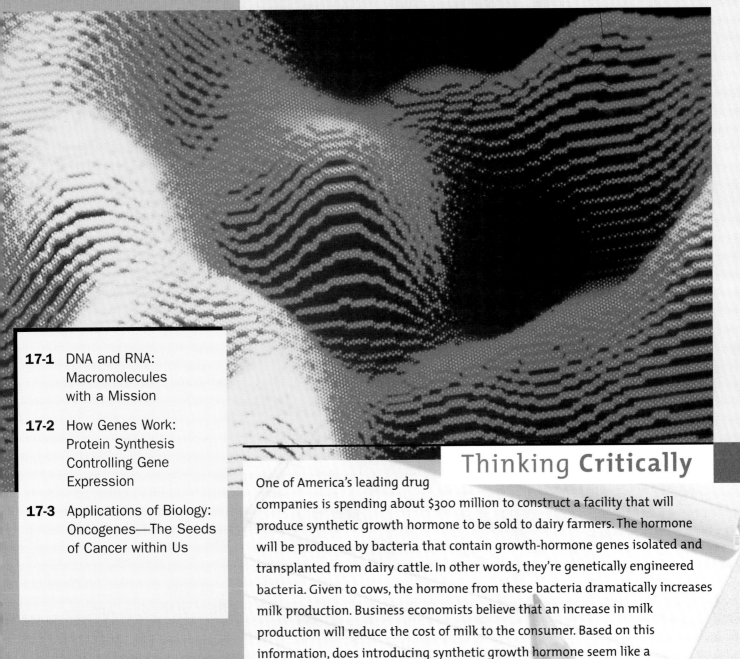

Thinking **Critically**

One of America's leading drug companies is spending about $300 million to construct a facility that will produce synthetic growth hormone to be sold to dairy farmers. The hormone will be produced by bacteria that contain growth-hormone genes isolated and transplanted from dairy cattle. In other words, they're genetically engineered bacteria. Given to cows, the hormone from these bacteria dramatically increases milk production. Business economists believe that an increase in milk production will reduce the cost of milk to the consumer. Based on this information, does introducing synthetic growth hormone seem like a good idea? ■

Tunneling electron micrograph of DNA.

In 1988, a U.S. military court sentenced a serviceman in Korea to 45 years in prison for rape and attempted murder. Ten days later, a Florida court convicted a man on two counts of first-degree murder. What makes these two convictions important is that prosecutors relied heavily on the results of a new technique known as "DNA fingerprinting."

In this procedure, which today is being used with more and more frequency, criminologists analyze the composition of the genetic material DNA in samples of hair, semen, or blood found at the scene of the crime. Then they compare the DNA in these samples with the DNA of the accused. If it matches, prosecutors can make a strong case for guilt. In fact, without this procedure, prosecutors believe, the two convictions cited above would not have been won.

Many people believe that DNA fingerprinting is revolutionizing criminal investigations. King County, Washington, in fact, has already begun taking DNA samples from all convicted sex offenders. Like fingerprints, the results of DNA analysis will be kept on file, readily available for future cases. The FBI is also using this technique in its work.

DNA fingerprinting holds great promise, say supporters, because there is only 1 chance of a mistaken identity in 4 or 5 trillion. In contrast, the best conventional methods, such as blood typing and blood-enzyme analysis, run the risk of error in about 1 in every 1000 cases.

Although DNA fingerprinting sounds promising, not all geneticists believe that it is as reliable as many think. In December 1991, in fact, two prom-inent geneticists published an article in the prestigious journal *Science* in which they assert that the probabilities (noted above) are based on improper assumptions (violating one of the critical thinking rules) and comparatively little scientific data on the genetic composition of populations.

DNA fingerprinting is one of many offshoots of research in genetics. This chapter covers some of the basic research that led to the discovery of this technique. You will learn about the structure of DNA and RNA, how genes work, and how genes are controlled in body cells.

Section 17-1

DNA and RNA: Macromolecules with a Mission

In 1953, James Watson, an American biologist, and Francis Crick, a British biologist, proposed a model for the structure of the DNA molecule. This model was based on research by Rosalind Franklin, Maurice Wilkins, and many other scientists, as outlined in Scientific Discoveries 15-1.

In 1962, Watson, Crick, and Wilkins, a British biophysicist, received the Nobel Prize in Physiology and Medicine for their model, a discovery that opened the doors to a new and infinitely fascinating field of study known as molecular genetics. **Molecular genetics** is the study of the structure and function of RNA and DNA at the molecular level. It brings us as close as we can get to the roots of inheritance. We turn first to the structure and the synthesis of DNA.

DNA Is the Molecular Basis of the Gene and Consists of a Double Helix Held Together by Hydrogen Bonds

DNA consists of two strands that intertwine to form a double helix, a structure that resembles a spiral staircase (**FIGURE 17-1**). Each strand of the double helix contains millions of smaller molecules, or nucleotides.

FIGURE 17-1 DNA DNA consists of two intertwined polynucleotide chains that form a double helix. Sugars and phosphates form the backbone of each chain, with the bases projecting inward. The bases on opposite strands are connected by hydrogen bonds.

DNA double helix

Phosphate
Sugar
Backbone

Base

Hydrogen bond

One nucleotide

Like several other important biological molecules, then, DNA is a polymer.

Each nucleotide consists of three smaller molecules: a nitrogenous base, a phosphate group, and a monosaccharide, deoxyribose (**FIGURE 17-2**). The nucleotides join by covalent bonds to form polynucleotide chains. As shown in **FIGURE 17-1**, nucleotides unite by covalent bonds between the sugar molecules and phosphates.

The two polynucleotide chains of DNA are held together by hydrogen bonds that form between the bases. As shown in **FIGURE 17-1**, the bases of the nucleotides of each chain project inward and therefore lie inside the helix. Hydrogen bonds between the bases are indicated by the dotted lines in **FIGURE 17-1**. These bonds are much weaker than covalent bonds and can be easily broken so the molecule can unzip for replication.

DNA contains two types of nitrogen-containing bases. They are the purines (PURE-eens) and pyrimidines (pa-RIM-a-DEENS) (**FIGURE 17-2**). The **purines** consist of two fused rings. The **pyrimidines** contain only one ring.

In DNA, you will find two purine bases. They are **adenine** (A) (AD-ah-neen) and **guanine** (G) (GUAN-neen). The pyrimidines in DNA are **cytosine** (C) (sigh-toe-seen) and **thymine** (T) (thigh-mean). My genetics prof came from the agricultural college of my university, and, evidently proud of his roots, gave us the mnemonic "pure AG" to remember these.

Purines on one strand bind (via hydrogen bonds) to pyrimidines on the opposite strand. But the relationship between the two is even more specific. If you look at **FIGURE 17-3B**, you will see that the adenine binds only to the pyrimidine thymine. Guanine binds only to the pyrimidine cytosine. Adenine and thymine are therefore said to be complementary bases, as are guanine and cytosine. As you will soon see, this unalterable coupling, called **complementary base pairing,** ensures the accurate replication of DNA and the reliable transmission of the genetic information from a parent cell to its daughter cells during cell division.

DNA Replication Takes Place on the Individual Polynucleotide Strands After the Double Helix "Unzips"

As noted in Chapter 3, before a cell can divide, it must first make an exact copy of all of its DNA. DNA replication ensures that a cell about to divide has two identical sets of genetic information, one for each daughter cell.

During the S phase of interphase, cells replicate their DNA by unzipping each DNA double helix along the hydrogen bonds that unite the complementary bases. Each polynucleotide strand then serves as a template (described

FIGURE 17-2 Nucleotides Containing Purine and Pyrimidine Bases All nucleotides consist of three subunits: a phosphate group; an organic, nitrogen-containing base; and a five-carbon sugar. DNA nucleotides contain the sugar deoxyribose. Two types of bases are found: purines and pyrimidines. *(a)* The purines are adenine and guanine. *(b)* The pyrimidines are cytosine and thymine.

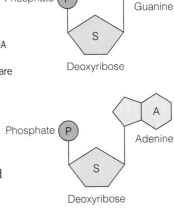

(a) DNA nucleotides containing purine bases

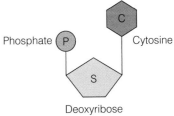

(b) DNA nucleotides containing pyrimidine bases

below) on which a new strand is produced (**FIGURE 17-3A**). The new strand is called a **complementary strand.** The template is called the **original strand.**

DNA replication is referred to as a semiconservative process because each polynucleotide chain of the DNA double helix serves as a template for the production of a new strand of DNA.

DNA replication during the S phase begins when special enzymes start to pull apart, or unzip, the DNA double helix. As the two strands are separated, the bases of the polynucleotide chains are exposed. They are then free to form hydrogen bonds with complementary nucleotides in the nucleoplasm (**FIGURE 17-3**). Because adenine binds only to thymine and guanine binds only to cytosine, the original strands, the templates, are said to direct the synthesis of new strands. Synthesis on the DNA templates occurs one base at a time, and the accuracy of replication is ensured by complementary base pairing.

During replication, incoming nucleotides must first be aligned properly so that the hydrogen bonds can form between complementary bases and so that the phosphate group of the incoming nucleotide can bond to the sugar of the nucleotide already in place, as illustrated in **FIGURE 17-4**. Alignment and attachment are aided by an enzyme known as **DNA polymerase** (PUL-yi-merr-ace) (**FIGURE 17-4**). DNA polymerase slides

P = phosphate

S = sugar

A = adenine

G = guanine

C = cytosine

T = thymine

DNA double helix

Original strands (template)

Replication underway

New strands

Replication completed

Original strands

New strands

(a)

(b)

FIGURE 17-3 DNA Replication DNA replication is semiconservative. *(a)* Each double helix unwinds, and each half of the helix serves as a template for the production of a new strand of DNA. When replication is complete, each new helix contains one old and one new strand. *(b)* Nucleotides attach to the template one at a time and are joined together with the aid of enzymes.

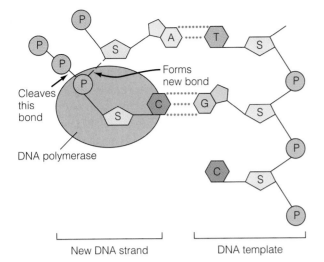

FIGURE 17-4 Role of DNA Polymerase DNA polymerase binds loosely to the DNA template and to the nucleotide, aligning it for insertion. The enzyme catalyzes the formation of the bond between the phosphate of the new nucleotide and the sugar of the one previously inserted. The enzyme also cleaves off two phosphates of each nucleotide.

TABLE 17-1

Role of RNA Molecules

Molecule	Role
Messenger RNA (mRNA)	Carries the genetic information that is needed to make proteins in the cytoplasm from the nucleus
Transfer RNA (tRNA)	Binds to specific amino acids, transports them to the mRNA, and inserts them in the correct location on the mRNA
Ribosomal RNA (rRNA)	Component of the ribosome

FIGURE 17-5 RNA RNA is a single-stranded molecule consisting of many RNA nucleotides. A small section of an RNA molecule is shown here.

along the template, aligning nucleotides one at a time, then linking each new nucleotide to the one already in place. As noted above, the enzyme joins the phosphate group of one nucleotide to the deoxyribose molecule (sugar) of its neighbor.

When DNA synthesis is finished, two new DNA molecules exist, each of which consists of a double helix. Each double helix, in turn, contains one strand from the original molecule and one new polynucleotide chain. The chromosome, once a single molecule of DNA and protein, now consists of two molecules with associated proteins. As noted in Chapter 15, each strand of DNA and associated protein is called a chromatid. The two chromatids of each chromosome are joined at their centromeres after synthesis.

Three Types of RNA Exist, Each of Which Is Involved in Protein Synthesis

DNA contains the genetic information, which determines the structure and controls most of the functions of cells. Like a commander in the army, DNA does not exert its influence directly. Its work is carried out by other molecules, notably RNA. Three types of RNA are involved in this process: ribosomal RNA (rRNA), messenger RNA (mRNA), and transfer RNA (tRNA). Each has a unique function in protein synthesis (**TABLE 17-1**). Despite major functional differences in these molecules, all three RNA molecules are biochemically similar. In humans, for example, all RNAs are single-stranded molecules, and all are polynucleotides (**FIGURE 17-5**). RNA nucleotides consist of three molecules: a sugar, a nitrogenous base, and a phosphate group. Unlike the DNA nucleotides, however, the RNA nucleotides contain the sugar ribose instead of deoxyribose and the pyrimidine

uracil instead of thymine. **TABLE 17-2** summarizes the key differences between RNA and DNA.

RNA Synthesis Is Called Transcription and Takes Place on a DNA Template in the Nucleus of the Cell

Unlike DNA, which is self-replicating, all three types of RNA must be synthesized on DNA templates. The synthesis of RNA on a DNA template permits the genetic information coded in the DNA to be transferred from the DNA molecule to RNA. As you will soon see, the genetic code in DNA is transferred to only one of the three types of RNA, and that's messenger RNA. Messenger RNA is free to leave the nucleus but DNA is

TABLE 17-2

Differences Between RNA and DNA in Prokaryotic and Eukaryotic Cells

DNA	RNA
Double-stranded	Single-stranded
Contains the sugar deoxyribose	Contains the sugar ribose
Contains adenine, guanine, cytosine, and thymine	Contains adenine, guanine, cytosine, and uracil
Functions primarily in the nucleus	Functions primarily in the cytoplasm

FIGURE 17-6 RNA Synthesis on DNA Template. RNA is synthesized on a DNA template. As shown, the DNA double helix unwinds, but only one strand serves as a template for the production of RNA. Complementary base pairing determines the exact sequence of bases in the RNA molecule.

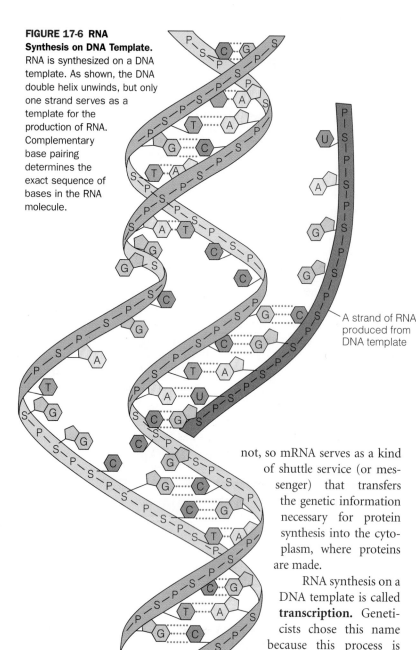

A strand of RNA produced from DNA template

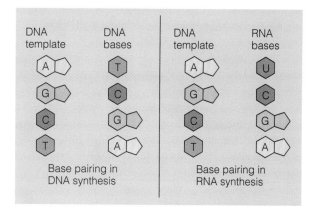

FIGURE 17-7 DNA and RNA Base Pairing The sequence of bases on the DNA template determines the sequence of bases on the complementary strand of DNA and RNA.

not, so mRNA serves as a kind of shuttle service (or messenger) that transfers the genetic information necessary for protein synthesis into the cytoplasm, where proteins are made.

RNA synthesis on a DNA template is called **transcription.** Geneticists chose this name because this process is much like the transcribing process students perform in lecture where they transfer information from one medium (speech) to another (written form). In this case, genetic information housed in the DNA is simply written in another form, RNA.

Transcription occurs during all three phases of interphase of the cell cycle at more or less the same rate. During transcription, small sections of the DNA helix unzip temporarily with the aid of special enzymes. This creates a DNA template on which RNA can be made (**FIGURE 17-6**). But RNA is produced on only one of the DNA strands, and only a small portion (less than 1%) of a cell's DNA is

used to make RNA. (This helps explain why most mutations in the DNA have no effect on cell function.)

During RNA synthesis, an enzyme called **RNA polymerase** helps align the RNA nucleotides on the DNA template in much the same way that DNA polymerase functions during DNA synthesis. RNA polymerase also catalyzes the formation of covalent bonds between ribose and phosphate groups, forming a polynucleotide chain. When the synthesis is complete, the RNA molecule is released from the DNA template, and the two strands of the DNA molecule reunite, reforming the double helix. RNA is then free to leave the nucleus.

During the synthesis of RNA, base pairing ensures the proper sequence of nucleotides on the RNA strand. **FIGURE 17-7** shows which bases pair up during RNA synthesis. The only difference between RNA and DNA synthesis is that adenine on the DNA template pairs with uracil.

Section 17-2

How Genes Work: Protein Synthesis

The information required to synthesize protein is transported out of the nucleus on one type of RNA, known as messenger RNA (mRNA). In the cytoplasm, mRNA serves as a template for protein synthesis, which may occur either on the endoplasmic reticulum or free within the cytoplasm, as noted in Chapter 3. The synthesis of protein on an mRNA template is called **translation** (**FIGURE 17-8**). In effect, the RNA message (the genetic code) is translated into a new "molecular language"—that of the protein.

Protein synthesis requires two additional "players," transfer RNA (tRNA) and ribosomes. **Transfer RNA** molecules are relatively small strands of RNA that bind

FIGURE 17-8 The Central Tenet of Molecular Genetics The DNA controls the cell through protein synthesis—that is, the production of enzymes and structural proteins. RNA serves as an intermediary, carrying genetic information to the cytoplasm, where protein is synthesized.

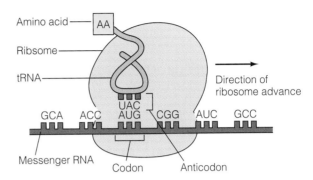

FIGURE 17-9 Messenger RNA The mRNA, either free within the cytoplasm or bound to the endoplasmic reticulum, serves as a template for protein synthesis. The codons, each consisting of three bases on the mRNA, determine the sequence of amino acids by binding to complementary anticodons on the tRNA molecules. Each tRNA, in turn, delivers a specific amino acid to the mRNA template. The ribosome provides binding sites for tRNA–AA molecules, catalyzes the formation of the peptide bonds, and slides down the mRNA template to permit chain elongation.

to specific amino acids in the cytoplasm and transport them to the mRNA, where they are incorporated into the protein that's being constructed on the mRNA molecule (**FIGURE 17-9**). A tRNA molecule bound to an amino acid is generally written like this: tRNA–AA.

Ribosomes, mentioned briefly in Chapter 3, are small granular structures found in the cytoplasm of cells. These structures play an important role in the production of protein, as you shall soon see. They are composed of **ribosomal RNA (rRNA)** and protein. Ribosomes consist of two subunits, a small one and a large one. The subunits are often detached in the cytoplasm, joining for protein synthesis on the mRNA template.

Protein synthesis consists of three stages: (1) chain initiation, (2) chain elongation, (2) and chain termination. During chain initiation, the small subunit of the ribosome attaches to the mRNA at a specific site called the **initiator codon** (COE-dawn). The initiator codon is a sequence of three bases on the mRNA molecule that marks where protein synthesis should begin. After the small subunit attaches, the large subunit of the ribosome links up. As shown in **FIGURE 17-10A**, the ribosome now contains two binding sites for tRNA–AA.

Soon after the ribosome attaches to the mRNA, a tRNA bearing a specific amino acid enters the first binding site. But how does the cell know which amino acid to insert? At the base of all tRNA molecules is a sequence of three bases. Called an **anticodon,** it contains complementary bases that pair with the bases of the initiator codon of the mRNA template.

After the first tRNA–amino acid is in place, a second tRNA–AA enters the scene, inserting itself into the second binding site on the ribosome. The second binding site is located above the next codon, the next three bases on the mRNA template (**TABLE 17-3**, page 401). In the example shown in **FIGURE 17-10**, the codon CGG

binds to the tRNA with the anticodon GCC. This tRNA, in turn, binds to only one amino acid, arginine. The cell therefore ensures the proper sequence of amino acids through two mechanisms: (1) complementary base pairing between codons (mRNA) and anticodons (tRNA), and (2) the specificity (matching) of tRNA molecules for (with) amino acids.[1]

Once the two amino acids are in place, the next step is to link them via a peptide bond. This occurs with the assistance of an enzyme in the ribosome (**FIGURE 17-10C**). After the peptide bond is formed, the first tRNA (minus its amino acid) leaves the binding site. It is then free to retrieve another amino acid for use later on. As illustrated in **FIGURE 17-10C**, the dipeptide formed during the first reaction is now attached to the second tRNA attached at the second binding site.

In order for the chain to grow, the ribosome must move down the mRNA strand. This is accomplished with the aid of a contractile protein in the ribosome. This protein permits the ribosome to slide along mRNA one codon at a time.

As illustrated in **FIGURE 17-10D**, after the first tRNA is released, the ribosome moves down the mRNA, and

---

[1]This process is a little more complicated than presented here, but it has been simplified for ease of comprehension. In reality, there are 64 codons that can be read from the mRNA, but only 40 distinct types of tRNA molecules. The reason is that some tRNA anticodons can pair with two or three different mRNA codons that specify the same amino acid.

FIGURE 17-10 Protein Synthesis

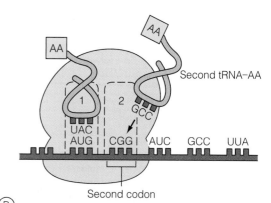

A
The ribosome binds to the mRNA template. The tRNA binds to a specific amino acid in the cytoplasm.

B
The tRNA–amino acid (tRNA-AA) complex binds to the first codon and is held in place by the first binding site. A second tRNA-AA complex binds to the second codon.

C
The ribosome contains an enzyme that catalyzes the formation of a peptide bond between the two amino acids.

D
The dipeptide is then attached to the second tRNA. This frees up the first tRNA, which vacates the first binding site.

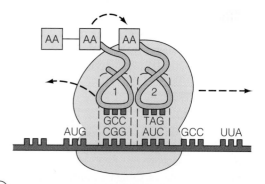

E
The ribosome next slides down the mRNA, transferring the tRNA–dipeptide to the first binding site and opening up the second binding site to a third tRNA–amino acid.

F
The dipeptide is then linked by a peptide bond to the third amino acid, forming a tripeptide. This frees the tRNA in the first binding site. The ribosome next slides down one more codon, exposing the second binding site and freeing it up for the addition of another tRNA-AA. This process repeats itself until the terminator codon is reached.

TABLE 17-3

Codons on mRNA and Their Corresponding Amino Acids

Codon	Amino Acid	Codon	Amino Acid	Codon	Amino Acid	Codon	Amino Acid
AAU AAC	Asparagine	CAU CAC	Histidine	GAU GAC	Aspartic acid	UAU UAC	Tyrosine
AAA AAG	Lysine	CAA CAG	Glutamine	GAA GAG	Glutamic acid	UAA UAG	Terminator codon*
ACU ACC ACA ACG	Threonine	CCU CCC CCA CCG	Proline	GCU GCC GCA GCG	Alanine	UCU UCC UCA UCG	Serine
AGU AGC AGA AGG	Serine Argenine	CGU CGC CGA CGG	Arginine	GGU GGC GGA GGG	Glycine	UGU UGC UGA UGG	Cysteine Terminator codon* Tryptophan
AUU AUC AUA AUG	Isoleucine Methionine	CUU CUC CUA CUG	Leucine	GUU GUC GUA GUG	Valine	UUU UUC UUA UUG	Phenylalanine Leucine

*Terminator codons signal the end of the formation of a polypeptide chain.

the dipeptide is shifted to the first binding site. This frees up the second site, permitting it to accept another tRNA–AA. A new tRNA–AA then enters the vacant site and is joined to the dipeptide, thus forming a tripeptide.

Chain elongation takes place by the addition of one amino acid at a time, but this does not mean that protein synthesis is a slow process. Quite the contrary, protein synthesis occurs with remarkable speed. In bacteria, many proteins containing numerous amino acids are synthesized in 15–30 seconds. In humans, the large alpha and beta chains of the very large hemoglobin molecule are synthesized in 3 minutes.

As the peptide chain is formed, hydrogen bonds between amino acids on different parts of the chain cause it to bend and twist, forming the secondary structure of the protein or peptide, described in Chapter 3 (**FIGURE 17-11**). When the ribosome reaches the terminator codon, the sequence of bases that signals the end of the protein chain, the protein is released. If the protein is produced on mRNA on the surface of the rough endoplasmic reticulum, it is transferred into its interior. The protein may then be chemically modified and packaged into transport vesicles, which pinch off and transport their cargo to the Golgi complex. If protein synthesis

FIGURE 17-11 Protein Synthesis As the protein is synthesized on the mRNA, it begins to coil and bend, forming its secondary structure. Several ribosomes may "work" a single strand of mRNA simultaneously.

Scientific Discoveries that Changed the World 17-1

Unraveling the Mechanism of Gene Control

Featuring the Work of Jacob and Monod

One of the questions that intrigued geneticists for many years—and still does—is how the genetic information contained in a cell's DNA is controlled. Many experiments have been performed over the years in an attempt to answer this question, but

FIGURE 1 Jacob and Monod These two French scientists proposed the operon hypothesis.

none so important as those of two French molecular geneticists, Francois Jacob and Jacques Monod, on the common intestinal bacterium *E. coli* (**FIGURE 1**). Today, much of what is known about gene regulation in bacteria and most of the terms that describe the process come from their studies.

Working at the Pasteur Institute in the late 1950s, Jacob and Monod focused much of their attention on the bacterial uptake and breakdown of lactose, a disaccharide also known as milk sugar. *E. coli* absorb lactose and catabolize it with the aid of an enzyme known as galactosidase (ga-lack-TOSE-uh-DACE). The catabolic breakdown of lactose results in the release of energy and carbon atoms useful in bacterial biosynthesis.

E. coli living in a lactose-free medium, however, contain very little galac-

tosidase. It is only when lactose is added that the enzyme is synthesized.

The introduction of lactose also increases the production of a carrier molecule (galactoside permease) that resides in the plasma membrane and transports lactose into the bacterium. In addition, the presence of lactose increases the intracellular concentration of another enzyme, which may play a role in lactose catabolism, but which is not essential to the process. The carrier protein and two enzymes are part of an inducible enzyme system—that is, their production is induced by the presence of lactose.

Mapping studies have shown that three adjacent genes on the bacterial DNA are responsible for the production of these proteins. These studies led Jacob and Monod to hypothesize that the three genes belong to a sin-

---

occurs on mRNA molecules in the cytoplasm, the protein is released into the cytoplasm.

Protein synthesis is quite involved and perhaps a little confusing at first glance, but once you've mastered it, you'll probably agree: It's one of the most fascinating processes you've ever encountered.

Section 17-3

Controlling Gene Expression

In the previous material, you've seen how RNA and protein are produced. In this section, we look at yet another fascinating bit of molecular wizardry: the mechanism that controls the synthesis of both messenger RNA and their proteins. In other words, we'll be looking at how genes are controlled.

After decades of research, molecular geneticists have a remarkably good understanding of the molecular mechanism responsible for gene regulation, although it is still not completely understood. But why, you ask, is this so important to know?

Besides the fact that it's likely to be covered on your next exam, understanding gene control is important because it could help scientists discover new ways to treat, or even cure, diseases such as cancer that originate in the genes of an organism. As you may recall from the last chapter, scientists are working on ways to control tumor suppressor genes. To begin our study of gene control, we first look to the bacteria. Insight gained here will provide a basis for understanding human gene regulation.

Bacterial Genes Consist of Three Interdependent Segments of DNA: the Regulator Gene, Control Regions, and Structural Genes

As explained in Scientific Discoveries 17-1, two French researchers, Francois Jacob and Jacques Monod, worked out the details of bacterial gene control based on their studies of a common intestinal bacterium with a tongue-twisting name, *Escherichia coli* (ESH-ur-EE-shee-ah KOLL-eye), or *E. coli* for short (**FIGURE 17-12**). *E. coli* inhabits the large intestine of humans and other gle unit, which they called an *operon*. They defined an operon as a cluster of genes with related functions that is regulated in such a way that all the genes in the group are activated and inactivated simultaneously.

In a paper published in 1961, the researchers proposed a mechanism by which these genes might be controlled, creating the model you studied in this chapter. This intriguing model is "one of the truly important conceptual advances in biology," according to University of Wisconsin cell biologist Wayne Becker. The bulk of the evidence in support of the model came from genetic analysis of mutant bacteria.

Extensive studies of the mutants and how they responded to lactose helped Jacob and Monod piece together a picture of gene regulation in *E. coli*. In these studies of the inducible *lac* operon, the researchers found that structural gene mutations resulted in an alteration of one specific protein. If the bacterium had a mutation in the *y* gene, one of the structural genes, the permease molecule would not be produced when the inducer was added to the system. Galactosidase was formed, but very little lactose could enter the cell. If it had a mutation in the *z* gene (another structural gene), galactosidase would not be produced, but permease would be. The bacterial cell could absorb lactose; it just could not do much with it.

In contrast, mutations in the regulatory regions affected all of the structural genes and proteins they produced. A defective operator site, which binds the repressor, for example, resulted in the production of galactosidase and permease whether or not the inducer, lactose, was present. (This response was due to the fact that RNA polymerase was free to move down the *lac* operon.)

Bacteria with a mutation in the regulator gene, the segment that codes for the production of mRNA that gives rise to the repressor protein, also produced galactosidase and permease. They did so because this mutation blocked all repressor protein production, letting RNA polymerase wander freely down the *lac* operon, transcribing the genes.

Data from these and other mutants helped the scientists piece together a model. As a testimony to the thoroughness of their work, the original model has undergone very little change in over 30 years.

FIGURE 17-12 *E. coli* A micrograph of the bacterium *E. coli*, a common inhabitant of the large intestine of mammals.

mammals, where it lives off undigested and unabsorbed food matter—not a glamorous existence for an organism that has contributed so much to science and our well-being.

Jacob and Monod's research led to a detailed understanding of bacterial gene control. One of their chief discoveries was that bacterial genes consist of three parts: structural genes, regulator genes, and control regions. (I use the letters SRC to remember them.)

Structural genes, shown in light blue in **FIGURE 17-13,** code for the production of mRNA, which serves as a template for the synthesis of enzymes and other proteins. Regulator genes are shown in a slightly darker shade of blue. They and the control regions, which are shown in yellow and green, govern the structural genes.

In the model proposed by Jacob and Monod, then, the structural genes do the work—that is, produce the mRNA—and the regulator genes and control regions, as their names imply, control the process. It's a little like a government work crew, with one set of workers and two sets of supervisors.

Jacob and Monod's research led them to hypothesize that the control regions (yellow and green) and structural genes (light blue) responsible for producing the enzymes of a single metabolic pathway are located side by side on the chromosome (**FIGURE 17-13**).

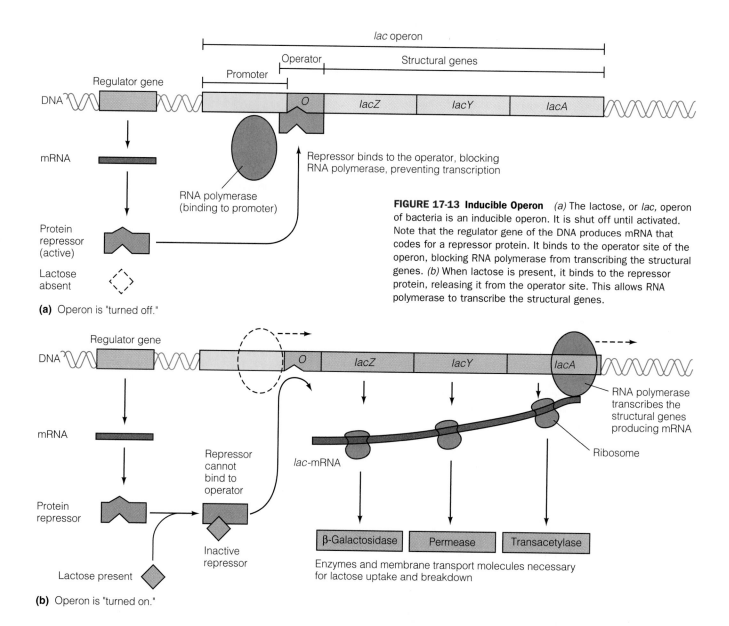

FIGURE 17-13 Inducible Operon *(a)* The lactose, or *lac*, operon of bacteria is an inducible operon. It is shut off until activated. Note that the regulator gene of the DNA produces mRNA that codes for a repressor protein. It binds to the operator site of the operon, blocking RNA polymerase from transcribing the structural genes. *(b)* When lactose is present, it binds to the repressor protein, releasing it from the operator site. This allows RNA polymerase to transcribe the structural genes.

Together, the structural genes and the control regions form a functional unit known as an **operon** (OP-ur-on). The regulator genes are located some distance from the operon. Using our analogy of government workers, the regulator gene is the big boss, who stays in the office downtown. The control region is the job foreman.

Based on the results of many experiments, Jacob and Monod proposed two types of operons: inducible and repressible. Let's look at each one in more detail.

Inducible Operons Are Switched On When Enzymes Are Needed. Most people don't turn on lights

in a room unless they're needed. Many bacterial genes operate by the same efficiency principle. For example, although *E. coli* is capable of producing many enzymes needed to digest leftover foodstuffs in our intestines, the organism only produces these enzymes when they're needed. That is, it produces them on demand. It does so by activating inducible operons. An **inducible operon** is a set of structural genes and accompanying control regions that remains off until activated or induced.

The operon we will examine to understand induction is called the ***lac* operon.** It is responsible for the production of three different proteins associated with the uptake and metabolism of lactose (milk sugar) in *E. coli.*

When lactose is absent, this operon is inactive. (Like a light bulb in a room, it is kept off until needed.) When lactose is present in the digestive system, small quantities diffuse into the bacteria. These molecules activate the *lac* operon. Lactose is therefore said to be an inducer. Inducers activate the operon. It then begins producing mRNA. The mRNA acts as a template for the production of proteins involved in the transport and metabolism of lactose.

Repressible Operons Provide a Steady Supply of Enzymes and Other Proteins and Remain On Until Switched Off. Bacteria require a steady supply of some enzymes to produce molecules, such as amino acids, necessary for cellular metabolism. During evolution, another strategy for controlling genes evolved to meet this demand. It is the **repressible operon.** Unlike the inducible operon, the repressible operon remains active unless turned off.

The repressible operon contains the same components as the inducible operon. But there's a big difference. In repressible operons, end products of chemical reactions build up inside cells, turning off the genes. When they're switched off, the production of mRNA needed to make proteins that catalyze chemical reactions in question is halted.

In Humans, Genetic Expression Is Controlled at Four Levels

Humans are a bit more complicated than your average bacterium and, as you might expect, the control of genes in human cells is also a bit more involved. Although inducible and repressible systems are present in human cells, most human genes are inducible. But several other mechanisms are also present. For simplicity, these can be divided into four major categories: (1) control at the chromosome level, (2) control at transcription, (3) control after transcription before translation, and (4) control at translation (**FIGURE 17-14**).[2]

Control at the Chromosome: Access to the Genes Is Controlled by Coiling and Uncoiling of the Chromosomes During Interphase. Chapter 15, you may recall, noted that chromatin fibers in the nucleus condense and become inactive during prophase of mitosis. In the condensed state, they cannot produce RNA

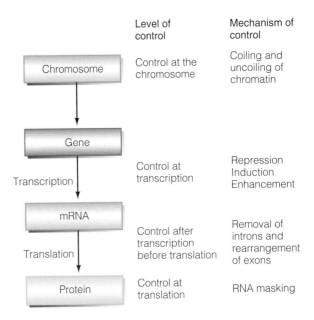

FIGURE 17-14 Gene Expression In humans, gene expression is regulated at four levels.

or new DNA. Condensation essentially shuts down the DNA as the cell prepares for nuclear division.

Cells also selectively inactivate some of their chromatin during interphase. Why? Most cells have far more DNA than they need. Muscle cells, for instance, don't need all of the genes that a liver cell needs, and vice versa. But since it can't discard this unnecessary DNA, it inactivates it.

Inactivated chromatin in the interphase nucleus is tightly coiled, or compacted, and appears as dark clumps called **heterochromatin.** Some heterochromatin remains in this state throughout the cell cycle, except during replication (S phase). The remaining chromatin in the interphase nucleus is diffusely organized—consisting of fine threads unraveled in the nucleus. It is called **euchromatin** ("true chromatin"). Euchromatin is metabolically active.

Chromosomal condensation or coiling provides a crude way of regulating genetic expression. More precise controls occur at other levels.

Three Control Mechanisms Operate at the Level of Transcription: Induction, Repression, and Enhancement. In humans, transcription (RNA production) can be controlled by the induction and repression of operons, similar to that which occurs in bacteria. Human cells also control gene activity via a third mechanism, known as enhancement.

---

[2]Bacteria also control gene expression at these levels.

Enhancement is a process in which already active genes increase their production of mRNA. This occurs as a result of the action of nearby segments of the DNA called **enhancers.** Research suggests that certain protein molecules bind to enhancer regions of the chromosome. These proteins, in turn, increase RNA production by the structural gene. Thus, enhancers do not turn nearby structural genes on and off like inducers or corepressors, they simply amplify their activity. An enhancer is therefore a little like the accelerator in your car—it doesn't turn the engine on, it simply speeds it up.

Genetic Expression Can Be Controlled by Altering the Structure of mRNA.

Genetic studies show that eukaryotic DNA contains two types of genetic material: sections that are used to produce mRNA and sections that are not. As **FIGURE 17-15** shows, the noncoding segments of DNA are called **introns** and are interspersed within the functional segments of DNA (functional genes), the **exons.** The name *intron* signifies that these are *intro*vening segments of noncoding DNA. Exons are *ex*pressed segments—sections of the DNA that can be used to produce the mRNA that is used to make protein.

Both the introns and exons are transcribed during the cell cycle, producing an RNA transcript that is a complete "readout" of the DNA. Eukaryotic cells process the transcript, cutting out the introns, then join the exons together to produce a functional mRNA molecule. Although this seems like a lot of work, it is necessary because in humans and other eukaryotes the structural genes that code for the enzymes of a metabolic pathway are not lined up next to one another as they are in bacteria. In order for a functional mRNA molecule to be synthesized, it must be "cut and pasted" together.

Control at Translation Occurs by Masking mRNA.

Eukaryotic cells can also control gene expression at the level of translation (protein synthesis). Messenger RNA, for example, which is produced in the nucleus, may be transferred to the cytoplasm in an inactive state. The mRNA is said to be **masked.** Masking allows the cell to build up large supplies of mRNA in preparation for a sudden burst of protein synthesis. When the time is right, the mRNA is activated and begins producing large quantities of protein. This phenomenon occurs in the human ovum, the female sex cell produced in the ovaries. The ovum produces an enormous amount of masked mRNA as it awaits fertilization. When the sperm arrives and fertilizes the ovum, the mRNA that has accumulated in the cytoplasm is unmasked, and there is an explosion of protein synthesis necessary for subsequent cell divisions.

In closing, gene expression in humans and other eukaryotes is a complex phenomenon. Like the cell cycle, it is no doubt under the influence of many controlling factors.

FIGURE 17-15 Posttranscriptional Control of Human Genes
One key mechanism of control occurs after transcription. DNA contains noncoded segments (introns) and useful segments (exons). An mRNA transcript is produced from the DNA, and the segments produced by introns are removed. The final product is a strand of mRNA containing only RNA copies of the exons. The exon copies can be linked differently, producing slightly different products.

Applications of Biology: Oncogenes—The Seeds of Cancer Within Us

Chapter 15 introduced you to the disease called cancer. You learned that cancer actually consists of over 100 different diseases such as liver cancer, lung cancer, breast cancer, and prostate cancer. Cancer, you may recall, is caused by numerous biological, chemical, and physical agents in a two-step process. The first stage, brought on by co-carcinogens, results from **mutations,** that is, alterations of parts of the genetic material. The second process, development and progression, is brought about by a promoter.

Broadly defined, mutations include (1) alterations of the DNA, such as the deletion or addition of a purine or

FIGURE 17-16 Hazardous Wastes The careless dumping of hazardous materials in rivers and lakes, in abandoned fields, along highways, and in abandoned warehouses creates a health hazard to humans and many other species and results in costly cleanup efforts. Thankfully, new laws have put tighter controls on hazardous waste disposal, although some industries and waste disposal companies still violate the law.

pyrimidine base; (2) alterations of the chromosome, such as missing segments; and (3) alterations in the chromosome number—that is, too many or too few chromosomes.

Mutations may occur in germ cells, the sperm and ovum, or in body cells. Germ cell mutations may result in genetically defective offspring or cancers in early life. This section concerns itself with mutations in body cells, or somatic cells, that involve changes in the structure of the DNA.

Mutations in the DNA (1) can improve cellular function; (2) may be neutral, having neither a positive nor a negative effect; or (3) may affect vital sections of the genome, killing the cell outright or releasing the cell on the rampage of growth called cancer—but only if the right genes are mutated. It is the mutations that may lead to cancer that will concern us here. In most instances, mutations in the DNA of somatic cells are rapidly repaired by enzymes in the nucleus. This helps ensure cellular homeostasis. Despite the presence of remarkably efficient repair mechanisms, some somatic mutations simply escape repair.

Researchers have made a startling discovery about such mutations that may explain the cause of most cancers. They have found that humans and other organisms contain a group of genes called **proto-oncogenes** (pro-toe-ON-co-JEANS). Proto-oncogenes control functions related to cellular replication, among them cell adhesion and the production of the plasma membrane receptors that bind to growth factors or hormones. When mutations in these genes are not repaired, the result can be uncontrolled cellular proliferation, cancer. (For a discussion of methods used to assess carcinogenicity, see the Point/Counterpoint.)

Certain viruses also cause cancer. Cancer-causing viruses fall into two groups. Some viruses stimulate cancer by activating proto-oncogenes in body cells. Others contain cancer-causing genes themselves, which they insert into the DNA of the nuclei of infected cells. These genes are known as **oncogenes.** After being inserted into a cell's DNA, oncogenes turn on the cell's genes that control division.

The discovery of proto-oncogenes and viral oncogenes has resulted in a quantum leap in our understanding of cancer. Some scientists believe that the key to treating cancer may ultimately lie in finding ways to turn off activated proto-oncogenes or repair tumor suppressor genes. Such changes could halt replication of cancer cells. Who knows, maybe someday you or someone you know will benefit directly from this idea. (For more on cancer treatment, see Health Note 15-2.)

Health, Homeostasis, and the Environment

Hazardous Wastes and Mutations

Thousands of mutations occur in each cell of your body every day, many of which could lead to serious problems, including cancer. As noted earlier, the cells of your body fortunately repair much of the damage. This repair is brought about by special enzymes in the nucleus that "snip off" damaged sections of the DNA, then rebuild the molecule, thus helping to ensure normal cell function.

Remaining healthy, though, requires that we not stretch that resiliency to the breaking point. And yet some individuals fear that modern industrial society may be doing just that. Today, 80,000 chemical substances are in commercial use. The National Academy of Sciences notes that few of these substances have been adequately tested for their ability to cause mutations, cancer, and birth defects.

The extensive use of chemicals and the widespread publicity over the ill effects of some have created a chemical paranoia—sometimes referred to as chemophobia—among some members of our society. New research suggests that while the threat is real, many

Point/Counterpoint

Are Current Procedures for Determining Carcinogens Valid?

Animal Testing for Cancer Is Flawed

Philip H. Abelson

Philip Abelson was the Deputy Editor of Science. *This essay is excerpted from "Testing for Carcinogens with Rodents,"* Science 249: September 21, 1990. Copyright © 1990 by the American Association for the Advancement of Science.

The principal method of determining potential carcinogenicity of substances is based on studies where huge doses of chemicals are administered daily to inbred rodents for their lifetime. Then by questionable models, which include large safety factors, the results are used to extrapolate the effects of minuscule doses in humans. Resultant stringent regulations and attendant frightening publicity have led to public anxiety and chemophobia. If current ill-based regulatory levels continue to be imposed, the cost of cleaning up phantom hazards will be in the hundreds of billions of dollars with minimal benefit to human health. In the meantime, real hazards are not receiving adequate attention.

The current procedures for gauging carcinogenicity are coming under increasing scrutiny and criticism. A leader in the examination is Bruce Ames, who with others has amassed an impressive body of evidence and arguments. Ames and Gold summarized some of their recent data and conclusions in *Science* (31 August 1990, p. 970). Three articles in the *Proceedings of the National Academy of Sciences* provide an elaboration of the information with extensive bibliographies. The articles also provide data about other pathologic effects of natural chemicals.

A limited number of chemicals tested, both natural and synthetic, react with DNA to cause mutations. Most chemicals are not mutagens, but when the maximum tolerated dose (MTD) is administered daily to rodents over their lifetime, about half of the chemicals give rise to excess cancer, usually late in the normal life span of the animals. Experiments in which synthetic industrial chemicals were administered in the MTD to both rats and mice resulted in 212 of 350 chemicals being labeled as carcinogens. Similar experiments with chemicals naturally present in food resulted in 27 of 52 tested being designated as carcinogens. These 27 rodent carcinogens have been found in 57 different foods, including apples, bananas, carrots, celery, coffee, lettuce, orange juice, peas, potatoes, and tomatoes. They are commonly present in quantities thousands of times as great as the synthetic pesticides.

The plant chemicals that have been tested represent only a tiny fraction of the natural pesticides. As a defense against predators and parasites, plants have evolved a large number of chemicals that have pathologic effects on their attackers and consumers. Ames and Gold estimate that plant foods contain 5,000–10,000 natural pesticides and breakdown products. In cabbage alone, some 49 natural pesticides have been found. The typical plant contains a total of a percent or more of such substances. Compared with the amount of synthetic pesticides we consume, we eat about 10,000 times more of the plant pesticides.

It has long been known that virtually all chemicals are toxic if ingested in sufficiently high doses. Common table salt can cause stomach cancer. Ames and others have pointed out that high levels of chemicals cause large-scale cell death and replacement by division. Dividing cells are much more subject to mutations than quiescent cells. Much of the activity of cells involves oxidation, including formation of highly reactive free radicals that can react with and damage DNA. Repair mechanisms exist, but they are not perfect. Ames has stated that oxidative DNA damage is a major contributor to aging and to cancer. He points out that any agent causing chronic cell division can be indirectly mutagenic because it increases the probability of DNA damage being converted to mutations. If chemicals are administered at doses substantially lower than MTD, they are not likely to cause elevated rates of cell death and cell division and hence would not increase mutations. Thus, a chemical that produces cell death and cancer at the MTD could be harmless at lower dose levels.

Diets rich in fruits and vegetables tend to reduce human cancer. The rodent MTD test that labels plant chemicals as cancer-causing in humans is misleading. The test is likewise of limited value for synthetic chemicals. The standard carcinogen tests that use rodents are an obsolescent relic of the ignorance of past decades. At that time, extreme caution made sense. But now tremendous improvements of analytical and other procedures make possible a new toxicology and far more realistic evaluation of the dose levels at which pathological effects occur.

Current Methods of Testing Cancer Are Valid

Devra Davis

The vast majority of the scientific community endorses the conduct of experimental studies in order to try to identify those materials that could cause disease and prevent harmful exposures. In the typical toxicologic study of 50 rodents, each animal is a stand-in for 50,000 people. Because rodents live about 2 years on average, they are usually exposed to amounts of the suspect agent that approximate what a human would encounter in an average lifetime of 70 years.

Some have argued that the use of the maximum tolerated dose (MTD) in these studies produces tissue damage and cell proliferation, which, in turn, lead to cancer. This is biological nonsense that ignores a fundamental characteristic of cancer biology that has been known for more than 50 years: cancer is a multi-stage disease, with multiple causes, which arises by a stepwise evolution that involves progressive genetic changes, cell proliferation, and clonal expansion. Thus, swamping of tissues with high doses alone may well kill an animal or damage its tissues, but high doses alone are not sufficient to cause cancer. A 2-year study at the National Institute of Environmental Health Sciences (NIEHS) by David Hoel and colleagues provides good evidence on this point. They looked for signs of damage in tissues taken from rats and mice used in cancer studies. Cancers occurred in organs that did not show apparent damage, and some damaged organs were completely free of tumors.

In addition, most compounds tested do not cause cancer only in the highest dose group tested but typically produce a dose-response relationship, where the amount of cancer developed is proportional to the dose administered. Some chemicals cause toxicity only, others cause only cancer. Not all of those that cause cancer do so through organ toxicity. In fact, almost 90% of the substances shown to cause cancer in the National Toxicology Program do so without producing any increased cellular toxicity, and they also cause cancer at both lower and higher doses.

Animal studies are evolving and being further refined, as is our understanding of differences between species that need to be taken into account in conducting these studies. Every compound known to cause cancer in humans also produces cancer in animals, when adequately tested. For 8 of the 54 known human cancer-causing agents, evidence of carcinogenicity was first obtained in laboratory animals; in many cases, the same target organs and doses have been involved in producing cancer in both animals and humans.

The NIEHS has carried out nearly 400 long-term rodent studies, which have been published following peer review by specialists in the field. Chemicals nominated for testing usually represent a sample of potentially "problematic" materials. About 40% of the "suspect" pesticides evaluated to date have been found to cause cancer. As to the role of so-called natural pesticides, rodent diets are also loaded with many of these materials. Nevertheless, a number of test compounds added to these diets markedly increase the amount of tumors produced. Thus, animals are more sensitive to certain synthetic compounds than to the background level of natural materials. Humans are also likely to have acquired some resistance to these natural materials through evolution.

To date, only about 20% of all synthetic organic chemicals have been adequately tested for their potential human toxicity. Those who must set public policy on the use of chemicals need a rational basis on which to stake their actions. Continued advances in animal testing provide an important contribution to environmental health sciences and to public health efforts to predict, and then prevent, the development of environmentally caused disease.

In summary, the current system should be used until it can be replaced by a demonstrably better one. There is no scientific basis for rejecting the MTD as capable of inducing cancer.

Devra Davis *is a senior adviser in the office of the Assistant Secretary for Health, Department of Health and Human Services.*

Sharpening Your Critical Thinking Skills

1. Summarize each author's main points and supporting data. Do you see any inconsistencies or examples of faulty logic in either essay? If so, where?

2. Why is it that two scientists can disagree on an issue such as this?

3. Given the disagreement, what course of action would you recommend?

Visit *Human Biology's* Internet site for links to web sites offering more information on this topic.

people are overreacting to it. In fact, numerous studies suggest that naturally occurring chemicals in our food, like one type of mold that grows on peanut butter, probably cause more cancer than pesticide residues. (For a debate over chemical contamination and the relative importance of pesticides and other industrial chemicals on human health, see the Point/Counterpoint in Chapter 18.)

Some critics argue, however, that the debate over human health is misleading, for it ignores the potentially widespread effects of toxic chemicals on plants, animals, and microorganisms that share this planet with us. Nowhere has the impact on humans and other organisms been more noticeable than around toxic waste dumps, where for decades companies have disposed of highly dangerous substances, often in cardboard containers or steel barrels that rust within a few years of burial (**FIGURE 17-16**, page 407).

Love Canal in the city of Niagara Falls, New York, was the scene of one of the nation's worst toxic nightmares. In an abandoned canal, Hooker Chemical Company dumped over 20,000 metric tons of highly toxic and carcinogenic wastes from 1947 to 1952.[3] In 1952, the city of Niagara Falls began condemnation proceedings on the site. But their intention was not to shut down the operation. It was a legal maneuver to seize the land to permit the construction of a school and housing. Under pressure from the city, Hooker sold the land to the city for $1 in exchange for a release from future liability.

A few years later, bulldozer operators preparing the site for construction of the school removed the protective clay lid that Hooker had placed over the site, but they didn't remove the hazardous wastes. In the late 1950s, after the construction was complete, rusty barrels began to work their way to the surface. Toxic chemicals oozed out of the site, killing trees and gardens and causing chemical burns in children. Some children even died.

The problem came to a head in the 1970s. After a period of heavy rainfall, toxic wastes began to leak into basements of local residents, and the chemical stench became unbearable. Over 80 different chemical substances turned up in studies of water, air, and soil. Many of the chemicals were known or suspected carcinogens. A New York State Health Department study showed that one of every three pregnant women who lived in the area had miscarried. The miscarriages could have been caused by chemically induced mutations in the early embryos or in the germ cells of the parents. Birth defects

were present in one of every five children, far in excess of the expected rate. Birth defects may have resulted from chemically induced mutations.

The chemical substances emitted from the old dump site irritated lungs, gave residents headaches, and resulted in convulsions in some people. Genetic studies showed mutations in the chromosomes of residents.

Nearly 1000 families were evacuated from the vicinity over the years. The homes nearest the contaminated canal were demolished or moved. Much of the contaminated dirt has been stripped off by bulldozers, then incinerated. A clay cap has been placed over the contaminated site. Wastes that escape from the contaminated canal via water are collected along the periphery and treated. Homes outside the contaminated site have been deemed habitable and sold. The area is now resettled, a fact that worries many individuals.

Cleaning up past mistakes like Love Canal has proved costly. Approximately $270 million has been spent so far to clean up the Love Canal area. What is even more startling, though, is that some experts estimate that there are nearly 10,000 hazardous waste sites, some worse than Love Canal, in the United States in need of cleanup. Government estimates put the cost of cleaning up the mess at $100 billion. Critics believe that the actual cost will be far greater. Adding to the problem however, are the more than 200 million metric tons of hazardous materials that American industry generates annually—nearly a ton of hazardous waste for every man, woman, and child each year! While much of it is now recycled and reused, significant amounts of hazardous waste are still being released into the environment.

Improper hazardous waste disposal now pollutes groundwater in many areas. That concerns public health officials because half the people in the United States get their drinking water from wells. By one estimate, more than 10 million Americans drink tap water contaminated with pollutants in excess of EPA standards. Because of years of careless waste disposal, groundwater contamination is expected to grow worse. Even if we stop polluting now, the problem will linger for many years.

A healthy population requires clean water. But how do we get it? Many changes are needed. Especially important are ways to reduce hazardous waste production. By redesigning chemical processes, for example, manufacturers can make significant reductions in their waste output. They can also reuse and recycle hazardous wastes. A waste product from one process may actually become the raw material for another process. These steps are preventive and can help avoid the problems of disposal altogether.

---

[3]A metric ton is 2240 pounds.

FIGURE 17-17 A Theromax solar water heater Solar energy is one way people can help ensure a healthy planet.

Individuals can also help reduce hazardous waste by reducing unnecessary consumption. Because hazardous waste is produced by many manunfacturing processes, the less you consume, the less waste will be produced. Individuals can also help by using nontoxic alternatives to common products. Environmentally safe cleaning agents, for example, help reduce pollution. Environmentally friendly insecticides can be used in gardens. Using energy and other resources more frugally and recycling household waste, including paper, aluminum, glass, and plastics can also make substantial inroads into hazardous waste production.

Truly, individual actions can have a profound effect on the production of toxic waste and the health of the environment and us. The health of the planet and the health of people depend on it (**FIGURE 17-17**).

Summary

DNA and RNA: Macromolecules with a Mission

1. *DNA* houses the genetic information. DNA is a molecule that consists of two polynucleotide strands joined by hydrogen bonds between purine and pyrimidine bases on the opposite strands. The strands produce a *double helix.*

2. Each nucleotide in the DNA molecule consists of a purine or pyrimidine base, the sugar deoxyribose, and a phosphate group. The nucleotides are joined by covalent bonds between phosphate groups and deoxyribose molecules.

3. *Complementary base pairing* is an unalterable coupling in which adenine on one strand of the DNA molecule always binds to thymine on the other and guanine always binds to cytosine.

4. Complementary base pairing ensures accurate replication of the DNA and accurate transmission of genetic information from one cell to another and from one generation to another.

5. To replicate, DNA must first unwind with the aid of a special enzyme. After unwinding, the strands provide templates for the production of complementary DNA strands, a process aided by the enzyme *DNA polymerase.*

6. The cell contains three types of *RNA:* transfer RNA, ribosomal RNA, and messenger RNA. All play a role in the synthesis of protein in the cytoplasm.

7. All three RNA molecules are single-stranded polynucleotide chains. RNA nucleotides contain the sugar ribose instead of deoxyribose, which is found in DNA. RNA nucleotides contain four bases: adenine, guanine, cytosine, and uracil (instead of thymine).

8. RNA is synthesized in the nucleus on a template of DNA. The synthesis of RNA is called *transcription.*

How Genes Work: Protein Synthesis

9. The genetic information contained in the DNA molecule is transferred to *messenger RNA*. Messenger RNA molecules carry this information to the cytoplasm, where proteins are synthesized.

10. Messenger RNA serves as a template for protein synthesis. Ribosomes are required to produce proteins on the mRNA template.

11. *Transfer RNA* molecules deliver amino acid molecules to the mRNA and insert them in the growing chain. Each tRNA binds to a specific amino acid and delivers it to a specific *codon,* a sequence of three bases on the mRNA. Thus, the sequence of codons determines the sequence of amino acids in the protein.

12. Proteins are synthesized by adding one amino acid at a time.

13. During protein synthesis, the ribosome first attaches to the mRNA at the *initia-tor codon.* Soon after, the large subunit attaches. A specific tRNA bound to an amino acid binds to the initiator codon and the first binding site of the ribosome. A second tRNA–amino acid then enters the second site.

14. An enzyme in the ribosome catalyzes the formation of a peptide bond between the two amino acids. After the bond is formed, the first tRNA (minus its amino acid) leaves the first binding site.

15. The ribosome moves down the mRNA, shifting the tRNA bound to its two amino acids to the first binding site and opening the second site for another tRNA–amino acid. This process repeats itself many times in rapid succession.

16. As the peptide chain is formed, hydrogen bonds begin to form between the amino acids, and the chain begins to bend and twist, forming the secondary structure of the protein or peptide. When the ribosome reaches the terminator codon, the peptide chain is released.

Controlling Gene Expression

17. Bacterial DNA contains functional units called *operons,* which consist of three parts: structural genes, regulator genes, and control regions. *Structural genes* code for the production of enzymes and other proteins and are controlled by the *regulator genes* and the *control regions.*

18. Two types of operons are present: inducible and repressible.

19. *Inducible operons* are switched off until needed. In an inducible operon, the regulator gene produces a *repressor protein.* The repressor protein binds to the *operator site* next to the structural genes and prevents the transcription of the structural genes by blocking RNA polymerase. When an inducer substance is present, it binds to the repressor, causing it to release from the operator site and permitting the transcription of the DNA.

20. *Repressible operons* are generally continuously activated but can be switched off by the presence of a chemical substance, usually an end product of a metabolic pathway.

21. Gene control in humans occurs at four levels: at the chromosome, at transcription, after transcription but before translation, and at translation.

22. At the chromosome: Condensation, or coiling, of the chromatin fibers inactivates genes. How the cell condenses a segment of the chromatin is not clearly understood.

23. At transcription: Research shows that inducible and repressible systems are present in human cells. Research also shows that certain segments of the DNA, called *enhancers,* can greatly increase the activity of nearby genes. Geneticists think that protein molecules bind to enhancer regions of the chromosome and increase gene activity.

24. After the production of RNA before translation: Human DNA contains far more genetic material than it needs. Those segments of the DNA used to produce the RNA that will be used to make protein are called *exons.* The intervening segments of noncoding DNA are called *introns.*

25. Both the introns and exons are transcribed during the cell cycle. The cell, however, removes the RNA from the introns and joins the RNA fragments produced by exons to create a functional mRNA molecule.

26. The exon-produced RNA can be spliced together in different ways; the resulting mRNAs produce different proteins.

27. At translation: Messenger RNA may be transferred to the cytoplasm in an inactive, or masked, state. Masking permits the cell to build up large supplies of mRNA in preparation for a sudden burst of protein synthesis.

28. Most cancers arise from mutations. Mutations include three basic changes: (a) alterations of the DNA itself, (b) alterations of the chromosome, and (c) alterations in the chromosome number.

Applications of Biology: Oncogenes—The Seeds of Cancer Within Us

29. Humans and other organisms contain specific genes, called *proto-oncogenes,* that when mutated lead to cancerous growth. Proto-oncogenes are normal genes that code for cellular structures and functions, such as cell adhesion, mitotic proteins, and the production of plasma-membrane receptors for growth factors or hormones.

30. Chemical, physical, and biological agents can mutate these genes, resulting in uncontrolled cellular proliferation (cancer).

31. Viruses can also cause cancer. Some viruses, for example, possess *oncogenes,* which enter human body cells and are incorporated in the cell's genome, stimulating uncontrolled cellular division. Other viruses carry genes that stimulate cancer by activating human proto-oncogenes.

Health, Homeostasis, and the Environment: Hazardous Wastes and Mutations

32. Numerous chemicals are released into the environment from factories, farms, automobiles, and other sources. Many chemicals now in common use have not been tested to determine their ability to cause cancer and birth defects.

33. New research suggests that people may be overreacting to the threat of low-level chemical pollutants. Naturally occurring chemicals in our food, in fact, may cause more cancer than pesticide residues.

34. In some locations, such as toxic waste dumps, chemicals are present in extremely high concentrations. Decades of improper waste disposal have left a legacy of pollution, ill health, and contaminated groundwater.

35. Reducing the contamination of our environment by hazardous wastes will require concerted efforts on the part of governments, businesses, and individuals. Especially important are ways to reduce the production of toxic waste by redesigning processes, recycling and reusing wastes, and finding substitutes.

www.jbpub.com/humanbiology

Connect to this book's web site: www.jbpub.com/humanbiology
The site features eLearning, an online review area that provides quizzes, chapter outlines, and other tools to help you study for your class. You can also follow useful links for in-depth information, research the differing views in the Point/Counterpoints, or keep up on the latest environmental and health news.

Critical Thinking

Thinking Critically— Analysis

This Analysis corresponds to the Thinking Critically scenario that was presented at the beginning of this chapter.

After you have thought about it for a while, consider some additional facts. The U.S. dairy industry already produces an excess of milk. The federal government buys the surplus, dehydrates some of it, and makes cheese out of the rest. The government stockpiles dehydrated milk and cheese at considerable cost to taxpayers. Does this change your view?

Before you draw a firm conclusion, however, remember that cheese and dehydrated milk are given to the needy. The food is not going to waste. Will increasing the surplus produce more food for the poor?

Again, before you draw any conclusions, consider another factor—the effects on small dairy operations of increasing the surplus of milk. Many owners of small dairy herds believe that the large producers will be the primary beneficiaries of the hormone. It will allow them to increase their milk production. As noted earlier, this increase will probably drive down the cost of milk and milk products, and it could put many small dairy farmers out of business. This loss could adversely affect the economies of many rural regions.

Some consumer groups are concerned about the potential health effects of using synthetic growth hormone. A trace of growth hormone is present in milk produced normally. Will the use of synthetic growth hormone increase this concentration in milk? What effect will that have on your health or the health of children?

Make a list of the pros and cons of using synthetic growth hormone. Then make a list of questions—those that you can answer and those that you cannot answer. Do you need more information to decide?

If you are able to make up your mind, what factors swayed your opinion? Did the concerns of one group outweigh the concerns of another? What critical thinking rules did you use in this exercise?

Test of Concepts

1. What is the genetic code? How is the genetic code, housed in the DNA, translated into instructions the cell can understand?
2. Describe how DNA is synthesized. How does the cell ensure the accurate replication of DNA?
3. List the three types of RNA, and briefly describe their function in protein synthesis.
4. In what ways are RNA and DNA similar? In what ways are they different?
5. Describe, in detail, the production of protein on mRNA. Be sure to note the enzymes involved and the role of the ribosome.
6. Discuss how bacterial cells control their genes. In what way does an end product of a metabolic pathway control genes? In what way does a starting material control the genes?
7. Discuss the various levels at which human genes are controlled. Give an example of each.
8. What is a proto-oncogene? How is it affected by a mutagen, a chemical or physical agent that causes mutation?

Genetic Engineering and Biotechnology
SCIENCE, ETHICS, AND SOCIETY

Thinking Critically

A chef at a famous restaurant in New York City organized fellow chefs in the city to protest genetically engineered produce, such as tomatoes. His main concern is that the government has refused to require tomato producers who are growing genetically engineered tomatoes to label their products. Consumers, among them chefs, therefore won't know if they're getting a genetically engineered vegetable or one produced naturally. How would you analyze this issue? What critical thinking rules might apply? ■

Recombinant DNA insulin.

In the movie *Jurassic Park,* scientists removed DNA from dinosaur blood found in the gut of mosquitoes preserved in amber (hardened sap of pine trees) during the age of the dinosaurs. They took this DNA and inserted it into the nuclei of frog cells and produced living, breathing, lawyer-devouring dinosaurs.

Although this scenario is pure science fiction, it illustrates the kinds of genetic manipulations that scientists are engaged in. This procedure, in which a segment of the DNA of one species is cut out and transferred to another species, is popularly referred to as **genetic engineering.** For reasons explained shortly, scientists typically refer to it as **recombinant DNA technology.**

Although we like to think of genetic engineering as a modern invention, it is not new at all. In fact, plants, animals, and microorganisms have been "performing" their own genetic experiments for at least 3.5 billion years. They've been undergoing mutations, exchanging segments of genes (via crossing-over), and combining genes in new ways through sexual reproduction. These manipulations were obviously not the product of conscious thought, but were the product of natural processes—evolutionary processes. Nonetheless, the outcome has been the same: new genetic combinations. Over the course of evolution, nature's genetic tinkering has resulted in a diverse array of life-forms.

Humans took genetic experimentation a step further by **selective breeding**—intentionally crossing certain plants or animals to produce offspring with desirable traits. Domestic animals, such as dogs, came about by selective breeding, as have cattle, cats, fancy pigeons, and other animals (**FIGURE 18-1**). Crops, such as corn and tomatoes, are here today thanks to the efforts of early geneticists who selected plants with desirable traits

FIGURE 18-1 Fancy Pigeon This beautiful bird barely resembles its relative the rock dove, or common pigeon. Selective breeding produced this bird, as it has many other new genetic combinations.

and then pollinated them from other plants with similar traits. The goal in all of this was to produce offspring with good-tasting fruits and seeds.

Some consider genetic engineering, the newest method of genetic manipulation, to be nothing more than an advanced form of the genetic tinkering that occurs in nature and in human societies through selective breeding. Others see it as an intrusion into the natural process of evolution. Still others view it as a dangerous gamble, a perilous flirtation with ecological disaster. They're often worried about potential health effects. Some opponents warn that genetically engineered organisms could spread throughout the world, causing disease and ecological disruption.

Yet another growing controversy has to do with a process called **cloning.** In this technique, cells from an organism are used to develop another, genetically identical organism—a clone. Nuclei from the cells of prize-winning cattle, for example, can be transferred to enucleated eggs. The eggs are then transferred to other cows, where they develop. The result is a genetically superior offspring.

In 1997, much furor arose when a Scottish researcher reported the birth of a cloned sheep. The clone, named Dolly, was derived from a cell taken from the mammary gland of another sheep. Although there is some suspicion about this being a true clone, the announcement stirred considerable controversy, as people began to wonder whether this technique would be used for humans. In 1998, scientists announced yet another clone—this one in mice.

In 2000, the first cloned cow was sold at auction. Produced by a company in Wisconsin, called Infigen, this cow was an exact copy of a prize-winning Holstein. It was produced when an ear cell from the mother was fused with an enucleated egg, then activated using a chemical that stimulates the release of calcium in the egg, causing it to divide. The newly "fertilized" egg was transplanted into another cow, where it developed fully.

Researchers at Texas A & M University have used cloning to produce a disease-resistant cow. They used genetic material from a bull that was naturally resistant to several common diseases. These diseases not only affect cattle, they can be passed to humans in uncooked beef or unpasteurized milk. One of the things that was remarkable about this feat is that the donor cells from the disease-resistant bull had been frozen 15 years earlier!

Cloning has also been used to produce an Asian gaur, a endangered oxlike animal native to the bamboo forests of India and Burma (**FIGURE 18-2**). A skin cell from the gaur was fused with an enucleated egg cell. Researchers hope that this technique may help increase

FIGURE 18-2 Asian Gaur Scientists are using cloning to help increase the numbers of this and other endangered species.

populations of endangered wildlife and may even bring back recently extinct species. Researchers are beginning cloning work to help the Giant Panda, another species in danger of extinction. They're hoping that eggs of black bears will prove to be up to the task.

This chapter examines recombinant DNA technology and its real and potential applications. It also outlines the basic controversy over the use of this technology.

Recombinant DNA Technology: Slicing, Splicing, and Cloning Genes

Genetic engineering got its start nearly 30 years ago as the result of research by Stanley Cohen at Stanford University and Herbert Boyer at the University of California at San Francisco. In 1973, these scientists cut segments of DNA from one bacterium using a special enzyme and

FIGURE 18-3 DNA Scissors Restriction endonucleases extracted from bacteria selectively slice through different segments of the DNA double helix, producing a staggered cut as shown here.

spliced them into the genetic material of another. The recipient bacterium then multiplied and, in the process, produced many copies of the altered genetic material. The process Cohen and Boyer pioneered still provides the basis for much of the genetic engineering research and development being done today. To understand how it works, let's look at the individual steps, beginning with the slicing of a piece of DNA from a chromosome.

Enzymes Are Used to Excise Segments of Genes and Insert Them into Foreign DNA Molecules

Genetic engineering was made possible by the discovery of a group of enzymes that snip off segments of the DNA molecule. Known as **restriction endonucleases,** these enzymes cut through both strands of the DNA, as shown in **FIGURE 18-3**.

Restriction endonucleases are found in many species of bacteria. In bacteria, these enzymes serve a protective function, destroying the DNA of viruses that enter bacterial cells. In so doing, they prevent these cellular pirates from taking over. To date, scientists have discovered hundreds of different restriction endonucleases, each one specific for a particular sequence of bases on the DNA.

As illustrated in **FIGURE 18-3**, these enzymes do not make a nice neat cut across the double helix; they create staggered cuts. Fortunately for geneticists, this "sloppy job" of cutting creates a gap in the DNA into which another piece of DNA can be inserted. All that's necessary for a segment of another DNA molecule to fit in is for its bases to match with those exposed by the enzyme.

Scientists can cut DNA from a bacterium and any other organism they'd like—for example, a human cell. If they use the same enzyme in both instances, they'll end up with segments of human DNA whose cut ends contain complementary base pairs to those in the bacte-

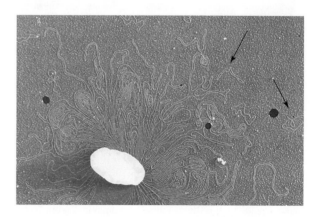

FIGURE 18-4 Plasmids Rupturing a bacterium releases circular chromosome and numerous plasmids, indicated by arrows.

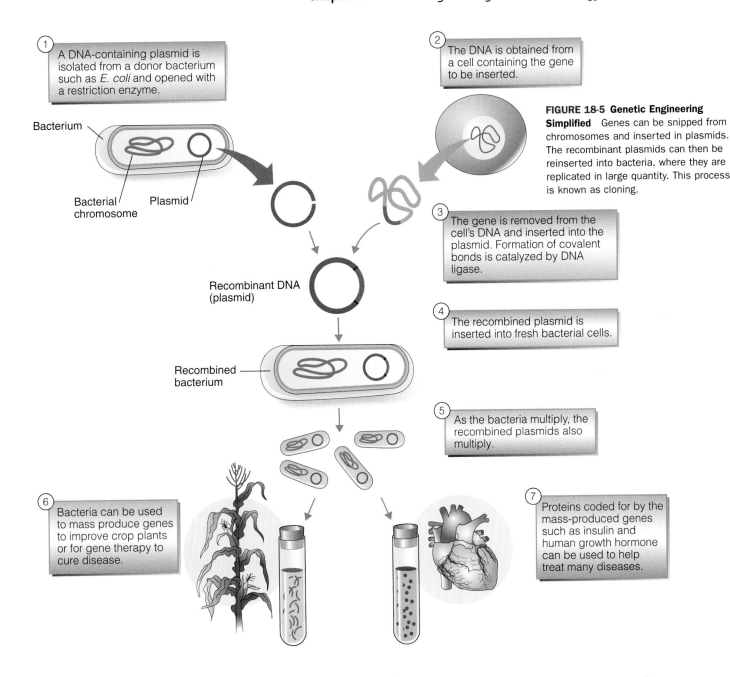

① A DNA-containing plasmid is isolated from a donor bacterium such as *E. coli* and opened with a restriction enzyme.

② The DNA is obtained from a cell containing the gene to be inserted.

Bacterium

Bacterial chromosome   Plasmid

Recombinant DNA (plasmid)

Recombined bacterium

FIGURE 18-5 Genetic Engineering Simplified Genes can be snipped from chromosomes and inserted in plasmids. The recombinant plasmids can then be reinserted into bacteria, where they are replicated in large quantity. This process is known as cloning.

③ The gene is removed from the cell's DNA and inserted into the plasmid. Formation of covalent bonds is catalyzed by DNA ligase.

④ The recombined plasmid is inserted into fresh bacterial cells.

⑤ As the bacteria multiply, the recombined plasmids also multiply.

⑥ Bacteria can be used to mass produce genes to improve crop plants or for gene therapy to cure disease.

⑦ Proteins coded for by the mass-produced genes such as insulin and human growth hormone can be used to help treat many diseases.

rial DNA. Thus, the human segments can be inserted into bacterial DNA.

After a slice of DNA is added to the bacterial DNA, a new enzyme is used to seal it in place. This enzyme is called **DNA ligase.** At this point, the DNA splicing is complete. Geneticists have formed a **recombinant DNA molecule**—a molecule that contains DNA from two different organisms (a combination of DNAs).

Plasmids Can Be Used to Clone DNA Fragments

As noted earlier, recombinant DNA technology began with experiments in bacteria. As noted in Chapter 3,

bacteria are prokaryotes with a single, circular "strand" of DNA (**FIGURE 18-4**). But bacteria also contain smaller circular strands, called **plasmids** (PLAZ-mids). Plasmids carry a few genes—such as those that confer antibiotic resistance to bacteria. They also replicate independent of the chromosome. Plasmids, being smaller than bacterial DNA and also relatively easy to extract, are often used in genetic engineering as a vector—a carrier of foreign genes.

As **FIGURE 18-5** illustrates, plasmids can be sliced with restriction endonucleases. This opens up the circular DNA. Foreign genes can be inserted into the gap in the plasmid and sealed in place with DNA ligase. This

mRNA transcript

mRNA extracted from cell and used as a template for DNA synthesis (reverse transcription)

mRNA-cDNA hybrid

Alkaline solution used to dissolve mRNA

Single cDNA strand

Single strand of cDNA used as template to produce double-stranded DNA molecules

Double stranded cDNA

FIGURE 18-6 Making Genes from mRNA In this process, mRNA is extracted and then used as a template for the production of a complementary strand of DNA (cDNA), a process called reverse transcription. The mRNA molecule is then destroyed, leaving behind a single-stranded molecule of cDNA, which is then used to produce complementary cDNA.

creates recombinant plasmids—plasmids containing foreign genes.

Plasmid carrying foreign genes can then be added to culture dishes containing bacteria or yeast cells. In culture, the plasmids are taken up by the new hosts. Then, as the host cells divide, the plasmids replicate. This produces multiple copies of the gene, which is then said to be **cloned.** Cloning produces numerous identical copies of the foreign gene. These can be used to produce useful products, such as hormones.

Cloning Is One Type of Gene Amplification

Geneticists can produce multiple copies of DNA in other ways, too. One common way of doing this is by extracting messenger RNA from cells and making copies of DNA from them. But wait a minute, you say, that's impossible! RNA can't produce DNA, it works the other way around!

In one of those interesting quirks of nature, there is an enzyme that can make DNA from messenger RNA. This process is called **reverse transcription** because it is the reverse of transcription. It relies on an enzyme called **reverse transcriptase,** which comes from certain viruses.

To make DNA, then, geneticists remove mRNA from a cell and add reverse transcriptase (**FIGURE 18-6**). This enzyme then builds a single strand of DNA on the mRNA template. The hybrid DNA/RNA molecule is then treated with a chemical that destroys the RNA, leaving a single strand of DNA. Additional enzymes convert the single-stranded DNA to a double-stranded

molecule. DNA molecules copied from mRNA are referred to as **cDNA.**

Perhaps the most widely used method of gene amplification is called the **polymerase chain reaction**, the brain child of biochemist Kary Mullis. Basically, it boils down to this: Geneticists extract a segment of the DNA double helix from a cell's nucleus. They then split the DNA molecules into two strands by heating them. Next, they cool the solution and add DNA polymerase enzymes. These enzymes catalyze the formation of complementary DNA molecules.

The DNA molecules are then split again with heat and more DNA polymerase is added. The new polymerase triggers another round of DNA replication. This procedure, which is carried out by machine, permits scientists to produce a million or more copies of the original DNA.

Mass production permits scientists to produce large quantities of DNA, which are needed to chemically analyze the DNA of various species. In so doing, geneticists can determine the exact sequence of bases that comprise the various genes. This procedure has helped scientists map the entire 100,000 or more genes of the human **genome** (JEAN-ome), as discussed in Chapter 16. An interesting finding of this study is that the human genome contains many genes found in other organisms, such as bacteria, mice, and snakes. This finding supports evolutionary theory.

Knowing the sequence of bases in a gene permits scientists to synthesize genes. Manufacturing genes permits geneticists to create normal copies of human genes, which can be inserted into human cells to correct genetic defects.

Mass-producing genes also gives scientists the needed material to mass-produce gene products—notably, proteins. This topic is discussed in the next section.

Applications of Recombinant DNA Technology

Recombinant DNA technology and other related techniques have resulted in a number of practical, though sometimes controversial, applications. This section looks at several potentially useful applications, beginning with one of great practical importance to medicine: the large-scale production of hormones and other proteins to treat diseases.

Hormones and Other Proteins Mass-Produced in Microorganisms Can Be Used to Treat a Variety of Disorders

By removing the human genes that code for hormones and transferring those genes into bacterial cells, scientists can create biological factories that generate huge quantities of hormones and other human proteins (such as blood clotting factors) missing in some individuals. This technique has resulted in a dramatic increase in the supply of protein hormones such as insulin and growth hormone for medical use. **TABLE 18-1** lists some of the products and their uses. So what's so important about this?

Consider an example: Human growth hormone used to treat people with glandular defects was once extracted from the pituitary glands of human cadavers. In order to extract enough growth hormone for one dose, technicians had to remove glands from 50 human cadavers. This process was not only costly, but time-consuming.

Pituitaries from pigs have also been used to obtain growth hormone. Although pig growth hormone acts like human growth hormone, it is different enough chemically to evoke an immune reaction in some patients. Recombinant DNA technology offers an opportunity to produce a

TABLE 18-1

Some Useful Products of Genetic Engineering

Products	Used to
Growth hormone	Treat patients with dwarfism
Insulin	Treat patients with diabetes
Tumor necrosis factor	Treat patients with cancer
tPA (tissue plasminogen activator)	Dissolves clots formed during heart attacks
Erythropoietin	Stimulates blood cell formation for patients with some forms of anemia
Clotting factors	Treat people with hemophilia
Surfactant	Treat babies with blue baby syndrome, caused by collapse of air sacs in lungs, which is caused by a lack of surfactant
Interferons	Treat some forms of cancer and some viral infections
Vaccines	To prevent hepatitis A, B, and C, as well as AIDS*, malaria*, and herpes*
DNA probes	Map human chromosomes, perform DNA fingerprinting, detect infectious diseases, and detect genetic disorders

*Under development, but not currently available.

growth hormone that is much safer than pig growth hormone, because it avoids potential immune reactions.

Protein hormones, like growth hormone, can also be produced for other uses, notably for livestock production. Cows, for instance, can be injected with bovine growth hormone produced by genetically engineered bacteria. This treatment greatly increases milk production. (For a discussion of the pros and cons of this, see the Thinking Critically section in Chapter 17.)

Recombinant DNA Techniques Can Be Used to Produce Vaccines. As noted in Chapter 8, vaccines consist of inactivated bacteria or viruses. When injected in an individual, a vaccine stimulates an immune response. This, in turn, protects a person for long periods from the infectious form of the bacterium or virus. Using genetic engineering, scientists can produce vaccines in large quantity and at a lower cost than is possible by conventional means.

Two types of genetically engineered vaccines are being produced. The first consists of proteins or polypeptides identical to those found in the capsid of viruses. These vaccines, produced from viral genes created by genetic engineering, stimulate an immune reaction and will very likely have little adverse effect.

The other type of genetically engineered vaccine consists of genetically modified viruses. These, too, stimulate an immune reaction. However, some researchers are concerned that the genetic changes could have unpredictable effects when the viruses are injected in humans. Such changes could also result in broader host species possibilities—meaning that the altered virus could affect other species not currently impacted by the viruses. There is also concern that the genetically altered viruses could exchange genetic material with live viruses with potentially adverse effects in humans.

At present, numerous vaccines are under development. One vaccine, for an infectious disease that strikes the liver (hepatitis B), has been produced via this method. But geneticists hope to develop others, perhaps even one for the AIDS virus.

Gene Splicing Can Be Used to Transfer Genes from One Organism to Another

In what some people view as a major intrusion into the evolution of life, scientists are now able to transfer single genes from one organism to another, creating a **transgenic organism.** These organisms don't differ much from their original form; they may, in fact, display only one new trait, such as a larger body size. One of the most successful attempts to date involves the transplantation of the human gene that codes for growth hormone into pigs and mice (**FIGURE 18-7**). When

FIGURE 18-7 Supermice The mouse on the right, pictured with its littermate, has received a gene for human growth hormone.

successful, this results in offspring that are much larger than their siblings who didn't receive the gene.

Researchers are looking for ways to re-engineer cows so that the milk they produce will be chemically more similar to human milk. Scientists, for example, have transplanted a human gene that codes for the production of a chemical found in mother's milk, called *lactoferin*, into cows. This substance helps babies fight off infections.

One of the most exciting developments is the production of mice containing genes identical to those that cause human diseases. This could advance medical research on diseases and speed the development of treatments and cures.

In 1997, scientists from the Medical College of Georgia announced the successful transplantation of genes that code for a green fluorescing protein into zebra fish. It turned the red blood cells green under blue light, allowing scientists to study blood cell formation in the zebra fish embryos. The scientists had performed the same process with nerve cells, and hope that this will allow them to study how nerve cells form connections in the developing brain.

Although such techniques sound simple, they're actually quite difficult. One can't just inject a foreign gene into a baby pig or mouse or cow. In order to successfully transplant a gene from one species into another, the gene generally has to be introduced at the embryonic stage when the organism is in the one-cell stage. This is accomplished by injecting genes into the nucleus of the ovum via tiny needles. Some nuclei incorporate the foreign gene, which is then transmitted from one cell to the next during embryonic development. Even so, there's no guarantee that the gene will end up in the proper location.

Scientists are also experimenting with ways to transplant normal genes into cancer cells or the cells lining the respiratory tract of people suffering from cystic fibrosis. In the latter case, they're inserting genes into viruses that infect the cells lining the respiratory passageways, hoping that it will become part of these cells' genome and correct the problems.

Transgenic Plants Are Easier to Produce Than Transgenic Animals, and Many Successes Have Already Occurred In This Area. Plants are easier to perform gene transplants on than animals. One of the first success stories involved the transplantation of a gene that codes for an enzyme called luciferase (lew-SIFF-er-

ace) into a tobacco plant. This enzyme is normally found in fireflies and is responsible for catalyzing a light-generating reaction. In the tobacco plant, the enzyme didn't do much unless the plant was sprayed with a chemical called luciferin. At this point, the plant glowed (**FIGURE 18-8**).

This experiment was not performed to create tobacco plants that glow in the dark so they could be harvested at night, but only to show that foreign genes could indeed be transplanted from one species to another. It opened up the door to more practical experiments—for instance, transplanting genes that make plants produce more nutritious seeds and fruit or that permit the roots of some plants to synthesize their own nitrogen fertilizer.

One of the more promising developments involves the introduction of genes that allow oats to grow in salty soil. Transplanting these genes into commercial crop species could allow farmers to use vast acreages in the United States and other countries idled by the buildup of salts. This is caused by the irrigation of poorly drained soils with water high in salts.

Researchers are also developing ways to make crop plants resistant to herbicides, chemicals applied to crops to control weeds. Although herbicides generally act only on weed species, they sometimes impair the growth of crop species. Proponents hope that herbicide-resistant crops will help farmers increase yields. Critics argue that if herbicide-resistant crops are used, farmers may apply larger amounts of herbicide to their fields. These chemicals, in turn, could be washed into nearby waterways, poisoning aquatic life. They could also poison soils, killing important bacteria and other microorganisms es-

FIGURE 18-8 Glow Little Tobacco Plant, Glimmer Glimmer This tobacco plant contains firefly genes for the enzyme luciferase. When the plant is sprayed with luciferin, the enzyme breaks it down, releasing light.

sential for the long-term health of the soil. (For a discussion, see the Point/Counterpoint in this chapter.)

Geneticists are also working on ways to alter plants themselves to increase their resistance to pests. By transferring the genes that protect wild species from insects into crop species, scientists may be able to produce many varieties that require little, if any, chemical pesticides.

Efforts are also underway to produce genetically engineered vegetables such as tomatoes. But critics fear that such experiments may result in unforeseen reactions such as allergies. There is some evidence to suggest that some people do indeed develop allergies to genetically engineered crops.

Transgenic Microorganisms Are Perhaps Some of the Most Controversial of All Applications. Genetic engineering began with microorganisms, and work in this area continues today. For example, scientists have successfully transplanted a bacterial gene that produces a toxin that kills insects into a species of bacteria that lives on the roots of crop plants. Root-eating insects ingest the lethal bacteria when they feed on roots of treated plants. This kills the insects and protects crops. This technique benefits the farmer, who has to use fewer chemicals to control root-eating insects, and also benefits the environment, because it reduces the use of potentially dangerous chemicals that could leach into groundwater or be washed into nearby lakes and streams.

Genetic researchers have also developed a bacterium that retards the formation of frost on plants. The genetic variant is found naturally in the environment, but not in sufficient quantities to protect crops. Thus, researchers have cloned the bacterium and have begun testing its efficiency in the field. Should it prove successful and safe, the bacterium could be sprayed on crops late in the growing season when frosts can be devastating, potentially saving farmers millions of dollars a year. Some environmentalists, however, worry that this bacterium and other genetically engineered creations could escape into the environment and displace normally occurring bacteria. Who knows what detrimental effects this might have on the function of natural systems?

Recombinant DNA Technology Can Be Used to Cure Genetic Disease, a Treatment Called Gene Therapy

As noted earlier, researchers are also tinkering with ways in which genetic engineering can be used to insert normal human genes into genetically defective body cells, thereby curing serious genetic diseases. This technique is called **gene therapy.**

Approximately 1 of every 100 children born in the United States suffers from a serious genetic defect, such as sickle-cell anemia or hemophilia. Thanks to advances in genetic engineering, scientists may soon be able to replace their defective genes with normal genes. Instead of simply finding a treatment, this technique will, if successful, permit doctors to cure diseases previously considered incurable. Many of these diseases cost our society millions of dollars and account for enormous human suffering. The largest obstacle, however, is getting the genes into body cells where they are missing. For instance, to cure a genetic defect in brain cells, the genes must somehow be delivered to the cells of the brain.

One promising means of delivering genes to sites where they're required is the bone marrow transplant. Consider an example. Krabbe's disease is a rare genetic disorder resulting from a deficiency in one enzyme in human brain cells. The absence of this enzyme allows fat to accumulate in the nervous system, causing nerve cells to degenerate. Seizures and visual problems occur early in life, and most victims die within the first 2 years of life.

To test a means of correcting this disease, scientists used a strain of mice that suffers from a similar condition. They injected them with bone marrow cells containing the gene that codes for the missing enzyme. Scientists found that the transplanted cells became established in the lungs and liver and restored enzymatic activity. Some even found their way into the brain!

Another potentially promising technique involves the use of microspheres—tiny lipid spheres. Called liposomes, these tiny lipid spheres can be packed with genes and coated with antibodies for specific target cells. If successful, this will allow the liposomes to deliver their contents to the correct cells.

Researchers have also developed a novel transplantation technique that could enable surgeons to introduce genetically engineered cells into specific organs in the human body. In laboratory studies, scientists have injected genetically altered liver cells into a foamlike material. The foam was then transplanted into rats after being impregnated with a hormone that stimulates the growth of blood vessels from nearby larger vessels. Within a week after implantation, the artificial tissue was riddled with a network of blood vessels. This technique could someday be used to introduce genetically normal cells into numerous tissues and organs of the body, providing a cure for disorders such as diabetes mellitus and Parkinson's disease.

DNA Probes Permit Analysis of DNA from Crime Scenes, Detection of Infectious Organisms and Genetic Disorders. Imagine that you're a police officer investigating a gruesome murder. The victim is a 29-year-old man who was found dead in his apartment. Unfortunately, the physical evidence is scant. There

Point/Counterpoint

Controversy over Herbicide Resistance Through Genetic Engineering

The Benefits of Genetically Engineered Herbicide Resistance

Charles J. Arntzen

Dr. Charles J. Arntzen *is a professor in the Alkek Institute of Biosciences and Technology in the Texas Medical Center in Houston, Texas. Dr. Arntzen was elected to the U.S. National Academy of Sciences in 1983 as a result of his pioneering research in photosynthesis and plant molecular biology. He was the chairman of the National Biotechnology Policy Board of the National Institutes of Health from 1991–1993, and is a member of the Editorial Board of* Science. *This article is adapted by the author from a 1991 publication entitled* The Genetic Revolution, Scientific Prospects and Public Perceptions *with the permission of the publisher, The Johns Hopkins University Press.*

One of the principal outcomes of plant genetic engineering has been a rapid expansion in our understanding of plant cell biology, genetics, and molecular controls over the structure and function of plants. This understanding is now helping to solve practical problems such as developing insect- and disease-resistant crops, thereby decreasing needs for chemical pesticides. Other approaches include creating herbicide-resistant plants, which will allow farmers more choices in weed control, and to switch to newer, rapidly biodegradable herbicides.

Herbicides are chemicals sprayed on crops to control weeds. Their effect is selective—that is, they kill weeds without significantly harming crops. All herbicides currently available to farmers began with an evaluation of the sensitivity of weeds and crops to experimental chemicals. This evaluation is accomplished by applying potentially useful chemicals to test samples of weed and crop seedlings. Compounds that kill weeds but not crops are then subjected to animal toxicology studies. Those deemed acceptable are developed for farmers' use.

The success of herbicides is based on the fact that crop species contain enzymes that convert chemical compounds, including herbicides, to inactive forms. These enzymes tend to be crop-specific. For instance, the enzymes that render soybeans immune to 30 or more commercial herbicides are different from the enzymes that make corn resistant to other herbicides. This can be a benefit when corn or soybeans are grown in rotation. In such instances, both the unwanted "volunteer" corn and weeds that germinate in a soybean field can be controlled by the soybean herbicide.

Interestingly, certain weeds have the same enzymes as the crop species they invade. This is often true when the weeds and crops are somewhat related, such as with wild oats in a field of wheat or barley. Thus, the oats are resistant to the same herbicides as the wheat or barley. Consequently, the farmer currently has few or no choices in chemical weed control since herbicides that would kill the weeds would also kill the crop.

Through genetic engineering, researchers have devised ways to make crops resistant to new classes of herbicides. That is, they have found ways to give crops such as soybeans additional enzymes to augment their natural herbicide resistance. By transferring genes that code for enzymes conferring herbicide resistance, scientists can give farmers a broader set of options when selecting herbicides. If successful, these options will solve problems where there is currently no weed control, or where the herbicides

available are prohibitively expensive or environmentally damaging.

This line of research may also give the farmer a simpler means to control weeds through the use of a single, more effective herbicide selected on the basis of several traits, including herbicide resistance, reduced cost, and, ideally, greater safety in the environment.

This explanation of the benefits of genetic research aimed at making crops more resistant to herbicides may not satisfy the reader who is asking, "Why don't they simply stop using all herbicides?" The main answer is economics. Weed control is essential for all crops. Left unchecked, weed populations can reduce crop yields to near zero. Prior to the 1950s, weeds were controlled strictly by mechanical means—that is, by cultivation or hand pulling. This was a labor-intensive and costly process. By the 1980s, more than 95% of all major row crops in the United States were produced using herbicides. Farmers based this decision (to apply herbicides rather than using a cultivator or a hoe) on costs. An application of herbicides at the time of planting, costing as little as $10 per acre, is many times cheaper than mechanical cultivation. Weed control through herbicides is a factor in the low food prices we enjoy in the United States. It also saves on energy use and, when properly used, does not harm the environment.

With the continuing development of herbicide-resistant crops as part of an integrated weed-control strategy, crop production costs can be held at low levels while new methods for weed control are being developed.

were no eye witnesses, no fingerprints, and no fragments of the perpetrator's clothing in the apartment. However, there is blood on the carpet and on the couch, which turns out to belong to two different

individuals—the victim and possibly the perpetrator. Some days later, an anonymous tip points you in the direction of a family member, a cousin. You take him into custody for questions, but he says he wasn't in town at

The Perils of Genetically Engineered Herbicide Resistance

Margaret Mellon

Environmentalists have been active in the debate about genetic engineering since the beginning. The current focus of environmental interest in genetic engineering is based on the prospect of commercial production of a broad range of genetically engineered organisms—for example, bacteria and viruses. These organisms could have direct and adverse impacts on our environment and our health.

Public concern over genetic engineering is also focused on indirect environmental consequences, the best example of which is herbicide-resistant plants. The development of major crops that are tolerant of chemical herbicides seems likely to lead to increased or prolonged use of these dangerous agricultural chemicals.

Herbicide-resistant crops, like most genetically engineered agricultural products, are being developed by large, transnational chemical companies. Worldwide, at least 28 enterprises have launched more than 65 research programs to develop herbicide-resistant crops. All of the major crop plants are involved, including cotton, corn, soybeans, wheat, and potatoes. Engineered crops being made resistant to a company's own herbicides will surely increase that company's market share in chemicals. Thus, industry analysts expect herbicide-resistant plants to be big business, mainly for pesticide and herbicide producers.

Herbicide-resistant products run directly counter to the promise of a reduced dependence on agricultural chemicals put forward by biotechnology advocates. Rather than weaning agriculture from chemicals, these crops will be shackled to herbicide use for the foreseeable future. Herbicides represent an estimated 65% of the chemical pesticides used in agriculture. By continuing to promote the use of herbicides, the biotechnology industry greatly restricts its potential for reducing overall chemical use.

While herbicide-resistant crops offer no hope of environmental benefits in agriculture, there are alternatives to these products that do promise substantial reduction in overall pesticide use. These alternatives fall under the rubric of sustainable agriculture.

Sustainable agriculture employs a variety of agricultural practices such as crop rotation, intercropping, and ridge tillage (that produce long ridges of soil on which plants are grown). These practices control pests without the application of synthetic pesticides and fertilizers. Used by knowledgeable farm managers, these techniques work to make farms more profitable and environmentally sound. Growing different crops in successive growing seasons, for example, dramatically reduces pests by sequentially removing the hosts on which the pests depend. With fewer weeds or insects to contend with, the farmers reduce the need for costly chemical pesticides. Once thought impractical, sustainable agriculture is rapidly gaining support in national policy forums, including the National Academy of Sciences.

The environmental advantage of such an approach is clear. Crop rotations that reduce pests reduce the need for pesticides now and into the future. Thus, developing sustainable practices should be the highest priority for agriculture as it moves toward the twenty-first century.

Although a minor part of the sustainable agriculture picture up to now, biotechnology could help by developing new crop varieties for use in sustainable systems—for example, faster germinating, cold-tolerant crop varieties could enhance low-input sustainable systems by enabling more effective weed control. Engineered products such as these would fulfill the promise of biotechnology, and would benefit farmers, the environment, and the rural economy alike.

Margaret Mellon *is the director of the Agriculture and Biotechnology Program at the Union of Concerned Scientists (UCS). UCS works at the interface of technology and society to promote sustainable agriculture and evaluate applications of biotechnology. Dr. Mellon lectures widely on biotechnology issues and has appeared frequently on television and radio talk shows.*

Sharpening Your Critical Thinking Skills

1. State the main thesis of each author in your own words.
2. List the data or arguments used to support each hypothesis and the data used by the authors to refute the other's point of view, if any.
3. Can you determine whether there are any flaws in the reasoning in either essay?
4. Which viewpoint do you agree with? Why?

Visit *Human Biology's* Internet site for links to web sites offering more information on this topic.

the time and has several people who will attest to his whereabouts. After you sample the blood of the cousin, though, you find that it matches that found in the apartment. Then you have the lab perform a genetic analysis of the alleged perpetrator's blood and find that it matches samples at the crime scene as well. In a court of law, this evidence alone may be enough to convict the cousin.

This technique of DNA matching is called **DNA fingerprinting,** and was introduced in Chapter 17. DNA fingerprinting relies on techniques derived from genetic engineering. In particular, it depends on **DNA probes,** small fragments of single-stranded DNA produced by machines called DNA synthesizers. Probes bind to complementary base pairs of DNA from samples taken at the scene of a crime and from suspected perpetrators. If you know the composition of the DNA probes, you can determine the sequence of bases in the DNA under study. Several probes are used to compare samples of blood as well as hair or semen.

DNA Probes Can Even Be Used to Help Geneticists Map Human Chromosomes

Geneticists have long been interested in mapping human chromosomes—that is, in determining which genes are on which chromosomes. For years, the mapping process has been rather crude, relying on studies of patterns of linked traits in families.

Another, more refined technique has also been used. In this procedure, scientists fuse a human cell with a mouse cell (**FIGURE 18-9**). The new hybrid cell containing 96 chromosomes divides, but when the cell divides, it begins to lose human chromosomes. The daughter cells divide again and lose more. Eventually, cells are produced with all mouse chromosomes and

one or two human chromosomes. By studying the resulting protein products, geneticists can associate certain genes with certain chromosomes.

Recombinant DNA technology has permitted yet another dramatic refinement in chromosome mapping. The DNA probe is helping geneticists determine not only what genes are on what chromosomes, but also their exact location on the chromosome.

Controversies over Genetic Engineering— Ethics and Safety Concerns

Although genetic engineering has spawned a great deal of enthusiasm, it also has its critics. And, despite the promises, genetic engineering is fraught with controversy over safety and ethics. In October, 1997, for instance, several scientists issued a worldwide alert asking all governments to ban import of a genetically engineered soybean from the United States. The soybeans were genetically altered to be resistant to a herbicide known as Roundup. The scientists are concerned that the use of this herbicide will increase the level of plant estrogens in soybeans, thus increasing

FIGURE 18-9 Mapping by Fusion This technique permits scientists to determine the chromosomal address of certain genes. Human and mouse cells are fused, creating a new cell with excess chromosomes. This cell divides and, in so doing, loses most of the excess chromosomes. Cells with one or two human chromosomes can be grown in culture. By determining the unique human proteins being synthesized in these cells and the chromosomes present, geneticists can determine the chromosomal "address" of certain genes. More precise techniques are needed to determine the exact location on the chromosome.

Human fibroblast (46 chromosomes)

Chromosomes

Cells fuse

Hybrid cell (96 chromosomes)

Cell divides

Cloned cell

Cloned cell

Mouse tumor cell (50 chromosomes)

| Human and mouse cells grow together in culture. | Cells are fused to create a hybrid. | After several cell divisions, hybrid loses most of the human chromosomes. |

the levels of these potentially harmful chemicals in humans.

In the year 2000, taco shells, tortillas, and numerous snack foods produced from an unapproved genetically engineered corn were recalled from U.S. markets as a result of health concerns. Approximately 300 types of taco shells, tortillas, and snack chips made by the Texas-based Mission Foods were affected by the recall with an estimated value of about $10 million. These products were made from a genetically engineered corn called Starlink that had not been approved because of questions about its ability to cause allergic reactions. Interestingly, "normal" corn growing in fields near farms where genetically engineered corn was also affected because pollen from the genetically engineered crops was dispersed by the wind into their fields, altering the neighboring corn crops.

At this time, many safety questions remain unanswered. As noted earlier, perhaps the greatest safety concern is the possibility of unleashing genetically altered bacteria or viruses. At least two studies now indicate that genetically engineered bacteria that are applied to seeds take up residence on the roots but migrate very little from the site of application in the short term. Critics, however, are concerned with long-term consequences. Some critics fear that a genetically altered strain could spread through the environment, wreaking havoc on ecosystems and, possibly, human populations. Once unleashed, it would be impossible to retrieve. The genetically altered bacterium that retards frost formation, for example, could enter the atmosphere on dust particles, reducing cloud formation and altering global climate. No one knows for sure how serious this threat really is. The Point/Counterpoint in Chapter 2 discusses the safety of genetically engineered food.

Other critics object to genetic tinkering, especially the transfer of genes from one species to another, on ethical grounds. Do humans have the right, they wonder, to interfere with the course of evolution?

Proponents of genetic tinkering argue that livestock and plant breeders have been selectively breeding hardy animals to produce genetically superior livestock and crops for hundreds, if not thousands, of years. In so doing, people have been performing a kind of genetic engineering—albeit a slow one—for millennia. Genetic engineering, say proponents, merely offers a quicker way of achieving the same goals.

To understand this debate, it is important to exercise one's critical thinking faculties by first defining the terms very carefully. When you do this, you find that genetic engineering and selective breeding do indeed achieve the same end points in some instances. Selective breeding simply alters gene frequencies—that is, the percentage of organisms in a population carrying a specific allele. Genetic engineering does the same, as in the case of the frost-retarding bacteria. In other words, geneticists are simply producing large quantities of a mutant already found in nature. But that in and of itself may be reason for concern. In nature, for reasons not well understood, the mutant is found in small quantity. Could shifting the allele frequency cause some ecological catastrophe?

In other instances, the two techniques produce quite different results. That is, in some cases, genetic engineering introduces new genes into species, producing genetic combinations never before encountered in life. Introducing the human growth hormone gene into cattle embryos is an example of this form of tinkering. This manipulation violates a fundamental law of nature: Different species do not interbreed. Is it ethical to blur nature's naturally maintained boundaries? Who can say? And can we put a lid on our ambition? Will we know when to stop?

Unfortunately, experience with genetic engineering is too limited to answer the safety concerns of critics. Preliminary work suggests that the dangers have been exaggerated and that genetically engineered bacteria are not a threat to ecosystem stability. Still, further research is needed to be certain that in our zeal to make life better, we don't do ourselves in. Ethical questions, like political questions that have been plaguing some countries for centuries, may never be answered to the satisfaction of everyone.

Another point, rarely mentioned in the debate, is the potential for wrong-doing—for creating superinfectious organisms that could wipe out huge numbers of people. Imagine for instance, the catastrophe that might arise if some mad scientist introduced the deadly AIDS virus genes into the genome of the flu virus, which is rapidly transmitted around the world.

Scientists who have been exploring designer pathogens, highly infectious agents, have found that most potential superbugs turn out to be less potent than their natural forms. Put another way, in these experiments, virulence was typically lost.

In 1998 and 1999, however, Australian researchers made a startling discovering, ironically, while working to find a way to render mice infertile, in an effort to protect world grain supplies. Mice and rats ravage grain supplies in many countries, reducing food available for people. The researchers had spliced a mouse immune system gene into the mousepox virus, which is similar to the human smallpox virus. Much to their surprise, the mice did not become infertile, they died—even mice that had been immunized against mousepox virus. The researchers published their work with a warning that this technique could potentially be used to produce deadlier forms of human pathogens for biological warfare.

Whatever the outcome of the debate, you can bet that genetic engineering is here to stay. Future disasters, should they occur, may compel us to prohibit certain forms of genetic tinkering, but in cases where genetic engineering reduces suffering, advances agriculture, and facilitates environmental cleanup, public support may be hard to thwart.

Summary

1. Genetic engineering, or *recombinant DNA technology*, is a procedure by which geneticists remove segments of DNA from one organism and insert them into the DNA of another.

2. Genetic manipulation is not a new phenomenon. Nature has been tinkering with genes for at least 3.5 billion years, yielding multitudes of new genetic combinations during evolution.

Recombinant DNA Technology: Slicing, Splicing, and Cloning Genes

3. Genetic engineering got its start over 20 years ago when scientists cut segments of DNA from one bacterium using a special enzyme and spliced them into the genetic material of another that was then permitted to replicate.

4. Geneticists use an enzyme called *restriction endonuclease* to excise segments of genes and insert them into foreign DNA molecules.

5. After a segment of DNA is transplanted, a second enzyme, *DNA ligase*, is used to seal it in place. At this point, geneticists have formed a *recombinant DNA* molecule—a molecule that contains DNA from two different organisms.

6. Bacteria contain small, circular strands of DNA, called *plasmids*, which are separate from the chromosome. Foreign genes can be spliced into plasmids, and the plasmid carrying a foreign gene can be reinserted into bacteria or yeast cells by adding them to culture dishes containing these microorganisms.

7. In culture, the plasmids are rapidly taken up by the new hosts. As these cells divide, the plasmids replicate. This produces multiple copies of the gene, which is then said to be *cloned*.

8. Cloning produces numerous identical copies of the foreign gene, which can be used for further studies in genetics or to produce useful products, such as hormones.

9. Geneticists can produce multiple copies in other ways, too. One of the most common ways of doing this is by extracting messenger RNA from cells and making copies of DNA from them using the enzyme *reverse transcriptase*.

10. The most widely used method of gene amplification is called the *polymerase chain reaction* in which DNA is alternately heated to split the double helix, then cooled. DNA polymerase enzymes are added to catalyze the formation of complementary DNA molecules.

Applications of Recombinant DNA Technology

11. Recombinant DNA technology and other related techniques have resulted in a number of practical and sometimes controversial applications.

12. Hormones and other proteins mass-produced in genetically engineered microorganisms can be used to treat a variety of disorders. Recombinant DNA techniques can be used to produce vaccines.

13. Gene splicing can be used to transfer genes from one organism to another, creating *transgenic organisms*. These organisms rarely differ much from their original form; they may, in fact, only display one new trait, such as a larger body size.

14. Transgenic plants are easier to produce than transgenic animals, and many successes can be enumerated. Attempts are being made to make plants that produce more nutritious products or are more resistant to herbicides and pests.

15. Recombinant DNA technology can be used to cure genetic disease, a treatment called *gene therapy*. In this procedure, scientists attempt to insert normal human genes into genetically defective body cells.

16. Although promising, gene therapy has two major barriers: delivering the gene to the proper cell and ensuring its incorporation into the DNA of that cell. Several techniques are under development to overcome these barriers.

17. Another practical outcome of research in recombinant DNA technology is the DNA probe. *DNA probes* are tiny segments of genes that bind to complementary base pairs of sample DNA—for example, hair, blood, or semen taken from crime scenes. DNA probes can also be used to detect infectious organisms and genetic disorders.

18. DNA probes are used in *DNA fingerprinting*.

19. DNA probes are being used to map human chromosomes—that is, to determine the location of genes on human chromosomes.

Controversies Over Genetic Engineering—Ethics and Safety Concerns

20. Although genetic engineering has spawned a great deal of enthusiasm, it does have its critics who are concerned with safety and ethical issues.

21. Perhaps the greatest safety concern is the possibility of intentionally or unintentionally releasing potentially dangerous genetically altered bacteria or viruses into the environment.

22. Some critics object to genetic tinkering, especially the transfer of genes from one species to another, on ethical grounds, wondering if we have the right to interfere with the course of evolution.

23. Unfortunately, experience with genetic engineering is too limited to answer the safety concerns of critics. Preliminary work suggests that the dangers have been exaggerated and that genetically engineered bacteria are not a threat to ecosystem stability. Further research is needed to be certain.

Critical Thinking

Thinking Critically— Analysis

This Analysis corresponds to the Thinking Critically scenario that was presented at the beginning of this chapter.

Before you accept or reject an argument, such as the one made by the chef, it's important to gather all the facts. Reading this chapter will give you some perspective on genetic engineering. I'd also suggest reading some specific articles on genetically engineered tomatoes. An excellent one was published in *Science News*, November 28, 1992. This article explains the ways that geneticists are trying to alter tomatoes, using genetic engineering. Upon careful analysis, it appears that several of the improvements they're seeking could have been acquired by selective breeding. In other words, they could have achieved the same results by cross-breeding tomatoes with desired traits with those with other traits, producing a "super" tomato with good taste, long shelf life, and other desirable features. In this instance, there's nothing magical about genetic engineering. It's just a faster way of getting desirable genes into a tomato.

But you'll also learn that geneticists are transplanting bacterial genes into tomato plants. One gene in particular retards the production of ethylene gas, which normally stimulates ripening. When the bacterial gene is present, it slows ripening, allowing farmers to leave the tomato on the vine several extra days. This increases the tomato's flavor with obvious benefits to anyone who has eaten a store-bought tomato and had the opportunity to compare it with one grown in a garden.

The questions here might be: Will this harm consumers? Can you think of any other concerns and ways to address them? Are the chefs merely reacting to the phrase "genetic engineering"? Could this be one of those thought stoppers described in the Critical Thinking section in Chapter 1?

Exercising Your Critical Thinking Skills

In an attempt to increase the supply of blood for surgery and medical emergencies and to avoid potential contamination from the AIDS virus, scientists are looking for blood substitutes. One group of scientists has successfully transplanted the human hemoglobin gene into pigs. About 10% of their hemoglobin is chemically identical to human hemoglobin. Using your critical thinking skills, analyze the potential of this discovery. Would you invest in this company? What obstacles lie in the way?

Test of Concepts

1. Describe the methods of recombinant DNA technology. Your answer should explain how genes are removed, spliced, and cloned.
2. Describe three methods of gene amplification.
3. What barriers lie in the way of creating transgenic organisms?
4. List and describe three practical applications of recombinant DNA technology.
5. List the major concerns for genetic engineering and describe each one.
6. Debate the statement: Genetic engineering is morally wrong and should be discontinued. It violates the laws of nature and gives humans a power beyond their control.

www.jbpub.com/humanbiology

Connect to this book's web site: www.jbpub.com/humanbiology
The site features eLearning, an online review area that provides quizzes, chapter outlines, and other tools to help you study for your class. You can also follow useful links for in-depth information, research the differing views in the Point/Counterpoints, or keep up on the latest environmental and health news.

Human Reproduction

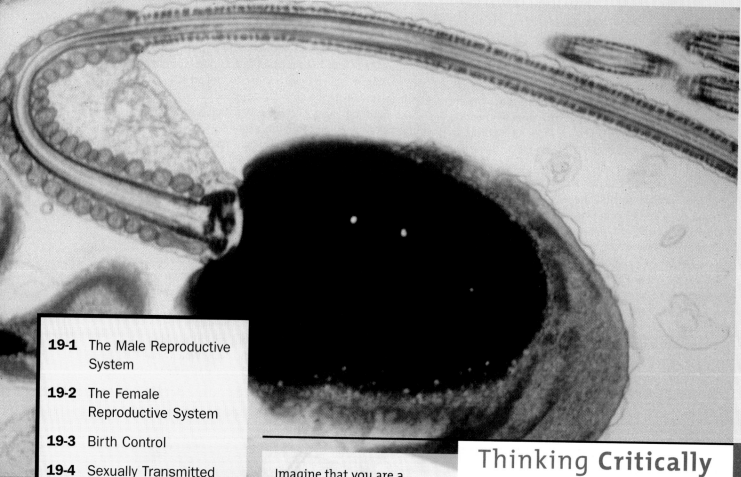

Thinking Critically

Imagine that you are a journalist for a major urban newspaper. One day, you receive a press release from a local medical school announcing that one of its researchers has discovered that a chemical found in a common household cleaning agent reduces fertility in rats and mice. Large doses were given to both males and females before conception. The results showed a statistically significant decline in the litter size as well as several physical abnormalities—misshapen legs and malformed skulls. The press release quotes the researcher who says that the chemical should be banned from use in homes. Using your critical thinking skills, what questions would you ask before writing your article? What other information would you seek out? ■

Human sperm, one of the most highly specialized cells in the body.

Sandra Collins woke one day with a terrible pain in her abdomen that persisted throughout the morning. Instead of calling her doctor, though, she shrugged off the pain and went Christmas shopping with her husband. A few hours later, while she was browsing through a bookstore, the pain grew worse and she blacked out. Her husband rushed her to the emergency room, where it was found that Sandra was suffering from severe internal bleeding caused by an ectopic (eck-TOP-ick) pregnancy—that is, a fertilized ovum that had developed in the upper part of her reproductive tract, outside the uterus.

Fortunately, physicians were able to counteract her blood loss with a transfusion. They then whisked her into the operating room, where they surgically removed the fetus, placenta, and surrounding tissue and repaired torn blood vessels.

Reproduction is one of the most basic body functions. However, as this account shows, it doesn't always operate smoothly. Like many other body functions, reproduction is controlled by the endocrine and nervous systems. This chapter describes human reproduction. We'll examine the male and female reproductive tracts as well as contraception and sexually transmitted diseases.

Section 19-1

The Male Reproductive System

In humans, the male reproductive system consists of seven parts: (1) the two **testes** (TESS-teas), which produce sex steroid hormones and sperm; (2) the two **epididymides** (EP-eh-DID-eh-mid-ees), which store sperm produced in the testes; (3) a pair of ducts, each known as a **vas deferens** (vass DEAF-er-ens), that conducts sperm from the epididymis of each testis to the urethra; (4) **sex accessory glands**, which produce secretions that make up the bulk of the ejaculate; (5) the **urethra** (yur-REETH-rah), which conducts sperm to the outside; (6) the **penis** (PEA-nuss), the organ of copulation; and (7) the **scrotum** (SCROW-tum), a sac that houses the testes (**FIGURE 19-1**; **TABLE 19-1**).

The Scrotum Helps Keep the Testes Cool

The testes are suspended in a pouch known as the **scrotum**. As **FIGURE 19-1** shows, the scrotum is attached to the body below the attachment of the penis.

Interestingly, the testes are not formed in the scrotum during development. Rather, they descend into the scrotum from their site of origin near the kidney before birth. In about 3 of every 100 boys, however, the testes fail to descend. In 2 of every 3 of these boys, the testes descend into

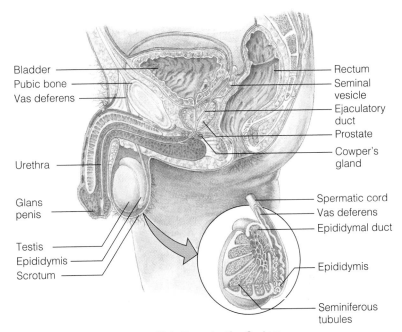

FIGURE 19-1 Anatomy of the Male Reproductive System

the scrotum during the first year. For those in which the testes do not descend, some corrective action must be taken. Drugs may be given to stimulate the release of male sex hormones that cause the testes to descend. If drug treatment is unsuccessful, surgery is required.

If the condition is not corrected, sterility may result. The reason for this is that sperm formation occurs at a temperature a few degrees below body temperature. The scrotum provides just the right temperature to permit normal sperm production. Inside the body cavity, the temperature is too high for sperm development.

The influence of body heat on sperm development is illustrated by the plight of male long-distance runners who run hundreds of miles a month. This level of exercise elevates their body temperature, and even though the testes are suspended in the scrotum, scrotal temperature may be so high that sperm formation declines.

TABLE 19-1

The Male Reproductive System

Component	Function
Testes	Produce sperm and male sex steroids
Epididymes	Store sperm
Vasa deferentia	Conduct sperm to urethra
Sex accessory glands	Produce seminal fluid that nourishes sperm
Urethra	Conducts sperm to outside
Penis	Organ of copulation
Scrotum	Provides proper temperature for testes

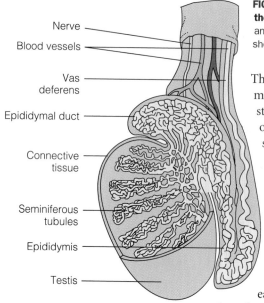

FIGURE 19-2 Interior View of the Testis The epididymal duct and seminiferous tubules are shown.

Thus, long-distance runners may become temporarily sterile. Tight-fitting pants or shorts can have the same effect.

Sperm Are Produced in the Seminiferous Tubules and Stored in the Epididymis

As **FIGURE 19-2** shows, each testis is surrounded by a dense layer of connective tissue. This layer is invested with numerous pain fibers, a fact to which most men will attest. Each testis contains numerous highly convoluted **seminiferous tubules** (SEM-in-IF-er-uss), in which sperm are formed. Stretched end to end, the seminiferous tubules of each testis would extend for about half a mile.

Sperm produced in the seminiferous tubules empty into a network of connecting tubules in the "back" of the testes. These tubules, in turn, empty into the **epididymal duct** (ep-eh-DID-eh-mal), where sperm are stored until released during **ejaculation**, the ejection of sperm. As **FIGURE 19-2** shows, the epididymal duct forms the **epididymis**. The epididymal duct empties into the **vas deferens** (plural, **vasa deferentia**, pronounced VAH-sah DEAF-er-en-she-ah). These ducts pass from the scrotum into the body cavity through the **inguinal canals,** small openings in the wall of the abdomen (**FIGURE 19-3A**).

As shown in **FIGURE 19-1**, the vasa deferentia empty directly into the urethra. Sperm therefore travel from the seminiferous tubules to the epididymal duct to the vas deferens to the urethra. The inguinal canals are potential weak spots in the abdominal wall. Loops of intestine can bulge through weakened canals of some men (**FIGURE 19-3B**). This condition, known as an **inguinal hernia,** can be corrected surgically. During surgery, an incision is made in the skin and fat. The loop of intestine is pushed back in the abdominal cavity. The weakened area is then repaired, usually by suturing the muscle together to close off the gap. In some cases, the weakened abdominal muscle is reinforced with a piece of synthetic mesh.

Semen Consists Mostly of Fluids Produced by the Sex Accessory Glands. During ejaculation, sperm are joined by fluids produced by the sex accessory glands. Located near the neck of the urinary bladder, the sex accessory glands include two seminal vesicles, the prostate gland, and two tiny Cowper's glands (**FIGURE 19-1**).

The sex accessory glands produce fluid. Together, these fluids make up 99% of the volume of the **ejaculate**, or **semen** (SEA-men). The remaining 1% consists of sperm produced in the seminiferous tubules.

Semen is therefore a fluid containing sperm and sex accessory gland secretions. The semen contains fructose, a monosaccharide that is used by sperm mitochondria to generate the energy needed to help propel the sperm through the female reproductive tract. Semen also contains a buffer that neutralizes the acidic secre-

FIGURE 19-3 The Inguinal Canal and Hernia *(a)* During development, the testis descends through the inguinal canal, an opening through the musculature in the lower abdominal wall. In adults, the inguinal canal provides a route for the vas deferens, blood vessels, and nerves that supply each testis. *(b)* Loops of intestine may push through the weakened musculature surrounding the inguinal canal.

FIGURE 19-4 Prostatic Nodules

tions of the female reproductive tract. Yet another component of the semen is prostaglandin, a chemical that causes the muscle of the uterus to contract, which is believed to be primarily responsible for the movement of sperm up the female tract. Interestingly, lymphocytes "patrol" the testes and seminal vesicles. If the lymphocytes are infected with the virus that causes AIDS, the disease can be spread to male or female sexual partners.

The paired **seminal vesicles** (SEM-in-al) empty into the vasa deferentia and produce the largest portion of the ejaculate. The **Cowper's glands** (COW-perz), a pair of small glands located below the prostate on either side of the urethra, are the smallest of the sex accessory glands.

The **prostate gland** (PROS-tate) surrounds the neck of the bladder and empties its contents directly into the urethra. Routine medical examinations of men over the age of 45 show that nearly all of them have enlarged prostates. This condition results from the formation of small nodules inside the gland. These nodules form by the condensation of prostatic secretions inside the gland (**FIGURE 19-4**). Although they usually cause no trouble, in some cases the nodules grow quite large and can block the flow of urine, making urination painful. In such cases, the prostate can be reamed out by a device inserted through the penis or can be removed through surgery.

The prostate is also a common site for cancer in men and should therefore be checked every year by a physician in men over 40. Prostate cancer typically remains undetected until either the tumor begins to press on the urethra, making urination difficult and painful, or metastases develop in tissues such as the bones, lymph nodes, and lungs. However, if a man over 40 receives an annual physical, physicians can detect prostate cancer early on.

Prostate cancers are detected by digit rectal exams that allow doctors to palpate the prostate. A blood test is also used to determine levels of prostate-specific antigen, that is, circulating levels of antigen produced by cancer cells. Ultrasound can be used to view the gland, and biopsies can be performed to remove tissue samples that are then examined under a microscope. If cancer is detected, further tests are done to see if the cancer has spread.

If cancer is confined to the gland, it will be removed surgically. Radiation can also be used to treat prostate cancer. If the cancer has spread, however, it may be too late. Hormone-blocking drugs, which inhibit testosterone's secretion or its actions, can be given to slow the growth of the tumor. The testes may also have to be removed to reduce testosterone secretion.

Sperm Are Formed from Stem Cells Known as Spermatogonia.

As noted previously, sperm are produced in the seminiferous tubules (**FIGURE 19-5A**). The lining of the wall of the tubule is known as the **germinal epithelium** because its cells give rise to sperm, the male germ cells. The formation of sperm is known as **spermatogenesis** (sper-MAT-oh-GEN-eh-siss) and involves two subprocesses: (1) a special type of cell division known as **meiosis** and (2) spermiogenesis (SPERM-ee-oh-GEN-eh-siss), a process of cellular differentiation (**FIGURE 19-5B**).

Spermatogenesis begins with **spermatogonia** (sper-MAT-oh-GO-nee-ah). Located in the periphery of the seminiferous tubule in the germinal epithelium, the spermatogonia divide mitotically and thus ensure a constant supply of sperm-producing cells. Some of the spermatogonia formed during cellular division, however, enlarge and become **primary spermatocytes** (sper-MAT-oh-sites). Two meiotic divisions follow in the formation of sperm.

As you may recall from Chapter 16, the first division in meiosis is meiosis I. During meiosis I, primary spermatocytes divide to form two **secondary spermatocytes** (**FIGURE 19-5B**). Each secondary spermatocyte contains 23 double-stranded chromosomes. During **meiosis II**, secondary spermatocytes divide, forming four **spermatids**. Each spermatid contains 23 single-stranded (unreplicated) chromosomes.

Spermatids soon develop into sperm (**FIGURE 19-5**). This process, called **spermiogenesis**, involves a dramatic transformation of the spermatid. During spermiogenesis, the round spermatid develops a tail. The nucleus condenses and the cytoplasm is eliminated. These changes streamline the cell so it is able to swim and to fertilize an ovum. It is another one of nature's most fascinating processes.

During spermiogenesis, the nuclear material of the spermatid condenses and most of the cytoplasm is shed to streamline the cell. The sperm tail also forms during this process from the centriole. Also during this amazing transformation, the mitochondria of the spermatid congregate around the first part of the tail, where they can provide energy for propulsion. The Golgi apparatus enlarges and forms an enzyme-filled cap that fits over the condensed nucleus like a stocking cap. This structure,

Each spermatogonium contains 46 single-stranded (unreplicated) chromosomes.

Each primary oocyte contains 46 double-stranded (replicated) chromosomes.

Each secondary oocyte contains 23 double-stranded chromosomes.

Each spermatid contains 23 single-stranded chromosomes.

FIGURE 19-5 The Seminiferous Tubules *(a)* A cross section through two seminiferous tubules showing the germinal epithelium and the interstitial cells. *(b)* Details of spermatogenesis.

the **acrosome** (ACK-row-sohm), will help the sperm digest its way through the coatings surrounding the ovum during fertilization.

The product of spermiogenesis is the **spermatozoan** (sper-MAT-oh-ZO-an), or mature **sperm**. It is a marvel of biological architecture—a true testimony of the marriage of structure and function. Rid of excess cytoplasmic baggage, it is streamlined for relatively swift movement.

On average, men produce 200–300 million sperm every day. The average 3-milliliter ejaculate contains 240 million or more—40 million short of the U.S. population. Such large numbers no doubt evolved because many sperm are required to ensure fertilization. In fact, nearly all sperm are eliminated as they travel through the female reproductive tract.

In humans, each sperm formed during meiosis contains 23 single-stranded (unreplicated) chromosomes—half the number in a normal somatic cell. Thus, when the sperm unites with an ovum (also containing 23 unreplicated chromosomes), they produce a **zygote** containing 46 single-stranded chromosomes. One-half of its chromosomes come from each parent. We'll examine its fate in Chapter 20.

Interstitial Cells Produce the Male Sex Steroid Testosterone

The testes do more than produce sperm. They also produce hormones, male sex hormones to be exact. These hormones are produced in cells found in spaces lying between the seminiferous tubules. Here you will find clumps of large cells known as **interstitial cells** (in-ter-STISH-al) (**FIGURE 19-6**). These cells produce a group of

Seminiferous tubule   Interstitial cells

FIGURE 19-6 Interstitial Cells Cross section of the wall of a seminiferous tubule showing the interstitial cells.

(a) Sebaceous glands associated with hair follicles secrete sebum, an oily substance that lubricates the skin.

Sebaceous gland

Hair follicle

Blockage

(b) A follicle may become blocked by excess sebum and dead skin cells. Unable to escape, the sebum builds up in the hair follicle.

Pimple

Pus

(c) Bacteria present on the skin may infect the sebum, causing inflammation; pus and swelling form an acne pimple.

FIGURE 19-7 Formation of an Acne Pimple *(a)* Testosterone stimulates oil production in the sebaceous glands. *(b)* If the outlet is blocked, sebum builds up in the gland and *(c)* the gland may become infected.

sex steroid hormones known as **androgens**, so named because they exert a masculinizing effect. The most important androgen is **testosterone**. Testosterone diffuses out of the interstitial cells and into the seminiferous tubules, where it stimulates spermatogenesis (prophase I) and spermiogenesis, the maturation of sperm. In the absence of testosterone, sperm cell production declines, then stops, and the walls of the seminiferous tubules shrink.

Testosterone is also transported in the bloodstream throughout the body, where it affects a variety of target cells. For example, it stimulates cellular growth in bone

and muscle and accounts in part for the fact that men are generally taller and more massive than women. In addition, testosterone promotes facial hair growth and thickening of the vocal cords, typically giving men deeper voices than women. Testosterone stimulates growth of the laryngeal cartilage, producing the prominent bulge called the *Adam's apple*. It also stimulates cell growth in the skin, making most men's skin slightly thicker than women's.

Testosterone affects the hair follicles on the heads of genetically predisposed men, causing pattern baldness. It is not the absence of testosterone, as some believe, but the presence of testosterone and certain genes that lead to this condition.

Testosterone also stimulates the sebaceous glands of the skin in both sexes. **Sebaceous glands** (seh-BAY-schuss) secrete oil onto the skin, moisturizing it (**FIGURE 19-7A**). During puberty (sexual maturation) in boys, testosterone levels rise dramatically, causing a marked increase in sebaceous gland activity. Dead skin cells may block the pores that normally carry the oil to the skin's surface (**FIGURE 19-7B**). As a result, sebum collects inside the glands. Bacteria on the skin often invade and proliferate in the small pools of oil, resulting in inflammation, pus formation, and swelling. The skin protrudes, forming an **acne pimple**.

Mild acne can be treated by washing the skin twice a day with warm, not hot, water and a mild, unscented soap. Be sure not scrub the skin. Wash gently. You should also apply a cream containing benzoyl peroxide daily to areas. Women should avoid makeup that has an oily base or use a nonoily type of foundation and wash their faces thoroughly each night. Sunlight also helps clear up acne, because it dries the oil on the skin and kills skin bacteria. Doctors may prescribe topical antibiotics. Pimples should not be picked either, as this may worsen the condition and cause scarring.

Moderate acne can be successfully treated with an oral antibiotic such as tetracycline or erythromycin. Severe acne can be treated by special ointments and antibiotics given by a dermatologist, skin doctor. One relatively new and fairly successful drug is Retin-A, a derivative of vitamin A.

The Penis Contains Erectile Tissue That Fills with Blood During Sexual Arousal

Sperm are deposited in the female reproductive tract with the aid of the **penis**. The penis consists of a shaft of varying length and an enlarged tip, the **glans penis** (**FIGURE 19-8**). The glans is covered by a sheath of skin at birth, the **foreskin**. The foreskin gradually becomes separated from the glans in the first 2 years of life. At puberty, the inner lining of the foreskin begins to pro-

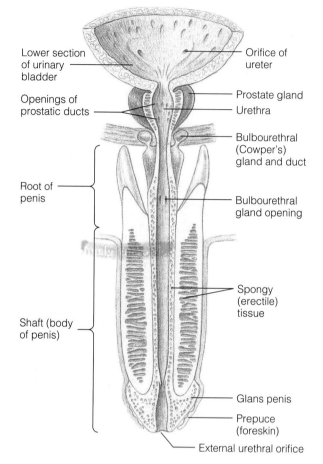

Lower section
of urinary
bladder

Orifice of
ureter

Openings of
prostatic ducts

Prostate gland

Urethra

Bulbourethral
(Cowper's)
gland and duct

Root of
penis

Bulbourethral
gland opening

Spongy
(erectile)
tissue

Shaft (body
of penis)

Glans penis

Prepuce
(foreskin)

External urethral orifice

FIGURE 19-8 Anatomy of the Penis The penis consists
principally of spongy tissue that fills with blood during sexual
arousal. The urethra passes through the penis, carrying urine
or semen.

duce an oily secretion. Bacteria can grow in the protected, nutrient-rich environment created by the foreskin, so special precautions must be taken to keep the area clean.

Because of potential health problems or religious reasons, many parents opt to have the foreskin removed in the first few days of their son's life. The operation, called **circumcision** (sir-come-SIZH-un; literally, "to cut around"), may help reduce penile cancer in men and may also reduce cervical cancer in the wives or sexual partners of circumcised men, as explained in the Point/Counterpoint in this chapter.

For successful copulation, the penis must become rigid, or erect. During sexual arousal, nerve impulses in the parasympathetic division of the autonomic nervous system cause arterioles in the penis to dilate. Blood flows into a spongy **erectile tissue** (eh-REK-tile) in the shaft of the penis, making it harden. The growing turgidity (swelling) compresses a large vein on the dor-

sal surface of the penis, blocking the outflow of blood and further stiffening the organ.

Coursing through the penis is the urethra, a duct that carries urine from the bladder to the outside of the body during urination. The urethra also transports semen—sperm, and secretions of the sex accessory glands during ejaculation.

Some men lose their ability to achieve or to sustain an erection. This condition is known as **impotence** (IM-poe-tense). Most men experience impotence at some time in their life, but it is usually temporary. Persistent impotence, however, is more serious condition, and is more common in middle-age and elderly men.

Persistent impotence may be caused by psychological, physical, or physiological problems—often combinations of them. Marital conflict, stress, fatigue, and anxiety all contribute to impotence. Nerve damage may also cause impotence. Alcohol ingestion and some medications may contribute to the condition as well. Blockages in the arteries leading to the penis may be the cause in some cases. Low testosterone levels can cause this troubling disorder.

Smoking is also a major contibutor to impotence. In fact, 52% of all men from 40 to 60 years of age suffer from impotence; smokers are twice as likely to be impotent as nonsmokers because smoking causes arterioles in the penis to constrict, reducing blood flow. Smoking also causes the buildup of atherosclerotic plaque, which permanently blocks blood flow to this organ.

In cases of persistent impotence, medical care is highly recommended, though few men will see a doctor. If the problem is psychological, therapy is often advised. Rest and relaxation help, as will reductions in anxiety. If the problem is a result of atherosclerosis in the arteries supplying the penis, surgery can help. If the problem is a medication you're taking, a change of prescription might be beneficial. Patients with nerve damage, however, are likely to suffer permanent impotence. Nerve damage may result from diabetes mellitus or from a traumatic accident.

For patients with irreversible impotence, urologists can surgically insert an inflatable plastic implant in the penis. The implant is attached to a small, fluid-filled reservoir in the scrotum. The fluid is manually pumped into the implant, making the penis erect upon demand, thus permitting sexual intercourse. Other types of implants are also available. Vacuum pumps can be used, too. These devices use a plastic cylinder that is fitted over the penis. A hand-held pump is used to create a vacuum. Blood rushes into the penis, causing an erection. After the vacuum aspirator is removed, rubber bands are placed around the base of the penis to maintain an erection.

Stimulates

Inhibits

FIGURE 19-9 Hormonal Control of Testicular Function Testosterone, FSH, and ICSH participate in a negative feedback loop. The testes also produce a substance called *inhibin*, which controls GnRH secretion.

send impulses to the smooth muscle in the walls of the epididymis and vasa deferentia, causing them to contract. Muscle contraction, in turn, propels sperm into the urethra.

Nerve impulses from the spinal cord also stimulate the smooth muscle in the walls of the sex accessory glands to contract, causing these glands to empty their secretions into the vasa deferentia and the urethra. The sperm and secretions from the sex accessory glands combine in the urethra to form semen.

Semen is propelled onward by smooth muscle contractions in the walls of the urethra, which cause the sperm to be released in spurts.

The Male Reproductive System Is Controlled by Three Hormones: Testosterone, Luteinizing Hormone, and Follicle-Stimulating Hormone

As noted earlier, the testes produce sex steroid hormones—mainly, testosterone. Testosterone secretion, however, is controlled by a hormone from the pituitary gland. This hormone is known as **luteinizing hormone (LH)**. In males, LH is also known as **interstitial cell stimulating hormone (ICSH)**. It gets this name because it stimulates the interstitial cells to produce androgen hormones.

ICSH secretion is controlled by a releasing hormone produced by the hypothalamus, known as **gonadotropin releasing hormone (GnRH)**. As **FIGURE 19-9** shows, the secretion of GnRH and ICSH is controlled by testosterone levels in the blood in a classic negative feedback loop. When testosterone levels in the blood decline, chemoreceptors in the hypothalamus detect the change and signal an increase in GnRH secretion. This hormone flows in the blood to the anterior pituitary where ICSH is produced. GnRH stimulates the production and release of ICSH. It travels in the bloodstream to the testes, where it stimulates testosterone production. But when testosterone levels return to normal, GnRH release subsides, as does ICSH secretion.

The pituitary also produces the gonadotropin **follicle-stimulating hormone** or **FSH**. Like testosterone, FSH stimulates spermatogenesis (**FIGURE 19-9**). However, FSH does not act directly on the spermatogenic cells. Instead, it exerts its influence through another cell in the germinal epithelium of the seminiferous tubule, the Sertoli cell (ser-TOLL-ee). **Sertoli cells**, are large "nurse cells." The spermatogenic cells

A number of drug treatments are also available including the much-talked-about drug Viagra, which promotes erection when men are sexually aroused. Viagra works by causing the muscle in the walls of the arteries supplying the penis to relax. This permits blood to flow into the organ more readily when stimulated.

Ejaculation Is a Reflex Mechanism

Ejaculation occurs when the penis is erect and is a reflex. Here's how the reflex is triggered: Sexual stimulation results in the transmission of nerve impulses along sensory nerves. When it becomes intense, sensory nerve impulses traveling to the spinal cord activate motor neurons located in the cord. These neurons, in turn,

The Medical Debate over Circumcision

An Unnecessary and Costly Practice

Dr. Thomas Metcalf

Dr. Thomas J. Metcalf *is a clinical associate professor of pediatrics at the University of Utah and practices at Willow Creek Pediatrics in Salt Lake City.*

Routine neonatal circumcision continues to be performed on the majority of American boys. I remain convinced that routine circumcision of the newborn is not needed if adequate hygiene of the uncircumcised penis is maintained throughout life. Circumcision costs the American public a significant amount of money and remains a culturally motivated operation without a valid medical *raison d'etre*.

Circumcision for nonreligious reasons began in the United States in the 1870s when genital surgery of both sexes became established as a preventive and/or cure for masturbation. Though genital surgery of females declined, circumcision of males persisted in the United States, even as it fell into disfavor in Europe. In 1949, Gairdner and other authors began to speak out against routine newborn circumcision. The medical community gradually came to the position that "newborn circumcision has potential medical benefits and advantages as well as disadvantages and risks" (1989, American Academy of Pediatrics).

Eighty percent of the world remains uncircumcised. In the United States, however, 60%–90% of 1.9 million male newborns are circumcised annually. The cost for a newborn circumcision in Salt Lake City, Utah is $110; in other areas of the U.S. the cost is 2–3 times higher. Thus, the total annual cost to the American public for newborn circumcisions is between $209 million and $627 million. Are there compelling reasons to circumcise newborn boys at such an expense, in an era of burgeoning health care costs? Is circumcision a public health measure, an "immunization"?

Wiswell and others, in retrospective studies, have documented a greater incidence of urinary tract infections (UTIs) in uncircumcised male infants, roughly 1%–2% versus 0.1% in circumcised infants. A prospective, controlled study has not been published. The higher rate in uncircumcised males could be due to more frequent and heavier colonization of the periurethral area by pathogens. However, circumcision cannot be thought of as a protective "immunization" against UTI. If a male infant presents with a febrile illness for which no obvious source of infection is found, the physician must consider the possibility of a UTI in *either* a circumcised or uncircumcised male. Circumcision does not obviate the need for this evaluation, which currently costs $99 in Salt Lake City. Given a UTI incidence of 1%–2% in uncircumcised infants, the cost to prevent one UTI by performing 100 circumcisions is $11,000.

Circumcision largely prevents cancer of the penis, which has a mortality rate of up to 25%. This would seem a strong argument for neonatal circumcision as a preventive. However, other factors play a role. According to a report by the Task Force on Circumcision, in developed countries where circumcision is not routinely performed (and parents and boys are used to caring for the uncircumcised penis), the incidence of penile carcinoma ranges from 0.3 to 1.1 per 100,000 men per year, about half the incidence in uncircumcised U.S. men, but greater than that in circumcised men. In developing countries with lower standards of hygiene, the incidence is from 3 to 6 per 100,000 men per year. Thus, good hygiene may make up for the effect of circumcision, at a fraction of the cost. A recent case-controlled study in Washington and British Columbia showed only a 3.2 times greater risk for uncircumcised relative to circumcised men.

Sexually transmitted diseases (STDs) have been shown in some studies to be more prevalent in uncircumcised men. Parker et al. showed a significantly higher risk of four types of STDs among uncircumcised men in Australia. However, these authors did not recommend circumcision to prevent STDs. They stated that "if these findings are confirmed in other studies, it would seem that attention should be directed to the improvement of personal hygiene among uncircumcised men." In the final analysis, physicians cannot promote circumcision as an effective way to prevent STDs.

Lack of circumcision appears to be associated with an increased risk of transmission of the AIDS virus. This correlation has been shown in both clinic-based studies and in a statistical study of male circumcision status in 37 African capital cities. The authors of the study suggest that lack of circumcision is a co-factor in HIV infection, not causative. They state that uncircumcised African males "are apparently at increased risk of developing chancroid and other genital-ulcer disease," which, in turn, facilitate infection with HIV; they also write that perhaps the intact foreskin enhances viral survival and, finally, that more frequent infection of the glans of the penis increases susceptibility to HIV. Again, while all this may be true, circumcision would not be an effective way of solving the AIDS epidemic and should not be promoted as such.

Complications of routine newborn circumcision are indeed infrequent, and most are easily treated. The use of xylocaine for local anesthesia, while inflicting its own pain, renders the remainder of the circumcision procedure painless in 80% of cases.

Studies in the United States and New Zealand have shown more problems in caring for the uncircumcised penis in the first few years of life, but data from Europe suggest that the uncircumcised penis presents few problems for parents and boys used to dealing with it. In any event, problems that arise during care of the circumcised *or* uncircumcised penis are generally minor, requiring only one medical visit for correction.

In summary, there is an increasing body of evidence for the medical benefits of newborn circumcision. However, this data is insufficient to support advocating circumcision, and its cost, as a national public health measure. Even in an individual case, a physician could never say, "Circumcise your newborn and he'll not have to worry about STDs, UTIs, penile cancer, or AIDS." Thus, newborn circumcision remains a costly, painful, and unnecessary procedure.

A Safe and Beneficial Procedure

Dr. Thomas Wiswell

Sixty percent to 90% of newborn boys (1.2 to 1.8 million) are circumcised annually in the United States. Several issues have convinced me of the benefits of this procedure: (1) the prevention of urinary tract infections (UTIs) and complications from them; (2) the prevention of penile cancer; (3) the lower incidence of sexually transmissible diseases in uncircumcised males; (4) the low risk for complications from the operation; (5) the greater incidence of penile problems among "intact" boys; and (6) recent evidence showing that circumcision protects against AIDS.

Circumcised boys are 10–39 times less likely to have UTIs during infancy. From population studies involving more than 600,000 children, there are nine investigations that have confirmed the increased risk for UTIs among uncircumcised male infants. In addition, three other studies have found older boys and adult males who are uncircumcised to be more likely to develop these infections. Urinary tract infections are not benign. More than 36% of 88 boys below 1 month of age with a UTI had concurrent infection in their bloodstream. Furthermore, three of these infants had concomitant meningitis, two had renal failure, and two died. Littlewood has reported that 11% of children with a UTI during the first month of life may die. There are longer-term effects of UTIs in children. In infected infants, 10%–15% will subsequently demonstrate kidney scarring. Approximately 10% of these infants will develop high blood pressure, and 2%–3% will ultimately require dialysis or kidney transplantation.

Penile cancer is the only malignancy that can be prevented categorically by a prophylactic procedure, neonatal circumcision. Of the more than 60,000 cases of penile cancer that have occurred in the United States since 1930, fewer than 10 have been in circumcised men. More than 1000 men develop penile cancer each year, and

225–317 die from it annually. The basic therapy for this malignancy is amputation of the penis.

Virtually all sexually transmissible diseases (STDs) have been found to occur more frequently among uncircumcised men. There are more than 70 references that have found STDs to occur more often among "intact" individuals. I am struck by the paucity of contrary reports. There is only one report of a venereal disease (nongonococcal urethritis) being more common in circumcised men. However, in this population, more than 60% of the cases of another STD (gonorrhea) occurred in uncircumcised men.

Serious complications from routine foreskin removal are infrequent and relatively minor. We have recently examined a population of more than 100,000 circumcised boys and found complications in fewer than 2 per 1000. Two other large investigations reported complications from circumcision in 0.06% and 0.20% of circumcised boys, respectively. The majority of the complications are easily treated bleeding and minor infections. Atypical complications of the procedure (glans loss, staphylococcal scalded skin syndrome, etc.) occur infrequently and receive note due to their uniqueness. Death rarely occurs as a complication of circumcision. To date, there have been a total of three reported deaths in the United States since 1954 that can be ascribed to neonatal circumcision. This contrasts sharply with the potentially preventable 7500–11,500 deaths from penile cancer that occurred during the same period.

Herzog and Alvarez found uncircumcised boys aged 4 months to 12 years to be more likely to have "penile problems" than were circumcised boys. Fergusson et al. similarly described uncircumcised boys as having more problems than their circumcised counterparts during the first 8 years of life. In both investigations, the "problems" largely consisted of balanitis (infection in and around the head of the penis) and phimosis (an abnormal constriction

of the foreskin that prevents urine from being excreted). Recent investigations have confirmed that adult uncircumcised men will have more "penile problems" (the majority of which are balanitis and phimosis) than their circumcised counterparts. Finally, we found the risks from circumcision during the first month of life to be fewer than the risks from the uncircumcised state.

Dr. Thomas E. Wiswell *is a professor of pediatrics and director of Neonatal Research at Thomas Jefferson University in Philadelphia.*

Over the past six years, at least eight investigations from the United States and Africa have found uncircumcised men to be 4 to 12 times more likely to become infected with the human immunodeficiency virus (HIV—the AIDS virus).

As a pediatrician, I am a child advocate. I have pondered this issue for many years. I understand that we would have to circumcise "the many" to protect "the few." However, we have no way of identifying "the few." Neonatal circumcision is a rapid and generally safe procedure that must be performed by experienced caretakers. With the low complication rate and the many benefits of the procedure, I personally believe we should routinely circumcise newborn boys.

Sharpening Your Critical Thinking Skills

1. Summarize the key points of each author, then list the data they use to support their main points.

Visit *Human Biology's* Internet site for links to web sites offering more information on this topic.

FIGURE 19-10 Anatomy of the Female Reproductive Tract   *(a)* Frontal view. *(b)* Midsagittal view.

(a)

(b)

(spermatogonia, spermatocytes, and spermatids) divide and differentiate within folds in the plasma membrane of the Sertoli cell, moving slowly to the surface of the germinal epithelium. The spermatids produced during spermatogenesis remain attached to the Sertoli cells, where they differentiate into sperm.

FSH stimulates the Sertoli cells to produce a cytoplasmic receptor protein that binds to testosterone. Called **androgen-binding protein**, this receptor concentrates testosterone within the Sertoli cell. Testosterone, in turn, stimulates spermatogenesis.

FSH secretion is controlled by GnRH and a peptide hormone called **inhibin**, which is produced by Sertoli cells. Inhibin gets its name from the fact that it inhibits the activity of FSH-secreting cells in the anterior pituitary and thus blocks the action of GnRH. When inhibin levels are high, FSH secretion is low.

Section 19-2

The Female Reproductive System

FIGURE 19-10 illustrates the **female reproductive system,** which consists of two parts: the external genitalia and the reproductive tract. We'll start with the internal structures of the female reproductive tract: (1) the ovaries, (2) the uterine tubes, (3) the uterus, and (4) the vagina. **TABLE 19-2** summarizes the role of each structure.

The Uterus and Uterine Tubes Are Hollow Muscular Organs That Connect the Vagina, the Site of Sperm Deposition, with the Ovaries Where the Ova Are Produced

The **uterus** or **womb** is a pear-shaped organ about 7 centimeters (3 inches) long and about 2 centimeters

TABLE 19-2

The Female Reproductive System

Component	Function
Ovaries	Produce ova and female sex steroids
Uterine tubes	Transport sperm to ova; transport fertilized ova to uterus
Uterus	Nourishes and protects embryo and fetus
Vagina	Site of sperm deposition, birth canal

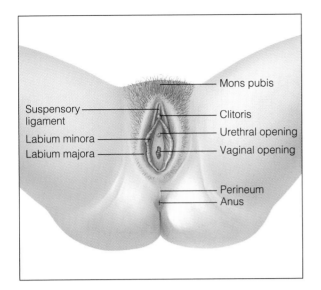

Mons pubis

Suspensory ligament

Clitoris

Urethral opening

Labium minora

Labium majora

Vaginal opening

Perineum

Anus

FIGURE 19-11 Female External Genitalia

(less than 1 inch) wide at its broadest point in nonpregnant women.[1] The wall of the uterus contains a thick layer of smooth muscle cells, the **myometrium** (MY-oh-ME-tree-um). The uterus houses and nourishes the developing fetus.

Attached to the uterus are two hollow, muscular tubes, known as the **uterine tubes** (YOU-ter-in), or **oviducts** (OH-va-ducts). In humans, the uterine tubes are often referred to as the **Fallopian tubes** (fal-OH-PE-ee-an). As **FIGURE 19-10A** shows, the ends of the uterine tubes are widened like a catcher's mitt and fit loosely over the ovaries. The **ovaries** (OH-var-ees) are paired, almond-shaped organs. Currents created by cilia in the lining of the uterine tubes draw the ova inside and down the tubes to the uterus.

Fertilization occurs in the upper third of the uterine tubes. The fertilized ovum is then transported down the uterine tubes to the uterus. Inside the uterus, the fertilized ovum attaches to the lining, or the **endometrium** (EN-doh-MEE-tree-um), and embeds itself there, remaining for the duration of pregnancy.

At birth, the baby is expelled from the uterus through the **cervix** (SIR-vix), the lowermost portion of the uterus. As **FIGURE 19-10** shows, the cervix protrudes into the vagina (vah-GINE-ah). The **vagina** is a distensible, 3-inch, tubular organ that leads to the outside of the body.[2] Although it is quite narrow, the cervix stretches considerably at birth to allow the passage of the baby into the vagina. The vagina also serves as the receptacle for sperm during sexual intercourse. To reach the ovum, sperm must travel through a tiny opening and narrow

canal of the cervix that leads into the uterus. From here, sperm move up both uterine tubes.

The **external genitalia** are the externally visible parts of the female reproductive system. They consist of two flaps of skin on either side of the vaginal opening (**FIGURE 19-11**). The outer folds are the **labia majora** (LAY-bee-ah ma-JOR-ah). These large folds of skin are covered with hair on the outer surface and contain numerous sebaceous glands on the inside. The inner flaps are the **labia minora** (meh-NOR-ah). Anteriorly, they meet to form a hood over a small knot of tissue called the **clitoris** (CLIT-er-iss). The clitoris consists of erectile tissue and is a highly sensitive organ involved in female sexual arousal. It is formed from the same embryonic tissue as the penis. In fact, some women are born with greatly elongated clitorides (plural).

The Ovaries Produce Ova and Release Them During Ovulation

During each menstrual cycle, one ovary releases an **ovum**, the female gamete. This process is called ovulation (OV-you-LAY-shun).[3] The ovum or egg is drawn into the uterine tube.

The release of an ovum occurs approximately once a month in women during their reproductive years—from puberty (age 11–15) to menopause (age 45–55). Ovulation is temporarily halted when a woman is pregnant and may be suppressed by emotional and physical stress.

The structure of an ovary is shown in **FIGURE 19-12**. As illustrated, several ovarian landmarks are visible. One is the female germ cells—immature ova or **oocytes**. Oocytes develop from **oogonia** (oh-oh-GO-knee-uh), cells akin to the spermatogonia of the seminiferous tubules. Oogonia, however, are only found in fetal ovaries. Well before birth, they enter meiosis I but do not complete it. At birth, all oogonia have therefore been converted into primary oocytes. Each primary oocyte contains 46 chromosomes and undergoes two meiotic divisions. This process is called **oogenesis** (oh-oh-GEN-eh-siss). Meiosis is similar in oogenesis and spermatogenesis. However, oogenesis produces only one ovum, whereas spermatogenesis produces four sperm. How does this happen?

During each meiotic division in oogenesis, the nucleus divides in half, but the cytoplasm doesn't (**FIGURE 19-13**). Thus, the first meiotic division produces

---

[1]The uterus is slightly larger in women who have had children, and it enlarges considerably during pregnancy to accommodate the growing fetus.

[2]The vagina is often called the *birth canal.*

---

[3]The release of the ovum is not an explosive event, although many women feel a sharp pain when it occurs.

FIGURE 19-12 Structure of the Ovary   *(a)* This drawing illustrates the phases of follicular development and also shows the formation and destruction of the corpus luteum (CL). Antral follicles give rise to the CL. A fully formed CL and antral follicle would not be found in the ovary at the same time. *(b)* A recently ovulated follicle showing the corona radiata and zona pellucida.

(a)

(b)

only one cell, the **secondary oocyte**, and a small package of discarded nuclear material containing 23 double-stranded chromosomes. This structure is called the **first polar body** and contains a tiny amount of cytoplasm.

During the second meiotic division, the nucleus divides again, but the cytoplasm doesn't. This "unequal division" results in the formation of an ovum, containing 23 single-stranded chromosomes and yet another "nuclear discard," the **second polar body**.[4]

Germ cells are housed in the ovary in special structures called *follicles* (**FIGURE 19-12A**). A **follicle** consists of a primary oocyte surrounded by one or more layers of **follicle cells**, which are derived from the loose connective tissue of the ovary.

FIGURE 19-13 (right side) illustrates the growth and development of follicles. Each month, a dozen or so follicles begin to develop. During early development, the oocyte enlarges. The follicle cells divide and grow, first forming a complete layer around the oocyte, then forming many layers.

In the largest follicles, a clear liquid begins to accumulate between the follicle cells. The fluid creates small spaces among the follicle cells, which enlarge as additional fluid is generated. Eventually, the cavities coalesce, forming one central cavity. At this point, the follicle is called an **antral follicle** (AN-tril). Although a dozen or so follicles begin developing during each cycle, as a rule only one makes it to ovulation. The rest stop growing and degenerate.

The follicle (or follicles) that survives continues to enlarge by accumulating more fluid. As the fluid builds up, the antral follicle begins to bulge from the surface of the ovary, not unlike a pimple. The pressure exerted on the outside of the ovary causes the ovary's surface to stretch. Blood vessels supplying the tissue may be com-

[4]Note that the second meiotic division occurs only after a sperm penetrates the secondary oocyte. Additionally, in humans and virtually all other animals, the first polar body usually does not divide.

FIGURE 19-13 Oogenesis and Follicle Development

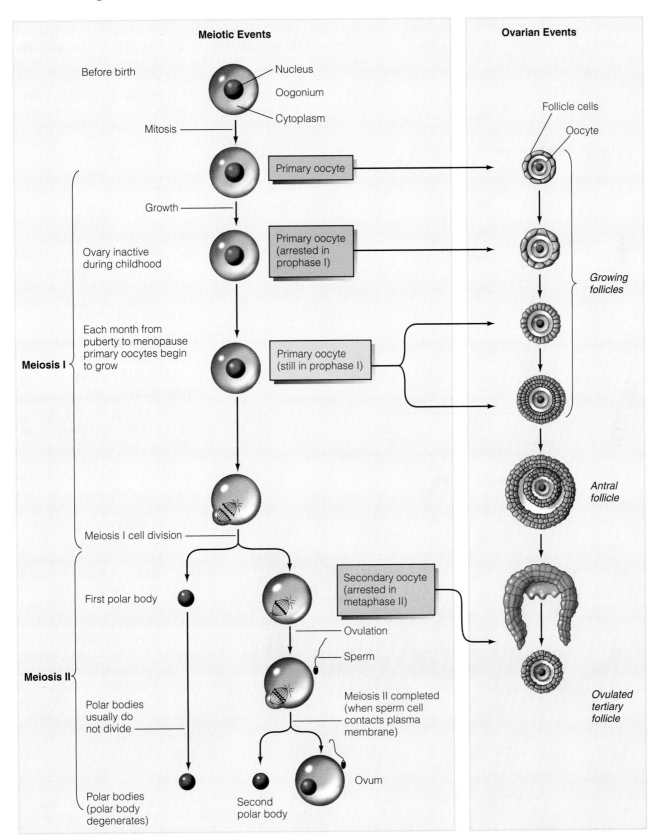

pressed, resulting in a region of cellular necrosis (neh-CROW-siss). Necrosis means death. This weakens the wall. Enzymes released from ovarian cells in the region then begin to digest the tissue at the weak point. Eventually, the wall of the follicle breaks down, and the oocyte is released.

Around the time of ovulation, the primary oocyte in the antral follicle completes the first meiotic division (**FIGURE 19-13**). It is then called a **secondary oocyte**. As **FIGURE 19-12B** shows, the secondary oocyte is surrounded by a fairly thick layer of gel-like material called the **zona pellucida** (pell-LEW-seh-dah) (**FIGURE 19-12B**). It is surrounded by a layer of follicle cells.

During ovulation, the oocyte and surrounding cells are expelled from the ovary, and the ovulated follicle collapses. The collapsed follicle forms the **corpus luteum** (CORE-puss LEU-tee-um; "yellow body") or **CL** for short—so named because of the yellow pigment it contains in cows and pigs (**FIGURE 19-14**).

The CL is a transient endocrine gland that produces two sex hormones, estrogen and progesterone. The fate of the CL ultimately depends on the fate of the oocyte. If the oocyte is fertilized, the CL remains active for several months, producing the estrogen and progesterone needed for a successful pregnancy. If fertilization does not occur, the CL soon disappears. (More on this in Chapter 20.)

Cyclic Changes in Pituitary Hormones in Women Are Responsible for the Menstrual Cycle

Women of reproductive age undergo a series of interdependent hormonal, ovarian, and uterine changes each month known as the **menstrual cycle** (MEN-strell). The length of the menstrual cycle varies from one woman to the next. In some it lasts 25 days, and in others it may last 35 days. The length of the menstrual cycle may also vary from month to month in the same woman. On average, however, the cycle repeats itself every 28 days. Ovulation usually occurs approximately at the midpoint of the 28-day cycle, or about 14 days before the onset of menstruation.

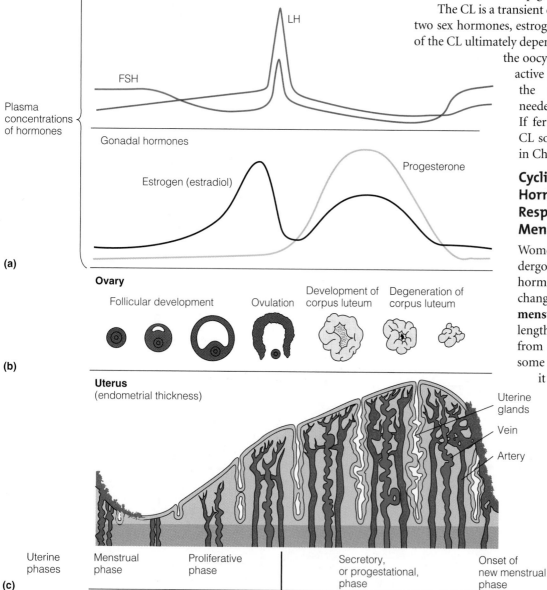

FIGURE 19-14 The Menstrual Cycle
(a) Hormonal cycles. (b) The ovarian cycle. (c) The uterine cycle.

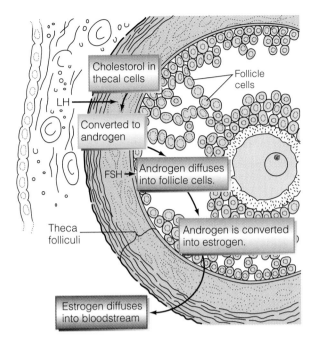

FIGURE 19-15 Estrogen Production in the Ovary

As noted above, the menstrual cycle involves three interdependent cycles (**FIGURE 19-14**). The first is a hormonal cycle. The hormonal cycle, in turn, produces cyclic changes in the ovary (the ovarian cycle) and the uterus (the uterine cycle). Understanding the menstrual cycle is easiest if we begin with the hormonal and ovarian cycles.

The Hormonal and Ovarian Cycles. The first half of the menstrual cycle is known as the follicular phase, because it is during this time that the follicles grow toward ovulation. The second half is called the **luteal phase** (LU-tee-al), so named because the corpus luteum forms during this time. To understand what drives these changes, let's turn our attention first to the pituitary gland, a small, pea-shaped endocrine gland suspended from the hypothalamus by a narrow stalk.

The pituitary releases two gonadotropic hormones, FSH and LH. These hormones peak in the middle of the menstrual cycle, just before ovulation. As its name implies, FSH stimulates follicular development by stimulating the mitotic division of the follicle cells. FSH's counterpart, LH, stimulates estrogen production by follicles. Estrogen, in turn, stimulates mitotic division of follicle cells, promoting growth.

As illustrated in **FIGURE 19-15**, estrogen production occurs in cells on the periphery of the antral follicles, known as **thecal cells.** These cells biochemically convert cholesterol to androgen under the influence of LH. Androgen, in turn, diffuses into the follicle cells, where it is converted to estrogen.[5]

LH and FSH secretion are controlled in a classical negative feedback mechanism involving estrogen and GnRH, which is produced by the hypothalamus. As a result, throughout most of the follicular phase, LH and FSH levels are low and fairly constant. Just before ovulation, however, LH and FSH secretion by the pituitary increases dramatically. These surges in LH and FSH secretion are the result of one of the body's rarest events, a positive feedback loop. Here's how it is triggered.

As **FIGURE 19-14A** shows, during the follicular phase of the menstrual cycle, the amount of estrogen in a woman's blood creeps up fairly slowly. When estrogen reaches a certain critical level, however, both the hypothalamus and the anterior pituitary respond with a sudden outpouring of LH and FSH.

The LH surge has at least four effects: (1) It causes the primary oocyte to complete its first meiotic division, forming a secondary oocyte. (2) It stimulates the release of the enzymes that break down the ovarian wall, resulting in ovulation. (3) It stimulates estrogen production and release. (4) It converts the collapsed follicle into a corpus luteum. The role of the preovulatory surge of FSH, if any, is not known.

During the second half of the menstrual cycle, the luteal phase, LH secretion gradually declines (**FIGURE 19-14A**). The small amount of LH that is present during this stage, however, stimulates the corpus luteum to produce estrogen and progesterone. If pregnancy does not occur, the CL stops producing hormones and degenerates (**FIGURE 19-14B**). Only a hormonal signal (discussed later) from the newly formed embryo can save it.

The Uterine Cycle. The uterine lining, or endometrium, also undergoes cyclic changes during the menstrual cycle (**FIGURE 19-14C**). These changes result from cyclic changes in ovarian hormones, which, as just discussed, are controlled by changes in pituitary hormone secretion. Before we examine the details of this process, take a moment to study **FIGURE 19-14C**. As illustrated, the endometrium thickens throughout much of the cycle in preparation for pregnancy. In the absence of fertilization, most of the thickened endometrium is shed, a process called **menstruation** (MEN-strew-A-shun).

To understand how the endometrium responds to hormonal changes, we begin on day 1 of the average 28-day menstrual cycle. Day 1 of the cycle marks the first day of menstruation. During the next 4 or 5 days, the uterine lining is shed—that is, the tissue that formed in the previous menstrual cycle sloughs (sluffs) off from the lining. It then passes out of the uterus into the vagina along with a considerable amount of blood—on average, about 50–150 milliliters. Incidentally, the loss

---

[5]FSH is also necessary for this conversion.

of blood during menstruation is the reason that women are more prone to develop anemia than men and why women should take iron supplements or eat iron-rich foods.

As soon as the endometrium has been shed, the lining of the uterus begins to rebuild—to prepare for the possibility of a pregnancy in the new cycle. Initial regrowth in the follicular phase is stimulated by ovarian estrogen. Estrogen stimulates the growth of glands (**uterine glands**) in the endometrium and also promotes cell division in the basal layer (deepest layer) of the endometrium—all that is left after menstruation. During the first half of the cycle, also called the **proliferative phase**, the uterine glands begin to fill with a nutritive secretion that will nourish an embryo should fertilization occur.

After ovulation the endometrium continues to thicken under the influence of estrogen and progesterone. The uterine glands become distended with a glycogen-rich secretion. The last half of the uterine cycle is therefore called the **secretory phase**.

If fertilization does not occur, the uterine lining starts to shrink approximately 4 days before the end of the cycle, then begins to slough off, starting menstruation. The shedding of the uterine lining (menstruation) is triggered by a decline in estrogen and progesterone concentrations in the blood. When progesterone levels fall, the uterus begins to undergo periodic contractions. That's because progesterone inhibits smooth muscle contraction in the myometrium. These contractions propel the detached endometrial tissue out of the uterus and are responsible for the cramps that many women experience during menstruation.

If fertilization occurs, the newly formed embryo produces a hormone called **human chorionic gonadotropin** (KO-ree-ON-ick), or **HCG**. HCG is an LH-like hormone that stimulates the corpus luteum, maintaining its structure and function. When HCG is present, estrogen and progesterone continue to be secreted by the CL. As a result, the uterine lining remains intact. When the newly formed embryo arrives in the uterus, it attaches to the thickened lining. It then embeds in the endometrium from which it derives its nutrients.

HCG shows up in detectable levels in a woman's blood and urine about 10 days after fertilization. If the ovum is fertilized and the zygote successfully embeds in the uterine lining, HCG will maintain the CL for approximately 6 months.

FIGURE 19-16 Home Pregnancy Test

Pregnancy tests available through a doctor's office or drugstore detect HCG in a woman's urine, and thus allow a woman to determine if she is pregnant. The tests use a commercially prepared antibody to HCG, which binds to the hormone (**FIGURE 19-16**). The home pregnancy tests are relatively inexpensive, fairly reliable, and fast.

Estrogen and Progesterone Exert Numerous Effects. Like testosterone in boys, estrogen secretion in girls increases dramatically at puberty. As the levels of estrogen in the blood increase, the hormone begins to stimulate follicle development in the ovaries. Estrogen also stimulates the growth of the external genitalia and the breasts as well as internal structures including the uterus, uterine tubes, and vagina.

Estrogen's influence extends far beyond the reproductive system. For example, estrogen promotes rapid bone growth in the early teens. Because estrogen secretion in girls usually occurs earlier than testosterone secretion in boys, girls typically experience a growth spurt before similarly aged boys. However, estrogen also stimulates the closure of the growth zones of the bones, known as the *epiphyseal plates*. This puts an end to the female growth spurt fairly early. Thus, most girls reach their full adult height by the age of 15–17. Boys experience their most rapid growth later in adolescence and continue growing until the age of 19–21. Finally, estrogen stimulates the deposition of fat in women's hips, buttocks, and breasts, giving the female body its characteristic shape.

Premenstrual Syndrome Is a Condition Afflicting Many Women

For reasons not yet fully understood, many women suffer from irritability, depression, fatigue, and headaches just before menstruation. Many also complain of bloating, tension, joint pain, and swelling and tenderness of the breasts.[6] These complaints are symptomatic of a condition known as **PMS**, or **premenstrual syndrome**.

Premenstrual syndrome is a clinically recognizable condition characterized by one or more of the symptoms noted above. Four of every 10 women of reproductive age experience PMS in varying degrees. Despite the prevalence of PMS, it may be years before scientists can pinpoint its cause or causes. Nevertheless, dozens of "cures," ranging from massive doses of progesterone to vitamin B-6, have been prescribed by clinics specializing

---

[6]All told, women report more than 150 different physical and psychological symptoms that emerge before menstruation begins.

in PMS. Buyers beware, however, for very little good scientific evidence is available to indicate which, if any, of the "cures" really work. Most of the evidence consists of testimonials—individual accounts. The critical thinking skills you learned in Chapter 1 suggest that anecdotal information such as this is no substitute for controlled studies.

Fortunately, work is now under way to test various treatments to see if any consistently bring relief. In the meantime, physicians recommend that women suffering from PMS see their family doctor to be certain that the symptoms are not caused by some other medical problem. Doctors recommend relaxation and avoidance of stress to help avoid or relieve PMS. Light exercise may help, as may warm baths. More frequent light meals with plenty of carbohydrates and fiber may be beneficial, too. Reductions in salt intake and avoiding excess chocolate consumption are also recommended. Cutting out caffeine drinks and taking vitamin B6 supplements are also generally advised.

Menopause Is the Cessation of Menstruation

The menstrual cycle continues throughout the reproductive years. However, after a woman reaches 20, her ovaries very gradually begin to become less responsive to gonadotropins. As responsiveness declines, estrogen levels gradually decline (**FIGURE 19-17**). In time, ovulation and menstruation become increasingly erratic and eventually stop. This complete cessation of these functions is called **menopause**—literally a cessation of the menses or menstruation.

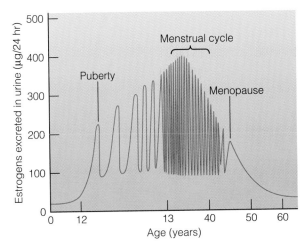

FIGURE 19-17 Ovarian Hormone Secretion Notice that at about age 20, ovarian estrogen secretion begins a gradual decline. Adapted with permission from A. C. Guyton, *Textbook of Medical Physiology*, 7th ed. (Philadelphia: W. B. Saunders Company, 1986), Figure 81–8, p. 979.

Menopause is attributed to a reduction in the number of ovarian follicles. At about age 45, most of the follicles that were in the ovary at puberty have been stimulated to grow and have either degenerated or ovulated. Consequently, FSH and LH from the pituitary have no target cells to stimulate. Not surprisingly, the production of ovarian estrogen plummets.

Menopause generally occurs between the ages of 45 and 55, but can occur earlier. The dramatic alteration in the hormonal climate results in several important physiological changes. For example, the decline in estrogen secretion causes the breasts and reproductive organs such as the uterus to begin to atrophy (shrink). Vaginal secretions often decline, and, in some women, sexual intercourse becomes painful.

The decline in estrogen levels may also result in behavioral disturbances. Many women, for instance, become more irritable and suffer bouts of depression. Very noticeable physical changes also occur. Three quarters of all women suffer "hot flashes" and "night sweats" induced by massive vasodilation of vessels in the skin. Fortunately for all people concerned, these symptoms usually pass.

As noted in Chapter 13, declining estrogen levels also accelerate osteoporosis, a softening of the bone due to a reduction in calcium. To counter osteoporosis due to the natural decline in ovarian function, physicians often prescribe small amounts of estrogen or, more commonly, a combination of estrogen and progesterone. This is known as **hormone replacement therapy**. They may also recommend a program of exercise and a diet rich in calcium and vitamin D to prevent osteoporosis (see Health Note 13-1). Hormone replacement therapy helps relieve other symptoms of menopause as well, including hot flashes and vaginal dryness. Hormones are administered via pills, skin patches, or both. Vaginal creams containing estrogen can also be used to treat vaginal dryness. Most women are treated for 5 to 10 years after the onset of menopause, but not longer for long-term treatment may increase the risk of breast cancer.

<hr>

Section 19-3

Birth Control

Few topics in modern society generate as much controversy as birth control. **Birth control** is any method or device that prevents births. Birth control measures fit into two broad categories: (1) **contraception**, ways of preventing pregnancy, and (2) **induced abortion**, the deliberate expulsion of a fetus.

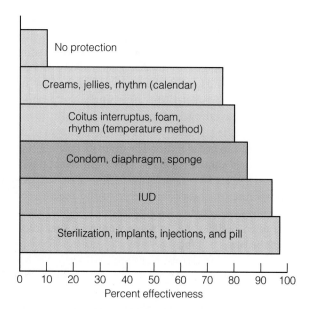

FIGURE 19-18 Effectiveness of Contraceptive Measures
Percent effectiveness is a measure of the number of women in a group of 100 who will not become pregnant in a year.

Contraceptive Measures Help Prevent Pregnancy

FIGURE 19-18 summarizes the effectiveness of the most common means of contraception. Effectiveness is expressed as a percentage. A 95% effectiveness rating means that 95 women out of 100 using a certain method in a year will not become pregnant.

Abstinence. Not listed in the figure is a form of birth control that many of us forget to talk about, **abstinence,** refraining from sexual intercourse. This form of birth control is appropriate for many people and should not be overlooked as a strategy of reducing unwanted pregnancy and preventing the transmission of AIDS and other diseases (discussed later).

Sterilization. Except for complete abstinence, sterilization and the pill (discussed shortly) are the most effective birth control measures (**FIGURE 19-18**). In 1982, sterilization became the leading method of contraception practiced by married couples in the United States.

In women, sterilization is performed by cutting the uterine tubes. This technique is called **tubal ligation** (TWO-bal lie-GAY-shun) (**FIGURE 19-19A**). Surgeons usually make two small incisions in the abdomen just beneath the navel or belly button. An instrument called a laparoscope (LAP-er-ah-scope) is inserted through each incision. With the aid of a specially lighted viewing lens in the **laparoscope**, the surgeon locates and cuts the uterine tubes. The cut ends are either tied off or cauterized—that is, burned using an electrical current. In some cases, surgeons clamp the uterine tubes shut with plastic or metal rings.

Male sterilization requires a far less traumatic surgical procedure called a **vasectomy** (vah-SECK-toe-me), which can be carried out in a physician's office under local anesthesia (**FIGURE 19-19B**). To perform a vasectomy, a physician makes a small incision in the scrotum. Each vas deferens is exposed, then cut, and the free ends are tied off or cauterized.

Vasectomies only prevent the sperm from passing into the urethra during ejaculation. They do not impair sex drive, and because they do not block the flow of the sex accessory glands, which produce 99% of the volume of the ejaculate, they have virtually no effect on ejaculation.

Vasectomy and tubal ligation are essentially irreversible. However, special surgical methods, called **microsurgery**, can be used to reconnect the uterine tubes and the vasa deferentia. This procedure is costly and not always successful.

The Pill. The **birth control pill** is the most effective temporary means of birth control available (**FIGURE 19-20**). Birth control pills come in several varieties, but the most common is the combined pill. It contains a mixture of synthetic estrogen and progesterone. These hormones inhibit the release of LH and FSH by acting on the pituitary and hypothalamus. The lack of LH and FSH, in turn, inhibits follicle development and ovulation. A minipill containing progesterone alone is also available. Even though it is less effective than the combined pill, the minipill is more suitable for some women because it results in fewer side effects.

FIGURE 19-19 Sterilization Methods *(a)* In a tubal ligation, the uterine tubes are cut, then tied off or cauterized. *(b)* In a vasectomy, the vasa deferentia are cut, then tied off.

Birth control pills must be taken throughout the menstrual cycle. Skipping a few days may release the pituitary and hypothalamus from the inhibitory influences of estrogen and progesterone, resulting in ovulation and possible pregnancy.

Although effective, birth control pills have some adverse health effects worth noting. Even though the incidence of these adverse side effects is small, a woman considering different birth control options should study them carefully before making a decision.

One rare side effect is death. **TABLE 19-3** compares the risk of death from taking birth control pills (and using other contraceptives) with a number of common risk factors. As shown, the risk of a nonsmoker dying from taking birth control pills is 1 in 63,000 in any given year, whereas the risk of dying in an auto accident is 1 in 6000.

Deaths from the use of birth control pills may result from heart attacks, strokes, or blood clots. The incidence of these life-threatening side effects is lowest in nonsmoking women under the age of 30. To reduce this risk even more, pharmaceutical companies have dramatically lowered the estrogen content of the combined pill, because estrogen is responsible for most of the adverse side effects.

FIGURE 19-20 The Birth Control Pill The pill consists of synthetic estrogen and progesterone, taken throughout most of the menstrual cycle to block ovulation.

Early studies showed a positive correlation between the use of birth control pills and cancers of the breast and cervix (see Health Note 19-1). More recent studies suggest that the new generation of low-estrogen pills is less likely to cause cancer of the breast or cervix.

Even with reduced estrogen levels, however, women who take birth control pills are more likely to develop cervical cancer than women who do not. Physicians therefore recommend annual Pap smears for women on the pill.

During a **Pap smear**, the cervical lining is swabbed. The swab picks up cells sloughed off by the epithelium, which are later examined under a microscope for signs of cancer (**FIGURE 19-21**). This

FIGURE 19-21 The Pap Smear
(a) A photomicrograph of a normal Pap smear showing large, flattened cells.
(b) A photomicrograph of a cancerous smear, showing many small cancer cells.

TABLE 19-3

Risks Involved in Some Voluntary Activities in the United States

Activity	Annual Risk of Death
Smoking	1 in 200
Motorcycling	1 in 1000
Automobile driving	1 in 6000
Power boating	1 in 6000
Rock climbing	1 in 7500
Using tampons (toxic shock syndrome)	1 in 350,000
Contracting reproductive tract infections through sexual intercourse	1 in 50,000
Preventing pregnancy:	
Oral contraception—nonsmoker	1 in 63,000
Oral contraception—smoker	1 in 16,000
Using intrauterine devices (IUDs)	1 in 100,000
Using barrier methods	None
Using natural methods	None
Undergoing sterilization:	
Laparoscopic tubal ligation	1 in 20,000
Hysterectomy	1 in 1600
Vasectomy	None
Pregnancy:	1 in 10,000
Nonlegal abortion	1 in 3000
Legal abortion:	
Before 9 weeks	1 in 400,000
Between 9 and 12 weeks	1 in 100,000
Between 13 and 16 weeks	1 in 25,000
After 16 weeks	1 in 10,000

(a)

(b)

Health Note 19-1

Breast Cancer: Early Detection Is the Key to Survival

Breast cancer is one of the most common cancers affecting women in the United States. Each year, an estimated 180,000 cases of breast cancer are detected in this country. Although men can develop breast cancer, it is very rare. (Less than 1 percent of the cases are in men.)

Breast cancer is a fairly lethal disease. One of every five women who contracts breast cancer will die from it. As you shall soon see, if breast cancer is detected early on, a woman's chances of survival increase dramatically.

Doctors and medical researchers do not know what causes breast cancer, but they have uncovered many risk factors associated with this disease. Age is of the one of the most important. Numerous studies show that the risk of breast cancer increases as a woman ages. In fact, the risk doubles every ten years of woman's life. Most women who are diagnosed with breast cancer are in their 50s; the disease is very rare in women under 30 years of age.

Studies also indicate that estrogen is a risk factor for breast cancer. Estrogen is the female sex hormone produced by a woman's ovaries. Generally speaking, the longer a woman is exposed to estrogen, the higher her chances of developing breast cancer.

The early onset of menstruation is another risk factor, as is the late onset of menopause. If a woman begins menstruating (and ovulating) before the age of 11, for example, her chances of developing breast cancer

rise. If she enters menopause late, her risks increase as well. Both of these risk factors are thought to be related to overall estrogen exposure.

Obesity also increases a woman's risk. Excess body fat causes an increase in estrogen. Weight control is therefore not only good for a heart, it reduces a woman's chances of developing breast cancer.

For reasons not completely understood, the age of a woman at the time of her first child's birth also affects her risk of developing breast cancer. If her first child is born after a woman's 30th birthday, her chances of breast cancer are two times higher than one whose first child was born before age 20. If she never has children, her chances of developing breast cancer are also twice as high as a woman who gives birth to a child before age 20.

Estrogen in birth control pills may also slightly increase a woman's chances of developing a cancerous breast tumor. Estrogen given to post-menopausal women for ten years or more can elevate a woman's risk, too. Such treatments, however, reduce symptoms of menopause but also reduce osteoporosis, a softening of the bones caused by a loss of calcium.

Some women inherit a higher risk for breast cancer. There are at least two abnormal genes that can be linked to this disease. Women who inherit these genes often elect to have their breasts removed as a kind of pre-emptive strike. Artificial implants,

discussed in Health Note 20-1, can be used to restore their appearance.

Researchers have also discovered factors that help reduce the risk of breast cancer. A low animal-fat diet is one of them. Breast feeding for two years or more also seems to lower risk.

Early detection is a key to beating this disease. The earlier it is detected, the more likely a woman is to survive. Because of this, many doctors recommend that women over 40 have a routine **mammogram**, an X-ray of the breast, every 1 to 2 years. Women over 50 should have a mammogram every year (**FIGURE 1**).

FIGURE 1 Mammogram showing a small breast tumor.

procedure helps physicians in diagnosing cervical cancer early, which increases a woman's chances of survival.

Smoking increases the likelihood of side effects from birth control pills. If a woman is a smoker and takes the pill, for example, she is four times more likely to die from a heart attack or stroke than a nonsmoker. The risk of side effects also increases with age. To reduce the chances of developing serious side effects, women over the age of 35 who smoke should either use an alternative method of birth control or give up smoking. Birth control pills are also not advised for women with a medical history of blood clots, high blood pressure, diabetes, uterine cancer, and cancer of the breast.

Women should also perform regular self-exams. Regular breast self-exams allow a woman to become familiar with the normal feel of the internal tissues as well as the outward appearance of the breast. If changes occur, they're more likely to be noticed.

The best time to perform a self-exam is immediately after a menstrual period. Looking in a mirror, a woman should first examine the appearance of her breasts and nipples (**FIGURE 2**). Look for changes in the shape of the nipple or changes in the skin over the breast. Widespread dimpling of the skin, for instance, may indicate the presence of a breast tumor. The breast will appear textured like an orange peel. A woman should also be on the lookout for any changes in the size or shape of the breast.

Then, lying down with one arm behind her head, a woman should press firmly on the breast using small circular motions. Each breast should be systematically examined. In addition, a woman should check out the armpit for the presence of any lumps or increases in the size of existing lumps.

Most lumps are harmless, but they should be checked out by a physician at once. If a suspicious lump is detected, a physician may order an ultrasound or mammogram to examine the lump more closely. A **biopsy**, a small tissue sample, of the lump may be taken and examined under a microscope. X-rays of

the chest and bones may be ordered to see if the tumor has spread to these organs.

Breast cancer is typically treated by surgery. If the tumor is small, the surgeon will remove it along with some of the surrounding tissue. This procedure is known as a *lumpectomy*. If the tumor is large, or if there are multiple tumors, all of the tissue in the breast will be moved. This procedure is known as a *mastectomy* (mass-teck-toe-me). The surgeon usually removes a few lymph nodes from the armpits as well. They're examined under the microscope for signs of the spread of cancer.

Although studies show that mastectomies are not warranted when there is a single small tumor, some women still elect to have it done to provide a level of assurance. The breast can be reconstructed using an artifical implants; these are discussed in Health Note 20-1.

Surgery is typically followed up by radiation therapy, especially if the tumor was large or if it had spread to the lymph nodes. In most cases, treatment commences a month after surgery and continues five days a week for six weeks.

Women with estrogen-sensitive tumors are typically treated with the drug tamoxifen. This drug blocks estrogen's effect, and causes the tumor to shrink. Treatment usually lasts at least 5 years. In other instances, doctors may recommend chemotherapy.

FIGURE 2 Indentation of the nipple as shown here is one sign of breast cancer.

As noted earlier, one in five women diagnosed with breast cancer dies from it. *The earlier the tumor is detected, the greater one's chances of survival, and the less likely a tumor is to recur.* Studies show that a combination of drug treatment and surgery enhance a woman's chances of survival. Nine of every ten women whose tumors are detected early and treated immediately survive ten years or more. If a tumor has spread to other organs, however, chances of survival are much lower.

Visit *Human Biology's* Internet site for links to web sites offering more information on this topic.

Birth control pills do have beneficial effects, not the least of which is that they prevent pregnancy. National statistics show that one of every 10,000 women who becomes pregnant and delivers will die from complications, usually during delivery. Thus, even with the risks associated with the pill, using this mode of contraception is six times safer than pregnancy.

Birth control pills also reduce the incidence of ovarian cysts, breast lumps, anemia, rheumatoid arthritis, osteoporosis, and pelvic infection. Although birth control pills may increase the risk of cervical and breast cancer, they apparently protect a woman from cancer of the ovary and uterus.

Intrauterine Device. The next most effective means of birth control is the **intrauterine device (IUD)** (**FIGURE 19-22**). The IUD is one of the least used birth control measures. It consists of a small plastic or metal object with a short string attached to it. IUDs are inserted into the uterus by a physician, usually during menstruation, because the cervical canal is widest then and because menstrual bleeding indicates that the woman is not pregnant.

No one knows exactly how the IUD works. Some researchers think that the IUD increases uterine contractions, making it difficult for the early embryo to attach and implant in the wall of the uterus. Others think that the IUD creates a local inflammatory reaction in the uterine lining, resulting in an inhospitable environment for a newly formed embryo. As a result, implantation is blocked. It is possible that both mechanisms are operating.

Like other forms of birth control, IUDs have adverse effects. In some cases, the uterus expels the device, leaving a woman unprotected. Expulsion usually occurs within a month or two of insertion. The IUD may also cause slight pain and increase menstrual bleeding. These effects, however, are minor compared with two much rarer complications: uterine infections and perforation (a penetration of the uterine wall by an IUD). Women with IUDs are more likely to develop uterine infections than women practicing other forms of birth control. If not treated quickly, infections can spread to the uterine tubes, where scar tissue develops. This can block the transport of sperm and ova, causing sterility. Perforation of the uterus is a life-threatening condition requiring surgery to correct.

The Diaphragm, Condom, and Sponge. The next most effective means of birth control are the barrier methods—the diaphragm, condom, and vaginal sponge—all of which prevent the sperm from entering the uterus. The **diaphragm** (DIE-ah-FRAM) is a rubber cup that fits over the end of the cervix (**FIGURE 19-23**). To increase its effectiveness, a spermicidal (sperm-killing) jelly, foam, or cream should be applied to the rim and inside surface of the cup.

Smaller versions of the diaphragm, called **cervical caps**, are also available. Fitting over the very end of the cervix, the cervical cap most often used is held in place by suction. When used with spermicidal jelly or cream, the caps are as effective as full-sized diaphragms.

Condoms are thin, latex rubber sheaths that fit onto the erect penis (**FIGURE 19-24**). Sperm released during ejaculation are trapped inside (in a small reservoir at the tip of the condom) and are therefore prevented from entering the vagina. Besides preventing fertilization, condoms also protect against sexually transmitted diseases, a benefit not offered by any other birth control measure except abstinence.

The newest condom on the market is for women. It fits into the vagina and is recommended by physicians to protect women against AIDS and other sexually transmitted diseases.

Yet another barrier method is the **vaginal sponge** (**FIGURE 19-25**). This small absorbent piece of foam is impregnated with spermicidal jelly. Inserted into the vagina, the sponge is positioned over the end of the cervix. The sponge is effective immediately after placement and remains effective for 24 hours. Cervical sponges can be purchased without a doctor's prescription. Like the condom, one size fits all.

Withdrawal. One of the oldest, but least successful, means of birth control is **withdrawal**, or **coitus interruptus** (COE-ee-tus), disengaging before ejaculation. This method requires tremendous willpower and frequently fails, for three reasons: because caution is often tossed to the wind in the heat of passion, because the penis is withdrawn too late, or because of preejaculatory leakage—the release of a few drops of sperm-filled semen before ejaculation. Accordingly, it is not an advisable method of birth control.

Spermicidal Chemicals. As mentioned earlier, spermicidal jellies, creams, foams, and films contain chemical agents that kill sperm but are apparently harmless to the woman. Spermicidal preparations are most often used in conjunction with diaphragms, condoms, and cervical caps. They can also be used alone but are only about as effective as withdrawal.

The Rhythm Method. Abstaining from sexual intercourse around the time of ovulation—the **rhythm,** or **natural, method**—can help couples reduce the likelihood of pregnancy. If a couple knows the exact time of ovulation, they can time sexual intercourse to prevent pregnancy more precisely.

To practice the natural method successfully, couples must first determine when ovulation occurs. One popular approach is the **temperature method.**[7] A woman's body temperature varies throughout the menstrual cycle, as shown in **FIGURE 19-26**. In most women, body temperature rises slightly after ovulation. By taking her temperature every morning before she gets out of bed, a woman can pinpoint the day she ovulates. By keeping a temperature record over several menstrual cycles, she

FIGURE 19-22 The IUD IUDs come in a variety of shapes and sizes and are inserted into the uterus, where they prevent implantation. Only one type is currently legal in the United States.

FIGURE 19-23 The Diaphragm Worn over the cervix, the diaphragm is coated with spermicidal jelly or cream and is an effective barrier to sperm.

FIGURE 19-24 The Condom Worn over the penis during sexual intercourse, it prevents sperm from entering the vagina.

FIGURE 19-25 The Vaginal Sponge Impregnated with a spermicidal chemical, the vaginal sponge is inserted into the vagina and is effective for up to 24 hours.

can determine the length of her cycle and the time of ovulation. Once the length of the cycle and the time of ovulation have been determined, days of abstinence can be determined. Erring on the safe side, some doctors recommend that couples refrain from sexual intercourse from the first day of menstruation until 4 days after ovulation. Translated, that means no sex for about 17 days of the 28-day cycle.

Another method used to time ovulation involves taking samples of the cervical mucus. Cervical mucus varies in consistency during the menstrual cycle. By testing its thickness on a daily basis, a woman can tell fairly accurately when she has ovulated. Because ova remain viable 12–24 hours after ovulation and sperm may remain alive in the female reproductive tract for up to 3 days, abstinence 4 days before and 4 days after the probable ovulation date should provide a margin of safety (**FIGURE 19-27**). As most people practice it, then the natural method of birth control requires about 8 days of abstinence during each menstrual cycle. This minimizes the chances of a viable sperm reaching a viable ovum. Unfortunately, some women experience the greatest sexual interest around the time of ovulation. Sexual intercourse after a period of abstinence may also advance the time of ovulation. (For a discussion of new methods of birth control, see Health Note 19-2.)

---

[7]The temperature method can also be used by women who want to get pregnant because it allows them to determine the time of ovulation.

Abortion Is the Surgical Termination of Pregnancy

Some couples may elect to terminate pregnancy through **abortion**. In the United States, approximately 1 million abortions are performed every year by physicians.

Abortion is not suitable or morally acceptable to all people. Pro-life advocates argue that abortion should be outlawed or severely restricted—that is, allowed only in cases of rape, incest, and threat to the life of the mother. These individuals advise unmarried women to abstain from sexual intercourse or, if they

FIGURE 19-26 Body Temperature Measurements During the Menstrual Cycle

become pregnant, to give birth and either keep the baby or put it up for adoption.

Pro-choice advocates, on the other hand, support abortion. They argue that women should have the freedom to choose whether to terminate a pregnancy or have a child. Abortion, they say, reduces unwanted pregnancies and untold suffering among unwanted infants, especially in poor families, and gives women more options than motherhood. Although pro-choice advocates view abortion as a legitimate means of family planning, many of them are quick to point out that it should not be practiced as a primary means of birth control. Contraception is less costly, less traumatic, and more morally acceptable.

In the first 12 weeks of pregnancy, abortions can be performed surgically in a doctor's office via **vacuum aspiration**. In this procedure, the cervix is first dilated by a special instrument. Next, the contents of the uterus are drawn out through an aspirator tube.

Vacuum aspiration is a fairly simple and relatively painless procedure. Usually no anesthesia is given. Although women bleed for a week or so after the procedure, they generally experience few complications.

Most abortions are performed by the end of the twelfth week of pregnancy. Vacuum aspiration may also be performed later—between 13 and 16 weeks. In such instances, physicians use a larger aspirator tube. In addition, they may need to scrape the lining of the uterus with a special instrument to ensure complete removal of the fetal tissue.

After 16 weeks, abortions are more difficult and more risky. Solutions of salt, urea, or prostaglandins, which stimulate uterine contractions, are injected into the sac of fluid surrounding the fetus to induce prema-

ture labor. The hormone oxytocin may be administered to the woman with the same effect.

In France, women can use a pill that prevents fertilized eggs from implanting in the lining of the uterus. Called RU486, or incorrectly the abortion pill, it pill is now legal in the United. (For more on RU486, see Health Note 19-2.)

In the United States, there is another chemical treatment that has the same effect. This pill restricts blood flow to the uterus. Two days after the initial pill is given, a second pill is taken. This regimen prevents the fertilized ovum from implanting. In the state of Washington, it is now legal for pharmacists to dispense emergency "morning-after" pills without a doctor's prescription.

In the controversy over abortion, it is important to remember that abortion is rarely an easy choice for anyone. Contrary to what many think, however, studies show that the majority of women who choose abortion do not suffer lasting emotional harm, especially if they have had counseling.

Section 19-4

Sexually Transmitted Diseases

Certain bacteria and viruses can be transmitted by sexual contact. These organisms can penetrate the lining of the reproductive tracts of men and women and thrive in the moist, warm environment of the body. These organisms cause **sexually transmitted diseases (STDs)**. Most of the infectious agents that cause STDs are spread by vaginal intercourse, but other forms of sexual contact such as anal and oral sex are responsible for their transmission. AIDS, for example, can be transmitted by anal sex as well as vaginal and (possibly) oral sex (Chapter 8). Syphilis is caused by a bacterium that is spread by oral, anal, and vaginal sex.

Although STDs pass from one person to another during sexual contact, the symptoms are not confined to the reproductive tract. In fact, several STDs, including syphilis and AIDS, are primarily systemic diseases— that is, they affect entire body systems.

One complicating factor in controlling STDs is that occasionally some diseases such as gonorrhea produce no obvious symptoms in many men and women. As a result, the disease can be transmitted without a person knowing he or she is infected. In others such as AIDS, symptoms may not appear for weeks or even years after the initial infection. Thus, sexually active individuals who are not monogamous can transmit the AIDS virus to many people before they are aware that they are infected. As noted in Chapter 8, new blood tests

			1	2	3	4
			Menstruation begins.			
5	6	7	8	9	10	11
					Intercourse leaves sperm to fertilize ovum.	
12	13	14	15	16	17	18 Ovum may still be present.
Ovum may be released.						
19	20	21	22	23	24	25
26	27	28	1			
			Menstruation begins.			

FIGURE 19-27 The Natural Method The yellow-shaded areas indicate an unsafe period for sexual intercourse, assuming ovulation occurs at the midpoint of the cycle.

are being used to detect HIV earlier and may help to reduce the spread of this deadly disease. In this section we will examine the most common STDs, except AIDS, which was discussed in Chapter 8.

Gonorrhea Is a Bacterial Infection That Can Spread to Many Organs

Gonorrhea (GON-or-REE-ah; referred to colloquially as the "clap") is caused by a bacterium that commonly infects the urethra of men and the cervical canal of women. Gonorrhea often causes no symptoms. When they do appear, painful urination and a puslike discharge from the urethra are common complaints in men. Women may experience a cloudy vaginal discharge and lower-abdominal pain. If a woman's urethra is infected, urination may be painful. Symptoms of gonorrhea usually appear about 1–14 days after sexual contact.

Gonorrhea is treated with antibiotics and clears up quickly, usually within 3 to 4 days, if treatment begins early. If left untreated, however, gonorrhea in men can spread to the prostate gland and the epididymis. They can be more difficult to treat. Moreover, infections in the urethra lead to the formation of scar tissue. This may narrow the urethra and make urination even more difficult. In some women, bacterial infection spreads to the uterus and uterine tubes, causing the buildup of scar tissue. In the uterine tubes, scar tissue may block the passage of sperm and ova, resulting in infertility.[8] Gonorrheal infections can also spread into the abdominal cavity through the opening of the uterine tubes. If the infection enters the bloodstream in men or women, it can travel throughout the body. Fortunately, gonorrhea can be treated by antibiotics, but early diagnosis is essential to limit the damage.

Syphilis Is Caused by a Bacterium and Can Be Extremely Debilitating if Untreated

Syphilis is a deadly STD caused by a bacterium that penetrates the linings of the oral cavity, vagina, and penile urethra. It may also enter through breaks in the skin. If untreated, syphilis proceeds through three stages. In stage 1, between 1 and 8 weeks after exposure, a small, painless red sore develops, usually in the genital area. Easily visible when on the penis, these sores often go unnoticed when they occur in the vagina or cervix. The sore heals in 1–5 weeks, leaving a tiny scar.

Approximately 6 weeks after the sore heals, individuals complain of fever, headache, and loss of ap-

petite. Lymph nodes in the neck, groin, and armpit swell as the bacteria spreads throughout the body. This is stage 2. It lasts for about 4 to 12 weeks.

As a rule, the symptoms of stage 2 syphilis disappear for several years. Then, without warning, the disease flares up again. This is stage 3. During stage 3, an autoimmune reaction occurs. Patients experience a loss of their sense of balance and a loss of sensation in their legs. As the disease progresses, patients experience paralysis, senility, and even insanity. In some cases, the bacterium weakens the walls of the aorta, causing aneurysms (Chapter 6).

Syphilis is diagnosed by the symptoms and by examing the pus under a microscope. Blood tests are also useful in stages 1 and 2. Syphilis can be successfully treated with antibiotics, but only if the treatment begins early. Suspicious sores in the mouth and genitals should be brought to the attention of a physician. In stage 3, antibiotics are useless. Tissue or organ damage is permanent.

Chlamydial Infections Are Extremely Common Among College Students

One of the most common sexually transmitted diseases, affecting 3 to 10 million people each year, and many of them college students, is known as **chlamydia** (clam-ID-ee-ah). Caused by a bacterium, this disease is characterized, in men, by a burning sensation during urination and a discharge from the penis. Women also experience a burning sensation during urination and a vaginal discharge. If the bacterium spreads, it can cause more severe infection and infertility. Like other STDs, many people experience no symptoms at all and therefore risk spreading the disease to others. Children born to mothers with chlamydia can develop eye infections and pneumonia.

Chlamydia bacteria often migrate to the lymph nodes, where they cause considerable enlargement and tenderness in the affected area. Blockage of the lymph nodes may result in tissue swelling in the surrounding tissue. Doxycycline and other antibiotics are effective in treating this disease.

Genital Herpes Is Caused by a Virus; It Is Extremely Common, and Essentially Incurable

Genital herpes (HER-peas) is another common sexually transmitted disease. Contracted by 200,000–300,000 people each year, genital herpes is caused by a virus that enters the body and remains there for life. The first sign of viral infection is pain, tenderness, or an itchy sensation on the penis or female external genitalia. These

---

[8]Sexually transmitted diseases are a leading cause of infertility in women.

Health Note 19-2

Advances in Birth Control—Responding to a Global Imperative

Every day of the year, 230,000 people join the world population. This translates into an annual rate of growth of about 80 million per year! Faced with resource depletion, environmental destruction, and a host of other problems, many countries recognize the need to stabilize population growth.

Concerns for providing adequate birth control are present in virtually all nations today. In wealthy, industrialized countries, many parents have already taken steps to limit their family size. For many parents in these nations, the decision to limit their family size is based on economics. Raising a single child to college age can cost as much as $85,000 in 1994 dollars. A recent study estimated that another $85,000 will be needed just to send a child born today to a public university. Considerably more is needed to send a student to a private university. Parents may also limit their family size to be able to provide more personal care for their offspring.

Some parents choose to have fewer children for environmental reasons. Consider some startling statistics: a child born in the United States today will require 16 pounds of coal, 3.6 gallons of oil, and 240 cubic feet of natural gas each day of his or her life. This heavy dependence on resources translates into an enormous amount of pollution and environmental dam-

age. Clearly, child rearing is an environmentally taxing activity.

Although most people tend to think of the need for family planning in the poorer, nonindustrial nations, it is just as important, perhaps even more so, in the United States and other developed countries because their impact on the environment is so great. Each American, for example, uses 20–40 times as much of the Earth's resources as a resident of India. In terms of environmental impact, then, the United States' 280 million people are equal to 5–11 billion Indians.

This is not to say that birth control is unimportant in Third World nations. Approximately, 90% of the more than 80 million people added to the global population each year are born into the Third World, where hunger and starvation abound. And these countries face environmental problems of epic proportions.

Family planning is making headway in Third World nations, but the task has only just begun. To facilitate this process, researchers are trying to develop safer, more convenient, and even more effective methods of birth control. For example, tests are under way on the effectiveness and safety of nasal spray contraceptives for women. Research is also proceeding quickly on transdermal contraceptive patches. These small, Band-Aid-like patches are impregnated with a blend of hormones and hormone analogs, including estro-

gen and progesterone, and are worn by a woman for a week, then replaced.

In many countries outside the United States, slow-acting, injectable contraceptives are now being used. Women are given a shot of crystalline progesterone under the skin. The crystals dissolve over a period of 3 months, blocking ovulation.

Another novel approach involves matchstick-sized capsules containing an even more potent progesterone implanted under the skin of a woman's arm; these prevent pregnancy for up to 5 years (**FIGURE 1**). Contraceptive implants have been approved for use in 13 countries, including the United States. Population experts hope that they will be widely used in Third World nations because they require virtually no effort on the part of the couple.

Researchers are also experimenting with biodegradable implants. Clinical trials are under way on a biodegradable material impregnated with progesterone that may prevent pregnancy for 18 months or more. The biodegradable material is broken down and gradually disappears.

Experimentation is continuing on "morning-after" pills, which can be taken after sexual intercourse to prevent pregnancy. At least two morning-after pills exist. One contains a synthetic estrogen called *DES* (diethylstilbestrol). DES stimulates muscle contraction in the uterus and uterine tubes, expelling the fertilized ovum

symptoms usually occur 6 days or so after contact with someone infected by the virus. Soon afterward, painful blisters appear on the external genitalia, thighs, buttocks, and cervix, or in the vagina (**FIGURE 19-28**, page 456).

The blisters break open and become painful ulcers that last for 1–3 weeks, then disappear. Unfortunately, the herpes virus is a lifelong resident of the body. New outbreaks can occur from time to time, especially when an individual is under stress. Recurrent outbreaks are

generally not as severe as the initial one, and, in time, the outbreaks generally cease.

Herpes can be transmitted to other individuals during sexual contact only when the blisters are present or (as recent research suggests) just beginning to emerge. When the virus is inactive, sexual intercourse can occur without infecting a partner.

Although herpes cannot be cured, physicians can suppress outbreaks with antiviral drugs such as *acyclovir* from the reproductive tract. DES is sometimes used in cases of incest or rape, but it is generally avoided because it causes vomiting and nausea.

A synthetic steroid called *RU486* is also in use in France and certain other countries, but not yet in the United States. RU486 binds to progesterone receptors in the uterus, blocking progesterone from binding. Because progesterone inhibits muscular contractions of the uterus, RU486 probably has the same effect as DES, causing an expulsion of the fertilized ovum. Vocal pro-life forces in the United States have taken a strong stand against the use of this method, calling it an abortion pill, but RU486 was recently approved for use.

You may have noticed that when it comes to birth control, there are few options for men. Why not develop a pill for men and shift some of the contraceptive burden to them?

To be effective, a pill would have to shut down spermatogenesis. Testosterone injections would do the job because this hormone blocks the release of pituitary FSH and LH. FSH is required for spermatogenesis, and its absence would depress sperm production. Unfortunately, testosterone injections may also cause aggressive behavior. Complicating matters, excess androgen in males is converted to estrogen, causing feminizing side effects. Finally, androgen treatments may depress spermato-

genesis, but not enough to lower sperm count to a level where a couple would feel confident.

Another route is to selectively inhibit FSH secretion. As noted in this chapter, the seminiferous tubules produce a substance called *inhibin,* so named because it inhibits the production of FSH by the pituitary gland. If inhibin could be produced and administered to men, it might give them a better chance to participate in birth control. It could be administered in contraceptive nasal sprays.

One thing is certain, the world's population problem will not be solved through new contraceptive technologies alone. What is required is a change in the attitudes of millions of men and women throughout the world. Controlling family size must be a conscious decision followed by conscientious action.

In Africa, where population is doubling in some countries every 17 years, modern contraceptive use is a paltry 18%. Worldwide, only about half the women of reproductive age are using modern contraceptives. It is crucial to involve more people as the world races to stem this tidal wave, which, if unchecked, could add 5 billion people to the world population in the next 40 years. Funds are needed to pay for education, contraception, and other family planning. When one condom costs more than the average person spends on medical care in a

FIGURE 1 Subcutaneous Progesterone Implant Inserted under the skin, this tiny device releases a steady stream of progesterone, blocking ovulation for months.

year, we can hardly expect widespread use. Many Third World countries, however, divert enormous amounts of money to pay for weapons and almost nothing to family planning. If the world population is to stabilize, if our children are to inherit a world worth living in, many experts agree that contraceptive use must increase.

Controlling population growth also requires improvements in education and job opportunities for men and women. Small-scale, sustainable economic development will give men and women options other than child bearing.

Visit *Human Biology's* Internet site for links to web sites offering more information on this topic.

(A-sigh-CLOE-ver). These drugs not only reduce the incidence of outbreaks, but also accelerate healing of the blisters.

Herpes is not a particularly dangerous STD, except in pregnant women. These women run the risk of transferring the virus to their infants at birth. Because the virus can be fatal to newborns, these women are often advised to deliver by cesarean section (an incision made just above the pubic bone) if the virus is active at the time of birth.

Nongonococcal Urethritis Is an Extremely Common Disease Caused by Several Types of Bacteria

Nongonococcal urethritis (YUR-ee-THRIGHT-iss), or **NGU** for short, is the most common sexually transmitted disease. Moreover, NGU is one of several STDs whose incidence is steadily rising in the United States. Caused by any of several different bacteria, this infection is generally less threatening than gonorrhea,

FIGURE 19-28 Genital Herpes Blisters on the External Genitalia and Inner Thigh

FIGURE 19-29 Genital Warts Genital warts on the penis are caused by infection of the skin by papilloma viruses. Genital warts can be removed by a variety of treatments but sometimes recur.

syphilis, and chlamydia, although some infections can result in sterility.

Many men and women often exhibit no symptoms whatsoever and can therefore spread the disease without knowing it. In men, when symptoms occur, they resemble those of gonorrhea—painful urination and a cloudy mucous discharge from the penis. In women, urination becomes painful and more frequent. NGU can be treated by antibiotics, but individuals should seek treatment quickly to avoid the spread of the disease and more serious complications.

Genital Warts Are Caused by Human Papillomavirus (HPV).

The vast majority of Americans carry a virus known as **human papillomavirus** (pap-ILL-oh-mah) or **HPV.** Transmitted by sexual contact, this virus can cause **gential warts.** Genital warts are benign growths that appear on the external genitalia and around the anuses of men and women (**FIGURE 19-29**). Warts also grow inside the vagina of women. Warts generally occur in individuals whose immune systems are suppressed, for example, after long periods of stress.

These warts can remain small or can grow to cover large areas, creating cosmetically unsightly growths. They may cause mild irritation, and certain strains of HPV are associated with cervical cancer in women.

Genital warts can be treated with chemicals or removed surgically—although rates of recurrence are quite high. In 20% to 30% of the cases, genital warts disappear spontaneously. Getting rid of the virus, however, is impossible, for it resides in the body forever.

Section 19-5

Infertility

A surprisingly large percentage (about one in six) of American couples cannot conceive. The inability to conceive (to become pregnant) is called **infertility.** According to some statistics, in about 50% of the couples, infertility results from problems occurring in the woman. Approximately 30% of the cases are due to

problems in the man alone, and about 20% are the result of problems in both partners. Can anything be done in such instances?

Fortunately, the answer is yes. If after a year of actively trying to conceive a couple remains unsuccessful, they can consult a fertility specialist who will first check obvious problems such as infrequent or poorly timed sex. Obviously, only intercourse around the time of ovulation is successful. If timing is not the problem, and it rarely is, the physician tests the man's sperm count. A low sperm count is one of the most common causes of male infertility and is easy to test.

A low sperm count may result from overwork, emotional stress, and fatigue. Excess tobacco and alcohol consumption can also contribute to the problem. Tight-fitting clothes and excess exercise, both of which raise the scrotal temperature, also tend to reduce the sperm count. The testes are also sensitive to a wide range of chemicals and drugs that reduce sperm production.

If infertility appears to be caused by a low sperm count, a couple may choose to undergo artificial insemination, using sperm from a sperm bank. These sperm are generally acquired from anonymous donors and are stored frozen. When thawed, the sperm are reactivated, then deposited in the woman's vagina or cervix around the time of ovulation.

If sperm production and ejaculation appear normal, a physician checks the woman's reproductive tract. First on line is a test of ovulation. If ovulation is not occurring, **fertility drugs** may be administered. Several kinds of drugs are available. One of the more common is HCG, which, as noted earlier, is an LH-like hormone that induces ovulation. Unfortunately, fertility drugs often result in superovulation (the ovulation of many fertilizable ova), leaving couples with a "litter" of 4–6 babies, instead of the one child they had hoped for. Most of the multiple births you hear about on the news are the result of fertility drugs.

If tests show that ovulation is occurring normally, the physician examines the uterine tubes to determine whether they are obstructed. In some instances, a previous gonorrheal or chlamydial infection that spread into the tubes may have caused scarring that obstructed the passageway. In such instances, couples may be advised to adopt a child or to try *in vitro* (in VEE-trow) fertilization.

During *in vitro* fertilization, ova are surgically removed from the woman and fertilized by the partner's sperm outside her body. The fertilized ovum is then implanted in the uterus of the woman where it can grow and develop successfully. Besides being expensive and time-consuming, this procedure has a low success rate. Repeated failures place heavy emotional demands on the couple.

Health, Homeostasis, and the Environment

The Sperm Crisis?

The human reproductive system is not essential to homeostasis or the survival of an individual. In the words of physiologist Lauralee Sherwood, "it is essential for sustaining the thread of life from generation to generation."

Like other systems, the reproductive system is susceptible to environmental conditions—to pollution and social and psychological conditions that create stress. In this section we will explore one crucial link between the environment and reproduction.

In September 1979, Professor Ralph Dougherty, a chemist at Florida State University, announced findings from a study of 130 healthy male college students. In his test group, the researcher found extremely low sperm counts of only 20 million per milliliter (ml) of semen, compared with an expected value of 60–100 million per ml. Biochemical analyses of the testes also revealed high levels of four toxic chemicals: DDT, polychlorinated biphenyls (PCBs), pentachlorophenol, and hexachlorobenzene.

An article in the Sierra Club's magazine describing the results proclaimed that America was facing a "sperm crisis" caused by toxic chemicals. But not everyone agrees. Health officials, in fact, have challenged these findings. Some officials contend that the low sperm counts that Dougherty recorded may have resulted from improved counting techniques. That is to say, over the years, advances in technology have allowed scientists to count sperm more accurately. As a result, estimates of the normal sperm concentration have been markedly lowered. Dougherty maintains that such improvements, while real, are not entirely responsible for the decline.

Other health officials argue that Dougherty's findings are not representative of the American public. Floridians, they say, are exposed to high levels of pesticides used on farms that contaminate the water supplies of urban and rural residents.

Additional studies in Florida and other states show that sperm counts in American men have indeed been falling since the 1950s. Prior to 1950, the average sperm count was about 110 million per ml. By 1980 and 1981, sperm counts had dropped to about 60 million per ml. Further studies show continuing decline to under 50 million in the late 1980s. Statistical studies suggest that the decline may be related to growing pesticide use, air pollution, and other factors.

Especially harmful may be chemicals in the environment that mimic the female sex hormone estrogen, such as dioxins, generated in paper production and waste incineration, and phthalates, which are used in many products including food and beverage containers. Research suggests that exposing males early *in utero*, a time at which they are extremely chemically sensitive, to such chemicals could have dramatic effects on their testes. At least 60 such chemicals have been identified to date.

Studies in Hawaii support the hypothesis that certain environmental chemicals are causing a decline in sperm count. These studies show that Hawaiian men have a considerably higher sperm count than men residing in the continental United States. This observation has been attributed to a generally cleaner environment. There are, say researchers, fewer factories on the Hawaiian islands than on the mainland. People are exposed to fewer agricultural chemicals, and frequent winds probably result in cleaner air. Reductions in sperm count are of concern to many people because a sperm count below 20 million per milliliter is generally insufficient for fertilization. Today, low sperm counts account for a significant percentage of all infertility in U.S. couples.

Human reproduction, like other bodily processes, depends on a healthy environment. Research shows that a wide range of factors—from drugs to radiation to industrial chemicals—are toxic, or potentially toxic, to human reproduction (**TABLE 19-4**). "There has been an explosion of spermatotoxins in the environment," says Dr. Bruce Rappaport, a fertility specialist. "The problem is environmental pollution." Today, at least 20 common industrial chemicals are known to be reproductive toxins. Ten commonly prescribed antibiotics can reduce sperm count. Tagamet, a drug that is used to relieve stress and treat excess stomach acidity, reduces sperm count by over 40%. By one estimate, at least 40 commonly used drugs depress sperm production. Thousands of other drugs and environmental pollutants have not been tested.

These facts do not necessarily mean that the United States is in a sperm crisis, but they do suggest the need for further research to determine the potential impacts, if any, of the many thousands of chemicals now commonly used or released into the environment. Research may prove that we need to clean up our act, or it may show that these fears are unwarranted.

TABLE 19-4
Some Agents Potentially Toxic to Male and Female Reproduction

Males	Females
Natural and synthetic androgens	Natural and synthetic estrogens
Heat	Natural and synthetic progestins
Radiation	Amphetamine
Dioxin	DDT
PCBs	Parathion (insecticide)
Vinyl chloride	Carbaryl (insecticide)
Ethanol	DES
Benzene	PCBs
DES (diethylstilbestrol)	
EDB (ethylene dibromide)	
Paraquat (herbicide)	
Carbaryl (insecticide)	
Cadmium	
Mercury	

Summary

The Male Reproductive System

1. The male reproductive tract consists of seven basic components: (a) testes, (b) epididymis, (c) vasa deferentia, (d) sex accessory glands, (e) urethra, (f) penis, and (g) scrotum.

2. The *testes* reside in the *scrotum*, which provides a suitable temperature for sperm development. Each testis contains hundreds of sperm-producing *seminiferous tubules*.

3. *Sperm* produced in the seminiferous tubules are stored in the *epididymis*. During *ejaculation*, sperm pass from the epididymis to the *vas deferens*, then to the *urethra*. Secretions from the *sex accessory glands* are added to the sperm at this time, forming semen.

4. Between the seminiferous tubules are the *interstitial cells*, which produce the hormone *testosterone*. Testosterone secretion is controlled by *luteinizing hormone (LH)* or *interstitial cell stimulating hormone (ICSH)* from the anterior pituitary. LH release is regulated in a negative feedback loop with testosterone.

5. Testosterone stimulates *spermatogenesis*, facial hair growth, thickening of the vocal cords, laryngeal cartilage growth,

sebaceous gland secretion, and bone and muscle development.

6. The *penis* is the organ of copulation. It contains *erectile tissue*, which fills with blood during sexual arousal, making the penis turgid.

7. Ejaculation is under reflex control. When sexual stimulation becomes intense, sensory nerve impulses travel to the spinal cord. There they stimulate motor neurons in the cord, which send impulses to the smooth muscle in the walls of the epididymis, the vasa deferentia, the sex accessory glands, and the urethra, causing ejaculation.

The Female Reproductive System

8. The female reproductive system consists of two basic components: the reproductive tract and the external genitalia.

9. The reproductive tract consists of (a) the uterus, (b) the two uterine tubes, (c) the two ovaries, and (d) the vagina.

10. The *external genitalia* consist of two flaps of skin on both sides of the vaginal opening, the *labia majora* and the *labia minora*.

11. Female germ cells are housed in follicles in the ovary. A *follicle* consists of a

germ cell and an investing layer of follicle cells.

12. A dozen or so follicles enlarge during each menstrual cycle, but most follicles degenerate. In humans, usually only one follicle makes it to ovulation.

13. The oocyte and an investing layer of follicle cells are released during ovulation and drawn into the uterine tubes.

14. The *menstrual cycle* consists of a series of changes occurring in the ovaries, uterus, and endocrine system of women.

15. The first half of the menstrual cycle is called the *follicular phase*. It is during this period that FSH from the pituitary stimulates follicle growth and development. LH stimulates estrogen production.

16. Estrogen levels rise slowly during the follicular phase, then trigger a positive feedback mechanism that results in a preovulatory surge of FSH and LH, which triggers ovulation.

17. The oocyte is expelled from the *antral follicle* at ovulation. The follicle then collapses and is converted into a *corpus luteum (CL)*, which releases estrogen and progesterone.

18. In the absence of fertilization, the CL degenerates. If fertilization occurs, how-

ever, HCG from the embryo maintains the CL for approximately 6 months.

19. During the menstrual cycle, ovarian hormones stimulate growth of the uterine lining, which is necessary for successful implantation. If fertilization does not occur, the uterine lining is sloughed off during *menstruation*, which is triggered by a decline in ovarian estrogen and progesterone.

20. Like testosterone levels in boys, estrogen levels in girls increase at puberty. Estrogen promotes growth of the external genitalia, the reproductive tract, and bone. It also stimulates the deposition of fat in women's hips, buttocks, and breasts.

21. Progesterone works with estrogen to stimulate breast development. It also promotes endometrial growth and inhibits uterine contractions.

22. Many women suffer from *premenstrual syndrome* or *PMS*, which is characterized by irritability, depression, tension, fatigue, headaches, bloating, swelling and tenderness of the breasts, and joint pain.

23. The menstrual cycle continues throughout the reproductive years, but after a woman reaches 20, the ovaries become progressively less responsive to gonadotropins. As a result, estrogen levels slowly decline as a woman ages. Ovulation and menstruation become erratic as a woman approaches 45.

24. Between the ages of 45 and 55, ovulation and menstruation cease. The end of reproductive function in women is known as *menopause.*

25. The decline in estrogen levels results in the atrophy of the reproductive organs and in behavioral disturbances. Many women become irritable, suffer bouts of depression, and experience hot flashes and night sweats induced by intense vasodilation of vessels in the skin.

Birth Control

26. Birth control refers broadly to any method or device that prevents births and includes two general strategies: *contraception* (measures that prevent pregnancy) and *induced abortion* (the deliberate expulsion of a fetus).

27. **FIGURE 19-18** summarizes the effectiveness of the various birth control measures.

28. The most effective form of birth control is abstinence. Another highly effective measure is sterilization—*vasectomy* in men and *tubal ligation* in women.

29. The pill is a highly effective means of birth control. The most common pill in use today contains a mixture of estrogen and progesterone that inhibits ovulation. In some women, however, estrogen causes adverse health effects.

30. The *intrauterine device* or *IUD* is a plastic or metal coil that is placed inside the uterus, where it prevents the fertilized ovum from implanting.

31. The diaphragm, condom, and vaginal sponge are less effective than the measures described above. The *diaphragm* is a rubber cap fitted over the cervix. To be fully effective, it must be coated with a spermicidal jelly, foam, or cream.

32. The *condom* is a thin, latex rubber sheath worn over the penis during sexual intercourse that prevents sperm from entering the vagina.

33. The *vaginal sponge* is a tiny, round sponge worn by the woman. It is impregnated with a spermicidal chemical.

34. One of the oldest, but least effective, methods of birth control is *withdrawal*, removing the penis before ejaculation. *Spermicidal chemicals* used alone are about as effective as withdrawal.

35. Abstaining from sexual intercourse around the time of ovulation, known as the *rhythm method*, is another way to prevent pregnancy. Statistics on effectiveness show that the natural method is one of the least successful of all birth control measures.

36. Some couples may elect to terminate pregnancy through an abortion.

Sexually Transmitted Diseases

37. Certain viruses and bacteria can be transmitted from one individual to another during sexual contact. Infections spread in this way are called *sexually transmitted diseases (STDs).*

38. *Gonorrhea* is caused by a bacterium that commonly infects the urethra in men and the cervical canal in women. Overt symptoms of the infection are frequently not present, so people can spread the disease without knowing it. If left untreated, gonorrhea can spread to other organs, causing considerable damage.

39. *Syphilis* is a serious STD caused by a bacterium that penetrates the linings of the oral cavity, vagina, and penile urethra. If untreated, syphilis proceeds through three stages. It can be treated with antibiotics during the first two stages, but in stage 3, when damage to the brain and blood vessels is evident, treatment is ineffective.

40. Chlamydial infections, an extremely common bacterial STD, resemble gonorrhea.

41. *Genital herpes* is also a very common STD. It is caused by a virus. Once the virus enters the body, it remains for life. Blisters form on the genitals and sometimes on the thighs and buttocks. The blisters break open and become painful ulcers. At this stage, an individual is highly infectious. New outbreaks of the virus may occur from time to time, especially when an individual is under stress.

42. *Nonspecific urethritis (NSU)*, the most common sexually transmitted disease, is caused by several different bacteria, but most commonly by chlamydia. It is less threatening than gonorrhea or syphilis. Many men and women show no symptoms of NSU and can therefore spread the disease without knowing it. Symptoms, when they occur, resemble those of gonorrhea.

43. Genital warts occur in men and women whose immune systems are suppressed and are caused by HPV.

Infertility

44. The inability to conceive is called *infertility.* Infertility can result from a variety of problems in men and women: poorly timed sex, low sperm count, failure to ovulate, or obstruction in the uterine tubes.

Health, Homeostasis, and the Environment: The Sperm Crisis?

45. A variety of drugs and chemical pollutants affect sperm development and may be causing a decline in the sperm count of American men.

Critical Thinking

Thinking Critically— Analysis

This Analysis corresponds to the Thinking Critically scenario that was presented at the beginning of this chapter.

Before writing your article, you might want to check the experimental design. Were adequate sample sizes used in the experiments? Did the researcher have proper con-

trol groups? Were the animals particularly prone to these abnormalities? What dosages were given? Are these at all similar to dosages people might be exposed to?

You might also want to see if these results have been reported elsewhere. Moreover, you would probably want to see whether there is any research data linking this chemical to human abnormalities. Having done this, you would have a strong base from which to piece together a good article.

Test of Concepts

1. You are a fertility specialist. A young woman arrives in your office complaining that she has been trying to get pregnant for 2 years but to no avail. Describe how you would go about determining whether the problem was with her, her husband, or both of them.

2. Describe the anatomy of the male reproductive system. Where are sperm produced? Where are they stored? What structures produce the semen?

3. Describe the process of spermatogenesis, noting the cell types and the number of chromosomes in each type.

4. Why is the first meiotic division called a *reduction division*?

5. List the hormones that control testicular function. Where are they

produced, and what effects do they have on the testes?

6. You are a family doctor. A man comes to your office complaining of impotence. What are the possible causes? How would you go about testing for the causes?

7. Trace the pathway for a sperm from the seminiferous tubule to the site of fertilization.

8. Describe the process of ovulation and its hormonal control.

9. What is the corpus luteum? How does it form? What does it produce? Why does it degenerate at the end of the menstrual cycle if fertilization does not occur?

10. What is menstruation? What triggers its onset?

11. Describe the effects of estrogen and progesterone on the reproductive tract and the body.

12. A woman comes to your office. She is 47 years old and complains of irritability and depression. She asks for the name of a reliable psychiatrist who could help her. She says that she wakes up in the middle of the night in a sweat. Would you give her the name of a psychiatrist? Why or why not? If not, what would you do?

13. Describe each of the following birth control measures, explaining what they are and how they work: the pill, IUD, diaphragm, cervical cap, condom, spermicidal jelly, and natural method.

14. Describe ways to prevent the spread of sexually transmitted diseases.

www.jbpub.com/humanbiology

Connect to this book's web site: www.jbpub.com/humanbiology
The site features eLearning, an online review area that provides quizzes, chapter outlines, and other tools to help you study for your class. You can also follow useful links for in-depth information, research the differing views in the Point/Counterpoints, or keep up on the latest environmental and health news.

CHAPTER 20

Human Development and Aging

Thinking Critically

"Thanks to improvements in medicine, people are living longer." You have heard this statement dozens of times in one form or another. The assertion is that advances in medicine are actually increasing how long you and I will live. This statement is repeated so often that most of us believe it implicitly. But is it true? ■

Human embryo showing the webbed fingers.

In a hospital room in a major city, two parents bring a newborn child into the world with the assistance of a nurse midwife. The wife holds their new daughter in the hospital bed while three floors up in the geriatric ward, an elderly man quietly passes away. Birth and death are two of life's most dramatic acts. They're the subject of this chapter. We will begin our journey with a discussion of fertilization, the beginnings of a new life, then study the development of the fertilized ovum into an embryo then into a fetus. We will conclude with a discussion of the other end of the human life cycle: aging and death.

Section 20-1

Fertilization

In sexually reproducing animals like us, life begins when the sperm and egg unite, forming a **zygote**. This process is called **fertilization**. In humans, fertilization occurs in the upper third of the uterine tube, close to the site of ovulation. In order for fertilization to occur, the sperm must undertake a rather rigorous and difficult journey up the female reproductive tract.

Their journey begins with **ejaculation**, the expulsion of the sperm from the male reproductive tract. Within a few minutes of ejaculation, the millions of sperm in the normal ejaculate enter the cervical canal, accessing it via a tiny opening that projects into the vagina. Thirty minutes later, those sperm that have successfully found their way into the cervical canal arrive at the junction of the uterus and oviducts or uterine tubes. Sperm then travel up the oviducts. In the upper portion of this long tubular structure, they may encounter an oocyte released from the ovary during ovulation.

Sperm face many obstacles along the way. The vagina, for example, often contains slightly acidic secretions. Although the ejaculate contains chemicals that neutralize these acids, many sperm die. Many sperm that survive the vaginal secretions simply can't find their way into the cervix. Those that make it into the cervix can get lost in the folds of the inner lining. The same fate faces sperm that enter the uterus.

Studies based on laboratory animals suggest that in humans only 1 in 3 sperm makes it through the cervical canal and 1 in 1000 makes it to the uterine tubes (**FIGURE 20-1**). The rest perish along the way. They're engulfed by cells in the lining of the female reproductive tract.

Movement through the reproductive tract of women relies on two processes. First is sperm motility, a feat permitted by the whiplike tail of the sperm. The second, and by far the most important mechanism for transporting sperm along the female reproductive tract, is muscular contraction occurring in the walls of the uterus and uterine tubes. These contractions are stimulated by prostaglandins, hormonelike substances in the semen.

Although sperm reach the site of fertilization an hour or so after ejaculation, they cannot fertilize an oocyte yet. They must wait around for 6 to 7 hours before they are able to accomplish this feat. The time spent swimming around in the fluids of the oviduct is required to remove a protective layer of cholesterol on their plasma membranes. This coat is derived from the secretions of the sex accessory glands. It stabilizes the sperm plasma membranes and protects these highly streamlined cells on their journey through the female reproductive tract. Removal of this coating renders the sperm's membranes fragile and disruptable, which you shall soon see is a prerequisite for fertilization.

After this process, the plasma membrane over the head of the sperm fuses with the outer membrane of the **acrosome**. First described in Chapter 19, the acrosome is a stocking-caplike structure pulled down over the head of the sperm. It is filled with digestive enzymes. Where the membranes of the acrosome and plasma membrane fuse, tiny openings develop. These tiny holes permit acrosomal enzymes to leak out (**FIGURE 20-2A**). These enzymes help the sperm dissolve its way through the layer of follicle cells that surrounds the oocyte. But sperm do not work in isolation. Rather, successful

Time of appearance (min after ejaculation)	Percent of ejaculated sperm*
30–60	0.001%
10–20	0.1%
1–3	3%
0	100%

Optimal site of fertilization

Ampulla of oviduct

Uterus

Ovary

Fimbria

Cervical canal

Vagina
400,000,000 sperm deposited

Penis

* Based on data from laboratory animals

(Sperm and ovum are enlarged.)

FIGURE 20-1 Sperm Transport in the Female Reproductive System Sperm move rapidly up the female reproductive tract of humans and other vertebrates principally as a result of contractions in the muscular walls of the uterus and uterine tubes. Notice the rapid decline in sperm number along the way.

fertilization relies on the action of acrosomal enzymes from many sperm swarming around the oocyte like so many bees around a hive. These enzymes dissolve the material that binds the follicle cells together (**FIGURE 20-2B**). After passing through this layer, known as the *corona radiata* (radiating crown), sperm must digest their way through another barrier. This one is the **zona pellucida** (the clear zone). The zona pellucidea is a clear gel-like layer immediately surrounding the oocyte. Sperm penetrate it with the aid of acrosomal enzymes, but at this stage it is each sperm for itself.

Sperm cells that traverse the zona pellucida enter the space between the plasma membrane of the oocyte and the zona. As a rule, the first sperm cell to come in contact with the plasma membrane of the oocyte will fertilize it; all other sperm are excluded.

Sperm are excluded by two mechanisms. The first is called the **fast block to polyspermy** (POLL-ee-SPERM-ee; "many sperm"). The fast block to polyspermy occurs when the sperm cell contacts the plasma membrane of the oocyte, triggering membrane depolarization. As you may recall from Chapter 11 on the nervous system, depolarization is a change in the resting potential of the plasma membrane. This change is caused by an influx of sodium ions that is triggered when the first sperm cell comes in contact with the plasma membrane of the oocyte. For reasons not well understood, depolarization blocks other sperm from fusing with the oocyte.

Sperm are also excluded by a **slow block to polyspermy**. When a sperm contacts the plasma membrane of a secondary oocyte, it triggers the release of enzymes from membrane-bound vesicles lying beneath the plasma membrane of the oocyte (**FIGURE 20-2A**). These enzymes cause the zona pellucida to harden, blocking other sperm from reaching the oocyte. These secretions may also cause the "extra" sperm that have attached to the plasma membrane of the oocyte to detach.

These two mechanisms are important evolutionary developments. They ensure that only one sperm penetrates an ovum. Without them, fertilized eggs might quickly overload with extra nuclear material, a condition that would likely impair subsequent cell divisions and result in embryonic death.

Sperm contact with the plasma membrane of the oocyte also triggers the second meiotic division, thus converting the secondary oocyte into an **ovum**. But the life of an ovum is short-lived, for once the sperm nucleus enters, the ovum is called a zygote.

Once inside the ovum, the sperm cell nucleus swells. At this stage, the nuclei of the ovum and sperm are called the male and female **pronuclei** (**FIGURE 20-3**). As you may recall from your studies of meiosis, the nuclei of the sperm and ovum contain 23 single-stranded chromosomes.

As the pronuclei move toward the center of the cell, the chromosomes in the pronuclei replicate. Each chromosome now contains two strands. A mitotic spindle also assembles. As you may recall from your studies of mitosis, the mitotic spindle is made of microtubules. It helps cells apportion their chromosomes during cell division.

After chromosome replication is complete, the chromosomes of the male and female pronuclei condense, and the nuclear envelopes of both pronuclei disintegrate. Some of the spindle fibers attach to the chromosomes. The chromosomes line up on the equatorial plate. The zygote is now ready for the first mitotic division, one of many billions of cell divisions that will occur in the long journey of human growth and development.

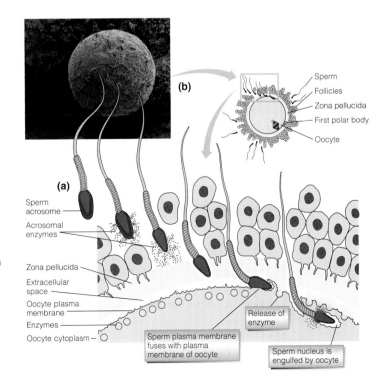

FIGURE 20-2 Fertilization *(a)* The plasma membrane of the sperm and the outer membrane of the acrosome fuse and the membranes break down, releasing enzymes that allow the sperm to penetrate the corona radiata. Sperm digest their way through the zona pellucida via enzymes associated with the inner acrosomal membrane. Sperm are engulfed by the oocyte plasma membrane. Cortical granules are released when the sperm cell contacts the membrane. These granules cause other sperm in contact with the membrane to detach. *(b)* Although many sperm gather around the egg, only one will enter. Fertilized sperm are phagocytized by the egg.

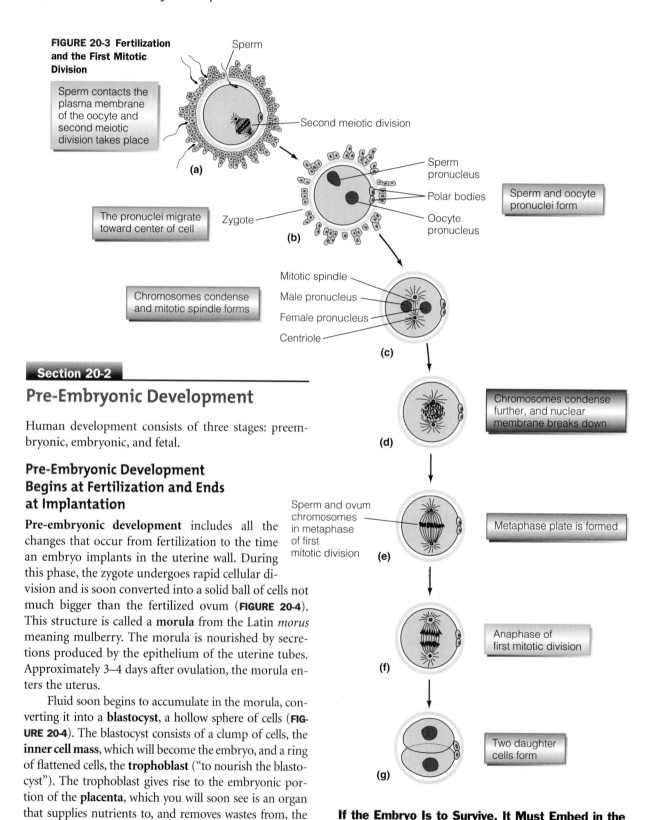

FIGURE 20-3 Fertilization and the First Mitotic Division

Sperm contacts the plasma membrane of the oocyte and second meiotic division takes place

Sperm

Second meiotic division

(a)

The pronuclei migrate toward center of cell

Zygote

(b)

Sperm pronucleus

Polar bodies

Oocyte pronucleus

Sperm and oocyte pronuclei form

Chromosomes condense and mitotic spindle forms

Mitotic spindle

Male pronucleus

Female pronucleus

Centriole

(c)

Chromosomes condense further, and nuclear membrane breaks down

(d)

Sperm and ovum chromosomes in metaphase of first mitotic division

Metaphase plate is formed

(e)

Anaphase of first mitotic division

(f)

Two daughter cells form

(g)

Pre-Embryonic Development

Human development consists of three stages: preembryonic, embryonic, and fetal.

Pre-Embryonic Development Begins at Fertilization and Ends at Implantation

Pre-embryonic development includes all the changes that occur from fertilization to the time an embryo implants in the uterine wall. During this phase, the zygote undergoes rapid cellular division and is soon converted into a solid ball of cells not much bigger than the fertilized ovum (**FIGURE 20-4**). This structure is called a **morula** from the Latin *morus* meaning mulberry. The morula is nourished by secretions produced by the epithelium of the uterine tubes. Approximately 3–4 days after ovulation, the morula enters the uterus.

Fluid soon begins to accumulate in the morula, converting it into a **blastocyst**, a hollow sphere of cells (**FIGURE 20-4**). The blastocyst consists of a clump of cells, the **inner cell mass**, which will become the embryo, and a ring of flattened cells, the **trophoblast** ("to nourish the blastocyst"). The trophoblast gives rise to the embryonic portion of the **placenta**, which you will soon see is an organ that supplies nutrients to, and removes wastes from, the embryo.

The blastocyst remains unattached in the uterine lumen for 2–3 days. During this period, it is nourished by secretions of uterine glands.

If the Embryo Is to Survive, It Must Embed in the Wall of the Uterus. The blastocyst eventually attaches to the uterine lining, that is, the endometrium. But this structure doesn't just stick to the endometrium, it actively digests its way into the layer using enzymes released by its cells. This process is called **implantation**. It occurs 6–7 days after fertilization. Take a moment to study **FIGURE 20-5** to view the events taking place during implantation.

Most embryos implant high on the back wall of the uterus. The cells of the trophoblast first contact the endometrium, then adhere to it, but only if the uterine lining is healthy and properly primed by estrogen and progesterone. If the endometrium is not ready or is "unhealthy"—for example, because of the presence of an IUD or an endometrial infection—the blastocyst cannot implant. Blastocysts may also fail to implant if their cells contain certain genetic mutations. RU 486 and other similar drugs described in Chapter 19 also prevent implantation. No matter what the cause, the blastocyst soon perishes. It is absorbed (phagocytized) by the cells of the endometrium or expelled during menstruation.

In cases where implantation occurs, the cells of the endometrium at and around the point of contact enlarge (hypertrophy). Enzymes released by the cells of the trophoblast digest a small hole in the thickened endometrium, and the blastocyst "bores" its way into the deeper tissues of the uterine lining (**FIGURE 20-5B**). During this process, the blastocyst literally "eats" its way into the layer of enlarged endometrial cells, feeding on nutrients liberated from the endometrial cells it destroys. Nutrients gained during this process sustain the blastocyst before the placenta forms.

By day 14, the uterine endometrium grows over the blastocyst, enclosing it completely and walling it off from

the uterine lumen (cavity). Endometrial cells respond to the invasion of the blastocyst by producing prostaglandins. These substances stimulate an increase in the development of uterine blood vessels, which ensures an ample supply of blood and nutrients for the blastocyst.

In yet another of life's most amazing feats, endometrial and embryonic tissue combine to form a structure known as the **placenta** (**FIGURE 20-6**). The placenta serves many functions. Three of the most important are the nourishment of the embryo and fetus, the provision of oxygen, and the removal of wastes produced by embryos and fetuses throughout their long residence in the uterus.

FIGURE 20-4 Formation of the Morula and Blastocyst During Pre-embryonic Development

FIGURE 20-5 Implantation *(a)* The blastocyst fuses with the endometrial lining. Endometrial cells proliferate, forming the decidua. *(b)* The blastocyst digests its way into the endometrium. Cords of trophoblastic cells invade, digesting maternal tissue and providing nutrients for the developing blastocyst. *(c)* The blastocyst soon becomes completely embedded in the endometrium.

(a)

(b)

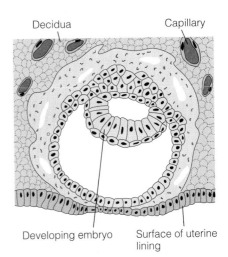

(c)

FIGURE 20-6 The Placenta
This organ, made from maternal and fetal tissue, helps nourish the developing fetus and remove wastes. It also produces important hormones.

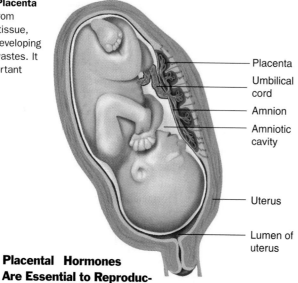

- Placenta
- Umbilical cord
- Amnion
- Amniotic cavity
- Uterus
- Lumen of uterus

FIGURE 20-7 Blood Levels of Placental Hormones Human chorionic gonadotropin levels peak in the second month of pregnancy, then drop off by the end of the third month. Levels of estrogen and progesterone, produced chiefly by the placenta, continue to rise.

Placental Hormones Are Essential to Reproduction.

Besides supplying oxygen and nutrients and getting rid of embryonic wastes, the placenta acts as a temporary endocrine gland, producing several hormones vital to the success of pregnancy. This section discusses three of the placenta's hormones: human chorionic gonadotropin (HCG), estrogen, and progesterone (TABLE 20-1).

FIGURE 20-7 shows blood levels of these three hormones during pregnancy. As illustrated, HCG levels peak at the beginning of the second month of pregnancy, then drop off by the end of the third month. In contrast, levels of estrogen and progesterone rise dramatically throughout gestation (the period between fertilization and childbirth).

As noted in Chapter 19, HCG is an LH-like hormone produced by the embryo early in pregnancy. One of its main functions is to prevent the corpus luteum (CL) in the ovary from degenerating when an embryo is

present. HCG also stimulates estrogen and progesterone production by the CL. These hormones are essential to maintaining pregnancy. However, as illustrated, HCG secretion from the embryonic tissue lasts only about 10 weeks. Because of the natural decline in HCG, the CL degenerates. At this time, estrogen and progesterone production shifts to the placenta.

Many women experience nausea (morning sickness) during the first 2–3 months of pregnancy. Although it often occurs in the morning hours, "morning" sickness in some women can last all day. The exact cause is not known, but some researchers think that HCG may be the culprit. They believe that HCG stimulates the brain directly, creating nausea. Other researchers blame the high levels of estrogen and progesterone. It may be high levels of all three hormones.

TABLE 20-1

Hormones Produced by the Placenta

Hormone	Function
Human chorionic gonadotropin (HCG)	Maintains corpus luteum of pregnancy
	Stimulates secretion of testosterone by developing testes in XY embryos
Estrogen (also secreted by corpus luteum of pregnancy)	Stimulates growth of myometrium, increasing uterine strength for parturition (childbirth)
	Helps prepare mammary glands for lactation
Progesterone (also secreted by corpus luteum of pregnancy)	Suppresses uterine contractions to provide quiet environment for fetus
	Promotes formation of cervical mucous plug to prevent uterine contamination
	Helps prepare mammary glands for lactation
Human chorionic somatomammotropin	Helps prepare mammary glands for lactation
	Believed to reduce maternal utilization of glucose so that greater quantities of glucose can be shunted to the fetus
Relaxin (also secreted by corpus luteum of pregnancy)	Softens cervix in preparation of cervical dilation at parturition
	Loosens connective tissue between pelvic bones in preparation for parturition

Estrogen and progesterone serve a number of functions essential for pregnancy. Together, estrogen and progesterone stimulate the growth of the uterine lining (endometrium), which is essential to successful pregnancy. Estrogen by itself also stimulates growth of the smooth muscle cells of the myometrium; this allows the uterus to expand to many times its original size during pregnancy. Smooth muscle growth not only accommodates the growing baby, it also provides additional propulsive force needed to expel the child at birth.

Progesterone has additional functions as well. For example, it calms the uterine musculature during pregnancy, preventing the premature expulsion of the embryo and fetus. Progesterone also stimulates mucous production by the cervix and the formation of a mucous plug that prevents bacteria from entering the uterus and infecting the growing embryo.

The Amnion Forms from the Inner Cell Mass. As the placenta begins to form, the inner cell mass (ICM) of the blastocyst undergoes some remarkable changes. Early in development, a layer of cells separates from the ICM to form the **amnion** (AM-knee-on). A small cavity, the **amniotic cavity**, forms between the ICM and the amnion. The amniotic cavity fills with a watery fluid called **amniotic fluid**. It forms a cushion around the baby during development, helping to protect it from injury[1] (**FIGURE 20-6**).

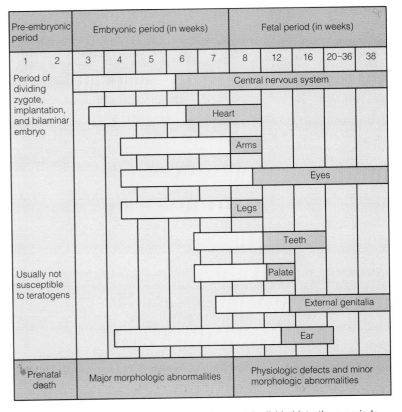

FIGURE 20-8 Organogenesis Human development is divided into three periods, or stages: pre-embryonic, embryonic, and fetal. Organogenesis occurs during the embryonic stage. Each bar indicates when an organ system develops. The yellow-shaded area indicates the periods most sensitive to teratogenic agents (agents that can cause birth defects).

Section 20-3

Embryonic Development

After the amnion forms, the cells of the inner cell mass differentiate, forming three distinct germ cell layers, the ectoderm, mesoderm, and endoderm. These are known as the **primary germ layers**. The formation of the primary germ layers marks the beginning of **embryonic development**.

---

[1]A portion of the amniotic fluid is produced by the fetus. The rest apparently comes from the amniotic membranes.

Embryonic Development Begins with Implantation and Ends When the Organs Are More or Less Formed

The primary germ layers of the embryo give rise to the organs of the body (**TABLE 20-2**) in a process called **organogenesis,** which begins about the third week of pregnancy (**FIGURE 20-8**). Organogenesis is the main event of embryonic development.

TABLE 20-2

End Products of Embryonic Germ Layers

Ectoderm	Mesoderm	Endoderm
Epidermis	Dermis	Lining of the digestive system
Hair, nails, sweat glands	All muscles of the body	Lining of the respiratory system
Brain and spinal cord	Cartilage	Urethra and urinary bladder
Cranial and spinal nerves	Bone	Gallbladder
Retina, lens, and cornea of eye	Blood	Liver and pancreas
Inner ear	All other connective tissue	Thyroid gland
Epithelium of nose, mouth, and anus	Blood vessels	Parathyroid gland
Enamel of teeth	Reproductive organs	Thymus
	Kidneys	

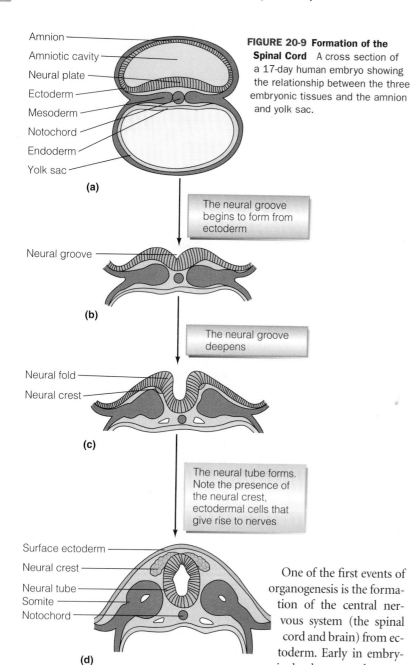

Amnion
Amniotic cavity
Neural plate
Ectoderm
Mesoderm
Notochord
Endoderm
Yolk sac

(a)

FIGURE 20-9 Formation of the Spinal Cord A cross section of a 17-day human embryo showing the relationship between the three embryonic tissues and the amnion and yolk sac.

The neural groove begins to form from ectoderm

Neural groove

(b)

The neural groove deepens

Neural fold
Neural crest

(c)

The neural tube forms. Note the presence of the neural crest, ectodermal cells that give rise to nerves

Surface ectoderm
Neural crest
Neural tube
Somite
Notochord

(d)

aggregations of ectodermal cells, which form the neural crest. As shown in **FIGURE 20-9D**, they lie on either side of the neural tube throughout most of its length. These cells sprout processes (axons) that extend into the body and attach to organs, muscle, bone, and skin. The ectoderm also gives rise to the outer layer of skin (the epidermis).

The middle germ layer, the mesoderm, gives rise to deeper structures—the muscle, cartilage, bone, and others. Much of the mesoderm first aggregates in blocks, called the **somites** (SO-mights), situated alongside the neural tube (**FIGURE 20-9D**). The somites form the vertebrae (the backbone) and the muscles of the neck and trunk. Mesoderm lateral to the somites becomes the dermis of the skin, connective tissue, and the bones and muscles of the limbs.

The endoderm, the "lowermost" germ layer of the ICM, forms a large pouch under the embryo, the **yolk sac** (**FIGURES 20-9A** and **20-10**). In birds, reptiles, and amphibians, the yolk sac nourishes the growing embryo, but in humans, nourishment comes from the placenta. The human yolk sac gives rise to blood cells and also primitive germ cells, known as **primordial germ cells**. During organogenesis, these cells migrate from the wall of the yolk sac via amoeboid motion to the developing testes and ovaries near the kidneys. They form high in the body cavity near the kidneys. The primordial germ cells become spermatogonia or oogonia, depending on the sex of the embryo. Finally, as shown in **FIGURE 20-10C**, the uppermost part of the yolk sac becomes the lining of the intestinal tract.

Section 20-4

Fetal Development

Fetal development begins in the eighth week of gestation and ends at birth. It involves two basic processes: (1) continued organ development and growth and (2) changes in body proportions—for example, elongation of the limbs.

Fetal Development Begins After the Organs Have Formed

The fetus grows rapidly during the fetal period, increasing from about 2.5 centimeters (1 inch) to 35–50 centimeters (14–21 inches) and increasing in weight from 1 gram to 3000–4000 grams. The fetus also undergoes considerable change in physical appearance, becoming more humanlike as each month passes. Organ development that commenced during the embryonic stage reaches completion during the fetal stage. Unfortunately, space limitations prevent a discussion of the development of each organ system, a fascinating subject that you may want to study on your own.

One of the first events of organogenesis is the formation of the central nervous system (the spinal cord and brain) from ectoderm. Early in embryonic development, the ectoderm along the back of the embryo invaginates or folds inward. This creates a long trench, the neural groove, that runs the length of the dorsal (back) surface of the embryo (**FIGURE 20-9B**). Over the next few weeks, the neural groove deepens and eventually closes off, creating the neural tube (**FIGURE 20-9D**). The walls of the neural tube thicken and eventually form the spinal cord. Anteriorly, the neural tube expands to form the brain.

As you may recall from your studies of the nervous system, numerous nerves attach to the spinal cord and brain. They're known as the spinal nerves and cranial nerves, respectively. Spinal nerves and cranial nerves form the peripheral nervous system; they develop from small

Sagittal (side) view

Frontal view

(b)

(a)

(c)

FIGURE 20-10 The Yolk Sac *(a)* A cross section of the embryo. The yolk sac forms from embryonic endoderm. *(b)* A longitudinal section showing how the upper end of the yolk sac forms the embryonic gut, *(c)* which will become the lining of the intestinal tract.

Section 20-5

Ectopic Pregnancy and Birth Defects

Pregnancy and embryonic development are rather complicated, involving hundreds of different processes, any one of which can go wrong. Two fairly common and potentially serious problems are ectopic pregnancy (ECK-TOP-ick) and birth defects.

Most Ectopic Pregnancies Occur in the Uterine Tubes

An **ectopic pregnancy** occurs when a fertilized ovum fails to be transported down the uterine tubes and instead develops outside the uterus, usually somewhere in the uterine tube itself.[2] Because of this, most ectopic pregnancies are also referred to as **tubal pregnancies**.

In a tubal pregnancy, the zygote actually implants in the lining of the uterine tube. However, placental development typically damages the uterine tubes, causing

internal bleeding and severe abdominal pain. Because the uterine tube cannot sustain the embryo, a tubal pregnancy cannot generally proceed to term. Surgery is required to remove the embryo.

About 1 in every 200 pregnancies is ectopic. Usually diagnosed within the first 2 months, tubal pregnancies generally occur as a result of defects in the uterine tubes or scar tissue from a previous infection, which impede the transport of the blastocyst to the uterus.

Embryonic and Fetal Development Can Be Altered by Outside Influences, Resulting in Birth Defects and Miscarriages

By several estimates, 31% of all conceptions (successful fertilizations) end in a miscarriage—that is, a **spontaneous abortion**. Fortunately, two of every three of these miscarriages occur before a woman is even aware that she is pregnant. Why such a high rate? Biologists hypothesize

---

[2]Ectopic pregnancies can also occur in the abdominal cavity.

FIGURE 20-11 A Common Birth Defect Scoliosis is a lateral curvature of the spine.

TABLE 20-3	
Known and Suspected Human Teratogens	
Known Agents	**Possible or Suspected Agents**
Progesterone	Aspirin
Thalidomide	Certain antibiotics
Rubella (German measles)	Insulin
Alcohol	Antitubercular drugs
Irradiation	Antihistamines
	Barbiturates
	Iron
	Tobacco
	Antacids
	Excess vitamins A and D
	Certain antitumor drugs
	Certain insecticides
	Certain fungicides
	Certain herbicides
	Dioxin
	Cortisone
	Lead

that early miscarriage is nature's way of "discarding" defective embryos. In other words, it is an evolutionary mechanism that helps ensure a healthier population.

Because nature generally eliminates defects, you might expect that most children born into the world would be free of defects. Unfortunately, this is not the case. Humans experience a surprisingly high rate of **birth defects**, physical or physiological abnormalities. By various estimates, 10%–12% of all newborns have some kind of birth defect, ranging from minor biochemical or physiological problems, which are not even noticed at birth, to gross physical defects (**FIGURE 20-11**).[3]

The study of birth defects is called **teratology** (TARE-ah-TOL-eh-gee). The word *teratology* comes from the Greek *teratos*, meaning "monster" and reflects some of the more gruesome or disfiguring birth defects. The term is an unfair characterization of most birth defects. Many are minor.

Although there is much to be learned about the causes of birth defects, scientists believe that most arise from chemical, biological, and physical agents, collectively known as **teratogens** (tah-RAT-uh-gens). **TABLE 20-3** lists known and suspected teratogens in humans.

The effect of a teratogenic agent on the developing embryo is related to three factors: (1) the time of exposure, (2) the nature of the agent, and (3) the dose. Consider time first. Because the organ systems develop at different times, the timing of exposure determines which systems are affected by a given teratogen. Organ systems are usually most sensitive to potentially harmful agents early in their development, as indicated by the yellow bars in **FIGURE 20-8** (page 467). The central nervous system, for example, begins to develop during the third week of gestation, or pregnancy. Because most women do not know they are pregnant for 3–4 weeks after fertilization, the central nervous system is at risk. In contrast, the teeth, palate, and genitalia do not begin to form until about the sixth or seventh week of pregnancy. Exposure to teratogens during the seventh week might therefore affect them but have little effect on the CNS, which has entered a less sensitive phase.[4]

The nature of the teratogen also influences the outcome of exposure. Some teratogens are broad-spectrum agents—that is, they affect a variety of developing systems. Others are narrow-spectrum agents, affecting only one system. Ethanol in alcoholic beverages, for example, is a broad-spectrum teratogen. Consequently, children who are born to alcoholic mothers—or even women who have consumed one or two drinks early in pregnancy—may have a variety of birth defects, including facial, heart, and skeletal defects. Behavioral problems and learning disabilities are also common in children of

---

[3]About 2% of all births show gross malformations.

[4]Note that the central nervous system is by no means fully formed at this time. Some teratogens, such as the rubella virus, can affect development through the first 3 months of gestation.

alcoholic mothers. These symptoms are part of a condition called **fetal alcohol syndrome**.

In contrast, other teratogenic agents are more selective, targeting only one system. Methyl mercury found in fish and shellfish, for instance, damages the CNS, creating abnormalities in the brain and spinal cord, but has little effect on other systems.

Finally, like most toxic substances, teratogens generally follow a dose-response relationship: The greater the dose, the greater the effect.

One of the best-known teratogens is not a chemical substance, but, rather, a biological agent. It is the virus that causes German measles or rubella (rue-BELL-ah). Rubella is less common and less contagious than ordinary measles. If a pregnant woman contracts the disease during the first 3 months of pregnancy, however, she has a one in three chance of giving birth to a baby with a serious birth defect. Deafness, cataracts, heart defects, and mental retardation are common. Moreover, 15% of all babies with congenital rubella syndrome die within one year of birth.

Many birth defects can be avoided. German measles vaccine given to young girls usually protects them throughout their childbearing years. Vaccinating boys also reduces the risk to society. As with many other diseases, prevention is the best policy.

Other precautions also help. For instance, during the first 8 weeks of pregnancy, women should avoid alcohol and other potential teratogens to protect the developing organ systems. As noted earlier, though, most women do not know that they are pregnant until 2–4 weeks after conception. Thus, a woman who is trying to get pregnant should carefully control what she eats and drinks.

Once the period of high sensitivity has passed, good nutrition and a healthy environment of course remain essential. This is because fetal development is also influenced by a number of physical and chemical agents in our homes and places of work. Toxic chemicals can stunt fetal growth and, in higher quantities, can even kill a fetus, resulting in a stillbirth. Proper nutrition is essential because nutrient, vitamin, and mineral deficiencies can retard growth.

Section 20-6

Childbirth and Lactation

For most expectant parents, the birth of a child is one of the most exciting events of their lives. Childbirth, also appropriately called *labor*, begins with mild uterine contractions. During labor, contractions increase in strength and frequency until the baby is born. What stimulates this process?

Uterine Muscle Contractions Are Stimulated by a Change in Hormonal Levels

Studies suggest that several factors play a role in stimulating uterine contractions. For instance, during the last few weeks of pregnancy, estrogen levels in the blood of a woman increase dramatically. This rise in estrogen levels is thought to stimulate the production of oxytocin receptors in the smooth muscle cells of the uterus. As you may recall from your study of the endocrine system, oxytocin is a hormone produced by the posterior pituitary. It causes contraction of the smooth muscle of the uterus, among other functions.

The increase in the number of receptors in the smooth muscle cells renders them increasingly responsive to the small amounts of oxytocin. But where does the oxytocin come from?

Interestingly, the fetal pituitary gland releases small quantities of oxytocin right before birth. Fetal oxytocin travels across the placenta and circulates in the mother's bloodstream. When it arrives at the sensitized uterine musculature, fetal oxytocin stimulates muscle contraction. Fetal oxytocin also stimulates the release of placental prostaglandins that act on smooth muscle. Together, these hormones stimulate more frequent and powerful uterine contractions.

Maternal oxytocin also plays an important role in childbirth. Scientists believe that uterine contractions and discomfort create stress that triggers the release of maternal oxytocin. It, in turn, augments muscle contractions caused by fetal oxytocin and prostaglandins (**FIGURE 20-12**). As uterine muscle contraction increases,

(4) Hypothalamus sends impulses to posterior pituitary

(5) Posterior pituitary releases stored oxytocin to blood; oxytocin stimulates mother's uterine muscle to contract

(6) Uterus contracts more vigorously

(3) Impulses to hypothalamus

(2) Receptors in cervix excited

(1) Baby moves further into mother's vagina

FIGURE 20-12 Oxytocin Positive Feedback Mechanism in Birth The mechanism continues to cycle until interrupted by the birth of the baby.

maternal oxytocin release increases. This stimulates even stronger contractions, resulting in additional oxytocin release, a positive feedback loop that continues until the baby is delivered.

Research also suggests that the high levels of estrogen at the end of pregnancy block the "calming" influence of placental progesterone. Consequently, the uterus begins to contract at irregular intervals.

Physicians (and expectant mothers) recognize two types of labor contractions. The first are **false labor contractions**. These irregular uterine contractions usually begin a month or two before childbirth and are also known as **Braxton-Hicks contractions**. As the due date approaches, false labor contractions occur with greater frequency, causing many anxious couples to race to the hospital only to be told to go home and wait for a few weeks for the real thing. In contrast, **true labor contractions** are more intense than those of false labor and occur at regular intervals.

Contractions are not all that's needed for childbirth. Some changes must also take place to enable the large baby to emerge from the uterus and pass through the uterus and vagina without causing severe damage.

Much of the success of parturition or birth depends on the hormone **relaxin**. Produced by the ovary and the placenta, relaxin is released near the end of gestation. As its name implies, relaxin softens the fibrocartilage uniting the pubic bones. This, in turn, allows the pelvic cavity to widen and thus greatly facilitates childbirth. Relaxin also softens the cervix, allowing it to expand so the baby can pass through it without causing severe damage. Without relaxin, delivery would be impossible.

Childbirth Occurs in Three Stages

FIGURE 20-13 illustrates the three stages of childbirth, dilation, expulsion, and placental.

Stage 1, the **dilation stage**, gets its name from the dilation of the cervix. This phase begins when uterine contractions start and generally lasts 6–12 hours; but it can last much longer.

At the beginning of stage 1, uterine contractions typically last only 30 seconds and may come every half hour or so. As time passes, however, contractions become more frequent and powerful. Uterine contractions generally rupture the amnion early in the dilation phase, causing the release of the amniotic fluid, an event commonly referred to as "breaking the water."

Uterine contractions push the infant's head against the relaxin-softened cervix, causing it to stretch and become thin (**FIGURE 20-13B**). By the end of stage 1, the

FIGURE 20-13 Stages of Labor *(a)* Position of the fetus near birth. *(b)* Dilation stage. Uterine contractions push the fetal head lower in the uterus and cause the relaxin-softened cervix to dilate. *(c)* Expulsion stage. Fetus is expelled through the cervix and vagina. *(d)* Placental stage. Placenta is delivered.

Placenta   Urinary bladder   Pubic bone

Vagina
Cervix
Rectum

(a)

Partially dilated cervix

(b) Dilation stage

(c) Expulsion stage

Placenta   Uterus   Umbilical cord

(d) Placental stage

cervix has dilated to about 10 centimeters (4 inches), approximately the diameter of a baby's head. During this phase, the baby is pushed downward by the uterine contractions and descends into the pelvic cavity. When its head is "locked" in the pelvis, the baby is said to be engaged.

Stage 2, the **expulsion stage,** begins after the cervix is dilated to 10 centimeters and the baby is engaged (**FIGURE 20-13C**). At this time, uterine contractions usually occur every 2 or 3 minutes and last 1–1.5 minutes each. For most first-time mothers, stage 2 lasts 50–60 minutes. If a woman is delivering her second child, it lasts about 20-30 minutes on average. The expulsion stage ends when the child is pushed through the vagina into the waiting hands of a doctor, midwife, proud father, or a bewildered cab driver.

To facilitate the delivery, physicians or midwives often make an incision in the skin to widen the vaginal opening. This procedure, called an **episiotomy** (eh-PEE-zee-AHT-oh-me), is performed when the baby's head enters the vagina in stage 2. The incision prevents unnecessary tearing and allows the infant to pass quickly. The incision is sutured immediately after the baby is born.

Once the baby's head emerges from the vagina, the rest of the body slips out quickly. However, the process isn't over yet. The newborn baby is still attached to the placenta via the umbilical cord. The cord pulsates for a minute or more, continuing to deliver blood to the newborn. Consequently, many health care workers wait about a minute before tying off and cutting the cord to allow the blood remaining in the placenta to be pumped into the newborn.

Most babies (95%) are delivered head first with their noses pointed toward the mother's tailbone (**FIGURE 20-13C**). Occasionally, however, babies may be oriented in other positions—making delivery more difficult, time-consuming, and hazardous for mother *and* baby.

The most common alternative delivery is the **breech birth**, in which the baby is expelled rear-end first. Because breech births require more time, they can cause extreme fatigue in the mother and brain damage in the baby. In breech babies, the umbilical cord sometimes wraps around the infant's neck during birth. This can cut off the fetus' blood supply, causing brain damage or death.

To avoid such complications, breech babies are often "turned" by physicians before birth by applying pressure to the woman's abdomen. If a fetus cannot be turned, the baby is usually delivered by a **cesarean section**, a horizontal incision through the abdomen just at the pubic hair line then through the uterus.

Cesarean sections are performed for other reasons as well—for example, if labor is prolonged or if the mother has an active infection caused by herpes or some other sexually transmitted disease that might be transferred to her child as it passes through the vagina.

The final stage of delivery is the **placental stage** (**FIGURE 20-13D**). It results in the expulsion of the placenta. The placenta remains attached to the uterine wall for a short while. It is then expelled by uterine contractions, usually within 15 minutes of childbirth. After the placenta is expelled, the uterine blood vessels clamp shut, preventing hemorrhage, although the mother continues to lose some blood for 3–6 weeks after delivery.

After delivery, the uterus gradually returns to its normal size. Uterine shrinkage (involution) results from the rapid decline in estrogen and progesterone, two hormones that had caused the uterus to grow in the first place. Shrinkage is accelerated by oxytocin released by the posterior pituitary after birth when a woman breast-feeds her baby. Complete involution in women who breast feed usually occurs within 4 weeks of pregnancy. In women who do not, the process usually takes 6 weeks.

The Pain Associated with Childbirth Can Be Relieved by Drugs and by Special Birthing Methods

The level of pain a woman feels during childbirth varies greatly and is partly governed by her level of fear and tension. Generally, the more tense a woman is, the more pain she feels. For this reason, many hospitals provide relaxation training to expectant mothers and comfortable birthing rooms. Drugs can also be given to reduce tension and pain, but they must be administered well before the birth of the baby to be effective. If given just before delivery, the drug offers little relief to the mother and may impair the baby's breathing.

Painkilling drugs can be injected into the wall of the vagina. This procedure, known as a **pudendal block** (pew-DEN-del), is performed if an episiotomy is likely or if forceps are going to be used to facilitate childbirth.

Many physicians routinely offer **epidural anesthesia** (ep-eh-DU-rel AN-es-THEE-zha). In this procedure, physicians inject an anesthetic agent into the bony canal that houses the spinal cord (just outside the dura mater). The drug temporarily deadens the sensory nerves leading from the vagina and lower body. The drug, however, not only blocks pain impulses, it blocks motor nerve impulses to the muscles of the abdomen, rendering a woman unable to push the baby out. In such cases, forceps may be required to facilitate the delivery, but forceps can damage a newborn and are generally avoided whenever possible.

Many couples and health care workers believe that drugs may be harmful to mothers and their babies. This belief and a desire to do things "naturally" have spawned the natural childbirth movement. **Natural childbirth** means different things to different people. In general, it refers to drug-free childbirth aided by relaxation and/or special breathing techniques.

The most popular natural childbirth method today is the **Lamaze technique** (lah-MAHZZ). Parents learn special breathing techniques to assist in the delivery. Shallow breathing, for example, commences when uterine contractions begin to keep the diaphragm from pressing down on abdominal organs, reducing tension and pain. It also ensures an adequate supply of oxygen to the fetus.

The second most popular method is the **Bradley method.** The Bradley method teaches women how to relax during uterine contractions, reducing pain and the need for drugs. No special breathing is required.

Milk Production, or Lactation, Is Controlled by the Hormone Prolactin

A baby emerges into a novel environment at birth. No longer connected to the placental lifeline, the newborn must now begin to breathe to obtain oxygen and dispose of carbon dioxide. It must also find a new way of

acquiring food. For most of human evolution, newborns have been fed milk from their mothers' breasts.

The **breasts** of a nonpregnant woman consist primarily of fat and connective tissue interspersed with milk-producing glandular tissue. The glands are drained by ducts that lead to the **nipple**, a surface structure where the milk ducts converge (**FIGURE 20-14**).

As noted earlier, during pregnancy the ducts and glands proliferate under the influence of estrogen and progesterone from the placenta and ovary. Milk production is itself stimulated by the hormone prolactin and a placental hormone, HCS (described below).

Prolactin secretion begins during the fifth week of pregnancy and increases throughout gestation, peaking at birth. The placenta also secretes a mild milk-producing hormone, **human chorionic somatomammotropin** (so-MAT-toe-MAM-oh-trow-pin) or **HCS**. Despite the presence of these lactogenic hormones, milk production does not begin until 2 or 3 days after birth. That's because the high levels of estrogen and progesterone throughout pregnancy necessary for breast development inhibit the action of the prolactin and HCS. When estrogen and progesterone levels decline after birth, HCS and prolactin exert their influence.

Although the breasts do not produce milk for 2 or 3 days, they immediately begin producing small quantities of colostrum. **Colostrum** (co-LOSS-trum) is a fluid rich in protein and lactose (a disaccharide), but lacking fat. Colostrum also contains antibodies that protect the infant from bacteria. A newborn subsists on colostrum for the first few days. (Health Note 8-1 describes the benefits of colostrum and breast-feeding.) Within 2–3 days, the breasts start to produce large quantities of milk.

Milk production relies on a hormone produced from the pituitary. It is known as *prolactin*. Prolactin's release is part of a neuroendocrine reflex. When a baby suckles her mother's breast, nerve impulses travel to a portion of the brain known as the hypothalamus. Cells of the hypothalamus release a hormone known as **prolactin releasing hormone (PRH)**. PRH travels to the pituitary in the bloodstream, where it stimulates the secretion of prolactin. Prolactin circulates in the blood to the breasts, stimulating milk production. Prolactin levels remain elevated for approximately 1 hour after each feeding. Each of these surges in hormone secretion stimulates the milk production needed for the next feeding.

Milk production continues as long as the baby suckles. If nursing is interrupted for 3 or 4 days, however, the breasts stop producing milk. In most women, milk production begins to decline by the seventh to ninth month of lactation, a time at which babies begin to feed on

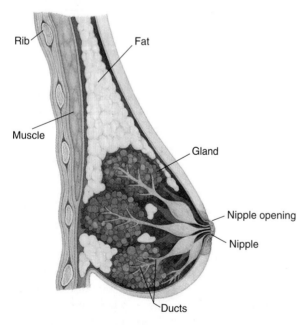

FIGURE 20-14 The Lactating Breast The glandular units enlarge considerably under the influence of progesterone and prolactin. Milk is expelled by contraction of musclelike cells surrounding the glandular units. Ducts drain the milk to the nipple.

Rib
Fat
Muscle
Gland
Nipple opening
Nipple
Ducts

semisolid food and breast-feed less frequently. The breasts decrease in size and may actually become smaller. (For a discussion of breast implants used to correct this condition, see Health Note 20-1.)

In order for milk to reach the nipple, it must be actively propelled from the glandular units and through the ducts. This is the function of oxytocin, the release of which is also controlled by a neuroendocrine reflex stimulated by suckling. Oxytocin, which is released from the posterior pituitary, causes muscles in the milk glands to contract and eject their milk. Neuroendocrine reflexes are important adaptations that provide hormones on demand. Such systems conserve energy and nutrients and contribute to the evolutionary success of mammals.

Aging and Death

Aging is a part of life, but it remains one of the great mysteries of biology. Technically, **aging** is defined as a progressive deterioration of the body's structure and function. One function whose deterioration is of extreme importance to us is homeostasis. As homeostatic mechanisms falter, the body becomes less resilient. Healing takes longer. Individuals become more susceptible to disease. Multiple breakdowns accelerate one's physical and mental deterioration.

The most notable changes occurring with age are physical shifts—wrinkling, loss of hair, and stooping. Less obvious is the gradual deterioration of the function of body organs. These often occur so slowly as to seem imperceptible (**FIGURE 20-15**). For example, as people age, their vision and hearing both decline, usually by small increments. Muscular strength also ebbs as a result of a decrease in the number of myofibrils (bundles of contractile filaments) in the skeletal muscles. Bones tend to thin, and joints often show signs of wear.

Aging is also accompanied by a gradual reduction in cardiac output and pulmonary function. The decrease in pulmonary function results from a reduction in the amount of air that can be inhaled and exhaled. As a result, oxygen absorption decreases. As we age, the number of functional nephrons in the kidney decreases, as does renal function.

The immune system also becomes less able to respond to antigens as we age. The nervous system does not escape the aging process, either. Memory deteriorates and reaction time decreases.

Although these changes are part of the aging process, not all of them begin at the same time. **TABLE 20-4**

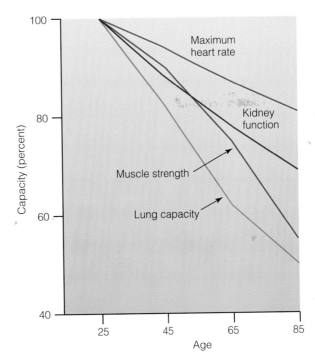

FIGURE 20-15 The Inevitable Slide   As we age, our bodies deteriorate. This graph shows the dramatic decline in four essential body functions.

(page 478) lists some important age-related changes in various organ systems along with their causes.

Aging May Be Brought About by a Decline in Cell Numbers and a Decline in the Function of Cells

The decline in homeostatic systems and general body function results from at least two factors: a decrease in the number of cells in the organs and a decline in the function of cells.

Cell number is determined by the balance between cell division and cell death. Laboratory experiments show that body cells grown in culture divide a certain number of times, then stop. The number of divisions a cell can undergo is directly related to the age of the organism from which the cell is taken: The older the organism, the fewer divisions are possible from that point in time on.

Laboratory studies such as these have also uncovered a correlation between the number of divisions in culture and the life span of the species from which the cells were taken. In other words, cells from species with long life spans undergo more divisions than cells from species with short life spans. These and other data suggest that the end of cell division and, therefore, aging, may be genetically programmed.

Health Note 20-1

Breast Augmentation: Balancing the Benefits and Risk

Marilyn Allbright is a 37-year-old mother of two children, both of whom she breast fed. After her second pregnancy, Marilyn noticed a dramatic decrease in the size of her breasts. After considering her options, she's decided to undergo breast augmentation surgery.

Marilyn is not alone. Each year, over 125,000 women in the United States undergo this procedure. The reasons for undertaking this surgery are several. Some women have implants to increase the size of their breasts, which like Marilyn's, have shrunk after breastfeeding or pregnancy. Others have implants because they feel their breasts are too small or because their breasts are markedly different sizes. Still others undergo the surgery because they've had breasts removed, either to halt an existing breast cancer or to prevent it. (Some women who have a high genetic risk for breast cancer opt to have their breasts removed pre-emptively.)

Breast implants were invented by two U.S. plastic surgeons, Drs. Cronin and Gerow in the early 1960s.

FIGURE 1. Implants.

Dow Corning developed the implant into a commercial product in 1962, and other companies began producing breast implants in the late 1960s.

Breast augmentation surgery was performed on a small number of women in the early 1960s and 1970s. In the 1980s and 1990s, increasing numbers of women have turned to this procedure for help.

Breast augmentation is most often performed on an outpatient basis under general anesthesia. In other words, women are operated on in clinics or surgical suites and they're completely "knocked out" during the operation. After surgery, they remain in the recovery room for a few hours. They're then given pain medication and driven home by a family member or friend that same day, although some women may be required to stay in the hospital overnight.

The breast implant is a soft, pliant roughly breast-shaped plastic bag made from an elastic-type silicone material (**FIGURE 1**). It is filled with one of four different solutions, usually saline (salt water). The implant is placed under the existing breast tissue, either directly under it or beneath the chest muscle, known as the *pectoralis majora.*

Most plastic surgeons and women agree that implants behind the muscle often turn out much better than those placed over it. There's little or no rippling of the skin and the breast is considerably softer and more natural looking. Moreover, this placement interferes little with routine mammography, X-rays of the breast to check for breast cancer.

In some instances, however, the implant is better placed over the

chest muscle. For example, if a woman is suffering from droopy breasts, the surgeon may remove some skin and then may place the implant directly over the muscle, creating a rounder, firmer breast.

Surgeons insert breast implants via an incision in the skin. Four main incision points are currently used: in the armpit or axilla, under the breast, at the outer margin of the areola (the darker skin surrounding the nipple), or, more recently, just above the belly button. The latter approach is known as a transumbilical insertion.

Transumbilical insertion is the latest technique, designed to reduce visible scarring. During this procedure, a tiny half-moon-shaped incision is made in the navel. Using a special device, the surgeon tunnels under the skin to reach the breast. Here, the surgeon creates a pocket for the breast implant, using a tissue separator. The empty implant is rolled up, inserted into the tunnel, and then moved into position. It is then filled with saline. When the surgeon removes the tube used to fill the implant, the plastic device self seals. The incision is sutured shut by a few absorbable stitches.

The transumbilical approach, which is only recently becoming popular in the United States, results in less scarring and, some pioneers of the technique claim, results in less pain and a faster recovery. It may also reduce the chances of damaging nerves that supply the breast, which can lead to a loss of sensation. The major drawback is that this approach can only be used to place an implant on top of the chest muscle.

As noted above, breast augmentation may correct a congenital absence of breasts, deformities, or loss of breast tissue. It can create symmetry and may add to a woman's breast size. Such accomplishments can have a positive effect on a woman's self-esteem.

Breast augmentation, however, is not without its downside. For one, breasts so modified do not appear normal. As a general rule, they tend to be rounder and firmer than natural breasts. (Some people think they're even better than what nature provided.) To address this complaint, some companies are now manufacturing tear-shaped breast implants that have a more natural appearance.

In some instances, for example, in the case of heavy, droopy breasts, the appearance of the breast after implantation may actually be much worse! Surgeons treating such women often advise them to pursue an alternative procedure, known as *mastopexy*. In this operation, the surgeon tightens the skin of the breasts, firming them up. Implants may or may not be used.

Breast augmentation, like any surgery, is also traumatic. After the operation, the breast and surrounding tissue swells. Some women report intense pain. Bruising, twinges, and pain may last for a couple of weeks. It may take a couple of months before the breasts look normal again.

Breast augmentation also carries certain risks. Swelling can be excessive. Infections can develop. Unforeseen complications may arise from anesthesia. One of the most common problems is that the body forms a connective tissue layer around the implant. It is called a *capsule* and consists primarily of scar tissue. Problems arise when the scar tissue shrinks. This causes a hardening of

the breasts and may cause the implants to deform. It can also be quite painful. As a result, the implant may need to be removed and replaced. To reduce this problem, some companies have begun producing implants that have a textured silicone shell.

Breast implants may also rupture. Although saline-containing implants are not considered to pose any threat, silicone-containing implants which were once commonly used are of greater concern.

Over the years, many women with silicone-filled implants have complained of unusual health symptoms, usually following the rupture of the implants. They have reported muscle spasms and pain, swollen and painful joints, rashes, and hair loss, among other symptoms. Although no one knows what causes these problems, some researchers think that they may be the result of low-grade infections that develop around the implants. Many of the women suffering from these problems joined a massive class action lawsuit against the maker of the silicone implants, Dow Corning, which settled the claim for $3.2 billion. (Incidentally, this caused the company to go into bankruptcy.)

Despite the success of the lawsuit, extensive clinical research studies do not show a correlation between adverse health effects and silicone breast implants. That is, the incidence of symptoms in breast implant patients is the same as in the general population of women.

Scarring is not generally a problem. If the incision is made around the areola, the scar is usually barely noticeable; if it is made under the breast, the breast itself hides any scar. Incisions in the armpit or axilla

are generally only noticeable when the arm is raised. However, sloppy surgery or skin that scars easily can result in rather ugly reminders. If a woman forms keloids, thick scars, breast scars can be quite noticeable. In about one in 20 women, scars are red or highly colored, thick, painful, and take several years to improve.

Some procedures result in a loss of sensation around the nipple and on the breast—for example, the insertion of the implant through an incision in the areola. Breast implants may also crinkle or crease around the edge, especially in women who had very little natural breast tissue at the outset. In addition, implants may need to be replaced at a later date. No one knows how long breast implants will last or how often they may rupture.

Like so many things in our lives, breast augmentation comes with benefits and risks. The decision should be made after considering many factors. Women considering a breast augmentation procedure should seek a competent surgeon with a good track record. Research options. Check out the web sites and publications. Ask questions. Seek several opinions. Be certain there are no health problems that could make this a costly a decision.

Visit *Human Biology's* Internet site for links to web sites offering more information on this topic.

TABLE 20-4

Age-Related Changes in the Body

Organ System	Change	Cause
Skin	Thinning	Reduced cell division in epidermis
	Loss of elasticity	Elastic fibers in dermis replaced by collagen fibers
	Wrinkling	Same as above plus loss of fat in hypodermis
	Drying	Loss of sweat glands and sebaceous glands
	Loss of body hair	Loss of hair follicles
Bones	Become weaker, more porous, and more brittle	Loss of calcium is the primary reason for this, but also caused by loss of collagen fibers
Joints	Often become difficult to move and sometimes arthritic	Deterioration of cartilage on bone surfaces
Muscles	Loss of mass and muscle strength	Loss of motor neurons which stimulate muscles and a loss of muscle protein; fat and collagen fibers tend to invade muscles
Respiratory	Decreased oxygen absorption	Breakdown of alveoli
Cardiovascular	Decreased ability to pump blood so less blood is supplied to other tissues and organs	Reduction in the amount of heart muscle
	Hardening of the arteries and high blood pressure	Loss of elastic fibers in arteries and deposition of calcium, fat, and cholesterol in arterial walls
Nervous	Brain shrinkage	Loss of nerve cells throughout life as a natural process and as a result of alcohol use and trauma
	Deterioration of short-term memory and longer time to process various forms of information	Same as above
Reproductive	Loss of menstrual cycle in women	Dramatic decline in estrogen secretion by ovaries
	Reduced fertility in men	Decline in testosterone production
Urinary	Urinary incontinence	Weakening of the muscles of the urinary sphincter in men and women and weakening of the muscles of the pelvic floor in women who have given birth in earlier years

If cells are programmed to divide a given number of times, why don't all humans live to be the same age? One answer is that people differ genetically, which may contribute to the differences in life span. In addition, people live markedly different life-styles and eat very different diets. Research shows that the better one lives, the longer one lives. Diet, exercise, and stress management are keys to a healthy life.

Scientists are beginning to discover why proper diet and exercise can increase life span. Laboratory studies, for instance, show that by manipulating the chemical environment of cells, one can produce more cell divisions than normal. For example, vitamin E in large quantities increases the number of cell divisions in tissue cultures and increases a cell's life span. Whether vitamin E extends a person's life is not known.

Aging also results from a decrease or deterioration of cellular function. To understand aging, scientists are looking at the cell itself to see what causes its function to deteriorate. Studies show that the decline in cell function results from problems arising in the DNA, RNA, and proteins. Cells are exposed to many potentially harmful factors in the course of a lifetime. Natural and human-produced radiation and other potentially harmful agents (such as chemicals in the home and at work) may damage cells and impair their function. The cells of the body also produce oxygen free radicals, which are oxygen atoms that carry unpaired electrons. These chemical species are natural by-products of cellular metabolism and can react with (oxidize) proteins, DNA, lipids, and other important molecules, causing damage. Studies of cells of various organs such as the skin, heart, brain, and others show that as we age, our cells accumulate oxidized lipids and oxidized proteins, including important enzymes, which are essential for normal cell function. Researchers have also found that mitochondrial DNA is particularly susceptible to free radicals. Damage to mitochondria would help explain the loss of cell function with aging.

Additional evidence shows that cells may lose the ability to repair DNA as they age, making matters worse. The impacts of this are many. Cells would, for instance, lose the ability to fix mutations in essential genes—ones that produce important structural and functional proteins such as enzymes. Cancer, the incidence of which increases with age, could result. As the damage accumulates, body function gradually deteriorates.

Some researchers think that aging is largely the result of a gradual decline in immune system function caused by a reduction in cell number and a loss of cell function. Although the immune system does falter, this decline surely cannot explain the other signs of aging.

Aging Is Often Associated with Certain Diseases, But the Likelihood of Contracting a Disease of Old Age Depends in Large Part on Life-Style

Many diseases are associated with old age. Osteoporosis, arthritis, atherosclerosis, Alzheimer's disease, and cancer are examples. Although these diseases are more prevalent in older people, they are emphatically not the inevitable consequence of aging. That is, they are not unavoidable signs of aging like gray hair. As previous chapters have shown, the likelihood of developing most of these diseases can be greatly reduced by exercise, diet, and other life-style adjustments. In other words, people can age in a healthy manner by living healthy lives. Although our bodies will eventually fail, we do not have to suffer chronic illnesses that plague so many people for so long.

One exception is **Alzheimer's disease.** Discussed in more detail in Chapter 11, Alzheimer's disease strikes older individuals in about one of every 10 families. Alzheimer's is an incurable nervous system disorder characterized by a progressive loss of memory and other intellectual functions such as reasoning and understanding. Individuals with Alzheimer's become increasingly confused and unaware of their surroundings. Conversations become more and more difficult as mental incapacitation progresses. Afflicted individuals become emotionally unstable and, at the end stages, a person's intellectual abilities and personality may distintegrate entirely.

The cause of Alzheimer's is not known, but researchers believe that it may be caused by the buildup of a plaque-like material called *beta-amyloid.* New research

suggests that beta-amyloid binds to nerve cells in the brains, then causes cell death. This leads to the loss of memory and other symptoms. The tangles of fibers found in the brains of Alzheimer's patients are believed to be remnants of the cells' proteins. They're formed when beta-amyloid binds to the nerve cells. Health Note 20-2 offers some additional information on efforts now underway to slow the process of aging.

Death Is the Final Chapter in Our Lives

Aging results in a deterioration of function that eventually leads to death. But death can also result from traumatic injury to the body—for example, severe damage to the brain or a sudden loss of blood—and many other causes. What is death?

When I began to research the subject of death for this book, I thought the task would be easy. After all, death occurs when a person ceases to be alive. What I found was that death is difficult to define precisely. Although we can all agree that death is the cessation of life, trouble begins when people try to define it in instances requiring life-support systems.

In 25 states, a person is considered dead when his or her heart stops beating and breathing ceases. In the remaining 25 states, however, death is more liberally defined as an irreversible loss of brain function. A person in a coma, for example, often shows little or no brain activity other than that needed to keep the heart beating and the lungs working. Is this person alive? In some states, she is; in others, she is not.

Maintaining a person on life support is extremely costly to a family and to society if, for example, the patient is receiving federal benefits through Medicare. The money spent on maintaining a life could arguably be used to save dozens of lives through preventive measures. These issues inevitably lead to another biomedical dilemma, the controversy over euthanasia, a word derived from the Greek meaning "easy death."

Euthanasia (you-thin-A-zah) refers to any act or method of causing death painlessly and may be either passive or active. **Passive euthanasia** consists of decisions and actions to withhold treatment that might prolong life. **Active euthanasia** consists of decisions and actions that actively shorten a person's life—for example, injecting a lethal substance to terminate a patient's life. The Michigan physician, Dr. Jack Kevorkian, has been engaged in active euthanasia and is currently serving time in jail for his actions.

Opinions on euthanasia vary widely, and the controversy will, no doubt, be debated for many years. (For a debate on physician-administered euthanasia, see the Point/Counterpoint in this chapter.) As a final note,

Physician-Administered Euthanasia

The Right to a Physician Who Will Not Kill

Rita Marker

Rita L. Marker *is director of the International Anti-Euthanasia Task Force and the author of* Deadly Compassion.

Should physician-administered euthanasia—the direct and intentional killing of a patient by a physician—be legalized? Common sense has always said NO. And laws have wisely banned euthanasia.

Now, however, an effort is underway to change these laws. Those who seek to legalize euthanasia have framed their arguments in terms of personal rights and freedom. They've clearly recognized the importance of words in molding public opinion: carefully crafted verbal engineering is being employed to transform the appalling crime of mercy killing into an appealing matter of patient choice.

Proposals appearing in state after state have such benign titles as "Death With Dignity Act," and the deceptively soothing term "aid-in-dying" is often substituted for "euthanasia."

As efforts of euthanasia activists increase, careful examination of what is at stake has become increasingly important. This examination should include answers to key questions.

Who will be the recipients of new "rights" if euthanasia is legalized? The law would benefit doctors, not patients. Competent adults already have the legal right to refuse medical treatment as well as the right to make their wishes known about such interventions for the future. Additionally, neither attempting nor carrying out the very personal and tragic decision to commit suicide is a criminal offense. Bluntly put, people can refuse medical care, or can kill themselves without a doctor's help.

Doctors, however, are prevented by law from killing their patients. Legalization of euthanasia would give doctors the right to directly and intentionally kill patients. An action that is now considered homicide would become a "medical service."

What about safeguards? Efforts to legalize euthanasia have failed in Washington and California. Opponents pointed out the real dangers inherent in the proposals. Advocates, however, insisted that their measures contained sufficient safeguards. Yet, after each version failed, proponents acknowledged the lack of necessary safeguards. It's as though each and every attempt to legalize euthanasia is treated as a dress rehearsal. Yet we're not dealing with a play or musical event. A "learn as you go" attitude in law and public policy could lead to the deaths of millions of vulnerable people.

What changes in law are now being promoted? Recognizing that the dangers of their initial proposals were too apparent, euthanasia proponents have repackaged their agenda, calling for changes that would allow physician "assisted" death. Often referred to as "assisted suicide" measures, these new proposals would permit a physician to prescribe medication with the express purpose that it be used to end a patient's life. Such a change would lead to classification of such an action as a medical intervention. The reality would be simple: The physician would have prescribed medication to kill.

Logic and common sense make it readily apparent that "prescribing" encompasses far more than writing a prescription that is taken to the corner drug store. Medication prescribed for a patient in a hospital or care facility is often provided by health professionals. The current "change" allowing "only" for the death prescription is yet another deception intended to mask reality in meaningless safeguards.

What has happened where euthanasia has been practiced? One need only look to the experience in Holland for a glimpse of where the euthanasia road leads. Although it is widely practiced in Holland, euthanasia remains technically illegal. Yet, even with "safeguards," which are far tighter than those which have been proposed in the U.S., a 1991 Dutch government study released horrifying information. The study found that in tiny Holland—a country with only one-half the population of the State of California—Dutch physicians deliberately and intentionally end the lives of more than 11,000 people each year by lethal overdoses or injections. And more than half of those killed had *not* requested euthanasia.

What will happen if euthanasia is legalized? With increasing emphasis being placed on cost containment, individuals who are disabled are particularly vulnerable. Leaders in the disability rights community are becoming increasingly alarmed by suggestions such as that of Jack Kevorkian that their "choice" of death would "enhance public health and welfare."

Euthanasia proponents have been clear in describing their goals. For example, Derek Humphry has called for expansion of euthanasia to include those who are physically and mentally disabled. He has also written that there would be a means for handling the dilemma of "terminal old age" once euthanasia is legalized. Jack has outlined plans for designated death zones with special clinics where "planned death" could be carried out.

Those who think that euthanasia, once unleashed, can be controlled are making a deadly mistake. Euthanasia is not a means of dying with dignity, nor is it a matter of liberty. It does not legislate compassion. It only legalizes killing.

The Right to Choose to Die

Derek Humphry

If we are truly free people and if our bodies belong to ourselves and not to others, then we have the right to choose when and how to die. Death comes to us all in the end, although modern medicine can often help us improve and extend our life spans. Thus, given today's high technology and ruinous cost of medicine, it is wise if we all give advance thought to the manner of our dying. Such decisions should be transferred to paper (a living will and durable power of attorney for health care), because 46 states now legally recognize one's wishes in respect to the withdrawal of life-support equipment.

Advance-declaration documents, of course, deal only with the legal and ethical problems of medical equipment and treatments. Less than half of dying people are connected to such equipment. For many more patients, technology does nothing for their terminal illness, so—in effect—there is no "plug to pull." Therefore, the cutting edge of the right-to-die debate in the twenty-first century centers on assisted death and voluntary euthanasia.

Hemlock Society supporters feel not only that hopelessly sick people should not only have an unfettered right to accelerate their end to save them pain, distress, and indignity, but also that willing doctors should be able to help them die. [To clarify some terms: *self-deliverance (suicide)* is ending your own life to be free of suffering; *assisted suicide* is helping another die; *euthanasia* is the direct ending of another's life by request. Currently, suicide in any form, for any reason, is legal, but assisted suicide and euthanasia are technically crimes.]

Most people at the close of life do not wish to suffer, desiring a quick and painless demise. The sophisticated pain-management drugs now available, when properly administered, control some 90% of terminal pain. But they do nothing to alleviate the indignities, the psychic pain, and the loss of quality of life associated with some debilitating terminal illnesses.

A complaint that any hastening of the end interferes with God's authority can be answered for many through a belief that *their* God is tolerant and charitable and would not wish to see them suffer. Other people have no faith in God. Pious people differ with this view, of course, and I respect that.

Numerous opinion polls in the United States and other Western countries indicate that two-thirds of people want the right to have a doctor lawfully assist them to die. People in the states of Washington, Oregon, Maine, Michigan, and California have engaged in political action to achieve this law reform. The proposed law in these states was called the Death With Dignity Act, and the broad outline of its purpose is as follows:

1. The patient wanting physician-assisted dying would have to be a mature adult suffering from a terminal illness likely to cause death within about 6 months.
2. People with emotional or mental illness (especially depression) could not get help to die under this law.
3. The request would have to be in writing, and the signature would have to be witnessed by two independent persons.
4. The physician could decline to help the patient die on grounds of conscience but would then cease to be the treating physician. The patient could then seek a physician who was willing.
5. The family would have to be informed and its views, if any, taken into account. But the family could neither promote nor veto the patient's request to die.
6. The physician would have to be satisfied that the patient was fully aware of his or her condition, had been informed of all possible alternatives, and was competent to make this request.
7. If the physician was unsure of the patient's mental state, a mental-health professional

could be called to make an evaluation.
8. The time and manner of the assisted dying would have to be negotiated between patient and physician, with the patient's wishes paramount.
9. At any time the patient could orally or in writing revoke the request for assisted dying.
10. Any person who pressured another person to get assistance in dying, who forged such a request, or who ignored a revocation would be subject to prosecution.
11. After helping the patient die, the physician would have to report the action in confidence to a state health agency.

The right-to-die movement feels that these conditions, plus others in the Death With Dignity Act too numerous to describe here, are an intelligent and humane approach to euthanasia with the necessary safeguards against abuse. Only Oregon has passed such a law.

Dying on one's own terms is not only an idea whose time has come, but also the ultimate civil and personal liberty.

Derek Humphry *was the principal founder of the Hemlock Society and its executive director from 1980 to 1992. He is the author of five books on euthanasia, including the best-seller* Final Exit *(1991). Web site: <www.finalexit.org>*

Sharpening Your Critical Thinking Skills

1. Summarize the key points of each author and their supporting arguments.
2. Which viewpoint corresponds to yours? Why?

Visit *Human Biology's* Internet site for links to web sites offering more information on this topic.

Can We Reverse the Process of Aging?

Suppose a drug were invented that would help you live to be 100. Would you take it?

If you are like most people, you probably would, as long as your additional years would be healthy and fairly trouble free. Because most of us would like to beat this aging thing that nature imposes on us, we secretly hope for a medical breakthrough that would prolong our lives.

Unfortunately, the search for a "cure" for old age has been fraught with frustration. Over the years, numerous treatments have been tried and have failed. As pointed out in the Critical Thinking section, although the average U.S. life span has increased, we really are not living much longer than our grandparents.

There is some encouraging news, however. Scientists recently discovered a protein called **stomatin** (stow-MA-tin), which they isolated from fi-

broblasts that have stopped dividing in tissue culture. Scientists hope that stomatin will stop other cells from dividing as well. If this turns out to be true, researchers may have discovered an important clue in the aging puzzle, the signal that ends cell division. Moreover, they may have found a way to prolong human life.

Their reasoning goes as follows. If this protein signals the end of cellular division, there must be a gene that controls its production. If the stomatin gene can be located, researchers may be able to find a way to inactivate the gene. A drug or genetically engineered chemical, for example, could be injected in people to block the gene. The tissues of these people, researchers think, might continue to regenerate beyond the genetically programmed life span.

Efforts to reverse the aging process have met with some success in

another arena as well—slowing down the aging of skin. Because age-related changes in the skin mirror those occurring in other aging tissues, scientists have long studied the skin to expand their understanding of the aging process. Their studies have shown that skin aging results from two processes: intrinsic or chronological aging—which may be genetically programmed, and extrinsic aging, which results from accumulated environmental damage from sunlight and other factors.

Many skin scientists doubt whether anything can be done about intrinsic aging. Their studies suggest that after a skin cell has lived out its lifetime, its plasma membrane receptors become insensitive to growth factors that stimulate DNA replication and cell division.

New research suggests, however, that extrinsic aging, especially that

---

individuals who want to save their relatives emotional and legal turmoil can sign a living will. This is a legal document stipulating conditions under which doctors should allow a person to die.

Health, Homeostasis, and the Environment
Video Display Terminals

Reproduction has nothing to do with maintaining homeostasis, but homeostasis is absolutely essential to normal reproduction, as this case study on the reproductive effects of computer monitors suggests.

Computer monitors, or video display terminals (VDTs), produce numerous types of radiation with frequencies ranging from X-rays to radio waves. Fortunately, manufacturers have installed protective shields that prevent most of this radiation from escaping and bombarding the user. It is the lower-frequency radiation (radio frequencies) that has people concerned. Why?

Laboratory experiments show that electromagnetic fields generated by extremely low-frequency radiation can alter fetal development in chickens, rabbits, and swine. In addition, researchers in Oakland, California, recently published results of a medical study on the incidence of miscarriage in nearly 1600 women. The study showed that women who sit in front of a computer monitor for more than 20 hours a week during the first 3 months of pregnancy are nearly twice as likely to miscarry as women in similar jobs not using computers. Researchers suspect that miscarriages result from radiation emitted from the VDTs, but believe that other factors may also be involved—for example, the stress of using a computer. Preferring to err on the conservative side, some scientists advise pregnant women to minimize their exposure to radiation from computer monitors. Should the link between radiation from VDTs and miscarriage be substantiated by further research, it would provide yet another link in the growing case for the importance of a healthy environment to human health.

induced by sunlight, is preventable and even reversible. Unknown to many, sunlight damages epithelial cells of the epidermis and the fibroblasts in the underlying dermis. When exposed to sunlight, molecules inside skin cells become electrically excited. The energy they absorb from the sun drives reactions with other molecules in the cell. These reactions, in turn, lead to the dissociation of chemical bonds, which can damage molecules essential for cellular function. Plasma membranes, in fact, can be damaged within a few minutes of exposure to sunlight (**FIGURE 1**). Sunlight energy can also be absorbed by oxygen in the tissue, resulting in the formation of oxygen free radicals, highly destructive chemicals that are primarily responsible for extrinsic aging.

In 1988, medical researchers found that Retin-A, a derivative of vitamin A used to treat severe cases of acne, reduces sunlight-induced wrinkling. A study of Retin-A that followed patients for 22 months or more after treatment showed that the drug reduces wrinkles, age spots, and roughness for at least 22 months as long as it is applied regularly.

Researchers do not know how the drug works, but studies suggest that it does indeed have several effects that could account for its success. For example, Retin-A stimulates the growth of new blood vessels in the dermis. This, in turn, may nurture the regeneration of damaged skin cells. Retin-A also detoxifies oxygen free radicals in tissues and can inhibit the destruction of collagen fibers in the dermis. Some researchers think that it may regulate genes that play a role in cell growth and differentiation.

Despite the discovery of stomatin and Retin-A, there is as yet no evidence that medical scientists can prevent or even retard the overall rate of aging. The best route to a long and healthy life is to live it well: Learn ways to reduce stress, eat well, exercise regularly, take alcohol in moderation or not at all, and avoid harmful practices such as smoking.

FIGURE 1 Beware: Skin Damage
A gorgeous tan may lead to premature skin aging.

Visit *Human Biology's* Internet site for links to web sites offering more information on this topic.

www.jbpub.com/humanbiology

Summary

Fertilization

1. The sperm and egg of sexually reproducing animals such as humans unite during *fertilization.*
2. In humans, fertilization usually occurs in the upper third of the uterine tube.
3. Sperm deposited in the vagina reach the site of fertilization with the aid of muscular contractions in the walls of the uterus and uterine tube.
4. Sperm dissolve away the cells surrounding the oocyte and then bore through the zona pellucida and contact the plasma membrane. The first one to contact the membrane fertilizes the oocyte. Further sperm penetration is blocked.
5. Sperm are engulfed by the oocyte. The chromosomes of the sperm and oocyte duplicate and merge in the center of the cell, where mitosis begins.
6. Human development during gestation is divided into three stages: preembryonic, embryonic, and fetal.
7. Sperm contact the plasma membrane of eggs and are phagocytized by them. The egg and sperm cell nuclei then fuse to form a diploid *zygote.*

Pre-embryonic Development

8. *Pre-embryonic development* begins at fertilization and ends at implantation. The zygote undergoes rapid cellular division and forms a morula.
9. The morula is then converted into a *blastula,* a structure with a hollow cavity, called a *blastocyst* in humans.
10. The morula arrives in the uterus 3–4 days after fertilization and is converted into a blastocyst, which implants in the uterine wall 2–3 days later.
11. The blastocyst consists of a clump of cells, the *inner cell mass* (*ICM*), which becomes the embryo, and the *trophoblast,* which gives rise to the embryonic portion of the placenta.
12. While the placenta is forming, a layer of cells from the ICM of the blastocyst separates from it and forms the *amnion.* The amnion fills with fluid and enlarges during embryonic and fetal development, eventually surrounding the entire embryo and fetus, protecting them during development.

Embryonic Development

13. After the amnion forms, the cells of the ICM differentiate into the three germ cell layers: ectoderm, mesoderm, and endoderm. The formation of the three primary germ layers marks the beginning of *embryonic development.*
14. The organs develop from the three basic tissues during organogenesis. **TABLE 20-2** lists the organs and tissues formed from each of the layers.

Fetal Development

15. *Fetal development* begins 8 weeks after fertilization. Because most of the organ systems have developed or are under development, fetal development is primarily a period of growth.
16. The *placenta* produces several hormones that play an important part in reproduction. *Human chorionic gonadotropin* maintains the corpus luteum during pregnancy. Progesterone and estrogen stimulate uterine growth and the development of the glands and ducts of the breast.

Ectopic Pregnancy and Birth Defects

17. About 10%–12% of all newborns enter the world with some form of birth defect. Birth defects arise from chemical, biological, and physical agents known as *teratogens.*

18. The effect of teratogenic agents is related to the time of exposure, the nature of the agent, and the dose. A defect is most likely to arise if a woman is exposed to a teratogen during the embryonic period when the organs are forming.
19. Many physical and chemical agents are toxic to the human fetus and, when present in sufficient quantities, can kill a fetus or retard its growth.

Childbirth and Lactation
20. *Labor* consists of intense and frequent uterine contractions that are believed to be caused by the release of small amounts of fetal oxytocin prior to birth. Fetal oxytocin stimulates the release of prostaglandins by the placenta. Oxytocin and prostaglandins stimulate contractions in the sensitized uterine musculature.
21. Emotional and physical stress in the mother may trigger maternal oxytocin release, augmenting muscle contractions.
22. As uterine contractions increase, they cause more maternal oxytocin to be released, which stimulates stronger contractions and more oxytocin release, a positive feedback that continues until the baby is born.
23. Labor consists of three stages, the *dilation*, the *expulsion*, and the *placental*.
24. The breasts of a nonpregnant woman consist primarily of fat and connective tissue interspersed with milk-producing glandular tissue and ducts.
25. During pregnancy, the glands and ducts proliferate under the influence of placental and ovarian estrogen and progesterone.
26. Milk production is induced by maternal prolactin and *human chorionic somatomammotropin* but does not begin until 2–3 days after birth.
27. Before milk production begins, the breasts produce small quantities of a protein-rich fluid, *colostrum*. A newborn can subsist on colostrum for the first few days; the baby derives antibodies from colostrum that help protect it from bacteria.
28. Suckling causes a surge in prolactin secretion. Each surge stimulates milk production needed for the next feeding.

Aging and Death
29. *Aging* is the progressive deterioration of the body's homeostatic abilities and the gradual deterioration of the function of body organs.
30. These changes result from at least two factors: a decrease in the number of cells in the organs and a decline in the function of existing cells.
31. Death results from aging, traumatic injury, or infectious disease.

Critical Thinking

Thinking Critically— Analysis

This Analysis corresponds to the Thinking Critically scenario that was presented at the beginning of this chapter.

Medical scientists measure longevity by a statistic called *life expectancy at birth*. Technically, it is the number of years, on average, a person lives after he or she is born. Life expectancy at birth has increased dramatically in the last century. In 1900, for example, on average, white American females lived only 50 years. Today, life expectancy is 81 years. For males, a similar trend is observed. In 1900, for example, the life expectancy of a white American male was 47 years; today, it is 74 years.

Most people take these statistics to mean that men and women are actually living to a much older age. In reality, something very different is happening: The increase in the life expectancy at birth is largely the result of declining infant mortality. That is, thanks to improvements in medicine, more children are living through the first year of life and this has dramatically increased life expectancy. In the early 1900s, 100 of every 1000 babies died during the first year of life. Today, that number has fallen to 12. The impact on average life expectancy is incredible.

This is not to say that all of the gain in life expectancy results from a decline in infant mortality. Medical advances have certainly increased life expectancy after infancy, but these changes are small in comparison to those brought about by lowering infant mortality. In fact, about 85% of the increase in life span in the last century is the result of decreased infant mortality.

Test of Concepts

1. Give an overview of the process of development in humans. Describe what happens during each stage.
2. The formation of the gastrula results in the formation of endoderm, mesoderm, and ectoderm and the rearrangement of cells. Why is this process so important to the future development of the embryo?
3. Describe the process of fertilization in humans. Use drawings to elaborate your points, and label all drawings.
4. Define the terms *inner cell mass* and *trophoblast*.
5. Where does the human embryo acquire nutrients before the placenta forms?
6. Describe the formation of the placenta in humans.
7. What are the major functions of the human placenta?
8. Describe the flow of blood from the placenta to the fetus and back. What is the role of the various shunts?
9. List and describe the function of the five placental hormones.
10. Discuss how the nature of a teratogenic agent and the time of exposure affect teratogenesis, the production of birth defects.
11. What factors trigger labor?
12. What factors are responsible for cervical dilation during labor?
13. Define the term *aging*, and describe some of the hypotheses that attempt to explain it.
14. Thanks to modern medicine, men and women are living longer, says a friend. Using your understanding of average life expectancy data and the reason for an increase in life expectancy in the last century, explain why this statement is not quite true.

CHAPTER 21

Evolution
FIVE BILLION YEARS OF CHANGE

This mosquito trapped in amber lived when the dinosaurs once ruled the Earth.

Thinking Critically

Nothing stirs the pot of controversy like a discussion of the theories of evolution and creationism. The theory of evolution says, in essence, that all life emerged from a common ancestry. It holds that the Earth is very old (about 4.5 billion years old, in fact) and that over time species changed—that is, evolved—through natural selection. Some species went extinct, and others gave rise to new species or entirely new taxonomic groupings.

Creationism, on the other hand, which proponents refer to as *Scientific Creationism*, says the Earth is very young, only about 6000 years old! This age is based on a study of the *Bible*. Furthermore, creationists argue that all species arose independently and therefore no species is related to any other.

Supporters of creationism argue that it should be taught in science classrooms in public schools alongside discussions of the theory of evolution. Imagine that you're a high school principal, and you get a letter from a parent who insists that creationism be taught along with Darwin's version of evolution. How would you answer this parent? ■

Scientists believe that the atoms that make up both the living world and the nonliving world (rocks, for example) once existed in outer space as a giant cloud of cosmic dust and gas. About 4.5 billion years ago, this huge cloud began to condense. No one knows what triggered the condensation, but some think that a nearby exploding star (supernova) may have been the catalyst. As the huge cloud condensed, scientists speculate, dust particles in the center compacted more rapidly than outlying particles. This region would eventually give rise to the sun. Scientists hypothesize that when the mass of the forming sun reached a critical density, heat and pressure began to cause hydrogen and helium in it to chemically combine to form larger atoms. This process, known as **fusion**, not only forms larger atoms, it releases large amounts of energy. This energy takes many forms including heat, light, X-rays, gamma rays, radio waves, and other radiation. The process continues today in our sun.

Cosmic dust lying outside the forming sun also condensed, creating the planets (Greek for "wanderers"). The third planet from the sun was the Earth, the only piece of real estate in our solar system that we know supports life.

When it originated, the Earth was a solid mass of rock and ice. Scientists believe that radioactive decay, intense solar heat, and other sources of heat caused the Earth to melt, turning it into a mass of molten material. As the Earth grew hotter, water and the lighter elements such as hydrogen escaped into the atmosphere.

In the millennia that followed, the Earth gradually cooled, and a thick, rocky crust formed around a molten core. As the Earth cooled, water in the atmosphere began to rain down from the skies, creating lakes and oceans. Today, the oceans cover nearly 70% of the planet. It is in these oceans, or on their shores, that life began.

In this chapter we will trace the emergence of life from the Earth's beginnings and examine evolution, the process responsible for the rich and varied life-forms on Earth.

Section 21-1

The Evolution of Life: An Overview

In the most general terms, **evolution** is a process in which existing life-forms change. As you will soon see, evolution also produces entirely new organisms.

The evolution of life on Earth can be divided into three phases. During the first phase organic molecules formed. During the second phase cells evolved. And during the third phase many-celled organisms arose. This section outlines the key events in each phase.

The Formation of Organic Molecules from Inorganic Molecules in the Earth's Primitive Atmosphere Is Called Chemical Evolution

When they first formed, the seas were lifeless bodies of water. The landmasses, so richly carpeted today with grasses, trees, and other plants, were barren rock. How could life have formed from such an unpromising start?

In 1924, a Russian scientist, A. I. Oparin, suggested one hypothesis (**FIGURE 21-1**). He conjectured that inorganic molecules in the Earth's early atmosphere reacted to form the very first organic molecules. **Organic molecules** are chemical compounds composed primarily of carbon and hydrogen. Oparin hypothesized that the organic molecules thus created combined to form **polymers**, long-chain molecules made of many smaller molecules. These chemical substances joined to form the very first primitive cells. The formation of organic molecules from the Earth's primitive atmosphere that Oparin hypothesized is now referred to as **chemical evolution**. As you shall soon see, there's pretty good evidence to suggest that Oparin's hypothesis was correct.

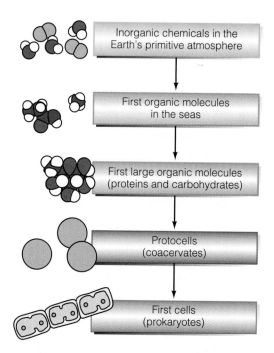

FIGURE 21-1 Oparin's Hypothesis   Oparin hypothesized that the organic molecules necessary for life formed from the Earth's primitive atmosphere. Today, this idea is called the *theory of chemical evolution* and is supported by a considerable body of evidence.

The figure shows a flow chart:

- Inorganic chemicals in the Earth's primitive atmosphere
- First organic molecules in the seas
- First large organic molecules (proteins and carbohydrates)
- Protocells (coacervates)
- First cells (prokaryotes)

Research suggest that chemical evolution began about 4 billion years ago or 500–600 million years after the Earth formed. At that time, the Earth's atmosphere contained a mixture of largely inorganic chemicals: water vapor, methane, ammonia, and hydrogen. It may also have included lesser quantities of nitrogen, carbon monoxide, and hydrogen sulfide, but it was devoid of oxygen. These molecules dissolved in rainwater and fell to the Earth. In the shallow waters of the newly formed seas, sunlight, heat from volcanoes, or lightning energized these molecules, causing them to react with one another in much the same way that molecules in a heated test tube react. These reactions produced a variety of simple organic molecules, including monosaccharides (simple sugars) and amino acids.

According to the theory of chemical evolution, these organic molecules, in turn, began to combine. In the process, they formed small polymers. As a result, primitive proteins and even rudimentary RNA or DNA molecules formed in the shallow waters of the seas. Little by little, and over tens of thousands of years, all of the organic molecules (monomers and polymers) necessary for life began to emerge. The polymers, in turn,

combined to form structures known as aggregates, or **protocells** (PRO-toe-cells; literally, "first cells"), the precursors of cells.

The Theory of Chemical Evolution Is Supported by Some Rather Convincing Experiments. The first direct evidence in support of the theory of chemical evolution came from an ingenious American graduate student, Stanley Miller. While studying for his Ph.D. in chemistry at the University of Chicago in the early 1950s, Miller devised an apparatus to test Oparin's hypothesis (**FIGURE 21-2**). To his closed, sterilized glass apparatus, Miller added three gases thought to have existed in the Earth's primitive atmosphere: methane (CH_4), ammonia (NH_3), and hydrogen (H_2). A sparking device that simulated lightning provided energy. Boiling water created steam that circulated through the device, carrying with it the reactant gases and the products of the reactions occurring inside.

Miller turned the apparatus on and sat back to see what would happen. After several days, the water in the apparatus turned brown. A chemical analysis of the brown, soupy liquid revealed the presence of several biologically important organic compounds, including amino acids, urea, and lactic acid (**TABLE 21-1**). In only a few days, Miller had created exciting evidence that supported the hypothesis that organic molecules could form abiotically (in the absence of life).

Although Miller's experiment did not prove Oparin's hypothesis, it created a groundswell of excitement and a flurry of research. Researchers soon found that a variety of organic molecules, including the building blocks of DNA and RNA (purines and pyrimidines), could be created abiotically. This work strongly supports the first part of Oparin's hypothesis, that the small molecules present in the Earth's early atmosphere combined to form the organic building blocks of life.

But what about the next step? Could these molecules join to form polymers? Researchers eagerly sought answers to this intriguing question and, to their delight, soon found that the organic building blocks produced

FIGURE 21-2 Miller's Apparatus This device showed that organic molecules could be produced from the chemical components of the Earth's early atmosphere.

TABLE 21-1	
Chemical Products Produced Abiotically in Miller's Experiment	
Glycine	Formic acid
Alanine	Lactic acid
Aspartic acid	Urea
Butyric acid	Succinic acid
Glutamic acid	Aldehyde
Acetic acid	Hydrogen cyanide

abiotically in the laboratory could indeed assemble into polymers in the absence of living organisms. One notable experiment was performed by Sidney Fox of the University of Miami. He found that when he heated amino acids in air, they joined to form small polymers, which he called **proteinoids** (PRO-teen-oids; meaning "like proteins").

This research led biologists to hypothesize that the dilute solutions of amino acids that formed during chemical evolution may have been splashed onto hot rocks or lava, where the amino acids polymerized. More recently, scientists have also hypothesized that polymerization may have taken place on clay particles, which tend to concentrate amino acids dissolved in water. Binding to the charged surface of the clay particles, amino acids united via peptide bonds.

Nucleic acids and polymers of carbohydrates have also been produced in similar experiments, thus supporting the second step in Oparin's hypothesis. Scientists next turned their attention to the third and final step, perhaps the most difficult of all to imagine—and to replicate—the formation of living cells from polymers.

The Theory of Cellular Evolution Suggests that the Precursors of Cells Were Aggregations of Polymers

The origin of the very first cells remains an enigma, but experimental evidence suggests a way in which these early cells could have formed from the mixture of organic molecules in the shallow coastal waters. Noteworthy again are the experiments of Professor Fox. He immersed the proteinoids he had produced abiotically (described above) in a boiling salt solution, then cooled the solution. This procedure resulted in the formation of tiny globules of protein, which Fox called **microspheres** (**FIGURE 21-3**).

Much to everyone's surprise, microspheres bore an eerie resemblance to bacteria. They not only looked like them, they behaved somewhat like bacteria. For example, Fox found that microspheres were capable

FIGURE 21-3 Microspheres Sidney Fox showed that his abiotically produced proteinoids formed small spherical structures that resemble cells. Could they have acquired genetic material and enzymes to become the first living cells?

of growing and reproducing. He found that when a microsphere reached a critical size, tiny protrusions formed, resembling buds. When they reached a certain size, they broke off, creating new microspheres. This process resembles budding, a form of asexual reproduction (Chapter 1).

Other experiments yielded similar results. Scientists found that simple life-like structures emerged. Microspheres and similar structures may have been the precursors of the Earth's first true cells. Some scientists hypothesized that some of the protein or RNA molecules in these precursor cells, or protocells, may have served as primitive enzymes. These primitive enzymes may have allowed the protocells to synthesize some of their own molecules and break down others to generate energy. Researchers also hypothesize that small molecules of DNA that formed during chemical evolution may have been incorporated into protocells, providing a primitive mechanism of heredity.

The Very First Cells Probably Acquired Nutrients from the Environment. Many biologists believe that the protocells gave rise to the first true cells. They also speculate that the first true cells probably received nourishment from organic molecules such as glucose that they absorbed from their environment. The emergence of these cells marks the beginning of the kingdom **Monera**, which today consists of bacteria (**FIGURE 21-4**).

Over time, biologists speculate, these bacterialike monerans gave rise to yet another a group of organisms, the **autotrophs**. Autotrophs are organisms capable of synthesizing their own food.

The very first autotrophs to evolve, however, were probably single-celled **chemosynthetic organisms**—organisms that produce their own organic molecules

FIGURE 21-4 The First Prokaryote A composite photograph of the first prokaryote fossil, discovered in western Australia. It is believed to be about 3.5 billion years old.

using energy from inorganic molecules in the environment. Some chemosynthetic bacteria can still be found today.[1]

Later on, another group of autotrophs arose. These were the more familiar photosynthetic organisms. They synthesize their own food from carbon dioxide, water, and solar energy. Plants and algae are modern-day representatives of this group. All of these organisms up to this point lived in an oxygen-free environment and are called *anaerobes*.

Although early forms of photosynthesis did not release oxygen, later forms did. The emergence of oxygen was probably the very first global pollution disaster and is responsible for a major turning point in evolution.

As populations of these oxygen-releasing organisms expanded, oxygen levels in the water and atmosphere increased. Many of the anaerobic organisms living at the time were probably unable to cope with the oxygen. They either perished or retreated to oxygen-free environments such as the mud or sediment beneath lakes and oceans. Many of their descendants (the anaerobic bacteria) remain in such locations today. Still others probably evolved mechanisms that allowed them to live in an oxygen environment. These organisms formed the aerobic monerans (aerobic bacteria). All of the organisms to date belonged to a group known as **prokaryotes**. As you may recall from Chapter 2 on cell biology, prokaryotes are cells that do not have true nuclei.

---

[1]Chemosynthetic bacteria on the seafloor live on hydrogen sulfide or natural gas.

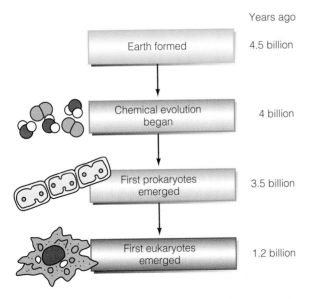

	Years ago
Earth formed	4.5 billion
Chemical evolution began	4 billion
First prokaryotes emerged	3.5 billion
First eukaryotes emerged	1.2 billion

FIGURE 21-5 Summary of the Evolution of the Earth and Life

Eukaryotes Probably Arose by Endosymbiotic Evolution.

After the emergence of the prokaryotes came the **eukaryotes**. These are cells with true nuclei. The very first eukaryotes to emerge during evolution were members of the kingdom **Protista** (pro-TEES-tah). As you may recall from Chapter 2, protista are all single-celled organisms like the ameba. (For a timetable of these events, see **FIGURE 21-5**.)

How eukaryotes arose during evolution is one of the most fascinating of all biological stories. Scientists believe that eukaryotes arose from preexisting cells approximately 1.2 billion years ago. They've formulated an elaborate and believable description of the process, known as the **theory of endosymbiotic evolution**. According to the theory, many of the organelles of eukaryotes arose when free-living organisms united to form a permanent relationship. In this section, we will consider the origin of mitochondria, the energy-producing organelle of eukaryotic cells, via endosymbiotic evolution. We'll also examine the origin of nuclei, which are believed to have emerged by an entirely different process.

According to the theory, mitochondria of the eukaryotes came into existence when an anaerobic host cell phagocytized a smaller, oxygen-respiring bacterium. The bacterium set up residence inside the host cell, where it consumed the oxygen that entered its host, much to the benefit of its host. As atmospheric oxygen levels increased, such unions may have conferred a selective advantage on this new biological composite. The theory of endosymbiotic evolution holds that as time went on, the relationship between host cells and their internal partners (the predecessors of mitochondria) became hereditary. Thus, when host cells divided, they passed the bacteria they contained to their daughter cells.

Unlike the mitochondrion, the nucleus of the eukaryote is believed to have evolved from infoldings of the plasma membrane that came to surround the DNA. The infoldings did not come from endosymbiosis. Evidence of them is found in some species of bacteria. In these species, the plasma membrane folds inward and envelops the DNA, forming packages called **mesosomes**. Although mesosomes remain attached to the plasma membrane, it is thought that similar structures may have formed during cellular evolution and lost their connection, giving rise to the true nucleus.

Like other aspects of the early evolution of life, evidence for endosymbiotic evolution is indirect. The first line of evidence can be classified as "proof by resemblance." Comparisons of mitochondria and free-living bacteria, for example, show several striking similarities. First, mitochondria contain circular DNA, similar to

FIGURE 21-6
The Five Kingdoms

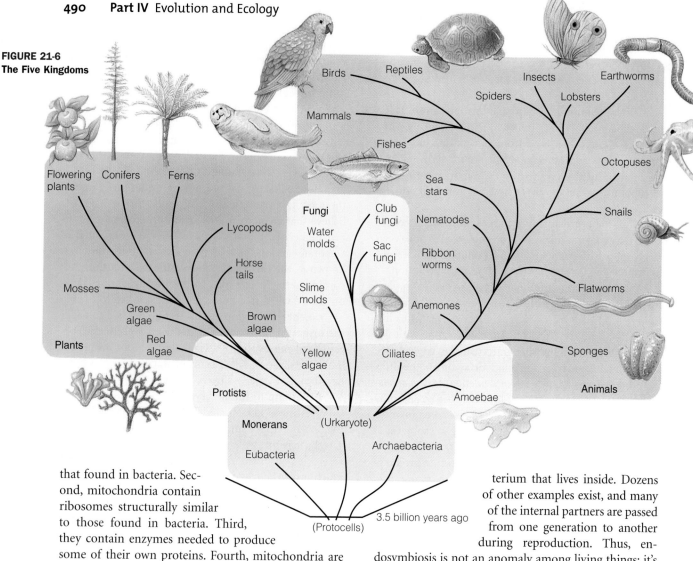

that found in bacteria. Second, mitochondria contain ribosomes structurally similar to those found in bacteria. Third, they contain enzymes needed to produce some of their own proteins. Fourth, mitochondria are capable of dividing. These similarities suggest that mitochondria may have been free-living, bacterialike organisms at one time.

Continuing along this same line, mitochondria also contain two membranes. Some biologists believe that the outer membrane may have been formed when the bacteria that gave rise to this organelle were first phagocytized by the host cells during endosymbiotic evolution many millions of years ago. The outer membrane may have been derived from the membrane of the host cell; the inner membrane may be the phagocytized bacterium's own plasma membrane.

Endosymbiotic evolution is also supported by the fact that endosymbiosis (one organism living inside another) is a rather common occurrence in biology. Termites, for example, contain a microorganism (a flagellate, pronounced FLAJ-eh-LATE) in their gut that digests the wood they eat. The flagellate living in the gut of the termite contains its own internal symbiont—a bac-

terium that lives inside. Dozens of other examples exist, and many of the internal partners are passed from one generation to another during reproduction. Thus, endosymbiosis is not an anomaly among living things; it's a common strategy for survival.

The anatomical evidence (resemblance) and the common occurrence of endosymbiosis do not *prove* that endosymbiotic evolution occurred. They do, however, strongly suggest that it is a plausible explanation for the emergence of eukaryotic cells.

However they evolved, the first eukaryotic cells, with their distinct organelles and membrane-bound nuclei, were the free-living, single-celled organisms that compose the kingdom Protista. Common members of the kingdom include such familiar examples as the amoeba and paramecium.

The previous discussion is not meant to suggest that scientists know all there is to know about chemical and cellular evolution. The truth is, we know very little about the origin of life and the emergence of prokaryotic and eukaryotic cells. We have many hypotheses, and this subject is one of the most controversial and open-ended in biology.

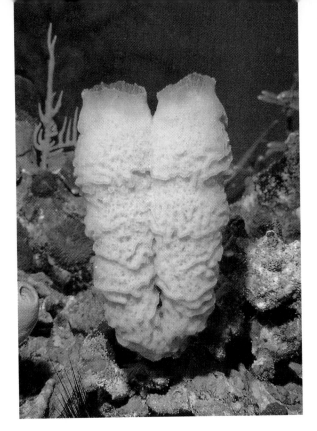

FIGURE 21-7 The Sponge Probably one of the first multicellular animals, the sponge consists of a central cavity into which it draws nutrients. The sponge exhibits a modest degree of specialization.

The Evolution of Multicellular Organisms Occurred Rather Rapidly Compared with Previous Stages

The evolution of eukaryotes from prokaryotes took an enormous amount of time and marked a major turning point in the history of life on Earth, for it opened the door to the evolution of multicellular eukaryotic organisms—plants, animals, and fungi. **FIGURE 21-6** shows the evolutionary relationship of these three kingdoms to monerans

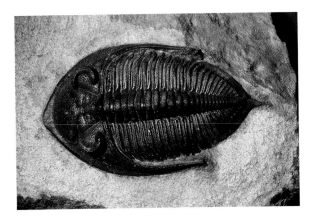

FIGURE 21-8 Early Sea Animals Trilobites were one of the most common life-forms in the ocean 600 to 500 million years ago.

and protistans. The next section offers a brief overview of the evolution of multicellular organisms.

The Evolution of Multicellular Life Began in the Sea. Because the first eukaryotic cells arose in the oceans and remained there for hundreds of millions of years, it should come as no surprise that the first multicellular plants also evolved in the seas.

The very first aquatic plants were the algae. Three types of algae exist today: brown, red, and green. Scientists believe that each form evolved from a different ancestor. Brown and red algae remained in the water. Green algae also remained in the water but are believed to have given rise to all land plants.

About the same time, between 400–600 million years ago, a variety of multicellular animals also evolved in the oceans. The fossil record suggests that many of them arose independently from early protists (single-celled eukaryotes). One of the first multicellular animals may have been the sponge (**FIGURE 21-7**). Sponges are sedentary (immobile) invertebrates (animals without backbones) that attach to rocks and other hard surfaces, usually in shallow water. Another early multicellular invertebrate was a soft-bodied organism that resembled modern-day jellyfish. Molluscs (shellfish) and arthropods (crabs and lobsters) also joined the extraordinary profusion of life (**FIGURE 21-8**).

Plants and Animals That Inhabited the Land Arose from the Seas. While life flourished in the seas, the Earth's continents were barren. Over time, though, plants and animals colonized the land and eventually formed an impressive array of terrestrial life-forms.

Scientists believe that the invasion of the Earth's barren landmasses was prevented for a long time in part by ultraviolet radiation from the Sun, which is lethal to plants and other unprotected organisms. The evolution of life on land may have been made possible in part by the emergence of the **ozone layer**, a thin layer of air containing a slightly higher concentration of **ozone molecules** (O_3) 10–20 miles above the Earth's surface. Ozone molecules absorb ultraviolet light, reducing the amount of harmful radiation that strikes the Earth by about 99%.

The ozone layer probably formed from oxygen released by photosynthesis. As noted earlier, oxygen first came from photosynthetic monerans, then from autotrophic protists, which evolved later. Oxygen molecules produced by organisms drifted into the atmosphere, where they reacted to form ozone molecules. Over time, the concentration of ozone in the upper atmosphere increased.

FIGURE 21-9 The First Land Animals Arthropods, perhaps the early ancestors of the scorpion, were the first to invade the land.

The colonization of the continents by plants occurred approximately 400–500 million years ago. The first land plants probably evolved from green algae. Soon after the terrestrial plants began to evolve, the first sea animals "invaded" the land. Evolutionary biologists believe that the previous emergence of plants provided the first land animals with an abundant supply of food.

(a)

FIGURE 21-10 The Dinosaurs
(a) Probably one of the most successful species ever to inhabit the land, the dinosaurs lived on Earth for about 125 million years. Why they disappeared remains a mystery.
(b) Alligators (shown here) and crocodiles are modern descendants of the dinosaurs.

(b)

The first animals to come onto land were probably the **arthropods.** Two well-known examples are insects and crustaceans. Arthropods have hard outer skeletons that reduce evaporation and provide support. This feature, which evolved in the ocean most likely as a protective measure, made the transition to terrestrial life much easier. Organisms with characteristics that make them suitable for other environments are said to be **preadapted** to the new environment. The very first terrestrial arthropods were probably the ancestors of the scorpion (**FIGURE 21-9**).

The arthropods had the land and its plants to themselves for millions of years. Meanwhile, in the seas and lakes of the newly forming world, fishes began to emerge. Evolutionary biologists believe that one group of fishes (the lobe-fins) gave rise to the amphibians. Modern amphibians include organisms such as frogs, toads, and salamanders, all of which are dependent on the land and water for their subsistence. Most amphibians must return to water to lay their eggs.

Reptiles (represented today by snakes, lizards, turtles, and alligators) evolved from amphibians many millions of years later. Ancient reptiles gave rise to the dinosaurs and many modern reptiles (**FIGURE 21-10**). Thanks to their thick, scaly skin and eggs covered by a thick, rubbery shell, reptiles survived nicely on land. One important reptile was the dinosaur. Although the dinosaurs perished after an impressive 125-million-year stay, many reptiles remained, among them alligators, crocodiles, snakes, lizards, and turtles.

Birds are believed to have evolved from reptiles about 225 million years ago at a time when the dinosaurs were beginning to diversify. Some scientists think the birds arose directly from early dinosaurs. Others believe they came from a separate reptilian ancestor.

Studies of the fossil record suggest that mammals probably also evolved from reptiles. Many mammal-like reptiles were present about 230 million years ago, around the time of the emergence of dinosaurs. The first truly recognizable mammals appear in rock about 180 million years old. Living among the dinosaurs for millions of years, the earliest mammals were rather small creatures that inhabited trees and were active principally at night.

Mammals are characterized by mammary glands and hair. Over time, body size increased greatly, and the limbs elongated and diversified, a feature that provides many styles of locomotion from flight (bats) to swimming (beavers, whales) to running (cheetahs, deer). Brain size also increased during evolution, and today mammals have the largest brains (relative to body size) of all organisms on Earth.

The primates, which include the apes and humans, are a group of mammals that evolved from a tree-dwelling mammal that lived among the dinosaurs. As you will see in Chapter 22, the early primates persisted long after the dinosaurs perished and gave rise to human beings. Contrary to many popular movies and cartoons like the *Flintstones*, dinosaurs and humans did not co-exist.

Section 21-2

How Evolution Works

Many life-forms have emerged over the millions of years of the Earth's history. And many have changed, or evolved, to produce a rich and diverse array of species. The theory of evolution presents a plausible explanation as to how life emerged, how it changed, and why it became so diverse. In other words, it explains the mechanisms behind these processes. This next section explains how evolution works.

Genetic Variation Is the Raw Material of Evolution

During evolution, the anatomical, physiological, and even behavioral changes that occur in species take place because of changes in the frequency of genes in populations of organisms.[2] Changes in gene frequency begin with random genetic changes in a population; these arise from one of five processes: (1) mutations, (2) crossing-over, or genetic recombination, (3) the independent assortment of genes during meiosis, (4) new genetic combinations produced during sexual reproduction (that is, the combination of genetically different gametes), and (5) gene flow. Of these sources of genetic variation, the only one that creates new forms of genes is mutations. The rest only shuffle existing genes, creating new combinations that may lead to favorable adaptations.

Mutations in the genes of organisms occur naturally and randomly. Many of these errors are corrected by the cells, but some remain. Mutations occur in the body cells (somatic cells) and germ cells. In the evolution of multicellular organisms, somatic mutations are meaningless, for they cannot be passed to future generations. It is germ cell mutations that are of importance.

Like somatic cell mutations, germ cell mutations can be harmful, even lethal. In fact, many human embryos that abort spontaneously are the result of harmful germ cell mutations in the sperm, the ovum, or both (Chapter 20).[3] These mutations end up in the cells of the embryo. For reasons not well understood, in some instances the presence of genetic mutations causes the embryo to be aborted.

Other germ cell mutations, however, are beneficial to the offspring. That is, they produce characteristics that give the offspring an advantage over other members of the population.

Genetically based characteristics that increase an organism's chances of passing on its genes are called **adaptations**. For example, a random mutation in the germ cell of a fish may make its offspring more efficient in food digestion. This efficiency, in turn, increases the likelihood that their offspring will survive and reproduce. Members of the same population that do not share this trait are less likely to survive and reproduce and will very likely produce fewer offspring. Over time, the better adapted fish will leave a larger number of offspring. Furthermore, these offspring are more likely than others to survive and reproduce. Over time, their success results in a shift in the gene pool so that future populations contain proportionately more offspring of the fish with the beneficial mutation. On a genetic level, then, the gene that gave some fish an advantage over others increased in frequency in the population.

Beneficial mutations, which produce genetic variation in populations, are often called the raw material of evolution, a fact that is true for sexually as well as asexually reproducing organisms (bacteria). In other words, mutations are a source of new alleles and thus a major source of **phenotypic variation** in a population—that is, differences in anatomical, physiological, and even behavioral characteristics.[4]

In sexually reproducing organisms, such as humans, genetic variation also results from recombination. **Recombination** is the formation of new combinations of genes during crossing-over in meiosis (Chapter 16). Crossing-over occurs when homologous chromosomes pair up and exchange segments. This reshuffling of genes results in new genetic combinations and thus produces variation in a population. If the new combination of genes produces advantageous adaptations, the genes may increase in frequency in the population.

The independent assortment of chromosomes during meiosis may be even more important than

---

[2]For our purposes, a species is a group of organisms whose members are anatomically and physiologically similar to one another. The members of a species interbreed successfully; that is, they produce viable, reproductively functional offspring.

[3]A mutation in a somatic cell in a morula or blastocyst can also lead to embryonic or fetal death and miscarriage.
[4]For bacteria and other organisms that reproduce asexually (by dividing or budding), mutation is the only source of variation.

crossing-over in producing new genetic combinations and phenotypic variation. Independent assortment, described in Chapter 16, simply means that maternal and paternal chromosomes in the forming germ cells segregate independently of one another during meiosis, creating new genetic combinations.

Still another source of genetic variation in population is the process of sexual reproduction. When male and female gametes combine, they produce new genetic combinations, some of which may provide advantageous adaptations.

The final source of genetic variation is called gene flow. **Gene flow** is the introduction of new alleles to a population by individuals from another population of the same species.[5] This process occurs when members of previously isolated populations mate. A male bird capable of flying long distances while using less energy than

other members of the population, for example, might cross a mountain range and mate with a female from a previously isolated population. Her offspring would then carry the gene that permits more efficient flight. Variation has been introduced into the population. This phenomenon is called *gene flow*.

Natural Selection Is a Process by Which Organisms Become Better Adapted to Their Environment

Sociologist Andrew Schmookler once wrote that "evolution employs no author, only an extremely patient editor." What he meant by that is that evolution is not directed. There is no author. Instead, mutations arise spontaneously. Mutations, recombination, gene flow, sexual reproduction, and new combinations from the independent assortment of genes and from sexual reproduction produce genotypic and phenotypic variants. If beneficial, the genetically based characteristics (adaptations) that arise from these sources tend to persist. The species changes over time, becoming better suited to its environment. In some cases, a whole new species may evolve.

The gene pool shifts because of evolution's patient "editor," a process called **natural selection**. **Charles Darwin**, a nineteenth-century British naturalist, and **Alfred Wallace** independently proposed the idea of natural selection. Darwin described it as a process in which slight variations, if useful, are preserved (**FIGURE 21-11**).

---

[5]The new genes are most likely to have arisen from a mutation.

FIGURE 21-11 "Evolutionary Voyage"
(a) Darwin as a young man proposed the theory of evolution by natural selection, helping solve one of the key puzzles of biology: how species evolve. *(b)* From 1831 to 1836, Darwin made a famous voyage on the *Beagle*, collecting and cataloging thousands of diverse species.

(a)

(b)

Thus, natural selection is a process by which organisms often become better adapted to their environment.

Two principal factors contribute to natural selection: **biotic factors**, or other living organisms, and **abiotic factors**, the physical and chemical environment (temperature, rainfall, and so on). Abiotic and biotic factors influence survival and reproduction by "selecting" the fittest—those best able to reproduce and pass on their genes. If these conditions change, those organisms best adapted to the new conditions tend to remain and pass their genes on to subsequent generations. This process causes a shift in the frequency of certain genes in a population.

In Darwin's time, evolution was widely discussed among naturalists and other scientists, but the mechanism by which it occurred remained a mystery. Darwin dedicated many years to the search for an answer, even traveling around the world by ship and cataloging species (**FIGURE 21-11B**). It was on this lengthy voyage that Darwin reportedly came up with the idea.

A careful scientist, though, Darwin spent the next 20 years looking for flaws in his own reasoning. In 1858, much to his surprise, Darwin received a paper from Wallace, a respected naturalist who had proposed the same concept. Darwin sent Wallace's paper to some of his colleagues and suggested that they publish it. Fortunately, Darwin's colleagues, who were aware of his own theory, prevailed on him to write a paper of his own. In 1858, Wallace's and Darwin's papers were both presented to the Linnaean Society. In 1859, Darwin published his now-famous book, *On the Origin of Species by Means of Natural Selection.*

As in the case of Mendel, Darwin's and Wallace's ideas took many years to be understood and accepted. Not until the 1940s, about 60 years after Darwin's death, did natural selection become widely accepted. Today, it is one of the central tenets of biology.

Natural Selection Ensures That the Fittest Organisms in a Population Survive and Reproduce.

Darwin used the phrase "survival of the fittest" to describe how natural selection worked.[6] Survival of the fittest is commonly interpreted as "survival of the strongest." To a biologist, however, **fitness** is a measure of reproductive success, which can be attributed to many different features, not just strength. Fitness does not necessarily result from speed, either. The ability to hide, digest food more efficiently, or use water more ef-

ficiently can be just as important, if not more important, than standard measures of strength.

Ultimately, fitness is a measure of the genetic influence an individual has on future generations. By definition, then, the fittest individuals leave the largest number of descendants. Their influence on the gene pool will be greater than that of their less-fit contemporaries.

Allele Frequencies Can Shift Because of Chance Events

Not all shifts in the gene pool result from natural selection. Some occur quite by chance. Imagine, if you will, a population of mountain goats in which 10 members—out of, say, 30—possess a slightly superior ability to climb extremely steep, rocky slopes. One day those ten animals climb a ridge to reach some food. The rest of their herd stays on lower ground. That afternoon a lightning bolt strikes the herd, killing most of less-talented climbers.

This chance event causes a shift in the frequency of alleles in the population, increasing the frequency of the gene that improved the ten goats' climbing ability. A shift in allele frequencies that is due to a chance occurrence is referred to as *genetic drift.* This process is most rapid when a population is small, as in the example above.

Over time, the population will increase in size as the remaining mountain goats breed. The number of skilled climbers will increase naturally. In this instance, the population that survived the electrical storm will establish or found a new, genetically different population. Evolutionary biologists call this phenomenon the **founder effect**. It occurs any time a small subset of a population founds a new genetically distinct population.

The founder effect is extremely important in the colonization of islands and other isolated habitats. It is also important when a few individuals of a species are introduced into new habitat.

Genetic drift and the founder effect occur in populations that are severely reduced through natural or human causes. In the late 1800s, for instance, the northern elephant seal was nearly hunted to extinction. The 20 or so remaining seals formed the basis of the new population, which today numbers more than 150,000 (near pre-exploitation levels). This much larger population has almost no genetic variation compared with other seal populations that have not gone through similar bottlenecks.

Genetic uniformity makes populations highly susceptible because they do not contain the genetic diversity vital to evolutionary change in the event that environmental conditions change. This is one reason why it is prudent not to let wild populations of any species be diminished. For an interesting view of a previous

---

[6]Herbert Spencer is thought to have coined the phrase.

FIGURE 21-12 Darwin's Finches All but one species (the Cocos Island finch) are believed to have evolved from a single ancestral flock that arrived on the Galapagos Islands within the past 500,000 years.

Plant-eating finch

Warbler finch

Swamp finch

Galapagos islands

Large insect finch

Small insect finch

Sharp-beaked ground finch

Medium insect finch

Small ground finch

Cocos Island finch

Woodpecker finch

Medium ground finch

Larger cactus ground finch

Smaller cactus ground finch

Large ground finch

hypothesis on the mechanism of evolution, see Scientific Discoveries 21-1.

The Evolution of New Species

Evolution is a process by which species change over time, becoming better adapted to their environment. As noted earlier, evolution can also produce new species.

New Species Evolve When Geographic Isolation Results in Reproductive Isolation

The evolution of a new species is called **speciation** (spee-sea-A-shun). New species arise in large part as a result of a phenomenon called **geographic isolation**. Geographic isolation occurs when members of a population of organisms are physically separated by some

barrier—a mountain range, a lake, an ocean, a river, or simply a great distance. In their separate habitats, the members of the subpopulations are exposed to different environmental influences. Over time, two distinct species may form, each adapted to its environment. If a population is separated into more than two subgroups, many new species may arise.

One of the best examples of this phenomenon occurred on the Galapagos Islands in the Pacific Ocean off the coast of Ecuador. On these islands, over a dozen species of finches (sometimes called Darwin's finches) evolved from a single population of seed-eating birds that arrived from South America sometime in the past 500,000 years (**FIGURE 21-12**). As the ancestral population settled on different islands, the birds began to evolve in different ways, primarily because of differences in food sources. Major changes took place in body size and the shape of the bill. The differences in beak size and shape correspond to different ways of obtaining food.

Darwin's finches illustrate how new species develop from a common ancestor. This phenomenon is called **divergent evolution**. The term refers to the fact that species diverge genotypically and phenotypically in response to differing environmental conditions.

FIGURE 21-13 shows divergent evolution among ancestral reptiles and ancestral placental animals that gave rise to a wide assortment of species, some adapted to life in the water, and others adapted to life on land or in the air. The term **adaptive radiation** is also used to describe the evolution of new species from a common ancestry, each of which is specially adapted to its environment. You can consider adaptive radiation and divergent evolution to be synonymous.

Certain genetic lineages may produce a number of new species over tens of millions of years. Others produce numerous species over a relatively short period. But how does geographic isolation "produce" new species?

One of the consequences of geographic isolation is that organisms that arose from the same population often lose the ability to interbreed, for reasons explained shortly. Biologists say that the members of the original population have become **reproductively isolated** from one another. New species emerge when geographical isolation results in reproductive isolation. When new species emerge in geographically separate regions, the process is called **allopatric speciation** (allopatric is derived from the Greek for "other" and "fatherland").

The first step in reproductive isolation in animal populations is the emergence of behavioral differences between the two groups. Courtship patterns, for example, may change so that females from one population no longer respond to males of the other. **TABLE 21-2** lists several additional reproductive isolating mechanisms that fall into one of two broad categories: (1) those factors that prevent mating such as different courtship behaviors and mating times; and (2) those that prevent the production of viable offspring and/or reproduction—for example, the inability of sperm to reach ova.

Interestingly, new species may also form without geographical isolation. This process is common in plants and is known as **sympatric speciation** ("same fatherland"). Sympatric speciation often occurs by polyploidy, the accumulation of one or more additional sets of chromosomes. This, in turn, results from complete nondisjunction of chromosomes during meiosis.

FIGURE 21-13 Divergent Evolution
From common ancestors, new species emerge, each adapted to its environment. Unrelated species often adapt to similar environments in similar ways, a phenomenon called convergent evolution.

TABLE 21-2

Reasons for Reproductive Isolation

Factors that prevent mating
   Mating occurs at different times.
   Different cues (songs and coloration) develop.
   Different courtship behaviors develop.
   Genital incompatibility develops.
Factors that prevent production of viable offspring and/or reproduction
   Sperm cannot reach ova.
   Hybrid offspring die in utero or shortly after birth.
   Hybrid offspring survive, but are sterile.
   Hybrid offspring survive, but have lower fitness.

Debunking the Notion of the Inheritance of Acquired Characteristics

Featuring the Work of Lamarck, Weismann, Castle, and Phillips

The eighteenth-century French naturalist Jean-Baptiste Lamarck argued that life had been created in a relatively simple state. Over time, he said, life-forms gradually improved as a result of an innate drive for perfection. He further hypothesized that this inherent drive was centered in nerve cells and that these cells released a "fluida" (chemical substance) that traveled to different body parts needing improvement.

Consider Lamarck's explanation of the evolution of the giraffe. According to him, the giraffe of years past was a short-necked animal. Over time, the elongation of the giraffe's neck resulted from the simple act of stretching of its neck—a feat required to feed on leaves that were out of the reach of other animals. The act of stretching, said Lamarck, directed fluida to the neck. This stimulus made the neck grow longer. What is more, the slightly stretched neck that an adult acquired was then transmitted to its offspring. The offspring, in turn, stretched their necks to reach food, causing further elongation. According to Lamarck

then, generation after generation of giraffes, each stretching to find food, led to the modern giraffe.

Lamarck proposed an evolutionary theory based on the "use and disuse" of organs. It stated that an individual acquired traits during its lifetime and that such traits were in some way incorporated into the hereditary material and passed to the next generation, thus explaining how a species could change over time. Conversely, disuse of organs led to their disappearance. The inheritance of acquired characteristics was doubted by many of Lamarck's contemporaries, in large part because he failed to support his hypothesis with observations or experiments.

Lamarck's concept is based on a fundamental fallacy, that is, the mistaken belief that all of the organs of one's parents produce the hereditary factors that form corresponding parts in the offspring. Thus, any change that occurred in an organ (an acquired characteristic) would result in the production of a hereditary factor that would reflect the altered organ. This

hereditary factor would then somehow be transmitted to the sperm of the male or egg of a female. Thus when a new offspring was formed, it would have the acquired characteristics. Put very simply, if you were lifting weights and had developed extensive musculature before the conception of your child, your muscles would transmit a hereditary factor to your sperm or egg, so you child would grow up to be brawny.

After the discovery of fertilization, it was assumed that the organs transmitted parcels of hereditary information to the gametes. In this way, acquired traits were passed on to the offspring.

August Weismann, a German scientist in the late 1800s, attempted to bring some sense to the debate in a series of extraordinary essays, based largely on the work of others, but also on his own ideas. Although Weismann did not perform experiments to disprove Lamarck's notions, his essays remain an important contribution to modern genetics. Among other things, he argued that the transmission of

Convergent Evolution Occurs Because Organisms Tend to Evolve Similarly When Faced with the Same Challenge

FIGURE 21-13 also illustrates a very interesting phenomenon—notably that unrelated species may adapt to similar environments in similar ways. In this example, ancestral mammals and reptiles both evolved flying forms (in fact, about 20% of all mammal species are bats). In addition, mammals and reptiles both gave rise to carnivores, as represented in the figure by the tyrannosaurus and the lion. The tendency for organisms to develop the same types of adaptations in response to similar environmental conditions is called **convergent evolution**.

Species Often Evolve in Concert with Each Other

So far, the discussion of evolution has focused principally on abiotic factors as agents of natural selection.

Abiotic factors such as climate are only part of the picture. Organisms are themselves agents of natural selection. Predatory pressure, for example, may act as an agent of natural selection in the evolution of prey populations. For example, owls hunt mice at night. Changes in the owls' ability to locate mice could have a profound effect on their prey population. If the eyesight of a population of owls improves, for instance, only the quickest mice will survive and reproduce, changing the mouse population over time.

Because biological organisms interact, two populations such as owls and mice evolve in concert. Owls can influence the evolution of mouse populations, and mouse populations, in turn, can influence the evolution of the owl. Changes in the ability of the mice to hide, for example, might eliminate all but the most skilled owl hunters. Over time, the owl population would "improve." As the owl population became better able to traits from one generation to the next depended on the sex cells. The sex cells, he said, are capable of reproducing all of the "peculiarities of the parent body in the new individual."

Furthermore, Weismann asserted that the cells of an organism did not dispatch small hereditary particles to germ cells from which the latter derived their power of heredity. Rather, he contended that heredity was brought about by the transference from one generation to another of a substance with a definite molecular constitution. He called it "germplasm" and agreed with others that it was probably found in the nucleus of germ cells. Today, we know it as DNA.

Although Weismann propagated a few erroneous ideas himself, his notion that a chemical substance contained the hereditary information responsible for the faithful transmission of traits profoundly influenced the thinking of many biologists and marked a turning point in our understanding of genetics. It also helped debunk Larmarck's notion of the inheritance of acquired characteristics

and his erroneous view that evolution was driven by such a mechanism.

One of the most rigorous tests of Weismann's hypothesis came about 20 years later in experiments by W. E. Castle and John C. Phillips. Castle and Phillips transplanted ovaries from black guinea pigs (homozygous dominant) into albino guinea pigs (homozygous recessive) whose ovaries had been removed. Later, the albino females were bred to albino males.

Previous studies had shown that matings between albino males and females resulted in 100% albino offspring. Therefore, if acquired characteristics were inherited, Castle and Phillips argued, the offspring of these matings should be white, having acquired their coloration from the host. When bred to an albino male, however, the females produced only black offspring. The young, they said, "are such as might have been produced by the black guinea pig herself, had she been allowed to grow to maturity and been mated with the albino male used in the experiment."

Lamarck did have many good ideas—for instance, that species changed over time and that the environment was a factor in this change. He also contributed to the science of biology in other ways. For example, he was the first scientist to distinguish between animals with backbones (vertebrates) and those without backbones (invertebrates). He went on to classify many invertebrates into the categories of arachnids, crustaceans, and echinoderms, and he also wrote a text on invertebrate systems and a seven-volume treatise on the natural history of invertebrates.

Unfortunately for Lamarck, he's best known for his erroneous concepts of inheritance and evolution. In fact, despite the general criticism of Lamarck's views, the twentieth-century Russian agronomist Trofim D. Lysenko adopted a Lamarckian viewpoint and, with Stalin's backing, established it as Soviet doctrine in genetics research and teaching. The result was a significant setback in genetic research in the former Soviet Union during the Stalinist era.

hunt and catch swift mice, the mouse population would change.

When members of two interacting species affect each other's gene pool, the species evolve in concert, a process called **coevolution**. In the example above, coevolution is like an arms race between predator and prey. Each improvement in a predator's ability to catch its prey is followed by an improvement in the prey's ability to avoid or resist attack. Coevolution occurs in relationships other than predator-prey interaction. Defense mechanisms in plants, for instance, may result in coevolutionary changes in insects that eat them. A toxic or noxious-tasting chemical, for example, may evolve in some plant species, persisting because it helps ward off hungry insects. In time, some insects may evolve enzymes capable of detoxifying the harmful chemical.

Section 21-4

A Modern Version of Evolutionary Theory

Darwin's theory of evolution by natural selection can be summarized in three principles. First, natural variations exist in all species. Second, which members of the species survive to reproduce and reproduce at a greater rate is determined by inherited (genetic) variations (adaptations). Third, natural selection "determines" which organisms survive and reproduce.

For many years, biologists thought that evolutionary changes occurred gradually over many millions of years, a process called **gradualism**. If gradualism does indeed occur, evolutionary biologists reason, the fossil record should contain many intermediate forms of plants and animals. In most cases, it doesn't.

(a)

(b)

(c)

FIGURE 21-14 Fossils (a) Dinosaur tracks made in a Texas streambed about 120 million years ago. (b) Imprint of a leaf. (c) Grasshopper embedded in amber about 40 million years ago.

As a rule, new species in the fossil record appear rather abruptly, persist for several million years, then vanish as abruptly as they arrived on the scene. Based on these and other data, Stephen Jay Gould of Harvard University and Niles Eldredge of the American Museum of Natural History have proposed an alternative hypothesis stating that evolution occurs in spurts. Their hypothesis is called **punctuated equilibrium**.

According to this theory, evolution consists of long periods of relatively little change (equilibrium) interspersed with (punctuated by) brief periods of relatively rapid change, although these periods are still many thousands of years long. During these periods of rapid change, some species become extinct, and new ones arise. Proponents of punctuated equilibrium believe that species undergo most of their morphological change when they first diverge from their parent species. Thus, a species will appear rather suddenly, then undergo little or no change for long periods. Recent genetic research suggests that only minor genetic changes are necessary to produce species dramatically different from their common ancestor.

Section 21-5

The Evidence Supporting Evolution

Evolution by natural selection is one of the central theories of modern biology. Although biologists may argue over some of the details, such as gradualism versus punctuated equilibrium, they agree about the basic tenets. From the outside, this bickering may appear to be evidence that the theory of evolution is on shaky ground. Nothing could be further from the truth. What is disputed is the time scale and other details, not whether evolution has occurred. The next section examines some of the evidence in support of the theory of evolution.

The Fossil Record Yields Some of the Best Supporting Evidence for the Existence of Evolution

Human knowledge of evolution comes from many sources. One of the most important sources is fossils. **Fossils** consist of the remains (wood from trees, bones and eggs from animals) or impressions of organisms that lived on Earth in times past.[7] Human interest in fossils dates back to 450 B.C. when Greek historian Herodotus discovered fossils of seashells in Northern Africa. It was not until the past 100 years or so that our understanding of fossils became firmly established. In this period, thousands of bones of dinosaurs and other animals have been excavated from sites all over the globe. How were these bones preserved?

The most common explanation is that animals that died in regions of rapid sediment deposition (shallow lakes, mud flats, and swamps) were quickly buried. Over time, the animal flesh decayed, leaving behind sediment-entombed bones.

In these sites, the minerals of the bones were often replaced by minerals in the water that seeped through them. (A similar process is responsible for the formation of petrified wood.)

Some creatures such as dinosaurs also left footprints in the mud that hardened into stone to become part of the vast body of fossil evidence of earlier life (**FIGURE 21-14A**). Imprints of leaves make up part of the fossil record (**FIGURE 21-14B**). Intriguingly, some ancient

---

[7]The word *fossil* comes from a Latin word meaning something "dug up."

FIGURE 21-15 Evolution of the Modern Horse

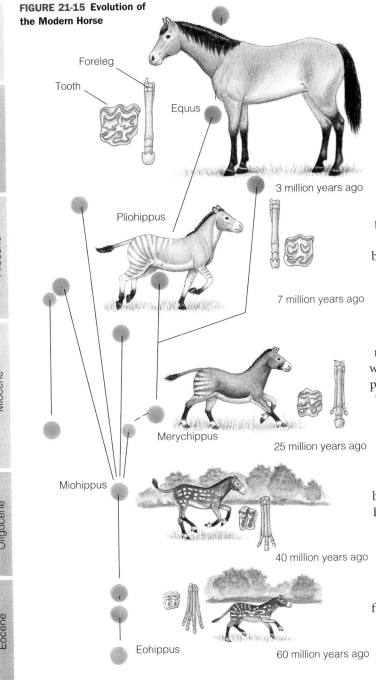

Recent

Pleistocene

Pliocene

Miocene

Oligocene

Eocene

Foreleg

Tooth

Equus

3 million years ago

Pliohippus

7 million years ago

Merychippus

25 million years ago

Miohippus

40 million years ago

Eohippus

60 million years ago

Studying when a species lived and tracking the types of life-forms present at different times during the Earth's history have permitted scientists to piece together an evolutionary history of the planet. These studies show that the oldest rock contains relatively simple single-celled organisms and that successively younger rock houses fossils representing increasingly more complex life-forms.

To date, scientists have discovered fossils belonging to about 250,000 species, most of them from rock formed within the last 600 million years. In this still-growing record, some lineages are nearly complete. The best records come from prehistoric environments such as shallow seas where sedimentation rates (and thus preservation) were high. Many other lineages are incomplete and may never be fully understood. This is particularly true of animals that lived on dry land. Land animals died and were probably eaten by scavengers. Their bones may have been devoured as well or scattered far and wide by hungry animals. Without sedimentation to bury them, the bones eventually crumbled into oblivion. Even in environments with rapid sedimentation, not all species left their mark. Many soft-bodied creatures, without bones, outer skeletons, or shells, could have perished without a trace.

FIGURE 21-15 shows a much simplified diagram of the evolution of the modern horse. This schematic used here is called an **evolutionary tree**. It and others like it are used to depict evolutionary relationships in species. They are based principally on the study of fossils and the anatomy of modern species.

An evolutionary tree for life on Earth shows the progression of life from simple to complex over a period of millions of years.

Evolutionary trees also show how various species are related to one another. As shown in **FIGURE 21-15**, horses evolved from dog-sized, woodland browsers (Eohippus) through a series of increasingly larger, plains-dwelling grazers. Structural similarities in the fossil remains of the horse's ancestors suggest that this progression is indeed real.

You will note in **FIGURE 21-15** that the evolution of horses was not a linear progression. A number of new

organisms (frogs, insects, and flowers) were preserved in amber, resins released by ancient trees (**FIGURE 21-14C**). Blocks of amber, like plastic blocks containing biological specimens, provide a window to our past. In fact, gas bubbles in amber have even been analyzed to determine the composition of the atmosphere in earlier times.

The fossil remains of species no longer in existence have intrigued humans for centuries, as noted earlier, and provide evidence in support of the theory of evolution. Because fossils and the rocks they come from can be dated using radioactive techniques, scientists can determine when different species lived.

FIGURE 21-16 Fossil of Early Amphibian This early amphibian resembles the lobe-fin fishes in many respects, suggesting an evolutionary relationship.

species arose from a common ancestor along the way, as indicated by the circles in the evolutionary scheme. All of these species became extinct, except, of course, the modern horse, which is doing very well.

The fossil record also suggests the origin of species or how new groups of organisms arose. As noted earlier, during evolution, a primitive fish probably gave rise to the amphibians. Amphibians gave rise to the reptiles. Birds and mammals evolved from reptiles. This progression is supported by two lines of evidence from the fossil record.

The first is structural evidence; that is, species thought to have given rise to new groups bear a remarkable resemblance to their supposed descendants. For example, the fossil remains of primitive fishes (lobe-fins) are remarkably similar to the fossil remains of the earliest amphibians (**FIGURE 21-16**). Similarly, the early rep-

tiles share many features in common with their amphibian ancestors.

The second line of evidence is chronological. That is, the amphibians, reptiles, mammals, and birds appear in the fossil record in this order. No one has ever found a mammal or a bird that predated the amphibians. Thus, the structural and chronological evidence can be interpreted to support evolutionary theory.

Common Anatomical Features in Different Species Support the Theory of Evolution

Today's organisms are adapted to a wide range of conditions and exhibit a dazzling diversity of appearance. Despite the diversity of life, many organisms exhibit similar anatomical features. Structures thought to have arisen from common ancestors are known as **homologous structures**. The presence of homologous structures among life's diverse forms represents yet another piece of evidence in support of evolution. **FIGURE 21-17** illustrates some homologous structures: wings, flippers, arms, and legs. As shown, the bones in the wing of a bird and bat, the flipper of a whale, the arm of a human being, and the leg of a horse and cat are quite similar, even though these appendages perform quite different functions. Similarities such as these correspond to what you would expect if birds and mammals evolved from a common ancestor.

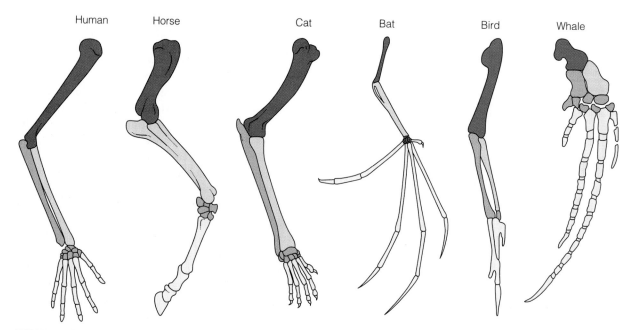

Human   Horse   Cat   Bat   Bird   Whale

FIGURE 21-17 Homologous Structures Among Vertebrates
The presence of homologous structures in vertebrates and other groups supports the theory of evolution.

Creationists, who believe that life on Earth was created by God, argue that the presence of common anatomical features among diverse organisms and the presence of analogous structures lend support to their beliefs. The common criticism from scientists is that creationism is not a science. It cannot be subjected to experimental method. It is, instead, based on faith.

Vestigial Structures Support Evolutionary Theory.

Vestigial structures (ves-TIJ-ee-al) serve no apparent purpose in an organism. An example is the pelvic bones of whales. The pelvis generally attaches an organism's legs to the axial skeleton, but because whales have no legs, the pelvis is useless. Then why are pelvic bones found in whales? Evolutionary biologists believe that whales evolved from terrestrial mammals that had four legs and an obvious need for pelvic bones. During evolution, whales retained the pelvic bones.

Vestigial structures are "evolutionary baggage." They support the notion of evolution. Had the whale been created through divine intervention, it is doubtful that a pelvis would have been included as standard equipment.

Humans contain many vestigial structures. Hair on the body, muscles that move the ears, the appendix, and the pointed canine teeth are examples. The presence of these structures should come as no surprise because we share so many genes with our ancestors.

Comparative Anatomy Permits Scientists to Determine Evolutionary Relationships

Studies of the anatomy of different species have long been used to determine "relatedness" among organisms, based on the belief that the more similar the internal structures of two species were, the more closely related they must be. Structural and functional similarities among species thus also allow scientists to classify organisms into groups.

The Common Biochemical Makeup of Organisms Also Supports the Theory of Evolution

Organisms as distantly related as roses and rhinos are made of the same basic biochemicals—ATP, DNA, RNA, and protein. All living organisms store genetic information in DNA, and all use ATP to collect, store, and transport energy. In addition, many biochemical pathways in organisms (such as those involved in producing energy) bear a remarkable similarity. Are these coincidental, or are they the result of evolution?

To many biologists, the common biochemistry of the Earth's diverse organisms lends further support to the notion of a common ancestry and thus to the theory of evolution. (To creationists, it supports the notion of a designer using similar blueprints.) Interestingly, although many species have similar enzymes and other proteins, differences do exist. Hemoglobin, for example, is found in vertebrate red blood cells, but differences in the composition of hemoglobin are common among vertebrates. These differences have proven quite useful to researchers. By comparing the amino acid sequence of certain proteins (such as hemoglobin) from different species, evolutionary biologists can determine how closely related they are. Chimpanzees and humans, for instance, share about 98% of the same genes, suggesting that they are indeed very closely related. The more differences, the more distant the evolutionary relationship.

Analysis of the amino acid sequence of proteins and the composition of the DNA have enabled evolutionary biologists to create their own evolutionary trees. Not surprisingly, the evolutionary trees they have developed correspond well to those created by comparative anatomists.

Biochemical analyses of DNA and protein have recently been expanded to extinct organisms (museum specimens) and even fossils. DNA extracted from the cells of extinct species can be cloned via genetic engineering. This process provides sufficient amounts of DNA to determine its sequence and make comparisons with other organisms, both living and dead, thus allowing evolutionary biologists to study the relationships among many more species.

Another Line of Evidence That Supports the Theory of Evolution Comes from Comparative Embryology

Studies show that the embryos of many different groups of organisms develop similarly. Thus, the embryos of chickens, turtles, mice, fishes, and humans—all vertebrates—bear a remarkable resemblance during their early stages of development. For example, each of them has a tail and gill slits, even though only adult fishes and amphibian larvae have gills.

One plausible explanation for the similarity of vertebrate embryos is that all of these species contain the genes that control the development of tails and gills and that these genes were passed on from a common ancestor. In humans, however, these genes are active only during embryological development. The structures they produce either become inconspicuous, as in the case of the tail (all that is visible is the tailbone), or become other structures, as in the case of the tissue lying between the gill slits. It forms various structures in the neck.

Health Note 21-1

Well Done, Please: The Controversy over Antibiotics in Meat

FIGURE 1 Feed Lot Cattle Antibiotics reduce infections in cattle in tight quarters and also accelerate growth. Microbiologists, however, worry that they may be stimulating the evolution of super strains of bacteria.

What does evolution have to do with how you have your meat cooked? Next time you order a steak or cook a hamburger over a grill, think about this: Approximately 50 years ago, livestock growers began adding antibiotics to cattle and pig feed to protect animals confined to pens from disease as they were being fattened for market (**FIGURE 1**). Antibiotics were first given to control disease, which can run rampant under crowded conditions. However, farmers soon found that the drugs had an unanticipated beneficial effect: For reasons still not fully understood, antibiotics accelerated the rate of body growth. That meant farmers could turn a higher profit.

Not surprisingly, today 70% of all cattle and 90% of all veal calves and pigs are reared on feed laced with penicillin or tetracycline. Nearly half of the antibiotics sold in the United States, in fact, are used for livestock feed. This practice is also popular in Europe.

The addition of antibiotics to feed has been sharply criticized by microbiologists and health officials who fear that widespread use could promote the evolution of superstrains of bacteria that are immune to antibiotics. In an editorial in the *New England Journal of Medicine,* a Tufts University microbiologist, Stuart Levy, noted that "every animal . . . taking an antibiotic . . . becomes a factory producing resistant strains" of bacteria. Resistant bacteria, in turn, could transfer their resistance to other bacteria, creating highly lethal strains that could infect humans. This is called the *crossover effect.*

Scientists are also concerned that some resistant bacteria in cattle (such as Salmonella) could be transmitted directly to people in meat or milk. The effects could be grave.

Medical researchers are also concerned that antibiotics in livestock grains may also end up in the meat of the animal. It may then be passed on to the meat-eating public. In humans, the antibiotics could result in the production of antibiotic-resistant bacteria, adding to the already growing problem caused by antibiotics used to treat infections (a problem discussed in Chapter 8).

Despite these concerns, efforts to reduce the use of antibiotics in feed have been soundly defeated. In 1978, for instance, the Food and Drug Administration, which controls food additives such as antibiotics, proposed cutting back on penicillin

Experimental Evidence Supports the Theory of Evolution by Natural Selection

A long list of experiments supports the theory of evolution by natural selection. An exhaustive series of field and laboratory studies, for example, shows how genetic differences in wild populations of fruit flies can be attributed to natural selection.

Health, Homeostasis, and the Environment
The Pesticide Treadmill

Evolution has resulted in the presence of many homeostatic mechanisms—in the bodies of organisms like us and in the environment upon which we depend. As pointed out previously, humans have adopted practices and tetracycline use in feeds. Livestock producers, feed producers, and the multimillion-dollar drug industry, however, fought vigorously. They argued that microbiologists' concerns had not been proven.

Scientific evidence is beginning to confirm the suspicions of the medical profession. Dr. Thomas O'Brien of the Harvard University School of Medicine published a study in the *New England Journal of Medicine* in 1982, showing that bacteria that commonly infect humans and other animals share genetic information quite freely through the exchange of plasmids, tiny segments of DNA separate from the bacteria's chromosomes. O'Brien argued that drug resistance could be transferred easily from bacterium to bacterium.

Another study, by researchers at the Centers for Disease Control, published in *Science* in 1984, confirmed the suspicion that antibiotic-resistant bacteria artificially selected by adding antibiotics to cattle feed could be transferred directly from meat to humans. This research showed that some of the outbreaks of illness caused by antibiotic-resistant Salmonella in the previous decade can be traced to meat from animals that had been fed antibiotic-treated grains. The research also showed that 20%–30% of the Salmonella outbreaks involved antibiotic-resistant strains. About 4.2% of the people con-

tracting the antibiotic-resistant bacteria died, compared with only 0.2% of the victims of the normal bacteria.

In 1999, a team of Minnesota researchers published a paper in the *New England Journal of Medicine* that provided additional evidence on the effects of antibiotics in feed. The researchers found that only 1.3% of bacteria isolated from humans in 1992 were resistant to a certain type of antibiotic, specifically the quinoline type. In 1998, three years after the drugs were approved for use in animal feed, 10.2% of the bacteria were resistant to the antibiotic. The researchers concluded that the practice of giving the drug to poultry "created a reservoir" of resistant bacteria. In 2000, Danish researchers found that antibiotic-resistant bacteria could be transmitted from meat to humans.

Richard Young, Advisor to the Soil Association, says, "We are facing a major epidemic of diseases which have developed multiple drug resistance. At least four of these (strains of *salmonella*, *E.coli*, *campylobacter*, and *enterococci*) arise directly as a result of the overuse of antibiotics in agriculture and there is evidence to suggest that further research would reveal agricultural links in other cases too."

Proponents of antibiotics believe that the link between antibiotics and

human disease is still weak and that further research is needed. Even if these findings are substantiated by further research, proponents believe, the benefits of using antibiotics outweigh the potential health effects. Banning antibiotics or cutting back on their use, they say, could have enormous economic impacts that must be weighed against sickness and loss of life. But health experts hope that the United States, like Europe, which strictly limited the use of antibiotics in animal feed in the early 1970s, will find the political will to end this activity.

Individuals can take direct action, too. You can buy "organically grown" beef—that is, beef fed a diet that contains no hormones or antibiotics. You can also change your eating habits. Instead of asking for rare meat or a half-cooked burger, you may want to consider asking for a well-done piece of meat. If ground beef has been heated in the center to over 160 °F, you are pretty safe; chicken and poultry need to be heated to more than 170 °F or until the fluids run clear.

Visit *Human Biology's* Internet site for links to web sites offering more information on this topic.

that inadvertently upset those mechanisms. One of these ways—the use of pesticides—has potentially far-reaching impacts.

During World War II, chemical pesticides became the cornerstone of modern agriculture. Chemical pesticides kill insects and other organisms that damage crops. To combat weeds and animal pests worldwide,

farmers, homeowners, and others spray 2.5 million metric tons of pesticides on the land each year. These chemicals cause a number of problems. First, many broad-spectrum pesticides kill beneficial insects that control pests naturally. Spider mites were once only a minor crop pest in California, but the heavy use of chemical pesticides to control them has killed the mites' natural predators, species that were more sensitive to spraying than the mites. As a result, spider mites today cause twice as much damage in California as all other insect pests combined. Pesticides have thus destroyed an important homeostatic mechanism in California's environment.

A second problem of great concern is genetic resistance. **Genetic resistance** results from genetic variation— the presence of a mutation that makes a small percentage (about 5%) of any insect population resistant to chemical pesticides. Therefore, when farmers spray their fields with chemical pesticides, they kill only the nonresistant insects.

Surviving the onslaught, the small subpopulation of genetically resistant insects breeds and produces a new population that is resistant to spraying. To kill it, farmers must apply additional pesticides or switch to another type. Once again, though, they find that a small segment of the population is genetically resistant to the higher dose or the new chemical preparation. That group survives the spraying, is selected for, and produces an even more resistant population, thus continuing an ever-escalating cycle often referred to as the "pesticide treadmill."

The pesticide treadmill is an excellent example of artificial selection at work. Some scientists warn farmers that they can never win in the battle against pests. Thanks to genetic variation in a population, no matter what pesticide they use, or how much they use, there will always be a resistant strain. Ever more powerful and ever more frequent applications at higher doses will be necessary just to stay even. As an example, a few decades ago, farmers in Central America applied pesticides about 8 times a year; today, 30–40 applications are the norm on any given field. Increased spraying pollutes the environment and kills fishes, birds, and other beneficial animals.

Unfortunately, farmers and chemical pesticide manufacturers have failed to take into account the existence of genetic variation and the selection process at work in the populations of insects. As a result, approximately 550 species of insects are resistant to one or more chemical pesticides. Twenty of the worst pests are now resistant to all types of insecticide. Even weeds develop resistance to herbicides.

Knowledge of this phenomenon suggests alternative strategies. One alternative is **crop rotation**. This practice successfully reduces damage by maintaining pest populations at manageable levels. Practiced years ago on many farms but now largely abandoned, crop rotation requires farmers to alternate the crops they plant in a given field. One year corn might be grown in the field, the next year, beans, and the third year, alfalfa. This practice not only maintains soil nutrient levels, but also effectively cuts down on pests. How does it work?

Many insect pests are specialists, preferring one crop over another. A field of corn, for example, provides an abundant supply of food for corn borers. At the end of the season, corn borers lay their eggs in the soil or in organic material on the surface. If the same crop is planted the next year, the newly hatched insects will have an abundant food supply. The insect population will increase quickly, causing considerable damage. If a different crop is planted the second year, however, the corn borer population will decline. Continued rotation helps hold down pests year after year without costly and potentially harmful pesticide applications.

Chemical resistance is a rather common occurrence in the modern world. As noted above, weeds also become resistant to herbicides; even microorganisms develop resistance to antibiotics, which is one reason many physicians prescribe antibiotics sparingly. They fear, and rightly so, that the more antibiotics we use in society, the more likely a resistant strain will emerge. Antibiotics are also used in livestock feed to protect closely housed animals and to stimulate growth; Health Note 21-1 discusses the problems that can arise from this common practice.

In sum, pesticide use upsets natural biological control mechanisms and puts us on a dangerous and costly pesticide treadmill. A little knowledge of genetics and natural selection can help farmers find alternative ways of controlling pests, ways that mimic nature's natural balance. These methods, many of them age-old practices that have been abandoned in recent times, can markedly reduce pesticide use and protect people and the many species that share this planet with us.

www.jbpub.com/humanbiology

Connect to this book's web site: www.jbpub.com/humanbiology
The site features eLearning, an online review area that provides quizzes, chapter outlines, and other tools to help you study for your class. You can also follow useful links for in-depth information, research the differing views in the Point/Counterpoints, or keep up on the latest environmental and health news.

Summary

The Evolution of Life: An Overview

1. Scientists believe that all atoms and molecules in our solar system came from the same source, an enormous cloud of cosmic dust and gas that gave rise to the Earth and the sun.

2. The Earth formed about 4.5 billion years ago.

3. The evolution of life probably began in the sea and can be divided into three phases: chemical evolution, cellular evolution, and the evolution of multicellular organisms.

4. *Chemical evolution*, scientists hypothesize, began about 4 billion years ago. At that time, the Earth's primitive atmosphere contained a mixture of water vapor and several gases. As rains drenched the Earth, the oceans formed. Dissolved in the waters of early seas were many inorganic molecules (from the atmosphere) that combined to form small organic molecules. Energy needed to drive the reaction may have come from sunlight or other sources. Over time, the small organic molecules combined to form polymers—small proteins and nucleic acids.

5. The theory of chemical evolution holds that organic polymers combined to form aggregates called *microspheres*. These aggregates exhibit structural and functional characteristics of living organisms and may have been the precursors of cells.

6. *Cellular evolution* is the evolutionary development of prokaryotic cells from cell precursors.

7. The first true cells probably contained primitive enzymes, rudimentary genes, and selectively permeable membranes. These cells may have derived nourishment from organic molecules they absorbed from their environment. They are thought to have been heterotrophic fermenters.

8. Autotrophs, organisms capable of synthesizing their own food, arose next. The earliest autotrophs were probably chemosynthetic bacteria that acquired energy from chemicals in the environment.

9. With the evolution of chlorophyll, photosynthetic autotrophs arose. The first form of photosynthesis, however, did not produce oxygen.

10. Over time, scientists believe, photosynthesis evolved further, and the new photosynthetic organisms began to produce oxygen. Oxygen was toxic to the organisms living in the oxygen-free environment of that time. As a result, many of the anaerobic organisms died. Others retreated to oxygen-free environments. Still others evolved ways to survive in an oxygen-rich atmosphere.

11. The theory of endosymbiotic evolution states that eukaryotes arose from prokaryotes when a host cell acquired an internal symbiotic partner (possibly a smaller, oxygen-respiring or photosynthetic bacterium). As atmospheric oxygen levels increased, these unions persisted, and, in time, the relationship became hereditary.

12. Prokaryotes emerged about 3.5 billion years ago, and eukaryotes evolved about 1.2 billion years ago. The evolution of eukaryotes opened the door for the evolution of multicellular organisms.

13. A variety of multicellular plants and animals evolved from single-celled eukaryotes in the oceans. As the ozone layer developed, life on land became possible.

14. The first species to invade the land were plants that thrived in moist environments. Soon after the land plants invaded, animals came ashore. The very first of these animals were probably scorpionlike creatures, which were preadapted to life on land.

How Evolution Works

15. Evolution has produced a great diversity of organisms.

16. Evolution takes place because of genetic variation and natural selection.

17. *Genetic variation* in a species arises from mutations, gene flow, recombination, independent assortment, and new combinations resulting from sexual reproduction. Genetic variation results in phenotypic variation. Some phenotypes confer a selective advantage on certain offspring, giving them a better chance of surviving and reproducing and passing the genes on to future generations.

18. Beneficial traits are preserved in a population by *natural selection*. Abiotic and biotic factors are the agents of natural selection.

19. It is important to remember that natural selection affects the survival and reproduction of individuals in a population, but that individuals do not evolve, populations do.

The Evolution of New Species

20. Natural selection results in a shift in the gene pool of a population and produces organisms that are better adapted to their environment. Dramatic changes in the gene pool may lead to the evolution of entirely new species.

21. *Geographical isolation* is one of the most common mechanisms by which new species evolve. It occurs when a population becomes physically separated. Subject to different environmental conditions, the populations may evolve independently. Over time, they may become *reproductively isolated*—that is, unable to interbreed. When this occurs, two different species are said to have formed.

22. Geographical isolation results in *divergent evolution*—the emergence of two or more species from a common ancestor. Another term that describes this phenomenon is *adaptive radiation*—the evolution of numerous related species, each of which is specially adapted to its environment.

23. Species often evolve in concert with each other, a phenomenon called *coevolution*. Predatory pressure, for example, may act as an agent of natural selection in the evolution of prey populations. Changes in the prey population may also affect the evolution of the predator population.

A Modern Version of Evolutionary Theory

24. Many evolutionary biologists believe that evolution occurs in spurts. According to the *theory of punctuated equilibrium*, long periods of relatively little change (equilibrium) are punctuated by briefer periods of relatively

rapid change, many thousands of years long.

The Evidence Supporting Evolution

25. The scientific knowledge in support of evolution is rich and varied. The fossil record, anatomical similarities in groups of organisms, the occurrence of vestigial structures, the common biochemical makeup of organisms, similar embryological development among many groups of organisms, and experimental evidence all support the theory.

Health, Homeostasis, and the Environment: The Pesticide Treadmill

26. Homeostasis at the organismic and environmental levels can be upset by pesticides. Pesticides upset ecological balances by destroying beneficial insects.
27. Pesticides also create a form of artificial selection that can be witnessed today in modern agriculture. Chemical pesticides used to control insects select resistant species. Farmers who spray their fields to kill insects leave behind a genetically resistant subpopulation that breeds and repopulates farm fields. A

second application at a higher dose or an application of another pesticide kills off more susceptible insects, but once again leaves behind another subset that often becomes a further pest, forcing farmers to use higher doses or switch to another pesticide. This escalation in the war against pests is called the *pesticide treadmill*.

28. Chemical resistance is a rather common occurrence in the modern world. Weeds can become resistant to herbicides, and even microorganisms develop resistance to antibiotics.

Critical Thinking

Thinking Critically— Analysis

This Analysis corresponds to the Thinking Critically scenario that was presented at the beginning of this chapter.

Begin by making a list of basic tenets of creationism and evolution. From this list, you may see that creationism is based on interpretations of the Bible. The Bible, although a powerful basis for a personal belief system, is not a systematic and methodical study of nature. In other words, creationism is based on faith,

not scientific fact. Evolution is based on interpretations of hard scientific data—a wide range of methodical and systematic observations and measurements. Although there are gaps in our knowledge of evolution, the data supporting this theory is quite impressive. In fact, there's not one iota of data that contradicts the theory of evolution.

One thing you may note about the creationist hypothesis is that it cannot be tested. You cannot perform experiments or test hypotheses to determine whether the events put forth by creationists really occured—another indication that it is based on faith. So, should it be taught in science classrooms? Most scientists believe that religion should not be taught in science classrooms. However, it may deserve some mention—similar to the one in this chapter. And, a comparison of evolutionary theory and creationism can be instructive. Finally, it might be useful to point out that many scientists have no conflict between science and religion. They do not see evolutionary theory as a refutation of the presence of a divine being.

Exercising Your Critical Thinking Skills

For more than a century, biology teachers have been relating a fascinating story of mimicry among butterflies that involves two colorful species, the monarch and viceroy (**FIGURE 21-18**).

The monarch larvae feed on milkweed and ingest a heart toxin (cardiac glycoside) produced by the plant, which remains in the bodies of the butterflies through adulthood.[8]

FIGURE 21-18 Monarch and Viceroy Butterflies New studies suggest that long-standing beliefs about the evolution of the viceroy butterfly may be wrong.

---

[8]Cardiac glycosides may have evolved to protect milkweed from herbivores.

Some birds that prey on the monarch die, but most simply become ill and from that point on avoid the monarch. According to common belief, birds also avoid similarly colored viceroy butterflies. Viceroys evolved from the tasty but drab-looking admiral butterfly. Over time, scientists thought, viceroys evolved a coloration similar to the monarch butterfly, and this coloration (mimicry) persisted because it protected the viceroy from predation.

Two researchers at the University of Florida in Gainesville, however, have recently challenged this classic explanation. They conducted an avian taste test, feeding the abdomens of seven different butterfly species, including viceroys and monarchs, to red-winged blackbirds. In their experiments, they found that viceroys were just as unappetizing as monarch butterflies.

This finding throws into question the belief that viceroys are Batesian mimics—otherwise palatable insects that, through evolution, acquired a protective coloration. (Henry Bates was the nineteenth-century British naturalist who studied the phenomenon.) Because the viceroy butterfly feeds on nontoxic willows, the Florida researchers hypothesized that this species must produce its own chemical defense. This hypothesis, if it turns out to be true, could dispel a long-held belief—that all butterflies depend on plant poisons for the protective chemicals they harbor.

This new research suggests that instead of being Batesian mimics—that is, exploiting another's protective mechanism—the viceroy is actually a Mullerian mimic (after zoologist Fritz Muller who first described the phenomenon). This type of mimicry evolves in two equally distasteful butterfly species, which gain greater protection from predators by evolving nearly identical coloration. Mullerian mimicry is therefore mutually beneficial to both species. A bird that eats either a viceroy or a monarch would very probably leave both species alone.

This is another example of a failure in critical thinking—notably, the failure of scientists to question underlying assumptions in the formulation of their theories. One key assumption in this instance was that the viceroy was a palatable species. Scientists knew that the viceroy evolved from the rather tasty admiral butterfly; therefore, if it came from a palatable species, it must be edible. When this assumption was finally tested, a classic biological hypothesis was called into question.

The second assumption that led scientists astray has to do with the evolution of color and wing pattern. Because the viceroy's ancestors are dark-colored and drab, scientists believed that the viceroy probably evolved to mimic the monarch. If the two species turn out to be Mullerian mimics, it may be that they evolved simultaneously, benefiting from similar wing and color patterns.

Test of Concepts

1. In 1924, the Russian scientist A. I. Oparin suggested that life arose from nonliving matter. Explain his hypothesis, and discuss the research supporting it.

2. Describe how the first cells may have arisen during evolution. What critical requirements must have been met for life to begin?

3. If life formed abiotically in the shallow waters of the sea, would you expect the process to be occurring now? Why or why not?

4. Describe the theory of endosymbiotic evolution and the evidence supporting it.

5. The development of photosynthesis and the emergence of eukaryotes were pivotal events in evolution. Why?

6. Numerous plants and animals had evolved in the sea before life emerged on land. Why?

7. A critic of evolution says, "Life-forms are too diverse to have come from a common ancestor." How would you respond?

8. What is meant by the phrase "the conservative nature of evolution"?

9. Over the course of the Earth's history, mountain ranges have risen and gradually worn down. Explain what might happen to a species population that was geographically isolated by the emergence of a mountain range.

10. How do random mutations in germ cells contribute to the evolutionary process?

11. Define the following terms: adaptation, variation, natural selection, biotic factors, abiotic factors, selective advantage, and fitness.

12. Discuss the following statement: natural selection is nature's editor.

13. Discuss the evidence supporting the theory of evolution.

14. How do crop rotation and heteroculture keep pest populations in check?

Tracing Our Roots

THE STORY OF HUMAN EVOLUTION

Humans have come a long way in their 3.7 million year evolutionary history.

Thinking **Critically**

The emergence of modern humans (people like us, *Homo sapiens sapiens*) is, like many other scientific issues, a matter of considerable debate among scientists. Two basic hypotheses exist: the Multiregional Evolution model (or Regional Continuity model) and the African Origins model.

The Multiregional Evolution model holds that modern humans derive from archaic human populations living in various regions of Europe, Africa, China, and Indonesia. That is to say, these archaic populations gave rise to existing populations. Thus, modern Chinese derive from archaic Chinese *(Homo erectus)*. In contrast, the African Origins model holds that, although regional archaic populations existed, they were displaced by a single population of humans that arose in Africa approximately 200,000 years ago. This new species supposedly spread into new territories replacing regional human populations living there.

The African Origins model is based on genetic analyses of mitochondrial DNA. In these analyses, scientists have found that only the African population exists in an unbroken maternal line. Other lineages of archaic peoples seem to have faded into oblivion.

Using your critical thinking skills, make a list of questions that might be useful in analyzing the African Origins model. ■

Humorist Will Cuppy once quipped that "all modern men are descended from a wormlike creature, but it shows more in some people." In reality, humans belong to a group or, more correctly, an order known as the primates. The primates are believed to have evolved not from worms, but from an insect-eating mammal that probably resembled the modern-day tree shrew of Southeast Asia (**FIGURE 22-1**).

This chapter examines the evolutionary development of the first primates, beginning with the mammalian insectivores. It then describes how human beings evolved. This chapter also highlights important evolutionary advances in primate evolution and concludes with a brief discussion of human cultural evolution, laying a foundation for an understanding of contemporary environmental problems.

FIGURE 22-1 Look Familiar? An organism resembling this tree shrew is believed to have been the early ancestor of the primates.

Section 22-1

Early Primate Evolution

Before you begin your study of primate evolution, it is important to spend a few minutes on terminology and some basic relationships. First, the order we call **primates** consists of two subgroups or suborders. They are the **prosimians** (pro-SIM-eeans) or premonkeys and a much larger group, **anthropoids** (AN-throw-POIDS). **FIGURE 22-2** shows the various types of anthropoids.

The **prosimians** were the very first primates to inhabit the Earth (**FIGURE 22-2**). Today, prosimians consist of tree shrews, lemurs, and tarsiers. **FIGURE 22-1** shows a tree shrew. **FIGURE 22-3** shows tarsier and a lemur. During the course of evolution, the prosimians gave rise to **anthropoids**. This group includes monkeys, apes, and humans.

Today, most primates—prosimians and anthropoids alike—inhabit tropical or subtropical regions where they live in forests, grasslands, and mixed woodlands (consisting of both grassland and forest). Most primate species are tree-dwellers. Humans are an important exception. Our kind ranges widely over the Earth, inhabiting virtually every available biome. We lead a largely terrestrial life.

Primates are characterized by several features, among them grasping hands, which permit them to pick up objects, and forward-directed eyes, which enhance three-dimensional vision. Primates also have the largest brains of all mammals in proportion to their body size.

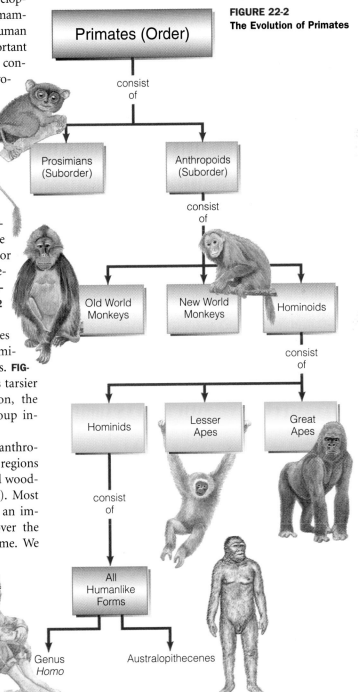

FIGURE 22-2
The Evolution of Primates

The Fossil Evidence of Primate Evolution Is Limited, Making it Difficult to Determine the Exact Progression of Early Human Ancestors

Unlike the dinosaurs, early primates did not live in habitats conducive to fossil preservation. Whereas the mud in swamps or along rivers preserved the bones of many a giant dinosaur, the forests and grasslands in which primates lived were not environments where bones of a dead animal would be readily covered with sediment and preserved. Thus, the primate fossil record is less than complete. Another reason for the scarcity of early primate fossils is that dead or dying animals were probably eaten by scavengers and their bones no doubt scattered across the landscape and even eaten.

Because the primate fossil record is incomplete, the origin of primates remains speculative. But this has not deterred many scientists from making tentative conclusions about primate evolution. The scheme presented here represents a synthesis of current thinking on the evolution of primates. Bear in mind, however, that new evidence could radically change the present interpretation.

The Prosimians Probably Evolved from Tree-Dwelling Mammals That Lived During the Age of the Dinosaurs

Approximately 80 million years ago, tree-dwelling insectivores (similar to tree shrews) lived in tropical regions. Over time, they gave rise to many nonprimate mammals, among them the ground-dwelling shrews, water shrews, moles, and bats. They also gave rise to the prosiminians or premonkeys mentioned earlier.

Although no one knows for sure, the earliest prosimians probably emerged about 65 million years ago. As a group, the early prosimians became quite abundant

FIGURE 22-3 Prosimians The prosimians (premonkeys) were probably the first primates. The earliest ones probably resembled modern-day *(a)* tarsiers and *(b)* lemurs.

and geographically widespread and lived for tens of millions of years. Approximately 55 million years ago, they gave rise to the modern-day prosimians: tree shrews, lemurs, and tarsiers (**FIGURES 22-2** and **22-3**).

The Fossil Evidence Suggests That One of the Early Prosimian Lines Gave Rise to the Anthropoids

Within the following 15 million years, the **anthropoids** (monkeylike primates) evolved from prosimian stock in Africa and possibly earlier in Asia. Technically, biologists divide the anthropoids into (1) the Old World monkeys; (2) the New World monkeys; and (3) another larger group, the **hominoids** (HAHM-eh-NOIDS). The hominoids consist of great apes (like gorillas), the lesser apes (like the gibbons), and humans (**FIGURE 22-2**).

The Old World monkeys occupy the tropical regions on the continents of Africa and Asia. They include ground-dwelling as well as arboreal species. The Old World monkeys have grasping hands, but lack prehensile (pre-HEN-sill) tails. Most monkeys in both groups live in bands and are active during the day. Some familiar examples are the baboon and rhesus monkey (**FIGURE 22-4**).

(a)

(b)

FIGURE 22-4 Old World Monkeys *(a)* Olive baboon and *(b)* Rhesus monkey.

(a)

(b)

FIGURE 22-5 New World Monkeys   *(a)* Squirrel monkey and *(b)* spider monkey.

The New World monkeys, which inhabit Central and South America, include the familiar squirrel and spider monkeys (**FIGURE 22-5**). All New World monkeys live in the trees and have prehensile tails.

The relationship between Old World and New World monkeys is not clearly delineated. However, most evolutionary biologists believe that Old World monkeys gave rise to the New World monkeys. First emerging in Africa and Asia, the Old World monkeys may have migrated across North America into Central and South America or may have arrived on rafts of logs or floating debris.

The hominoid line, which today consists of great apes, lesser apes, and hominids (all humanlike forms), diverged from the Old World monkeys over 20 million years ago. The very first hominoids were apelike creatures. Two distinct apes were present at this time and are considered to be potential ancestors of humans and modern apes.

The first family, the **dryopithecines** (dry-o-PITH-a-seens), originated about 20 million years ago in Africa and spread to Eurasia about 14 million years ago (**FIGURE 22-6**). Unfortunately, no complete skulls or skeletons of the dryopithecines have been found, and our knowledge of these animals is based on fragments of skulls, jaws, and limb bones. This evidence suggests that dryopithecines had relatively small brains and apelike teeth, jaws, and faces. The structure of their limbs suggests that dryopithecines walked on four legs, much like chimpanzees and gorillas, but spent most of their time in the trees.

The second possible ancestor of apes and humans lived slightly later—from about 17–7 million years ago. Called **ramapithecines** (ram-ah-PITH-o-seens), these creatures were similar to the dryopithecines in many respects.

Dryopithecines and ramapithecines may have been related or may have evolved separately. Unfortunately, fossil evidence is not complete enough to establish the relationship between them or to determine their exact relationship to apes and humans. For now, all we can do is content ourselves with knowing that these creatures existed and hypothesize that they represent a link between early primates and more modern primates, including gorillas, chimpanzees, and humans.

Evolution of the Australopithecines

Archaeological evidence suggests that the first **hominids,** the first humanlike primates, belonged to the genus *Australopithecus* (awe-STRAY-loh-PITH-eh-cuss; meaning "southern apeman") (**FIGURE 22-6**). The oldest known australopithecine skeleton was unearthed by Donald Johanson, Yves Coppens, and their co-workers in Africa and is about 3.5 million years old. The specimen named Lucy is one of the most complete fossils of early hominids yet found (**FIGURE 22-7**). Known as *Australopithecus afarensis* (afarensis means from the Afar region of Ethiopia), these hominids stood only about 3 feet high and had brains only slightly larger than those of apes. The skulls of *A. afarensis* have many apelike features, including massive brow ridges, low foreheads, and forward-jutting jaws. The shape of its pelvis suggests that *A. afarensis* walked erect.

About 3 million years ago, *A. afarensis* vanished and was replaced by another species, *A. africanus*, which lived for about 1.5 million years (**FIGURE 22-6**). *A. africanus* was slightly taller than its predecessor and had a slightly larger brain.

Studies of the fossil record suggest that about 2.3 million years ago another species of *Australopithecus* emerged, *A. robustus*—so named because it was heavier and taller and had a larger brain than *A. africanus* (**FIGURE 22-6**). About 2.2 million years ago, the fourth species, *A. boisei*, appeared. It was even more robust than *A. robustus*.

Members of the genus *Australopithecus* had many common features. For example, they were all **bipedal** (buy-PED-al)—that is, they walked on two legs—and they all ranged in height from 1 meter to 1.7 meters. Their brains were larger than those of chimpanzees, but considerably smaller than modern humans. The differences among the

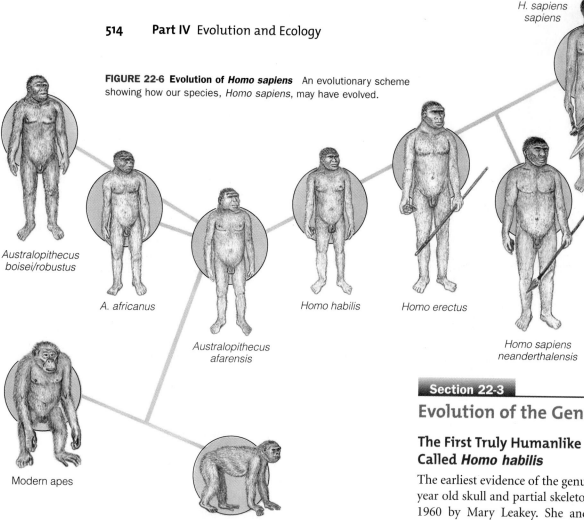

FIGURE 22-6 **Evolution of *Homo sapiens*** An evolutionary scheme showing how our species, *Homo sapiens*, may have evolved.

Australopithecus boisei/robustus

A. africanus

Australopithecus afarensis

Homo habilis

Homo erectus

Modern apes

Dryopithecus

H. sapiens sapiens

Homo sapiens neanderthalensis

Evolution of the Genus *Homo*

The First Truly Humanlike Creatures Were Called *Homo habilis*

The earliest evidence of the genus *Homo* is a 1.8 million year old skull and partial skeleton found in Tanzania in 1960 by Mary Leakey. She and her husband, Louis, called this species **Homo habilis** ("skillful man"). Archaeological evidence indicates that *Homo habilis* apparently made primitive tools from fractured rocks and butchered large animals.

What was *Homo habilis* like physically? The skull of *H. habilis* is like that of *Australopithecus*, suggesting an evolutionary relationship. However, the brain of *Homo habilis* is 50% larger than its presumed australopithecine relatives. The skeleton of *H. habilis* displays many apelike features, especially the relatively long

four species are relatively minor, mostly a matter of degree. As the genus evolved, their brains got larger, and their height increased. The enlarged brain is believed to be the result of natural selection.

FIGURE 22-8 indicates when the various species of *Australopithecus* lived. As illustrated, anthropologists believe that all three "younger" species coexisted, at least for a while, during the time span ranging from 1 million to 3 million years ago. Over 1 million years ago, however, australopithecines disappeared. Why they vanished no one knows.

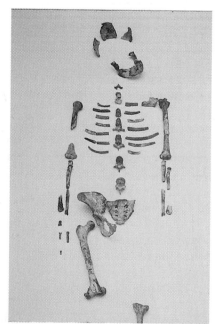

FIGURE 22-7 **Skeleton of *Australopithecus afarensis*** This skeleton, estimated to be about 3.5 million years old, is popularly known as Lucy.

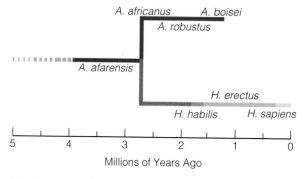

A. africanus   *A. boisei*

A. robustus

A. afarensis

H. erectus

H. habilis   *H. sapiens*

| 5 | 4 | 3 | 2 | 1 | 0 |

Millions of Years Ago

FIGURE 22-8 **Australopithecine Evolution** Conventional thinking holds that the genus *Homo* evolved from *Australopithecus afarensis*.

FIGURE 22-9 Skeleton of Homo erectus This, the most complete fossilized skeleton of *H. erectus* ever found, belonged to a boy who lived about 1.6 million years ago.

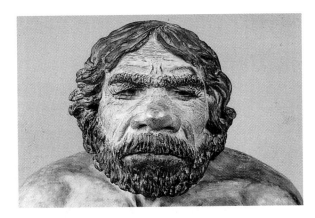

FIGURE 22-10 Neanderthal Notice the projecting brow ridges of this reconstruction of a Neanderthal man.

arms and small body. Because of this, some paleontologists contend that skeletons classified as belonging to *Homo habilis* are really members of the genus *Australopithecus*.

Homo habilis Gave Rise to *Homo erectus*

Two hundred thousand years after the emergence of *Homo habilis*, the first unmistakable member of the genus *Homo*, known as **Homo erectus** ("upright man"), arose (see **FIGURE 22-6**). Skeletons of *Homo erectus* appear in geological formations 300,000 to 1.6 million years old in the Old World. The most complete fossilized human skeleton to have been found is that of a 12-year-old boy (**FIGURE 22-9**).

Unlike *Australopithecus* and *H. habilis*, which remained in Africa, *H. erectus* first appeared in Africa, then spread to Europe and Asia (India, China, and Indonesia). *Homo erectus* appears to be the first hominid to leave the warmth and abundance of the tropics and subtropics and take up residence in the **temperate zone**, a region characterized by warm summers but cold winters.

Homo erectus stood about 5 feet tall, used fire, and made more sophisticated tools and weapons than its predecessor, *Homo habilis*. With a brain slightly smaller than ours, *Homo erectus* is believed to be the direct ancestor of *Homo sapiens*, the self-proclaimed "thinking man."

Modern Humans Belong to *Homo sapiens*

Homo sapiens emerged about 300,000 years ago. Homo sapiens consists of two subspecies in order of their appearance: **Homo sapiens neanderthalensis**, the Neanderthals, and **Homo sapiens sapiens**, modern humans (**FIGURE 22-6**).

Widely distributed in Europe and Asia, the Neanderthals lived in caves and camps. Their name comes from the Neander Valley in Germany, where the first specimens were discovered. Archaeological evidence shows that the Neanderthals gathered fruits, berries, grains, and roots and hunted animals with weapons. They cooked some of their food on fires. Neanderthals stood erect and walked upright. Evidence

also indicates that they lived in small clans and buried their dead in elaborate rituals.

Although the skeletons of the Neanderthals resemble those of humans, they differ in several ways. For example, the skulls of Neanderthals were, on average, larger than those of modern humans. Their skeletons were also more massive and heavily muscled than those of modern humans, and they had rather short lower limbs, much like Inuits (Eskimos) and other cold-adapted people.

Many people think of the Neanderthals as dim-witted and brutish, shuffling along bent over like an ape. This view is based on an interpretation of a Neanderthal skeleton found in 1908 in France. At the time of the discovery, however, the researchers failed to recognize that the skeleton under study was bent over because the individual suffered from arthritis of the hip and had diseased vertebrae. It is interesting, though, how this hasty conclusion from one observation spawned such a long-standing myth.

Some anthropologists wonder whether Neanderthals, despite many humanlike behaviors, should really be considered members of *Homo sapiens*. The differences in their physical appearance are quite striking. With broad faces, large projecting brow ridges, and heavily built bodies, they should perhaps be placed in a species all their own (**FIGURE 22-10**). Nonetheless, if one compares skeletons of australopithecines, early species of the genus *Homo*, and modern *Homo sapiens*, the Neanderthal does seem to fit well in the progression from *Homo erectus* to *Homo sapiens sapiens* (**FIGURE 22-11**).

Neanderthals disappeared approximately 40,000 years ago for reasons still not understood. Some archaeologists believe that they were replaced by the earliest known members of *Homo sapiens sapiens*, the **Cro-Magnons** (CROW-MAN-yens). Cro-Magnons first appeared in Africa and then spread out across Europe

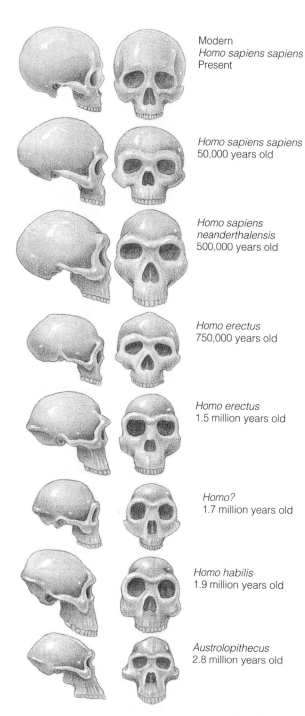

Modern
Homo sapiens sapiens
Present

Homo sapiens sapiens
50,000 years old

Homo sapiens neanderthalensis
500,000 years old

Homo erectus
750,000 years old

Homo erectus
1.5 million years old

Homo?
1.7 million years old

Homo habilis
1.9 million years old

Austrolopithecus
2.8 million years old

FIGURE 22-11 Evolutionary Progression in Skull Development
Notice the changes that occurred over time in the shape of the human skeleton, starting with the apelike *Australopithecus* at the bottom. The dates indicate age of skulls in the drawing, not the evolutionary emergence of each species.

and northern Asia, perhaps wiping out the Neanderthals or possibly interbreeding with them.

Archaeological evidence shows that Cro-Magnons used sophisticated tools and weapons, including the

FIGURE 22-12 Cro-Magnon Art

bow and arrow, and were highly skilled nomadic hunters, following great herds of animals during their seasonal migrations. They may have had a well-developed language. Cro-Magnons lived in caves and rock shelters, in groups of 50–75 people, and are best known for the elaborate artwork that adorned the walls of their caves (**FIGURE 22-12**).

Approximately 10,000 years ago, truly modern humans emerged, but the changes were not great. In fact, over the past 40,000 years, human evolution has produced little noticeable change in the physical appearance of humans. A Cro-Magnon on the streets of Los Angeles, in fact, would probably go unnoticed. Those 40,000 years have not been without change, however, for during this period, *Homo sapiens* has developed a rich and varied culture, complex language, and extraordinarily sophisticated tools.

Human Races Result from Variations Caused by Geographic Separation

As noted in Chapter 21, species that become subdivided into isolated populations undergo changes in response to their environment. If the changes are profound, the subpopulations often lose the ability to interbreed and produce new species.

Over the course of time, the human population has wandered far and wide on the planet and has fragmented into distinct subpopulations, living in very different environments. This fragmentation has resulted in the formation of a number of phenotypically distinct subpopulations, or **races** (**FIGURE 22-13**). It is important to remember, however, that races are not distinct species, just regional variants of the one species *Homo sapiens*.

Most of us are familiar with regional characteristics. We know, for instance, that Mexicans tend to have brown eyes, dark skin, and black hair and that Scandinavians tend to have blue eyes and blond hair. Many differences found in the races are undoubtedly adaptations to differing environmental conditions. The darker skin that evolved in tropical and subtropical populations, for instance, may be an adaptation

(a)

(b)

(c)

(d)

(e)

FIGURE 22-13 Human Races
Humans, no matter what they look like, belong to one species, *Homo sapiens.* The various races are phenotypic variants of that species. Many scientists recognize five distinct races: *(a)* Mongoloid, *(b)* Negroid, *(c)* Caucasian, *(d)* Native American, and *(e)* Australian Aborigine.

that protects people from harmful ultraviolet light.

How many races are there? Some scientists recognize three main ones: Mongoloids, Negroids, and Caucasians. Others recognize two others: Native Americans and Australian Aborigines (**FIGURES 22-13D** and **22-13E**). Still others recognize 30 different races. What all this tells us is that the races are arbitrary categories. As time goes on, the distinction among various races will probably decrease. Why? As people move about the planet and interbreed, the races are mixing, blurring the lines among the world's peoples.

Section 22-4

Trends in Primate Evolution

The evolutionary path that leads first to primates and then to humans is marked by a number of significant changes. One important change was the evolution of bipedal (two-legged) locomotion, which freed the front legs for other useful tasks. In other words, bipedal locomotion may have, among other things, facilitated the evolution of the highly mobile front limbs we call arms.

In order to understand the importance of highly mobile front limbs, consider the four-legged ancestors of primates, the earliest prosimians. In these quadrupeds, the limbs function primarily as a means of propulsion. The front limbs move back and forth, but cannot be rotated or spread very far from the body. In sharp contrast, the front limbs of monkeys, apes, and humans are highly mobile. In tree-dwelling primates, this evolutionary advance permitted free movement among the branches, and it has enabled humans to use tools and weapons.

The evolution of primates was no doubt accelerated by the increased mobility of the fingers. This mobility permitted monkeys to grasp branches and fruit and apes to manipulate objects and even primitive tools. Chimpanzees, for instance, use sticks to dig termites out of the ground. In humans, manual dexterity permits us to engage in intricate crafts, to play musical instruments, and to perform many other fine motor skills.

Yet another significant advance, related most likely to the arboreal life of the early primates, was the development of eyes on the front of the head. This placement permits three-dimensional vision, essential to the quick pace of life in the trees. Swinging from branch to branch, often jumping long distances, monkeys would be nearly helpless without three-dimensional vision.

Another important development during the evolution of primates to humans was the steady increase in brain size. Larger brains were probably selected for because they gave organisms an advantage over others. Precise hand-eye coordination afforded by a larger brain no doubt facilitated life within the trees. A larger brain has also been a boon to humans. Our large, highly capable brain combined with our extraordinary manipulative abilities have permitted humans to devise elaborately powerful tools to reshape the environment—sometimes with harmful consequences.

Health, Homeostasis, and the Environment
Human Cultural Evolution

This book has been organized around the concept of homeostasis, showing how important homeostasis is to human health and how human actions can upset homeostasis—in our bodies and our environment. As we have seen, upsets in both systems lead to human disease. To better understand why humankind finds itself in a growing environmental crisis, let us take an admittedly simplified look at human cultural evolution.

Human culture has evolved through three general phases: hunting and gathering, agricultural, and industrial. For 99% of human evolutionary history, humans

FIGURE 22-14 Hunters and Gatherers   Some anthropologists believe that the early hunters and gatherers acquired most of their food by gathering nuts, fruits, berries, roots, and seeds. Hunting may have provided a supplementary food source.

survived by gathering grains, fruits, nuts, berries, and roots and by hunting animals (**FIGURE 22-14**). Recent archaeological evidence suggests that our earliest ancestors were also scavengers, eating animals that died from natural causes. Our modern way of life and our modern agricultural practices, however, are really newcomers in human cultural evolution.

Based on studies of modern-day hunters and gatherers, whom some anthropologists call our "living ancestors," early hunter-gatherers were probably extraordinarily knowledgeable about the environment. For example, they very likely knew hundreds of edible and medicinal plants and were adept at locating insects, grubs, and other foods in nature's vast outdoor kitchen. Some studies also suggest that the lives of many hunters and gatherers, especially in warmer climates, were not as difficult as we often imagine. In many locales, they did not live in constant danger of starvation and did not spend a great deal of time finding food. Their lives were often leisurely and healthy.

Today, remaining hunters and gatherers live in relative harmony with nature, taking what they need and generally causing little ecological disruption, especially compared with the rest of humankind. Because of this, it is assumed that ancient hunting and gathering societies also lived in relative harmony. Their lack of environmental damage can be attributed to at least three facts of life: (1) many were nomadic, wandering in search of food and a favorable climate, (2) their numbers were small, and (3) their tools were primitive.

This is not to say that all hunter-gatherers were environmentally benign. Some North American Indians,

for example, set fire to the prairie to drive buffalo off cliffs. Their massive fires killed large numbers of animals. In addition, the extinction of several North American species such as the giant tree sloth and giant beaver parallels the migration of ancient hunters and gatherers across the continent.

New archaeological research suggests that many groups of hunters and gatherers grew their own food and raised animals to feed their people earlier than we previously thought. Some may even have engaged in trade with other groups. Over time, more and more of our early ancestors began to cultivate food crops, slowly giving rise to a new form of life, the agricultural society.

Agricultural societies emerged between 10,000 and 6,000 years ago. In the moist rain forests of Southeast Asia, farmers cleared small jungle plots to raise their crops. They grew a variety of vegetables and raised pigs and other domesticated animals for additional food.

Seed crops (grains like wheat) originated in a wider region, extending from China west to India and eastern Africa. In these regions, farmers cleared forests to plant crops and, with the advent of the plow, began to till the rich grassland soils.

The plow allowed for larger fields and higher grain production. Farming, which had generally supplied the immediate needs of a single family, began to change. Now a farmer could produce food for many families and with this development, towns and cities came into existence. People who were no longer needed on the farm congregated in cities and towns, where they began to engage in trades—making clothing, pots, tools, and weapons.

Several important changes in the human-environment interaction were also evident as agriculture grew. First, humans began to drastically modify the natural environment—sometimes on an enormous scale. Poor soil management, overgrazing, and heavy timber cutting destroyed large regions. The rich Tigris-Euphrates river valley, often referred to as the cradle of civilization and now part of Iran and Iraq, was once lush and productive. For several millenia now, much of this landscape has lain parched and unproductive because of human abuse. Further abuse continues today in many parts of the world, threatening long-term food production.

The second major change during the shift to agriculture came with an upsurge in commerce. Commerce demands natural resources—metals, energy, and stone. These materials came from the outlying countryside. The towns and cities, therefore, drew heavily on the surrounding land, often causing considerable environmental damage.

FIGURE 22-15 The Control of Nature Many forms of agriculture attempt to control or dominate the forces of nature, reshaping landscapes to human liking.

FIGURE 22-16 A Product of Cultural Evolution

The third change, possibly the most important of all, was a weakening of the link between humans and nature. As noted above, many hunter-gatherers took little from the land and lived within the bounds of nature. Agriculturalists, however, attempted to harness the forces of nature. Humankind began to see itself as separate from the environment, as nature's master (**FIGURE 22-15**). This profound change in attitude followed humans into the next phase of cultural evolution, the industrial society. With the advent of trade and commerce in agricultural societies, humans began to regard the natural world primarily as a source of wealth.

The industrial society is a recent occurrence in human history. In fact, if the Earth's history were condensed into a 1-year-long movie, the Industrial Revolution would occur in the last half-second of the film. The **Industrial Revolution**, the advent of mechanized production, began in England in the 1700s and in the United States in the 1800s. During the Industrial Revolution machines took over much of the manual production, greatly improving output and making goods more cheaply so they could be purchased by a larger number of people. However, machines required vast quantities of energy and produced enormous amounts of air and water pollution (**FIGURE 22-16**).

Mechanization swept the farms, too, in the industrial era. As a result, still fewer people were needed to raise food. Cities grew. Pollution increased. Streams once teeming with fish turned putrid with the stench of human and factory wastes. The countryside was often pillaged to provide energy and materials for factories. Pollution and species extinction were two of the principal environmental problems that arose during the Industrial Revolution.

Changes occurring during the agricultural and industrial revolutions planted the seeds of a dramatic increase in human population. Between 1850 and 2002, human population increased from 1 billion to 6.2 billion. This dramatic rise occurred for many reasons. The most important were (1) modern medicines, which lowered infant mortality; (2) improved sanitation, which stopped the spread of disease in the increasingly crowded urban environment; and (3) greater food production.

Humans' relationship with nature grew even more strained. Philosophers, economists, and some theologians argued that people needed to seek power over nature. Control became the byword. Survival, as many saw it, required complete domination of nature. Today, efforts at domination continue and have spawned serious global environmental problems. Some think they are a warning sign that we have pushed too far—that our culture is on a collision course with its future.

Current problems such as global warming and ozone depletion threaten to alter global climate and to create widespread species extinction. It is no exaggeration to say that the survival of humankind and the other species that inhabit this planet is in danger. Our health and survival on the planet depend on reestablishing a balance with nature. Today many people believe that to meet this challenge we must find sustainable ways of living and conducting business. Our future depends on finding ways to meet our needs without bankrupting the Earth and foreclosing on future generations and the millions of species that share this planet with us. In a sense, we need to construct a way of life that makes sense from both an economic and an environmental standpoint. We need a creative balancing of life-style and economics with the dictates of the Earth's ecological life-support systems.

Summary

Early Primate Evolution

1. Humans belong to the order called *primates*, which includes two suborders: the *prosimians* (premonkeys) and the *anthropoids* (monkeys, apes, and humans).

2. Today, most primates live in tropic and subtropic forests and are well adapted to an arboreal way of life. The main exception is humans, who inhabit a wide range of habitats.

3. Primates are characterized by grasping hands, forward-looking eyes, and large brains (in proportion to body size).

4. Based on fossil evidence, it appears that the primates evolved from a mammalian insectivore that resembled the modern-day tree shrew and lived about 80 million years ago.

5. The first primates to evolve were the tree-dwelling prosimians. Modern-day prosimians include the lemurs and tarsiers.

6. The prosimians gave rise to the *New World* and *Old World monkeys*. The *hominoids*, which today consist of the great apes, the lesser apes, and humans, diverged from the Old World monkeys over 20 million years ago.

7. The very first hominoids were apelike creatures. Two distinct apes present at that time are considered potential ancestors of humans and modern apes.

8. The first family, the *dryopithecines*, originated about 20 million years ago in Africa and spread to Eurasia about 14 million years ago. The scant fossil remains of these creatures suggest that they walked about on four legs, much like chimpanzees and gorillas, but spent most of their time in the trees.

9. The second possible ancestor of apes and humans lived slightly later, from about 17 million years ago to 7 million years ago, and are called *ramapithecines*.

Evolution of the Australopithecines

10. The first truly human primate belonged to the genus *Australopithecus* and may have evolved from either the dryopithecines or ramapithecines.

11. The oldest known australopithecine skeleton was unearthed in Africa and is believed to be about 3.5 million years old. It belongs to a group called *Australopithecus afarensis*.

12. *A. afarensis* stood only about 3 feet high and had a brain only slightly larger than an ape's, but it probably walked erect.

13. About 3 million years ago, *A. afarensis* was replaced by another species, *A. africanus*, which was slightly taller than its predecessor and had a slightly larger brain.

14. About 2.3 million years ago *A. robustus* emerged. It was taller and heavier and had a larger brain than its predecessors.

15. About 2.2 million years ago, the fourth species, *A. boisei*, appeared. It was even more robust than *A. robustus*.

Evolution of the Genus *Homo*

16. Many paleontologists believe that *A. afarensis* also gave rise to the genus *Homo*, the ancestors of modern humans, *Homo sapiens*. Others believe that the genus *Homo* may have evolved from an as-yet-unidentified ancestor.

17. The earliest discovered evidence of the genus *Homo* is a 1.8 million year old skull and partial skeleton found in Tanzania. It belongs to *Homo habilis*.

18. Two hundred thousand years after the emergence of *Homo habilis*, *Homo erectus* arose. Skeletons of *Homo erectus* appear in geological formations 300,000 to 1.6 million years old in the Old World.

19. Unlike *Australopithecus* and *H. habilis*, which remained in Africa, *H. erectus* moved from Africa to Europe and Asia.

20. *Homo erectus* stood about 5 feet tall, used fire, and made more sophisticated tools and weapons than its predecessors. With a brain slightly smaller than ours, *Homo erectus* is believed to be the direct ancestor of *Homo sapiens*.

21. *Homo sapiens* emerged about 300,000 years ago and consists of two subspecies: *Homo sapiens neanderthalensis* (the Neanderthals) and *Homo sapiens sapiens*.

22. The Neanderthals lived in caves and camps in Europe and Asia until approximately 40,000 years ago, when they disappeared. Some archaeologists believe that they were replaced by modern humans, the *Cro-Magnons*, the earliest known members of *H. sapiens sapiens*.

23. The Cro-Magnons first appeared in Africa and then spread across Europe and northern Asia, perhaps wiping out the Neanderthals or possibly interbreeding with them.

24. Over the course of time, the human population has wandered far and wide on the planet and come to inhabit a wide range of climatic zones. This has resulted in the formation of a number of phenotypically distinct subpopulations, or races. Many differences found in the races are thought to be adaptations to differing environmental conditions.

Trends in Primate Evolution

25. The evolutionary history that leads first to primates and then to humans is marked by significant developments, including (1) the evolution of bipedal locomotion, (2) an increase in brain size, (3) modifications of the hands that improve dexterity, and (4) the emergence of stereoscopic vision.

Health, Homeostasis, and the Environment: Human Cultural Evolution

26. Over the past 40,000 years, human evolution has provided little noticeable change in physical appearance but tremendous cultural change.

27. Human culture has evolved through three phases: *hunting and gathering*, *agriculture*, and *industry*. During that transition, humans have sought ways to control the environment, sometimes with disastrous consequences.

28. Today, our attempts to dominate nature continue. But current global environmental problems are warning signs that we may have pushed too far, that our society is out of balance with the natural world, threatening our own existence.

Critical Thinking

Thinking Critically— Analysis

This Analysis corresponds to the Thinking Critically scenario that was presented at the beginning of this chapter.

One of the first questions you might ask is this: Does the archaeological data support the genetic data? In other words, does the fossil record support the African Origins model? Or does it support the Multiregion Evolution model?

Some archaeological evidence suggests that the Multiregion Evolution model might be the most valid hypothesis. For example, studies of facial features of the Chinese skulls illustrate commonalities in modern and archaic Chinese. More importantly, these features are not present in the skulls of early modern Africans. One would expect the skulls of early modern Africans to resemble the Chinese skulls if the modern Chinese populations did indeed come from an ancestral African population. A similar study of skulls of modern and archaic European populations shows no similarities with either the earliest modern Africans or archaic African populations.

Another question that might be useful is this: Is there any archaeological evidence of the spread of African populations into other areas at the proper time? Again, the answer is no. Nor is there evidence of the spread of African culture (as witnessed by stone tools) as one might expect.

Given these facts, can you think of any reason to question the Multiregion Evolution model?

One common criticism of the Multiregion Evolution model is that archaeologists make many subjective judgments and often base their conclusions on small numbers of skulls. Geneticists wonder if such small samples are truly representative of an entire population. In contrast, the genetic data offers quantitative indicators of evolutionary change that are relatively free of biases.

Given the controversy, it is clear that neither hypothesis can be ruled out. More research is needed, and many years will no doubt pass before scientists can agree on which is correct.

Exercising Your Critical Thinking Skills

Some critics make a blanket statement that genetic engineering in humans allows scientists to tinker with our evolutionary process and should therefore be avoided. Using your knowledge of human evolution, genetics, and genetic engineering and your critical thinking skills, how would you analyze this statement?

Hint: You might want to start by examining what genetic engineering in humans attempts to do. Then determine whether it could affect our evolution as a species. Is there any possibility that it will help or hinder our evolution?

Test of Concepts

1. Why is the primate fossil record incomplete? What problems does this gap create in tracing the evolutionary history of primates?

2. Draw a flow diagram indicating the progression of primate evolution, beginning with the mammalian insectivores and ending with humans. Briefly describe each organism, and note how it differed from the early prosimians.

3. When you have finished Question 2, describe the major anatomical changes that have taken place over the course of primate evolution.

4. Describe the major changes that took place in human cultural evolution. How have they affected the health of the planet and the future of humankind?

www.jbpub.com/humanbiology

Connect to this book's web site: www.jbpub.com/humanbiology
The site features eLearning, an online review area that provides quizzes, chapter outlines, and other tools to help you study for your class. You can also follow useful links for in-depth information, research the differing views in the Point/Counterpoints, or keep up on the latest environmental and health news.

Principles of Ecology
UNDERSTANDING THE ECONOMY OF NATURE

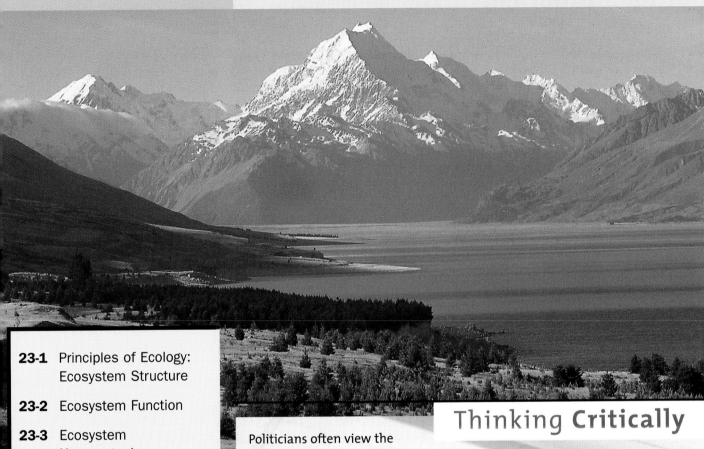

Thinking Critically

Politicians often view the environment as just another issue that must compete for limited funds with other issues such as crime. Furthermore, many people view expenditures on the environment as a detriment to economic health. They assert that investments in environmental protection automatically hurt the economy. Using your critical thinking skills, analyze this belief. Is it valid? Should environmental issues compete with other funds, or are they core issues that deserve maximum attention? Are there ways to achieve environmental goals without harming the economy? Or, better yet, are there ways to create a clean, healthy environment while fostering a strong economy? ■

Mount Cook in New Zealand, a cut above the rest.

Most of us live our lives seemingly apart from nature. We make our homes in cities and towns, surround ourselves with concrete and steel, and drown out the sound of birds with our noise. The closest many of us get to nature is a romp with the family dog on the grass in our backyard.

Raymond Dasmann, a world-renowned ecologist, wrote that despite what many of us may think, a human apart from nature is an abstraction. No such being exists. Human life depends heavily on the environment. The clothes we wear, our morning coffee, and even the breakfast cereal we eat are all products of nature. So is the oxygen we breathe. Without plants, which produce oxygen, humans and other animal species could not survive.

Nature provides other free services as well. For example, plants protect the watersheds near our homes, preventing flooding and erosion. Swamps help purify the water we drink. Birds control insect populations, and predators control rodent populations. Clearly, nature "serves" us well. Thus, although we may have isolated ourselves from nature, we have not emancipated ourselves. The ties that bind us cannot be broken without serious repercussions. This chapter will help you understand why.

This chapter discusses ecology. Technically, ecology is a branch of science. As ecologist Garrett Hardin once wrote, "ecology takes as its domain the entire living world." But its main focus is on interactions—how organisms interact with one another and how they are affected by the abiotic, or nonliving, components of the environment (like rainfall and temperature). It also looks at ways organisms affect their environment. An understanding of ecology provides many practical lessons. Throughout this chapter, I will point out our personal connections to the living world and ways we can lessen our impact on living systems.

Principles of Ecology: Ecosystem Structure

Ecology, like all disciplines in science, is a body of knowledge and a process of inquiry that seeks to understand the mysteries of nature. However, ecology probably ranks as one of the most misused words in the English language. Banners proclaim, "Save Our Ecology." Speakers argue that "our ecology is in danger," and others talk about the "ecological movement." These common uses of the word *ecology* are incorrect. Why?

Ecology is a scientific field of inquiry. It is not synonymous with the word *environment*. It does not mean the web of interactions in the environment. We can save our ecology department and ecology textbooks, but we cannot save our ecology. Our ecology is not in danger; our environment is. You cannot join the ecology movement, but you would be a welcome addition to the environmental movement.

The Biosphere Is the Zone of Life

The science of ecology, unlike many other branches of scientific endeavor, often focuses on systems. The largest biological system on Earth is the **biosphere** (BUY-oh-sfear). The biosphere can be thought of as the thin skin of life on the planet. As shown in **FIGURE 23-1**, the biosphere forms at the intersection of air, water, and land. All organisms consist of components derived from all three spheres. The carbon atoms in protein come from the carbon dioxide in the atmosphere that is captured by plants. The minerals in your bones come from the soil in which plants grow. Water comes from streams and lakes.

The biosphere extends from the bottom of the ocean to the tops of the highest mountains. Although that may seem like a long way, it's not—at least, in comparison with the size of the Earth. In fact, if the Earth were the size of an apple, the biosphere would be about the thickness of its skin. Although life exists throughout the biosphere, it is rare at the extremes, where conditions for survival are marginal.

The biosphere is a **closed system**, much like a sealed terrarium. By definition, a closed system receives no materials from the outside.[1] The only outside contribution is sunlight, which is vital to the health and well-being of virtually all life.

As noted previously in this book, sunlight powers almost all life on the planet. Even the energy released by the combustion of coal, oil, and natural gas, which we use to light our homes and run our factories, owes its origin to the sunlight that fell on the Earth several hundred million years ago. Coal, for instance, is made from ancient plants that lived in and along swamps. Leaves and other plant matter fell into the water and were covered by sediment. Over time, pressure and heat converted the plant matter to coal.

Because the Earth is a closed system, all materials necessary for life must be recycled over and over. The carbon dioxide you exhale, for instance, may be used by a rice plant during photosynthesis next week in Indonesia. Those carbon dioxide molecules will be incorpo-

---

[1]Cosmic dust settles on the Earth, but virtually all of the materials necessary for life come from the Earth itself.

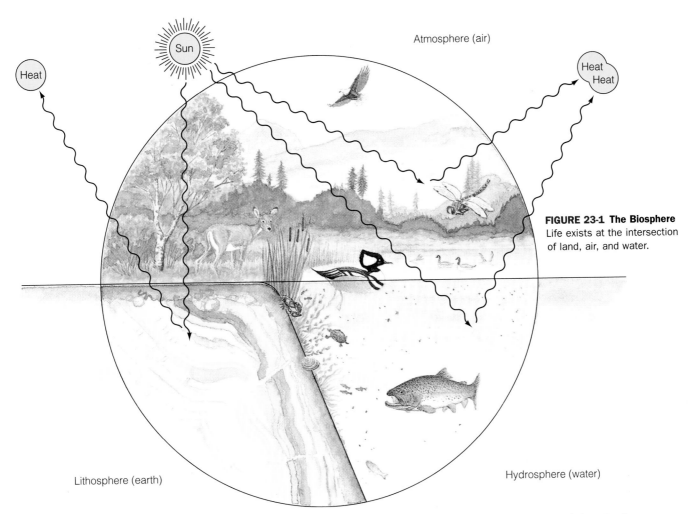

FIGURE 23-1 The Biosphere
Life exists at the intersection of land, air, and water.

rated in carbohydrate produced by the plant and stored in the seed. Consumed by an Indonesian boy, the carbohydrate will be broken back down during cellular respiration, and the carbon dioxide molecules will be released once again into the atmosphere to continue their never-ending cycle. Without this and dozens of other recycling processes, all life on the planet would grind to a halt. Part of the reason for protecting the environment is to protect the components of the global recycling systems on which we all depend.

The Biosphere Can Be Divided Into Distinct Regions Called Biomes and Aquatic Life Zones

Viewed from outer space, the Earth resembles a giant jigsaw puzzle, consisting of large landmasses and vast expanses of ocean. The landmasses, or continents, can be divided into large biological subregions or biomes (**FIGURE 23-2**). A **biome** is a region characterized by a distinct climate and a particular assemblage of plants and animals adapted to it. This section gives an over-

view of some of the major biomes of the North American continent. As illustrated in **FIGURE 23-2**, the North American continent contains seven biomes, five of which are discussed here.

Starting in the frozen north is the **tundra** (TON-drah), a region of long, cold winters and rather short growing seasons (**FIGURE 23-3A**). The rolling terrain of the tundra supports grasses, mosses, lichens, wolves, musk oxen, and other animals adapted to the bitter cold. Trees cannot grow on the tundra for at least two reasons. First, the growing season is quite short. Second, the subsoil (permafrost) remains frozen year-round, preventing the deep root growth necessary for trees.

Immediately south of the tundra lies the **taiga** (TIE-ga). It is also called the **northern coniferous**, or **boreal, forest** (**FIGURE 23-3B**). The taiga's milder climate and longer growing season result in a greater diversity and abundance of plant and animal life than exists on the tundra. Evergreen trees, bears, wolverines, and moose are characteristic species.

FIGURE 23-2 The Biomes

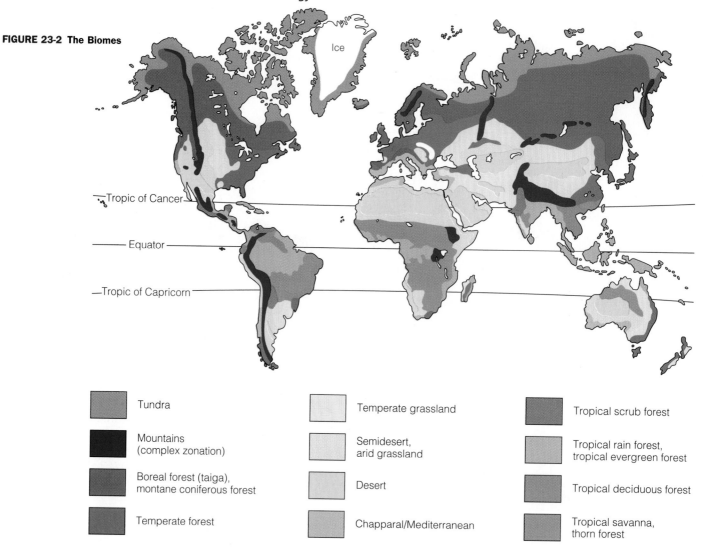

Tundra	Temperate grassland	Tropical scrub forest
Mountains (complex zonation)	Semidesert, arid grassland	Tropical rain forest, tropical evergreen forest
Boreal forest (taiga), montane coniferous forest	Desert	Tropical deciduous forest
Temperate forest	Chapparal/Mediterranean	Tropical savanna, thorn forest

East of the Mississippi River lies the **temperate deciduous forest biome,** characterized by an even warmer climate and more abundant rainfall (**FIGURE 23-3C**). Broad-leafed trees make their home in this biome. Opossums, black bears, squirrels, and foxes are characteristic animal species.

West of the Mississippi lies the **grassland biome** (**FIGURE 23-3D**). Inadequate rainfall and periodic drought prevent trees from growing on the grasslands, except near rivers, streams, and human habitation. Over the years, deep-rooted grasses evolved on the plains. These grasses could tolerate drought and withstand grazing and survive periodic fires. However, virtually all of the natural grasslands have been plowed under to make room for human crops. Coyotes, hawks, and voles are characteristic animal species.

In the Southwest, where even less rain falls, is the **desert biome** (**FIGURE 23-3E**). Contrary to what many people think, the desert often contains a rich assortment

of plants and animals uniquely adapted to the aridity and heat. Cacti, mesquite trees, rattlesnakes, and a variety of lizards all make their home in this environment.

The oceans can also be divided into subregions, known as **aquatic life zones.** Aquatic life zones are the aquatic equivalent of biomes. Like their land-based counterparts, each of these regions has a distinct environment and characteristic plant and animal life adapted to conditions of the zone. Four major aquatic life zones exist: coral reefs, estuaries (the mouths of rivers where fresh and salt water mix), the deep ocean, and the continental shelf.

Humans inhabit all biomes on Earth, a testimonial to our remarkable adaptability. Within these regions, humans benefit in numerous ways from the microbes, plants, animals, soil, water, and air that compose the biome. We tend to think of biomes, though, in terms of their natural resources (coal, timber, oil). Although vital to our economic health, these resources are but a

(a)

(b)

FIGURE 23-3 North American Biomes
(a) Tundra *(b)* taiga *(c)* temperate deciduous forest *(d)* grassland *(e)* desert.

(c)

(d)

(e)

fraction of the services we receive from the biome. Trees, for instance, not only provide oxygen and protect watersheds, they may remove certain pollutants from the air. Soil bacteria recycle nutrients on farms. Lest we forget, many other species also depend on these same services.

Ecosystems Consist of Organisms and Their Environment

The biosphere is a global **ecological system**, or **ecosystem**. The term *ecosystem* is used to describe a community of organisms and their physical and chemical environment. Innumerable interactions are possible within an ecosystem. For the sake of convenience, ecologists often limit their study to small ecological systems—for example, a pond, a rotting log, or a grassy meadow. Even in these small ecosystems, the number of organisms present and the number of possible interactions can be astounding. Reduced to a minimum, ecosystems consist of two basic components: abiotic and biotic.

Abiotic Components. The **abiotic components** of an ecosystem are the physical and chemical factors necessary for life. They include such things as sunlight, precipitation, temperature, and nutrients. Because abiotic conditions within most ecosystems vary, organisms must be able to survive a range of conditions. The range of conditions to which an organism is adapted is called its **range of tolerance.** As **FIGURE 23-4** (page 530) shows, organisms do best in the optimum range. Outside of that are the **zones of physiological stress**, where survival and reproduction are possible but not optimal. Outside of these zones are the **zones of intolerance,** where life for that organism is not possible.

Humans often alter the physical and chemical components of the environment. Changes can lead to serious biological impacts. If conditions change drastically, for instance, some species perish. Dams, for example,

create lakes in streambeds, changing the water temperature, water flow, and other abiotic factors. As a result, many fishes that live in the stream perish. Native razorback suckers and other species that once thrived in the Colorado River, for example, are now endangered species (in danger of extinction) because of the large dams constructed along the river (**FIGURE 23-5**, page 530). Cold water released from the bottom of huge reservoirs formed by these dams has changed the temperature of the river and wiped out most of the native fish. The Point/Counterpoint in this chapter gives two opposing views on human-caused extinction.

Although species are sensitive to all of the abiotic factors in their environment, one factor often turns out to be more important than others in regulating growth of an entire ecosystem. This factor, which ultimately regulates the growth of a population, is called a **limiting factor**.

In freshwater lakes and rivers, for example, dissolved phosphate is the limiting factor. Phosphate is required by plants and algae for growth, but phosphate

Point/Counterpoint

Why Worry About Extinction?

Humans Are Accelerating Extinction

David M. Armstrong

David M. Armstrong *teaches science for nonscientists at the University of Colorado at Boulder and has written several books on the mammals and ecology of the Rocky Mountain region.*

Evolution is the process of change in gene pools. When one gene pool becomes reproductively independent of another, a new species has formed. Such speciation generates species; extinction takes them away. Simply put, extinction is a failure to adapt to change, the termination of a gene pool, and the end of an evolutionary line.

Extinction is a natural process. Most of the species that have lived on this planet are now extinct. The 3–30 million species on Earth today are no more than 1%–10% of the species that have evolved since life began about 3.5 billion years ago. Given these facts, why are thoughtful people concerned about endangered species? After all, history makes it clear that—given enough time—all species will become extinct.

The basis for concern is that today the natural process of extinction is proceeding at an unnatural rate. Let us estimate by how much human activity has accelerated rates of extinction. The lifespan of species seems to average from 1 million to 10 million years. Assume (to be conservative) that the average longevity of a species of higher vertebrates is 1 million years. In round numbers (to make calculations easy), there are 10,000 species of birds and mammals. So, on average, one species ought to go extinct each century. However, between 1600 and 1980, at least 36 species of mammals and 94 species of birds became extinct. That is about 0.29 species per year, 29 times the natural rate.

What does it mean to increase a rate by 29 times? The speed limit is 55 miles per hour. Exceed the speed limit by 29-fold, and you are moving 1,595 miles per hour, over twice the speed of sound. The difference between natural rates of extinction and present, human-influenced rates is analogous to the difference between a casual drive and Mach 2! Is that a problem? You decide: concern is a moral construct, not a scientific one.

Several human activities have contributed—mostly inadvertently—to accelerating rates of extinction. The dodo and the passenger pigeon were extinguished by overhunting. Wolves and grizzly bears were exterminated over much of their ranges as threats to livestock. The black-footed ferret was driven to the verge of extinction because prairie dogs, its staple food, were poisoned as agricultural pests. The smallpox virus was exterminated in the "wild" (but survives in a half-dozen laboratories). This is the closest that humans have come to deliberate elimination of an organism, and note that thoughtful scientists with the power to destroy smallpox chose not to do so, electing instead to manage it with care.

Habitat change is the most important cause of endangerment and extinction. Clearing forests for agriculture has decimated the lemurs of Madagascar. Chemical pesticides led to the decline of the peregrine falcon. Introducing exotic species (like goats on the Galapagos and mongooses in Hawaii) displaces native animals and plants. Developing the Amazon Basin is a habitat alteration, and a cause of extinction, on an unprecedented scale.

Many urge saving species for their aesthetic value. Whooping cranes are beautiful, and part of the beauty is that they are products of a marvelous evolutionary process. Most concern about accelerated extinction, however, stresses economic value. A tiny fraction of Earth's seed plants are used commercially. Perhaps an obscure plant like jojoba will become a source of oil more reliable than that beneath the sands of Saudi Arabia.

Wild grasses have furnished genes that improved disease-resistance in wheat. Numerous wild animals (like musk ox, kudu, and whales) could contribute protein to the human diet. Wild species may have medical value; penicillin, after all, was once merely an obscure mold on citrus fruit. Some sensitive species are useful monitors of environmental quality, and the presence of healthy populations of many species may promote greater stability or resilience of ecosystems. Naturalist Aldo Leopold noted that we humans have a way of "tinkering" with the ecosphere to see how it works. Given that, we ought to remember the first rule of tinkering: never throw away any of the parts.

"Extinction is forever," and extinction impoverishes both Earth's ecosystems and the potential richness of human life. Borrowing again from Aldo Leopold, I believe we should be concerned about unnaturally rapid extinction because such concern is part of a "right relationship" between people and the landscapes that nurture and inspire them.

Biologist Sir Julian Huxley noted that "we humans find ourselves, for better or worse, business agents for the cosmic process of evolution." We hold power over the future of the biosphere, the power to destroy or to preserve. German philosopher George Hegel noted that freedom (including the power to destroy species) implies responsibility (to preserve them). I agree. The question of human-accelerated extinction boils down to a simple ethical question, "Does posterity matter?" Some of us have ethics that are human-centered. We ask simply, "Do my children deserve a life as rich, with as much opportunity, as mine?" If they do, then we have the responsibility to choose restraint. (Perhaps my life has been rich enough without the dodo, but I am reluctant to make that judgment for future generations.)

Extinction Is the Course of Nature

Norman D. Levine

Evolution is the formation of new species from preexisting ones by a process of adaptation to the environment. Evolution began long ago and is still going on. During evolution, those species better adapted to the environment replaced the less well adapted. It is this process, repeated year after year for millennia, that has produced the present mixture of wild species. Perhaps 95% of the species that once existed no longer exist.

Human activities have eliminated many wild species. The dodo is gone, and so is the passenger pigeon. The whooping crane, the California condor, and many other species are on the way out. The bison is still with us because it is protected, and small herds are raised in semicaptivity. The Pacific salmon remains because we provide fish ladders around our dams so it can reach its breeding places. The mountain goat survives because it lives in inaccessible places. But some thousands of other animal species, to say nothing of plants, are extinct, or soon will be.

Some nature lovers weep at this passing and collect money to save species. They make lists of animals and plants that are in danger of extinction and sponsor legislation to save them.

I don't. What the species preservers are trying to do is to stop the clock. It cannot and should not be done.

Extinction is an inevitable fact of evolution, and it is needed for progress. New species continually arise, and they are better adapted to their environment than those that have died out.

Extinction comes from failure to adapt to a changing environment. The passenger pigeon did not disappear because of hunting alone, but because its food trees were destroyed by land clearing and farming. The prairie chicken cannot find enough of the proper food and nesting places in the cultivated fields that once were prairie.

And you cannot necessarily introduce a new species, even by breeding it in tremendous numbers and putting it out into the wild. Thousands of pheasants were bred and set out year after year in southern Illinois, but in the spring of each year there were none left. Another bird, the capercaillie, is a fine, large game bird in Scandinavia, but every attempt to introduce it into the United States has failed. An introduced species cannot survive unless it is pre-adapted to its new environment.

A few introduced species are pre-adapted and some make spectacular gains. The United States has received the English sparrow, the starling, and the house mouse from Europe, and also the gypsy moth, the European corn borer, the Mediterranean fruit fly, and the Japanese beetle. The United States gave Europe the gray squirrel and the muskrat, among others. The rabbit took over in Australia, at least for a time.

The rabbit and the squirrel were successful on new continents because their requirements are not as narrow as those of species that failed. Today, adjustment to human-made environments may be just as difficult as adjustment to new continents. The rabbit and the squirrel have succeeded in adjusting to the backyard habitat, but most wild animals have disappeared.

Human-made environments are artificial. People replace mixed grasses, shrubs, and trees with rows of clean-cultivated corn, soybeans, wheat, oats, or alfalfa. Variety has turned into uniform monotony, and the number of species of small vertebrates and invertebrates that can find the proper food to survive has become markedly reduced. But some species have multiplied in these environments and have assumed economic importance; the European corn borer in this country is an example.

Would it improve Earth if even half of the species that have died out were to return? A few starving, ship-wrecked sailors might be better off if the dodo were to return, but I would not be. The small-pox virus has been eliminated, except for a few strains in medical laboratories. Should it be brought back? Should we bring panthers back into the eastern states? Think of all the horses that the automobile and tractors have replaced, and of all the streets and roads that have been paved and the wild animals and plants killed as a consequence. Before people arrived in America about 10,000 years ago, the animal-plant situation was quite different. What should we do? Should we all commit suicide?

Evolution exists, and it goes on continually. People are here because of it, but people may be replaced someday. It is neither possible nor desirable to stop it, and that is what we are trying to do when we try to preserve species on their way out. It can be done, I think, but should we do it to them all? Or to just a few, as we are doing now?

Norman D. Levine *is a professor emeritus at the College of Veterinary Medicine and Agricultural Experiment Station, University of Illinois at Urbana. His research interests cover parasitology, protozoology, and human ecology. This essay is from "Evolution and Extinction," BioScience 39:38, and is copyright © 1989 by the American Institute of Biological Sciences.*

Sharpening Your Critical Thinking Skills

1. Summarize the key points of both authors.
2. Do you see any flaws in the reasoning of either author?
3. Which viewpoint do you adhere to? Why?

Visit *Human Biology's* Internet site for links to web sites offering more information on this topic.

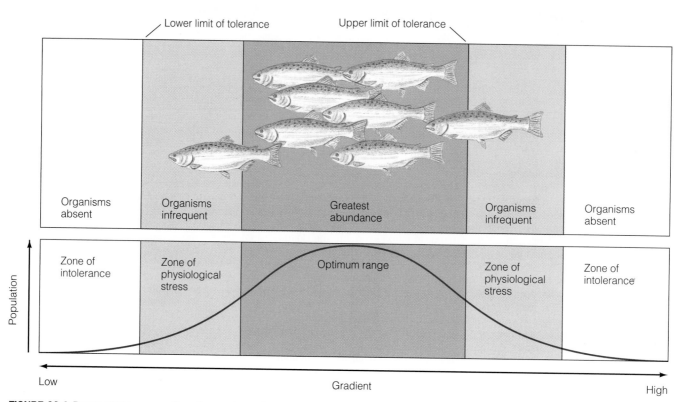

FIGURE 23-4 **Range of Tolerance**   Organisms tolerate a range of conditions but thrive within an optimum range.

concentrations are naturally low. As a result, plant and algal growth is held in check. When phosphate is added to a body of water, plants and algae proliferate. Algae often form dense surface mats, blocking sunlight (**FIGURE 23-6**). As a result, plants rooted on the bottom may die, and oxygen levels in the deeper waters may decline, killing fishes and other aquatic organisms.

Phosphate pollution in lakes and rivers comes from several sources. One of the major sources is the sewage-

treatment plant. The phosphates released by these plants come from detergents and human waste. People can lessen the problem by using low- or no-phosphate detergents. They can even use laundry disks to avoid detergents altogether. Laundry disks are plastic disks containing ceramic beads coated with silver and copper. They supposedly increase the ionization of water. In the same way that detergents act, water ions pull dirt off of clothes and keep them suspended in the water, so they can be removed.

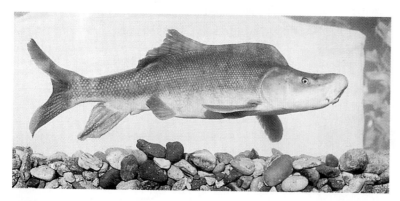

FIGURE 23-5 **Altering Native Fish Life Along the Mighty Colorado**   Dams on the Colorado River have changed the water temperature in the river below the dam. Extremely cold water flows out of the bottom of the reservoirs into the river and has nearly eliminated several native fish species, including the razorback sucker.

FIGURE 23-6 **Algal Bloom**   This pond is choked with algae due to the abundance of plant nutrients from human sources.

On land, precipitation tends to be the limiting factor. At any given temperature, the more moisture that falls, the richer the plant and animal life.

Biotic Components. The **biotic components** of an ecosystem are the organisms that live there. Within biomes and aquatic life zones, organisms of a given species often occupy very specific regions to which they are well adapted. A group of organisms of the same species occupying a specific region constitutes a **population**. The members of a population may remain together throughout all or much of the year. Bighorn sheep, for example, live in herds throughout the year. Other organisms such as the grizzly bear are solitary for the most part, keeping to themselves except for mating. In any given ecosystem, several populations exist together and form a **biological community**, an interdependent network of plants, animals, and microorganisms.

Competition May Occur Between Species Occupying the Same Habitat if Their Niches Overlap

If asked to give a brief description of yourself, you would probably begin by describing the place where you live. You would then likely discuss the work you do, the friends you have, and other important relationships that describe your place in society. A biologist would do much the same when describing an organism. He or she would start with a description of the place an organism lives—that is, its **habitat**. Next, he or she would describe how the organism "fits" into the ecosystem, its **ecological niche,** or simply **niche** (nitch). An organism's niche includes all of its relationships with its environment. For example, the niche includes what an organism eats, what eats it, its range of tolerance for various environmental factors, and other important facts.

Organisms in a community occupy the same habitat, but most of them have quite different niches. This phenomenon minimizes competition for resources and is a condition favored by natural selection. The fact that organisms occupy separate niches provides for a wider use of an ecosystem's resources, especially food.

Niches do overlap somewhat. For example, two species may feed on some of the same foods. The more two species' niches overlap, however, the more the organisms compete with each other. Just as in the human economy, competition in

the natural world can be a good thing, for it is an agent of natural selection that may lead to the evolution of new adaptations. When niches overlap considerably, competition becomes intense, and one species usually suffers. If two species occupy identical niches, competition will eliminate one of them. As a result, two species cannot occupy the same niche for long. This law of nature is called the **competitive exclusion principle.**

The concept of the niche is very important to us. For example, successful control of an insect pest is best achieved through an understanding of the pest's niche. Such an analysis might show that a particular species of bird or insect feeds on the pest. By simply encouraging these beneficial species—say, by providing trees for the birds—farmers can hold pest populations down and save themselves enormous sums of money on chemical pesticides. Individuals interested in saving species have also learned that to protect a plant or animal, you have to protect the ecosystem it lives in, efforts that help protect the species' niche.

Humans Have Become a Major Competitive Force in Nature

Humans compete with many other species for food and living space. However, humans possess a marked advantage provided, in large part, by our technology.

Already, commercial overfishing has depleted dozens of the world's fisheries (**FIGURE 23-7**). Such actions not only reduce our food supply, they also greatly

FIGURE 23-7 Depletion of North Atlantic Fisheries The dates on the map indicate the approximate time when various commercial fisheries were depleted by overfishing.

reduce the food supply of other species—notably, seals and other fish-eating animals.

On every continent and in every nation, humans are outcompeting the species that share this planet with us. According to estimates by various experts, 40–100 species become extinct every day, largely because of tropical deforestation, but also because of a loss of wetlands and coral reefs. Unless we do something, hundreds of thousands of species will become extinct in the next decade.

Saving other species is more than a humanitarian act. It is an act of self-protection. Cutting down the rain forests, for example, could alter global climate, making the Earth hotter. If conditions became bad enough, massive food shortages could occur.

Ecosystem Function

Life on land and in the Earth's waters is possible principally because of the existence of one group of organisms, the **producers** (**FIGURE 23-8**). Producers primarily include the algae and plants. These organisms absorb sunlight and use its energy to synthesize organic mole-

cules from atmospheric carbon dioxide and water. This process is called **photosynthesis.**[2] Organic molecules generated by photosynthesis not only nourish the producers, but also feed all the other organisms in the web of life. As a result, producers form the foundation of the living world.

Another large group of organisms is the **consumers.** They reap the benefit of the producers' photosynthetic work. Ecologists place consumers into four general categories, depending on the type of food they eat. Some such as deer, elk, and cattle feed directly on plants and are called **herbivores.** Others such as wolves feed on herbivores and other animals and are known as **carnivores.** Humans and a great many other animal species subsist on a mixed diet of plants and animals and are known as **omnivores.** The final group feeds on animal waste or the remains of plants and animals. These organisms are called **detritivores** (DEE-treh-TEH-vores), or **decomposers.**[3] This important group includes many bacteria, fungi, and insects.

---

[2]Some producers are chemosynthetic organisms—that is, organisms capable of using methane and hydrogen sulfide as a source of energy to produce organic molecules.
[3]Remember that detritus is waste material.

FIGURE 23-8 Simplified Food Chains
Two grazer food chains are shown, a terrestrial one and an aquatic one.

Grazer food chain

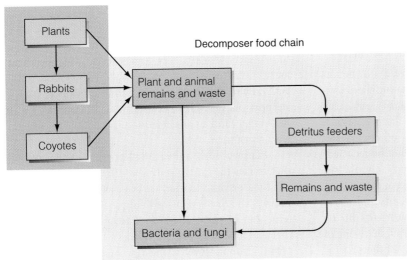

Decomposer food chain

FIGURE 23-9 Food Chains A grazer food chain and a decomposer food chain, showing the connection between the two.

known as **food webs** (**FIGURE 23-10**). Food webs present a complete picture of the feeding relationships in any given ecosystem.

Energy and Nutrients Flow Through Food Webs, But in Very Different Ways

Although we tend to think of food chains simply as a display of feeding relationships, they are much more. From an ecological perspective, food chains are conduits for the flow of energy and the cycling of nutrients through the environment. Let's begin with energy.

In the biosphere, almost all of the energy needed by organisms comes from the sun. Solar energy is captured by plants and algae and used to produce organic food molecules. Energy from the Sun is stored in the covalent bonds of these molecules. In the food chain, organic molecules pass from plants to animals, where they are broken down in mitochondria, which release stored solar energy. This energy is used to power numerous cellular activities.

Food and Energy Flow Through Food Chains That Are Generally Part of Much Larger Food Webs in Ecosystems

As scientists began to study the relationships between producers and consumers, they found that specific organisms fed on others. They called these feeding relationships food chains. Technically, a **food chain** is a series of organisms, each one feeding on the organism preceding it (**FIGURE 23-8**). Biological communities consist of numerous food chains. All organisms in the community are members of one or more food chains.

Biologists recognize two general types of food chains: grazer and decomposer. **Grazer food chains** begin with plants and algae, the producers. These organisms are consumed by herbivores, or **grazers**; hence the name *grazer food chain*. Herbivores, in turn, may be eaten by carnivores. **Decomposer food chains** begin with dead material—either animal wastes (feces) or the remains of plants and animals (**FIGURE 23-9**).

As in most things in nature, decomposer and grazer food chains are tightly linked and highly interdependent (**FIGURE 23-9**). For example, waste products from the grazer food chain enter the decomposer food chain. Nutrients liberated by the decomposer food chain enter the soil and water and are reincorporated into plants at the base of the grazer food chain. The survival of all living things depends on this linkage.

Food chains exist only on the pages of textbooks. In a biological community, all food chains are part of a much more complex network of feeding interactions

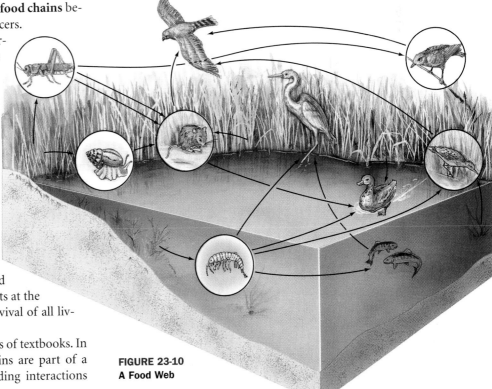

FIGURE 23-10
A Food Web

During cellular respiration, much of the energy stored in organic food molecules is lost as heat. Heat escaping from plants and animals is radiated into the atmosphere and then into outer space. It cannot be recaptured and reused by the Earth's organisms. Because all solar energy is eventually converted to heat, energy is said to flow unidirectionally through food chains and food webs. Put another way, energy cannot be recycled.

In sharp contrast, nutrients flow cyclically; that is, they are recycled over and over. Nutrients in the soil, air, and water are first incorporated into plants and algae, then passed from plants to animals. Nutrients in the food chain eventually reenter the environment by one of three paths: (1) the excretion of wastes, (2) the decomposition of dead organisms, and (3) the decomposition of waste.

Every time you exhale, for example, you release carbon dioxide. It reenters the atmosphere for reuse. Thus, through the act of breathing, you play an important role in the global recycling system that makes life possible.

Nutrients also reenter the environment through the decomposition of dead organisms. When a plant or animal dies, it decomposes. Decomposition is caused by bacteria and fungi. These organisms release enzymes that break down organic matter. Although these microorganisms absorb many nutrients released during this process, some nutrients escape, entering the soil and water for reuse. And, of course, when a bacterium dies, it too breaks down, releasing nutrients into its environment.

Finally, many nutrients reenter the environment through the decomposition of animal waste. The feces of a rhinoceros, for example, are broken down by bacteria, which liberate carbon dioxide, nitrogen, and numerous minerals.

One way or another, all nutrients eventually make their way back to the environment for recycling. Each new generation of organisms therefore relies on the recycling of material in the biosphere. The atoms in your body, for instance, have been recycled many times since the beginning of life on Earth. Who knows, some of those atoms may have been in the very first cell that lived in the shallow seas.

The Organisms of a Food Chain Exist on Different Trophic Levels

Ecologists classify the organisms in a food chain according to their position, or **trophic level** (TROE-fic; literally, "feeding" level). The producers comprise the base of the grazer food chain and are therefore members of the first trophic level. The grazers are members of the second trophic level. Carnivores that feed on grazers are members of the third trophic level, and so on.

Most terrestrial food chains are limited to three or four trophic levels. In fact, longer terrestrial food chains are quite rare. The reason for this is that food chains generally do not have a large enough producer base to support many levels of consumers. Put another way, in the longer food chains, less food is available for the top-level consumers. Why?

Plants absorb only a small portion of the sunlight that strikes the Earth (only 1%–2%), which they use to produce organic matter, or biomass. Technically, **biomass** is the dry weight of living material in an ecosystem. The biomass at the first trophic level is the raw material for the second trophic level. The biomass at the second trophic level is the raw material for the third trophic level, and so on.

Not all of the biomass produced by plants is converted to grazer biomass. Not all of the grazer biomass becomes carnivore biomass. At least three reasons account for the incomplete transfer of biomass from one trophic level to the next. First, some of the plant material such as the roots is not eaten. Second, not all of the material that the grazers eat is digested. Some of it passes through their intestinal tracts and is excreted as feces. Third, among animals, some of the digested material is broken down to produce energy and heat. It therefore cannot be used to build biomass in the grazers. As a rule, only 5%–20% of the biomass at any one trophic level can be passed to the next. (The amount varies depending on the organisms involved in the food chain.)

When plotted, the biomass at the various trophic levels forms a pyramid, the **biomass pyramid** (**FIGURE 23-11**). Because biomass contains energy (stored in the covalent bonds), the biomass pyramid can be converted into a graph of the chemical energy in the various trophic levels. This graph is called an **energy pyramid**.

In most food chains, the number of organisms also decreases with each trophic level, forming a **pyramid of numbers**. Knowledge of ecological pyramids will help you understand why people in many less developed countries generally subsist on a diet of grains (corn, rice, or wheat) rather than meat. **FIGURE 23-12** shows energy pyramids for two food chains. In the grain → human food chain on the right, 20,000 kilocalories of grain can feed 10 people for a day. In the grain → steer → human food chain, the 20,000 kilocalories fed to the cow produces only 2000 kilocalories of meat, barely enough to feed one person for a day (assuming a 10% transfer of biomass). Thus, the shorter the food chain, the more food is available to top-level consumers.

This simple rule has profound implications for the human race. The human population increases by about

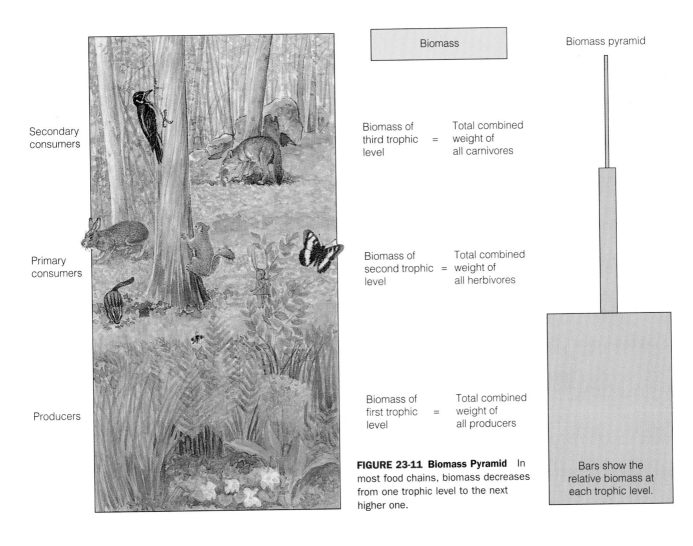

Secondary
consumers

Primary
consumers

Producers

Biomass

| Biomass of third trophic level | = | Total combined weight of all carnivores |

| Biomass of second trophic level | = | Total combined weight of all herbivores |

| Biomass of first trophic level | = | Total combined weight of all producers |

FIGURE 23-11 Biomass Pyramid In most food chains, biomass decreases from one trophic level to the next higher one.

Biomass pyramid

Bars show the relative biomass at each trophic level.

FIGURE 23-12 Energy Pyramids in Two Food Chains (a) The typical American diet. Note that the 20,000 kilocalories of corn fed to cows feeds only one American for a day. (b) In the shorter food chain in the Third World nations, the same 20,000 kilocalories will feed 10 people directly.

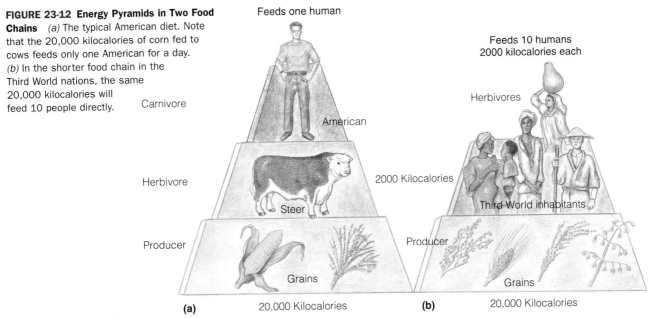

Feeds one human

Carnivore

American

Herbivore

Steer

Producer

Grains

(a) 20,000 Kilocalories

Feeds 10 humans
2000 kilocalories each

Herbivores

2000 Kilocalories

Third World inhabitants

Producer

Grains

(b) 20,000 Kilocalories

80 million people a year, and feeding these people poses an enormous challenge. How can new residents be fed most efficiently?

The most efficient food source will be crops such as corn, rice, and wheat that are fed directly to people. It is obviously far less efficient to feed corn and other grains to cattle and other livestock, which are then slaughtered for human consumption. Vegetarianism, say supporters, is not only good for your health but better for the environment, because it requires less grain production than a nonvegetarian diet. People, however, require an adequate intake of protein. Protein can be obtained by eating a mixture of legumes, as noted in Chapter 5. (Chapter 24 has more on feeding the world's hungry.)

Nutrient Cycles Consist of Two Phases, the Environmental and the Organismic

As noted earlier, nutrients flow from the environment through food webs, then are released back into the environment. This circular flow constitutes a **nutrient cycle**, also known as a **biogeochemical cycle**.

Nutrient cycles can be divided broadly into two phases: the environmental and organismic. In the **environmental phase**, a nutrient exists in the air, water, or soil or sometimes in two or more of them simultaneously. In the **organismic phase**, nutrients are found in the biota—the plants, animals, and microorganisms.

Dozens of global nutrient cycles operate continuously to ensure the availability of chemicals vital to all living things, present and future. Unfortunately, however, a great many human activities disrupt nutrient cycles. These activities can profoundly influence the survival of a species. This section looks at two of the most important nutrient cycles, the carbon and nitrogen cycles, and the ways they are being altered. (Solutions to the problems are described in Chapter 24.) Remember that the cycles mentioned here are only two of several dozen nutrient cycles essential to life.

The Carbon Cycle. The carbon cycle is illustrated in **FIGURE 23-13** in a simplified form. We begin with free carbon dioxide. In the environmental phase of the cycle, carbon dioxide resides in two reservoirs, which scientists often call *sinks*: the atmosphere and the surface waters (oceans, lakes, and rivers). **FIGURE 23-13** shows that atmospheric carbon dioxide is absorbed by plants and photosynthetic organisms and thus enters the organismic phase of the cycle. These organisms (autotrophs) convert carbon dioxide into organic food materials, which travel along the food chain from one trophic level to the next. Carbon dioxide reenters the environmental phase via cellular energy production (cellular respiration) of the organisms in the grazer and decomposer food chains.

For tens of thousands of years, most of our ancestors lived in harmony with nature. With the advent of the Industrial Revolution, however, human beings began to interfere with natural processes on a large scale. One of the victims of our technological development has been the global carbon cycle. The widespread combustion of fossil fuels, which releases carbon dioxide, and rampant deforestation (which reduces carbon dioxide uptake) have seriously overwhelmed the cycle.

FIGURE 23-13 The Carbon Cycle

Grazer food chain

Decomposer food chain

For many years before the Industrial Revolution, global carbon dioxide production equaled carbon dioxide absorption by plants and algae. Today, approximately 7 billion tons of carbon—in the form of carbon dioxide—is added to the atmosphere each year. Three quarters of the carbon dioxide comes from the combustion of fossil fuels such as the gasoline in our cars; the remaining quarter stems from deforestation. How does deforestation add carbon dioxide to the atmosphere?

Trees absorb enormous amounts of carbon dioxide for photosynthesis. As forests are cleared, the amount of atmospheric carbon dioxide they absorb declines. Making matters worse, many forests are burned after cutting, further adding to the carbon dioxide levels in the atmosphere.

In the past 100 years, global atmospheric carbon dioxide levels have increased 32.5%. In the atmosphere, carbon dioxide traps heat escaping from Earth and reradiates it to the Earth's surface. As carbon dioxide levels increase, global temperature may rise dramatically. Such a rise could have devastating effects on global climate. It could shift rainfall patterns, destroy agricultural production in many regions, and wipe out thousands of species. A rising global temperature might cause glaciers and the polar ice caps to melt, raising the sea level and flooding many low-lying coastal regions. Fortunately, there are many cost-effective strategies for greatly reducing our dependency on fossil fuel. The most notable are energy efficiency and renewable fuels—solar energy and wind, for example. (Global warming is detailed in Chapter 24.)

The Nitrogen Cycle. Nitrogen is an element essential to many important biological molecules, including amino acids, DNA, and RNA. The Earth's atmosphere contains enormous amounts of it. However, atmospheric nitrogen exists as nitrogen gas (N_2), which is unusable to all but a few organisms. To be incorporated into living organisms, atmospheric nitrogen must first be converted to a usable form—either nitrate or ammonia.

The conversion of nitrogen to ammonia is known as **nitrogen fixation**. As **FIGURE 23-14** shows, nitrogen fixation partly occurs in the roots of leguminous plants (peas, beans, clover, alfalfa, vetch, and others) in small swellings called **root nodules**. Inside the nodules live symbiotic bacteria that convert atmospheric nitrogen to ammonia. Ammonia is also produced by cyanobacteria that live in the soil. Once ammonia is produced, other soil bacteria convert it to

nitrite and then to nitrate. Nitrates are incorporated by plants and used to make amino acids and nucleic acids. All consumers therefore ultimately receive the nitrogen they require from plants.

Nitrate in soil is also produced indirectly from the decay of animal waste and the remains of plants and animals. As shown on the right side of **FIGURE 23-14**, this process returns ammonia to the soil for reuse. Ammonia is converted to nitrite, then to nitrate and reused. Some nitrate, however, may be converted to nitrite and then to nitrous oxide (N_2O) by denitrifying bacteria (**FIGURE 23-14**). Nitrous oxide is converted to nitrogen and released into the atmosphere.

Humans alter the nitrogen cycle in at least four ways: (1) by applying excess nitrogen-containing fertilizer on farmland, much of which ends up in waterways; (2) by disposing of nitrogen-rich municipal sewage in waterways; (3) by raising cattle in feedlots adjacent to waterways; and (4) by burning fossil fuels, which release a class of chemicals

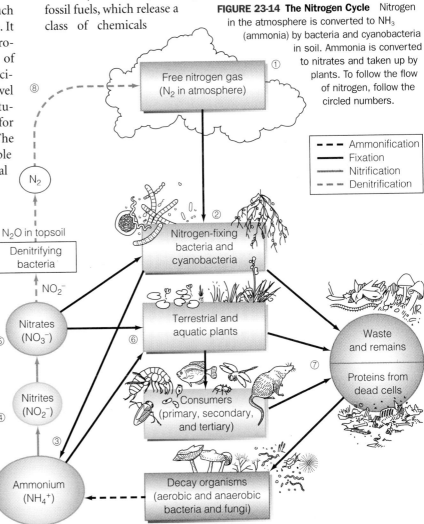

FIGURE 23-14 The Nitrogen Cycle Nitrogen in the atmosphere is converted to NH_3 (ammonia) by bacteria and cyanobacteria in soil. Ammonia is converted to nitrates and taken up by plants. To follow the flow of nitrogen, follow the circled numbers.

- - - - Ammonification
——— Fixation
——— Nitrification
- - - - Denitrification

Free nitrogen gas (N_2 in atmosphere) ①

N_2 ⑧

N_2O in topsoil
Denitrifying bacteria
NO_2^-

Nitrates (NO_3^-) ⑤

Nitrites (NO_2^-) ④

Ammonium (NH_4^+) ③

Nitrogen-fixing bacteria and cyanobacteria ②

Terrestrial and aquatic plants ⑥

Consumers (primary, secondary, and tertiary)

Decay organisms (aerobic and anaerobic bacteria and fungi)

Waste and remains ⑦
Proteins from dead cells

known as nitrogen oxides into the atmosphere. The first three activities increase the concentration of nitrogen in the soil or water, upsetting the ecological balance. Nitrogen oxides released into the atmosphere by power plants, automobiles, and other sources are converted to nitric acid, which falls with rain or snow. Acid rain and snow can have devastating effects on terrestrial and aquatic ecosystems, as you will see in Chapter 24.

Nitrogen, like phosphate, is a plant nutrient. It stimulates the growth of aquatic plants. Rivers and lakes may become congested with dense mats of vegetation, making them unnavigable. Sunlight penetration to deeper levels is also impaired by the growth of plants, causing oxygen levels in deeper waters to decline. In the autumn, when aquatic plants die and decay, oxygen levels can fall further, killing aquatic life.

Section 23-3

Ecosystem Homeostasis

In this book, I have repeatedly pointed out that human health requires internal balance. A breakdown of internal homeostasis can lead to disease and even death. Human health is also dependent on environmental homeostasis to maintain conditions conducive to life. I have used the word *environment* to include the physical, chemical, social, and psychological environments we are part of. As this chapter shows, the physical and chemical environments depend on the operation of homeostatic mechanisms like the carbon and nitrogen cycles operating in the biosphere to maintain proper conditions.

Homeostatic mechanisms operate to maintain ecosystem balance. **Ecosystem balance** is not a steady state, but a kind of dynamic equilibrium. In balanced ecosystems, for example, populations grow and decline in natural cycles (they are dynamic). But from year to year, they remain more or less the same (they are in a state of equilibrium).

Ecosystem Homeostasis or Balance Is the Result of Many Interacting Factors

Ecosystem homeostasis or balance results in large part from forces that act on individual populations within an ecological system (**FIGURE 23-15**). The first set of forces consists of those that cause populations to grow. I refer to them as **growth factors**. Favorable weather, ample food supplies, and a high reproductive rate are three of many factors that cause populations to increase. The second set of factors includes those that cause populations to decline, the **reduction fac-**

tors. Adverse weather, lack of food, disease, and predation, for instance, can cause populations to decline. Reduction factors collectively constitute **environmental resistance**—so named because they resist population growth.

Numerous growth and reduction factors operate simultaneously in ecosystems. As **FIGURE 23-15** shows, each set of factors has two components: abiotic and biotic. To understand how they work, consider a simplified example.

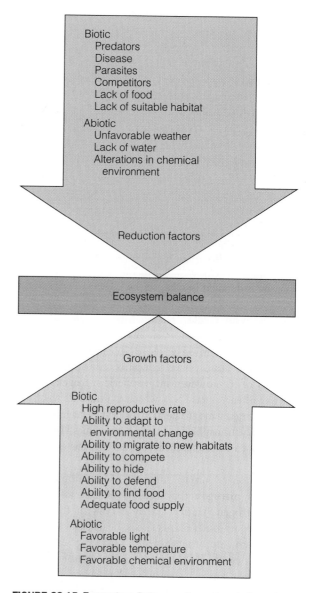

FIGURE 23-15 Ecosystem Balance Ecosystem balance is a complex equilibrium brought about by biotic and abiotic growth and reduction factors.

(a)

FIGURE 23-16 Aftermath of an Eruption *(a)* This lifeless landscape was created by an enormous volcanic eruption at Washington's Mount Saint Helens. Thousands of acres were destroyed. *(b)* Life soon began to take root in the volcanic ash, but complete recovery may take decades.

(b)

In the midwestern United States, grasses and other plants grow well during wet years. Because of the abundance of food, mice and other rodents that live there thrive and their populations increase. This increase, in turn, results in larger populations of hawks and owls, which feed on rodents. The more food that is available, the more owl and hawk young that will survive.

In this simplified chain of events, favorable weather conditions shift ecosystem balance. Conditions are partly restored, however, by the increase in the hawk and owl populations. Increased predatory pressure from these birds tends to decrease the mouse population. As the mouse population falls, the number of predators decreases.

Balance can also be restored by abiotic conditions. A harsh winter, for example, might cause the mouse population to plummet. Because the number of mice decreases, the owl and hawk populations fall.

This example illustrates some mechanisms by which slight ecosystem imbalances are corrected. Owls and hawks are biotic reduction factors that help maintain ecosystem stability. In contrast, adverse winter weather is an abiotic reduction factor that can offset the rise in the rodent population and even reduce the size of the hawk and owl populations.

Changes in abiotic and biotic conditions occur with great regularity in ecosystems. Minor fluctuations are of little consequence, however, as the simplified example above shows. As a rule, when minor changes occur, ecosystems appear to remain fairly resilient—capable of bouncing back. Unfortunately, in most instances, human intrusions are so severe that natural systems cannot offset them.

Succession Is the Progressive Development of Biological Communities, Either on Barren Ground or in Damaged Ecosystems

The ability of ecosystems to recover from minor changes gives them a measure of stability. The same is true in the human body. But not all changes in ecosystems (or our

bodies) can be quickly reversed. Thus, ecosystem balance can be drastically upset by natural forces such as volcanoes, or by human forces (**FIGURE 23-16**). In such instances, ecosystems may recover, but the recovery is quite slow. A deciduous forest that is cleared, then planted with crops, for example, will return to forest on its own if it is abandoned. However, a full recovery may require 70 years or more. This process of restoration, described more fully shortly, is an example of secondary succession and is a means by which natural systems are restored following severe disruption. In a sense, secondary succession is nature's healing process.

Succession, in general, is a process of sequential change in which one community is replaced by another until a mature, or climax, ecosystem is formed. A mature ecosystem is one that has reached a state of long-term dynamic balance. It is characterized by a stable level of species diversity (explained below). Two types of succession exist: primary and secondary.

Primary succession occurs where no biotic community previously existed—for example, when deep-sea volcanoes form islands. On volcanic islands in the tropics, a rich paradise can form on the barren rock, but it will take tens of thousands of years. Seeds for plants may be carried to the islands by waves or may be dropped by birds. Over time, the plants take root, then spread to cover the entire island. New species may arise as a result of genetic changes in these species (Chapter 21). Birds may settle on the island as well. In the ensuing years, new species may evolve from the old. The process of primary succession on rock exposed by the retreat of glaciers is shown in **FIGURE 23-17**. Take a few minutes to study this figure.

Secondary succession occurs when a biotic community that had previously existed is destroyed by natural forces or human actions. **FIGURE 23-18** shows secondary succession in an abandoned eastern farm field. As illustrated, crabgrass first invades the abandoned field. Crabgrass is well suited to life in open, sunny fields. Unlike many other plants, it can tolerate hot, sunny locations because it is capable of fixing atmospheric carbon dioxide when other plants have closed down their pores to conserve water.

In the next 2 years, grasses and other herbaceous plants take root from seeds in the soil. Seeds may also be blown in from neighboring fields or carried in by animals. Over the next three decades, pine seedlings take root and begin to grow. As they get larger, sun-loving pine trees produce shade—so much, in fact, that shade-tolerant hardwood trees begin to take root. Hardwoods eventually grow so large that they "shade out" many of the pine trees. In ecological terms, they outcompete the pines. Seventy years after this process begins, a mature, or climax, forest is formed, consisting mostly of hardwoods and an occasional pine. This is a climax forest, which exists in a state of dynamic equilibrium. It will remain more or less the same if it is not disturbed by fire, timber cutting, or some catastrophic event.

Secondary succession in the abandoned farm field illustrates some key principles of succession. One of those is that colonizers such as crabgrass and transitional species such as pines thrive in their new habitat because environmental resistance is low and the conditions necessary for growth (growth factors) are favorable. These same species, however, gradually alter the environment, creating conditions suitable for the growth of other species. The new species, in turn, alter environmental conditions so much that they eliminate the species that made their growth possible.

Secondary succession occurs much more rapidly than primary succession because soil is already present. In primary succession, soil must be formed from rock, gravel, or sand, and this can take 100–1000 years.

Just as damage to the human body cannot always be repaired, damage to ecosystems, if severe enough, also may not be remedied by secondary succession. In Vietnam, for example, thousands of acres of tropical forests were destroyed by allied forces who sprayed Agent Orange, a herbicide, on them from planes and helicopters in an effort to reduce the likelihood of ambush. Broadleaf trees are quite susceptible to Agent Orange and died quickly. Today the forests, however, have been invaded by a hardy brush that some scientists think may prevent mature forests from reestablishing.

Ecosystem Stability May Be Related to Species Diversity

Ecosystem stability results from the interplay of growth and reduction factors, which are part of nature's homeostatic mechanisms. Some ecologists believe that ecosystem stability may also result from species diversity. Generally speaking, **species diversity** is a measure

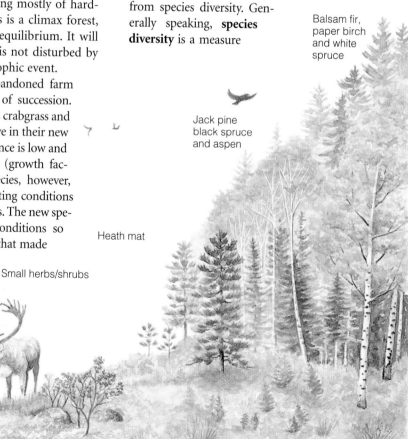

Balsam fir, paper birch and white spruce

Jack pine black spruce and aspen

Heath mat

Small herbs/shrubs

Lichens/ mosses invade

FIGURE 23-17 Primary Succession As rock is exposed by a retreating glacier, biological communities develop in a process that can take hundreds or thousands of years.

Exposed rocks

Pioneer community → Intermediate communities → Climax community

Abandoned farmland	10–30 years
0–1 years	Pine forest is established
Crabgrass colonizes first	
1–3 years	30–70 years
Tall grass/ herbaceous plants establish	Hardwoods invade
3–10 years	70+ years
Pines invade	Hardwood climax forest is formed
	Succession complete

FIGURE 23-18 Secondary Succession On an abandoned eastern farm (top left), nature begins the process of restoring a biotic community.

of the number of different species in a given community or ecosystem. The more species there are, the more diverse an ecosystem is said to be.

Ecologists who believe that species diversity leads to ecosystem stability support this contention with the following facts. First, extremely stable ecosystems such as tropical rain forests are characterized by a remarkably high species diversity. By various estimates, tropical rain forests cover about 10% of the Earth's land surface, but are home to about 60% of the world's species. In contrast, some ecosystems such as the tundra contain populations that tend to oscillate widely. Ecologists sometimes attribute this instability to their low species diversity.

A second fact that supports the notion that species diversity is related to ecosystem stability is that intentionally simplifying an ecosystem (removing species) tends to make it unstable. Farm fields are a good exam-

ple. Large fields containing one crop are known as **monocultures.** Monocultures are much more vulnerable to pests and disease than **heterocultures**—that is, fields containing several different crops. And both monoculture and heteroculture crops are more vulnerable than nature's heteroculture grasslands, which contain many more species of plants and animals.

To understand why scientists think diversity leads to stability, consider the simple models shown in **FIGURE 23-19.** As illustrated, in the simplified ecosystem, there are few species and few connections. Thus, the loss

FIGURE 23-19 Diversity and Stability (a) In a simplified ecosystem, the loss of one species generally has a more profound impact on the food web than the loss of one species in (b) a more complex ecosystem.

(a)

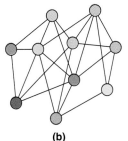

(b)

of one species—for example, a producer—in a simplified ecosystem would be far more noticeable than the loss of a producer in the much more diverse one where several producers are present.

Not all ecologists agree with the preceding ideas. Some say that diverse ecosystems such as tropical rain forests are stable because of their uniform climate, not because of their species diversity. Instability in the tundra could be a result of the volatile climate, not of the low level of diversity.

Despite differences of opinion, some generalizations can be drawn from the evidence. The most important is that intentionally reducing species diversity makes ecosystems unstable. That is important advice for farmers and foresters, who tend to convert diverse ecosystems into much simpler ones.

Scientists debate the concept of ecosystem stability with vigor these days because some recent research has cast doubt on the concept of a naturally maintained equilibrium. Some researchers believe that populations and ecosystems rarely, if ever, return to equilibrium once disturbed. The debaters agree on one thing though: A return to normal equilibrium depends in large part on the nature and severity of the disturbance. Evidence suggests that small perturbations like changes in rainfall or short-term drought are resisted or adequately compensated for. More severe alterations such as deforestation of the tropics may render a system unable to recover.

Unfortunately, the topic is so complex and so easily misconstrued that the debate is more confusing than edifying. What can be said at this time is that our understanding of ecosystem homeostasis is a long way from complete. As the critical thinking rules outlined in Chapter 1 suggest, sometimes a little uncertainty is necessary.

Health, Homeostasis, and the Environment

How We Alter the Environment

Over and over again in this section, I've shown that human health is dependent on a healthy environment. Environmental disturbances such as pollution affect homeostasis, which can then lead to disease. Creating an enduring human presence, therefore, depends on our achieving a better balance—a healthy balance. In order to understand how we can achieve such a balance, the topic of the next chapter, we must first look at the ways we impact our environment.

Humans impact the environment in two principal ways: (1) by altering the abiotic components and (2) by altering the biotic components.

FIGURE 23-20 Foreign Competitor Introduced to the United States Kudzu grows wild in the South, covering fields and homes.

Consider some examples of human tampering with abiotic factors—chemical and physical components. Chemical pollutants from factories, power plants, lawns, and even gardens enter streams and lakes. Here they alter the chemical environment, often killing fish and other aquatic organisms. Hot water from power plants and factories is yet another pollutant released in large quantities into lakes and streams where it alters the physical environment of these bodies of water, often killing aquatic life. Changing the physical and chemical environment has an impact on plants, nonhuman animals, and microorganisms, but it can also affect humans.

Human populations also directly impact the biotic components of the environment. Overfishing, for example, eliminates species of valuable aquatic food chains. In the Pacific Northwest, for example, overfishing of salmon reduces food available for seals and other sea mammals. Another important impact occurs when foreign species are introduced into an ecosystem. In their new home, these species often outcompete native species of plants and animals. An example is shown in **FIGURE 23-20**. The plant is known as *kudzu*. Intentionally introduced in the South to control soil erosion, kudzu literally takes over fields, growing over trees and covering abandoned homes.

It is important to point out that all organisms have an impact on their environment. That is to say, all living things alter the abiotic and biotic components of the ecosystem in which they live. But the impact of human populations is different from that of other organisms, for several reasons. First, our advanced technological development has given us incredible power to alter the face of the Earth. Second, the human population has reached unprecedented numbers. Today, more than 6 billion people live on the planet. The cumulative impact of all these individuals is enormous and may be endangering the biosphere. Chapter 24 examines the evidence behind this assertion and describes ways to reduce human impact and build a sustainable future.

The key to success, many experts believe, is restoring global ecosystem balances and building a relationship with nature that does not endanger the homeostatic mechanisms that maintain the planet's health and the health and well-being of the millions of species that make the Earth their home.

Summary

Principles of Ecology: Ecosystem Structure

1. Most of us see our lives as apart from nature. But in truth we depend heavily on our environment for food, oxygen, clothing, materials, and much else.

2. *Ecology* is the study of ecosystems. It examines the relationship of organisms to their environment and the many interactions between the abiotic and biotic components of ecosystems.

3. The living "skin" of the planet is called the *biosphere*. It extends from the bottom of the oceans to the top of the highest mountains.

4. The biosphere is a *closed system* in which materials are recycled over and over. The only outside contribution is sunlight, which powers virtually all biological processes.

5. The Earth's surface is divided into large biological regions, or *biomes*, each with a characteristic climate and characteristic plant and animal life.

6. The oceans can also be divided into biological regions, known as *aquatic life zones*.

7. An *ecosystem* consists of a community of organisms, its environment, and all of the interactions between them.

8. Organisms are adapted to a range of conditions in the ecosystem in which they live. This is called their *range of tolerance*.

9. Human activities can alter the abiotic and biotic conditions in an ecosystem, causing considerable harm.

10. In any ecosystem, one factor tends to limit growth and is therefore called a *limiting factor*.

11. A group of organisms of the same species living in a specific region constitutes a *population*. Two or more populations occupying that region form a *community*.

12. The physical space a species occupies is called its *habitat*. A species' *niche* includes its habitat, its position in the food chain, its range of tolerance, and so on.

Ecosystem Function

13. Virtually all life on Earth depends on the *producers*, organisms that synthesize organic materials from sunlight, carbon dioxide, and water. The major producers are the plants, photosynthetic protists (single-celled organisms like algae), and photosynthetic bacteria.

14. Organisms dependent on producers and other organisms for food are called *consumers*. Four types of consumers are present: *herbivores, carnivores, omnivores*, and *detritivores*.

15. All organisms are part of food chains. A *food chain* represents a feeding relationship in an ecosystem. Food chains that begin with plants consumed by grazers (herbivores) are known as *grazer food chains*. Those that begin with animal waste or the remains of plants, animals, and microorganisms are known as *decomposer food chains*.

16. Food chains are simplified components of larger networks, called *food webs*, that represent a truer picture of the feeding relationships in an ecosystem.

17. Food chains and food webs are a conduit for the one-way flow of energy through an ecosystem; they provide avenues for the cycling of minerals and other nutrients through the ecosystem.

18. The position of an organism in a food chain is called its *trophic level*. In a grazer food chain, plants (producers) are on the first trophic level; herbivores are on the second; carnivores are on the third.

19. Nutrients necessary for life are involved in *nutrient cycles*. Nutrients in the environment enter the organismic phase through producers. The nutrients are then shunted through the food chain (organismic phase of the cycle) and eventually reenter the environment (environmental phase), where they are generally available for reuse.

20. Humans can interrupt nutrient cycles, locally and globally. For example, the global *carbon cycle* is flooded with carbon dioxide from the worldwide consumption of fossil fuels. Deforestation also increases atmospheric carbon dioxide.

21. The *nitrogen cycle* is flooded with nitrogen from human sources (fertilizer, sewage, and animal waste) in towns, cities, and rural communities.

Ecosystem Homeostasis

22. Human health is dependent on homeostasis at two levels: within the environment and within ourselves. Healthy physical, chemical, social, and psychological environments are crucial to a healthy body.

23. The environment contains numerous homeostatic mechanisms. *Ecosystem balance* is the net result of the interplay of biotic and abiotic *growth* and *reduction factors*.

24. *Environmental resistance* is the sum of the reduction factors.

25. Ecosystems can recover from minor disturbances rather easily, but more significant changes may require more time. In some cases, damage may be so severe that recovery is impossible.

26. The term *succession* refers to a series of changes in an ecosystem in which one community replaces another until a mature, or climax, ecosystem is produced. Primary succession occurs where no community previously existed. Secondary succession occurs where a community was destroyed by natural or human events.

27. Ecosystem stability may also result from high species diversity or from favorable abiotic factors such as climate.

Health, Homeostasis, and the Environment: How We Alter the Environment

28. Humans change the environment by altering the abiotic and the biotic components.

29. All organisms have an impact on their environment. The impact of human populations, however, is different from that of other organisms because of our technological prowess and because our population has reached unprecedented numbers. Even small acts are now beginning to add up and may be putting many other species and our own population at risk.

Critical Thinking

Thinking Critically—Analysis

This Analysis corresponds to the Thinking Critically scenario that was presented at the beginning of this chapter.

At this point in your education, it may be hard to discern fact from fiction in the debate over the environment. But you do know from reading this book that the environment is extraordinarily important to our well-being and our long-term future. The environment is not just another issue. It is a make-it-or-break-it issue. What we do to the environment we do to ourselves.

But can environmental goals be achieved without harming the economy? If you listen to the news or read the newspaper on a regular basis, you've been exposed to a common misconception—notably, that environment and economics embody fundamentally conflicting goals. What you do to protect the environment will automatically harm the economy. This myth has been repeated so many times, in fact, that it may take some time to dislodge.

Fortunately, numerous examples show that we can meet, even in many cases exceed, both environmental and economic goals with alternative measures. These measures, in fact, often make extraordinary economic sense. For instance, by using energy more efficiently, we can greatly reduce air pollution and other environmental impacts. Energy efficiency measures generally cost a lot

less than new sources of energy. Cheaper energy as a rule results in a stronger economy. Numerous other examples also exist, each showing that environmental protection, rather than being an impediment to business, can represent a net gain. The missing element is often creativity and a willingness to examine alternative strategies.

Exercising Your Critical Thinking Skills

1. The following statements express the view of some citizens in this country: Technology can solve all problems. We don't need to worry about global warming, overpopulation, and other environmental problems because scientists will find technical answers to address them.

    This view is often labeled as pure technological optimism. Do you agree or disagree with the viewpoint expressed above? Why or why not? Give specific examples that support your case. Is bias entering into your opinion, and are your views based on solid facts?

2. You work for your state's Department of Natural Resources and are asked to comment on the proposed introduction of a deer from a remote part of the Soviet Union. The rationale behind the introduction is that it would enhance hunting in the state, and this would improve the economy of several rural areas. How would you evaluate the proposal? On what ecological criteria would you rely as you determine whether it is a good idea?

Test of Concepts

1. Humans are a part of nature. Do you agree or disagree with this statement? Support your answer.
2. Define the term *ecology*, and give examples of its proper and improper use.
3. The Earth is a closed system. What are the implications of this statement?
4. Define the following terms: biosphere, biome, aquatic life zone, and ecosystem.
5. Define the term *range of tolerance*. Using your knowledge of ecology, give some examples of ways in which humans alter the abiotic and biotic conditions of certain organisms, and describe the potential consequences of such actions.
6. Describe ways in which humans alter their own range of tolerance for various environmental factors.
7. What is a limiting factor? Give some examples.
8. Define the following terms: habitat, niche, producer, consumer, trophic level, food chain, and food web.
9. Explain why the biomass at one trophic level is lower than the biomass at the next lower trophic level.
10. Outline the flow of carbon dioxide through the carbon cycle, and describe ways in which humans adversely influence the carbon cycle.
11. Using what you have learned about ecology, describe why it is important to protect natural ecosystems and other species.
12. With the knowledge you have gained, explain why it is beneficial to set aside habitat to protect an endangered species.
13. Looking back over the principles you have learned in this chapter, write a set of guidelines for human society that would enable us to live sustainably on the Earth.

www.jbpub.com/humanbiology

Connect to this book's web site: www.jbpub.com/humanbiology
The site features eLearning, an online review area that provides quizzes, chapter outlines, and other tools to help you study for your class. You can also follow useful links for in-depth information, research the differing views in the Point/Counterpoints, or keep up on the latest environmental and health news.

CHAPTER 24

Environmental Issues
POPULATION, POLLUTION, AND RESOURCES

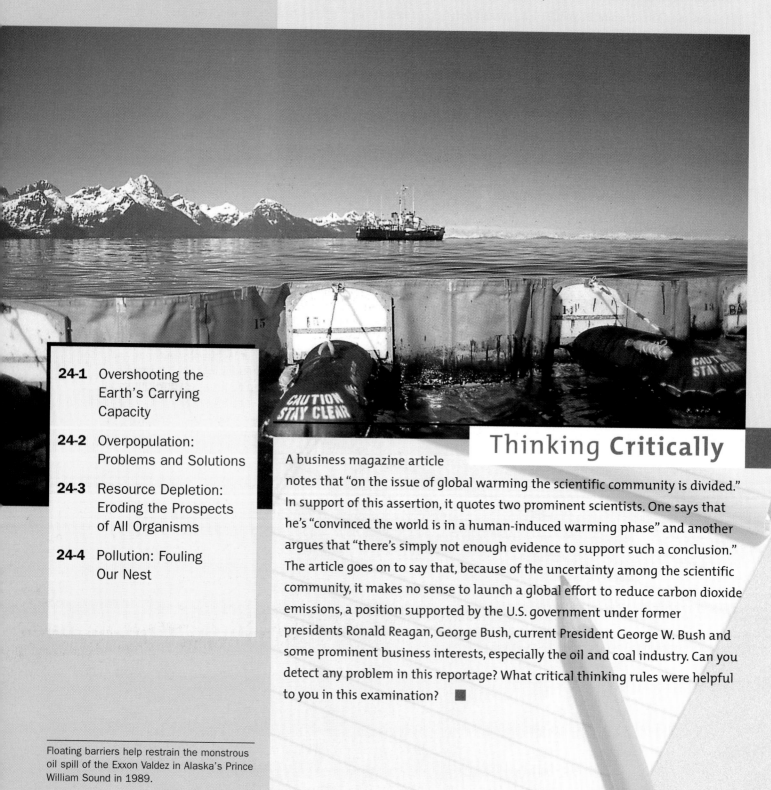

Thinking Critically

A business magazine article notes that "on the issue of global warming the scientific community is divided." In support of this assertion, it quotes two prominent scientists. One says that he's "convinced the world is in a human-induced warming phase" and another argues that "there's simply not enough evidence to support such a conclusion." The article goes on to say that, because of the uncertainty among the scientific community, it makes no sense to launch a global effort to reduce carbon dioxide emissions, a position supported by the U.S. government under former presidents Ronald Reagan, George Bush, current President George W. Bush and some prominent business interests, especially the oil and coal industry. Can you detect any problem in this reportage? What critical thinking rules were helpful to you in this examination? ■

Floating barriers help restrain the monstrous oil spill of the Exxon Valdez in Alaska's Prince William Sound in 1989.

The threat to the environment is commonly referred to as the "environmental crisis." To many people, the phrase "environmental crisis" seems like an exaggeration. But a close examination of trends in population growth, pollution, and resource use and depletion yields a disturbingly different view, and many experts who have studied the trends believe that the problems are severe enough to warrant the term "crisis."

This chapter grapples with a handful of the world's leading environmental problems, focusing primarily on overpopulation, resource depletion, and three pollution problems: acid deposition, ozone depletion, and global climate change. This chapter discusses a variety of solutions for individuals, businesses, and governments. These discussions will help you understand steps required to help human society onto a sustainable course—that is, a path that ensures long-term ecological stability on the planet, a condition essential for a healthy human existence.

Section 24-1

Overshooting the Earth's Carrying Capacity

Environmental problems of significant import occur in both the rich, industrialized nations and the poor, less-developed nations. Although the problems vary from one nation to another, they all are signs of a common root cause: human society is exceeding the Earth's carrying capacity.

Carrying capacity is the number of organisms an ecosystem can support indefinitely—that is, the number it can sustain. Carrying capacity for all organisms, including humans, is determined by at least three factors: (1) food production, (2) resource supply, and (3) the environment's ability to assimilate pollution. Let's look at each one.

In Many Places, the Human Population Is Exceeding Food Production

As the global human population grows, many nations are finding it more and more difficult to meet rising demands for food. Starvation abounds in the less developed nations. There, an estimated 12 million people, many of them children, perish each year from malnutrition and starvation or from diseases worsened by hunger. These are a sure sign of populations living beyond the local carrying capacity (**FIGURE 24-1**).

Many Resources Are in Short Supply and Will Be Depleted in the Near Future

Human populations require many resources such as fuel, fiber, and building materials. Those resources that are finite such as oil, natural gas, and minerals are known as **nonrenewable resources**. Resources that replenish themselves via natural biological and geological processes are called **renewable resources**. Wind, hydropower, trees, and fishes are examples.

Today, some important nonrenewable resources such as oil are on the decline, and some nonrenewable resources are just about used up. Renewable resources such as tropical forests are being depleted faster than they are being replanted. Such rapid depletion provides partial proof for the assertion that human populations are living beyond the Earth's carrying capacity. The rapid destruction of renewables also indicates that we're destroying the carrying capacity itself—that is, systematically eroding the life-support system of the planet.

Pollution from Human Activities Exceeds the Environment's Assimilative Capacity

The final determinant of carrying capacity is the capability of the environment to assimilate and degrade pollutants. In natural ecosystems, wastes are usually diluted to harmless levels and are recycled in nutrient cycles. Animal feces, for instance, are broken down by soil bacteria. These bacteria release carbon dioxide, nitrogen, and other nutrients into the environment for reuse. In nature, nutrient cycles ensure a steady supply of resources for all generations. Unfortunately, many human activities interrupt these vital cycles. Too much animal waste in an aquatic environment, for example, may shift the concentration of nitrogen and phosphorus, starting a series of changes that results in rapid growth of algae and aquatic plants; algae and plants decay in the fall, consuming oxygen in the process and killing fish.

Human populations produce enormous amounts of wastes that

FIGURE 24-1 Food Shortages Overpopulation, drought, political turmoil, and mismanagement of farmland are the chief causes of hunger and starvation. Children die by the thousands every day.

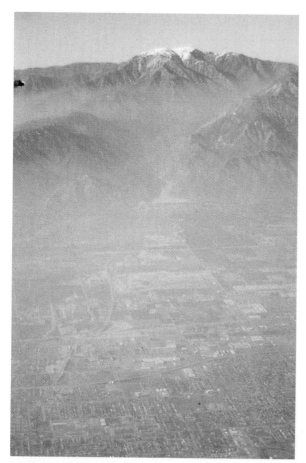

FIGURE 24-2 Air Pollution   Studies show that air pollutants in some locales can increase respiratory disease such as emphysema and lung cancer. Air pollution is aesthetically unappealing, and levels that do not directly affect human health can still cause considerable environmental damage.

overwhelm natural systems. The U.S. population represents only 4% of the world population but produces about 25% of the world's pollution. The environment can dilute some of this waste to harmless levels. It can break down other wastes, rendering them harmless, but in many locations, the environment's assimilative capacity is being severely overtaxed. In lakes, rivers, and oceans, pollution is taking a toll on fish and wildlife. Even though efforts have been made to reduce the amount of pollution our society produces, continued economic expansion and growing numbers of people often offset these gains.

The stress on the assimilative capacity of the atmosphere is evident around most cities with populations over 50,000. Polluted waters and skies are commonplace. Generally the larger the city, the greater the problem. These pockets of air and water pollution pose a threat to human health and to a great many species that make this planet their home (**FIGURE 24-2**). Today, over 100 million Americans live in cities whose air is deemed harmful to their health because of ground-level ozone pollution. Fifty million are exposed to unhealthy levels of particulate pollution.

The environmental crisis is clearly multifaceted. In all instances, the problem is basically the same: We humans are exceeding the Earth's carrying capacity. One of the main reasons for this is overpopulation.

Section 24-2

Overpopulation: Problems and Solutions

Overpopulation can be explained in six words: too many people, reproducing too rapidly. The world population is 6.2 billion and is increasing at a rate of 1.4% per year. Although the growth rate may seem small, it translates into 87 million new people every year or about 240,000 people being added to the world population every day. If the current rate continues, world population could reach 9 billion people by the year 2050. To understand this problem requires a little background information.

Overpopulation Is a Problem in Virtually All Countries, Rich and Poor

The annual **growth rate** of the world population is calculated by the following formula:

$$\text{growth rate} = \text{birth rate} - \text{death rate}$$

In 2000, the world birth rate was 23 per 1000. In other words, 23 children were born each year for every 1000 people living on the Earth. The global death rate was 9 per 1000. To calculate the growth rate, you simply subtract the death rate from the birth rate. The global growth rate was therefore equal to 23/1000 − 9/1000, or 14 per 1000. This means that 14 new residents are added to the planet each year for every 1000 people alive. To convert the growth rate (14/1000) to a percentage, simply multiply by 100. Thus, the growth rate is equal to 14/1000 × 100, or 1.4%.

Growth rates are important measures of population dynamics, but they can be deceiving. For this reason, **demographers** (scientists who study populations) often convert growth rates into **doubling time**, the time it takes a population to double. Doubling time is calculated by the following equation:

$$\text{doubling time} = \frac{70}{\text{growth rate (\%)}} = \frac{70}{1.4} = 50 \text{ years}$$

The figure 70 in this equation is a demographic constant. The global growth rate is an average of all coun-

TABLE 24-1

Growth Rate and Doubling Time

Region	Growth Rate (%)	Doubling Time (Years)
World	1.5	47
Developed countries	0.1	564
Less-developed countries	1.8	38
Africa	2.6	26
Asia	1.6	44
North America	0.6	117
Latin America	1.8	38
Europe	−0.1	—
Oceania	1.1	63

tries and thus masks regional growth differences. For example, the U.S. growth rate for the last 10 years has averaged about 0.9%. In other words, 9 new residents are added to the population each year for every 1000 people alive.[1] If this growth rate continues, our present population of 285 million people will double in 78 years. In contrast, in Africa the growth rate is 2.4%, yielding an alarming doubling time of 29 years!

Today, the most rapid growth is occurring on three continents: Africa, Asia, and Latin America (**TABLE 24-1**). In Europe, the population is actually shrinking.

---

[1]Population growth in any country is the result not only of the difference between birth rate and death rate, but also of the net migration—that is, the number of people entering or leaving the country. In the United States, about 40% of our annual growth results from legal and illegal immigration.

Most people view overpopulation as a problem of the less developed nations. Actually, overpopulation is a problem in all countries. It is as serious in the United States as it is in Bangladesh. The reason for this apparent irony is the fairly high standard of living in the rich, industrialized countries. Citizens of these nations have an enormous impact on the environment. In fact, each baby born in the United States will use 20–40 times as many resources as a baby born to a family in India. This means the 285 million Americans alive in 2000 caused as much environmental damage as 5.6 to 11.2 billion people in the Third World!

The Human Population Is Growing Exponentially

The human population has not always been so large, nor has it always grown so rapidly. As **FIGURE 24-3A** shows, it was not until the last 200 years that global human population began to skyrocket, and then only because of better sanitation, improvements in medicine, and advances in technology. As you may have noticed, the graph of human population growth in **FIGURE 24-3A** is J-shaped. This is an **exponential curve**.

What is exponential growth? To begin, consider an example. Suppose your parents invested $1000 in a savings account at 10% interest the day you were born. Suppose also that the interest your money earned was applied to the balance, so that it too earned interest. If this were the case, your bank account would be said to be growing exponentially. **Exponential growth** occurs anytime a value, such as population size, grows by a fixed percentage—but only if the interest (increase) is applied to the base amount.

(a)

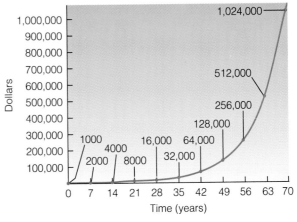

(b)

FIGURE 24-3 Exponential Growth of the World Population (a) World population. (b) Exponential growth of a bank account starting with $1000 at 10% interest.

TABLE 24-2

Global Population Growth

Population Size	Year	Time Required to Double
1 billion	1850	All of human history
2 billion	1930	80 years
4 billion	1975	45 years
8 billion (projected)	2017	42 years

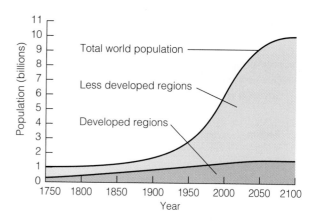

FIGURE 24-5 Human Population Growth The graph shows the relative size of the populations in the less developed regions and the developed regions and projected growth. Note that 90% of the growth is occurring in the Third World. Today, about one of every five people in the world lives in an industrialized country. By 2100, if current growth rates continue, the ratio will be about 1 to 10.

Exponential growth is deceptive. In this example, the growth in your account seems small at first. At 10% interest, the $1000 will double in 7 years, yielding $2000 (**FIGURE 24-3B**). It will double again in 7 years, yielding $4000. The next doubling, occurring when you are 21 years old, will give you $8000. By age 42, the account will have grown to $64,000. By the time you were 49, your account would hold $128,000. At age 56, you'd have over $250,000. If you waited 7 more years, the account would grow to over $500,000. In 7 more years, at 70 years of age, you'd be a millionaire.

What is deceptive about exponential growth is that it begins slowly, then seems to go wild, even though the rate of growth is constant throughout the entire period. In this example, it took 49 years for your account to grow from $1000 to $128,000. In the next 21 years, however, your account grew by $900,000. Why?

Although your account doubled every 7 years, it was not until the base amount was very large that the doublings amounted to much. Thus, once the base amount

reached a certain critical level, each doubling yielded what appeared to be incredible gains—even though the account grew at a steady 10% per year. The human population has taken over 3 million years to reach its current size of 6.2 billion, but because of exponential growth, it could increase by another 6.2 billion in the next 50 years, if current growth continues (**TABLE 24-2**).[2]

Pollution and resource demand will also grow exponentially as the human population skyrockets, and therein lies another concern. Even though supplies of many resources seem large, exponential growth could deplete them in a very short time. Just to show you how insidious exponential growth is, consider a resource with a billion-year life span at the current rate of consumption. If the rate of demand increases 5% per year, that billion-year resource will last only about 500 years.

Many People in Less Developed Nations Are Already Suffering Enormously as a Result of Overpopulation

In many countries, large segments of the population are living in extreme poverty. Many of these people do not have enough to eat. People live in makeshift homes or on the streets (**FIGURE 24-4**). An estimated 840 million people are chronically malnourished. About 2 billion people are on the edge of poverty, with barely enough to eat. Thus, nearly 5 of every 10 people on the planet are living in horrible conditions.

Because humans are living beyond the carrying capacity of the environment now, further growth will very

FIGURE 24-4 Poverty Abounds About three-fifths of the world's people live in poverty. Nearly one of every five people on this planet does not have enough to eat. Many live in makeshift shelters like these in Rio de Janeiro.

---

[2]Note that the human population has not been growing at 1.6% per year for the 3 million years.

TABLE 24-3

Some Solutions to Alleviate World Hunger

Reduce population growth.

Reduce soil erosion.

Reduce desertification.

Reduce farmland conversion.

Improve yield through better crop strains.

Improve yield through better soil management.

Improve yield through fertilization.

Improve yield through better pest control.

Reduce spoilage and pest damage after harvest.

Use native animals for meat production.

Tap farmland reserves available in some countries.

likely worsen problems. Unfortunately, little is being done to stem the swelling tide of humanity. Each year, in fact, about 87 million new residents are added to the world population. Approximately 9 of every 10 of these people are born in the poorer less developed nations, where hunger and poverty are often a way of life (**FIGURE 24-5**). In African nations such as Ethiopia where the human population is expected to double in 29 years, efforts aimed at keeping up the substandard food supplies will put enormous strains on the economy and the environment. Making improvements in diet to reduce starvation and persistent hunger seems impossible. In this struggle, many believe that nature will restore a more equitable balance—and already has. Evidence shows that in many African nations death rates are on the rise. Hunger, starvation, and diseases such as AIDS are beginning to take their toll. Millions of people will die unless something is done to reduce population growth and increase food supply.

Solving World Hunger and Living Sustainably on the Planet Require Many Actions

There is no easy answer to world hunger. Solving such a complex issue and learning to live sustainably on the Earth require a multifaceted response (**TABLE 24-3**).

Slowing the Rate of Growth. One of the most important steps is to reduce population growth. Most world leaders agree that greatly reducing the rate of increase will help less developed countries meet the demand for food and will improve the human condition. Reducing the rate of growth will also help industrial countries reduce their demand for resources and reduce

pollution, habitat destruction, and a host of other environmental problems. Population control measures will also reduce expenditures for social services in the less developed nations. Every birth averted through family planning, studies suggest, saves a less developed nation between $15 and $200 per year in social services.

Reducing Numbers Through Attrition. Judging from the state of the environment, today's population of over 6 billion people is well beyond the carrying capacity of our planet. Slowing the growth of human population, therefore, will not be sufficient to build a sustainable human presence. Over the next 50 years, it will very likely be necessary to reduce the size of the human population. This will permit human society to live within the Earth's carrying capacity. The principal means of reducing population size is through attrition—reducing the birth rate so that it falls below the death rate. Under such conditions, populations will begin to shrink. Attrition is safe, humane, and effective.

Reducing the Total Fertility Rate. Reducing the population size of a country, indeed the world, is not as difficult as many might believe, nor as undesirable. Already, approximately 50 countries in Europe have reached a stage of extremely slow growth, no growth, and even "negative" growth (shrinkage), among them Hungary, Denmark, Italy, and Austria. The decline in population growth is achieved, in large part, because couples are having smaller families. Globally, birth rates also appear to be falling dramatically, a very good sign. The decline in birth rates means that fewer children are being born to each woman of reproductive age.

The number of children a woman has in her lifetime is called the **total fertility rate**. For a population to remain stable in countries such as ours, the total fertility rate must be maintained at 2.1.[3] This means that each woman of reproductive age has, on average, 2.1 children. This level of fertility is called the **replacement-level fertility**. It is the number of children that will replace a couple when they die. A replacement-level fertility rate of 2.1 means that every 10 couples in a population must have 21 children to maintain a steady population size. The additional child accounts for typical mortality.

When the total fertility rate is below the replacement-level fertility, a population will decline, but only if there is no net immigration—that is, there are no newcomers from other countries. In the United States, the total fer-

---

[3]Assuming there is no immigration.

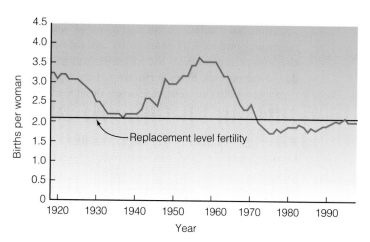

FIGURE 24-6 Total Fertility Rate in the United States Since 1972, the total fertility rate in the United States has been below replacement-level fertility. Yet overall population growth continues because of immigration and because of the large number of women having children.

tility rate has been below replacement-level fertility since 1972 (**FIGURE 24-6**). Despite this important development, the U.S. population continues to grow. Why?

One of the reasons for growth is the steady inflow of illegal and legal immigrants—over a million people each year. Growth also occurs because of the age structure of our population. **FIGURE 24-7** is a **population histogram**, or **population profile**, of the United States in 1960 and 1998. It shows the number or percentage of

males and females in each age group. As you can see, the profile for 1960 is bottom-heavy. There are more people in the lower age groups than in the upper ones. Many of the people in the lower age groups are products of the baby boom era; that is, they were born soon after World War II.

After the war, America's prospects looked bright. Judging from the rise in total fertility to well over 3, people must have been extremely optimistic and happy to be done with the brutal war. The large postwar families created a demographic phenomenon known as the baby boom (**FIGURE 24-8**). Now the baby boomers are having children of their own, and even though they are having far fewer children than their parents, the reproductive-age group is larger than it was after the war. The current growth in the U.S. population therefore occurs not because women are having more children, but because more women are having children.

If immigration quotas do not increase and if the total fertility rate remains the same, the U.S. population profile should become more boxlike, or stationary. At this point, the population would cease growing, reaching a steady state called **zero population growth**. However, Congress passed legislation in 1991 that greatly increases the number of legal immigrants and could again

FIGURE 24-7 Population Profiles for the United States
(a) In 1960, the U.S. population was growing; the broad base of the population profile reflects this fact. (b) In 1998, growth was slowing, and the population was beginning to stabilize; the profile is becoming more boxlike.

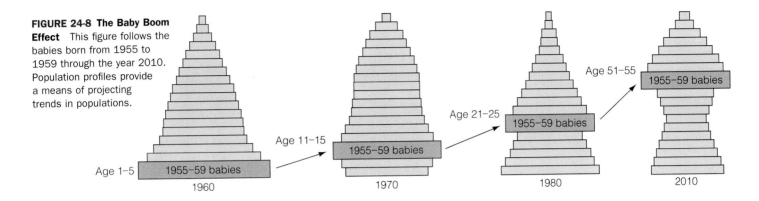

FIGURE 24-8 The Baby Boom Effect This figure follows the babies born from 1955 to 1959 through the year 2010. Population profiles provide a means of projecting trends in populations.

accelerate U.S. population growth. Current projections show that the U.S. population will increase from 280 to 390 million between the present and 2050.

Worldwide, the population profile today looks a lot like the U.S. population profile did shortly after the war—that is, the histogram is triangular, or expansive. The only difference is that the base of the histogram is even broader, meaning there are relatively more youngsters in the global population. Today, in fact, 33% of the world's people are under the age of 15. Soon, they will be entering the reproductive-age group and will start having families. Unless these children restrict their own reproduction, they will cause massive population growth in the next four decades.

Section 24-3

Resource Depletion: Eroding the Prospects of All Organisms

The human population depends on a variety of resources for its survival and well-being—among them, forests, soil, water, minerals, and oil. Today, however, many of these resources are in danger. This section describes the problems and some of the solutions.

Humanity Is Destroying the World's Forests, but Massive Replanting Efforts Could Reduce or Even Stop Deforestation

At one time, tropical rain forests covered a region about the size of the United States (**FIGURE 24-9**). Today, about half of those forests are gone. Because of an exponential increase in population size and the resulting timber harvests "needed" to provide a host of products, most of the remaining tropical rain forests could be destroyed within your lifetime. Along with them, thousands of species, perhaps as many as a million, would vanish. Making matters worse, in the tropics, only 1 tree is re-

planted for every 10 trees that are cut down. In tropical Africa, this ratio is 1 to 29.

The decline of the world's forests is not limited to the tropics. In the United States, for example, 45% of the forested land present when the eastern seaboard was first colonized has been converted to other uses. In the Pacific Northwest, 90%–95% of the old-growth forests, consisting of 250-to-1000 year-old trees, have been cut. India's forests decline by 1.5 million hectares (3.7 million acres) per year. On every continent, forests are in danger.

Because global deforestation exceeds reforestation and because population and demand for resources continue to climb, many scientists have little hope for the world's forests. Consequently, many environmentalists are urging sharp cutbacks in demand for timber and wood products and other strategies that will ease the pressure on forests. Smaller homes, paper recycling, widespread tree planting, and better forest management could all help avert a shortage of timber in the coming years and thereby protect remaining forests. Increasing the rate of paper recycling by 30% in the United States alone would save an estimated 350 million trees per year.

Saving forests is not just a matter of ensuring a steady supply of wood and wood products. Forest conservation also protects the habitat of wild species, helps purify air, and reduces carbon dioxide buildup in the atmosphere. It protects watersheds, reduces soil erosion, and protects recreational opportunities as well. Tropical forests are a potential source of new medicines and food plants that could help feed the world's people.

Destroying tropical forests also disrupts native cultures. Protecting forests is a way of protecting these people and their cultures. New efforts are now under way to save the forests by developing markets for sustainable products such as nuts and fruits. Several recent studies suggest that sustainable harvesting of the forest is far more profitable than timber harvesting and cattle ranching—and much better for the forest and its inhabitants.

FIGURE 24-9 Tropical Rain Forests *(a)* This map shows the steady decline in tropical forests and projected remaining trees in the year 2000. *(b)* Deforestation: a desperate effort to stave off poverty results in an environmental disaster. These farmers live near the Andasibe reserve in Madagascar, an island where the per capita income is less than $250 a year. Clearing the rain forest allows these impoverished farmers to plant rice and graze cattle. But the environmental price may be too steep. In Madagascar alone, 80% of the rain forest has been destroyed.

(b)

(a)

Tropical rain forests

▢ Original extent	▢ Present extent	▢ Year 2000 at current deforestation rate

Soil Erosion, Like Deforestation, Is Also a Worldwide Phenomenon

Although soil erosion occurs naturally, it is often greatly accelerated by human activities such as farming, construction, and mining (**FIGURE 24-10**). In the past 100 years, about one-third of the fertile topsoil on American farmland has been eroded away by water and wind, largely because of poor land management. According to U.S. Department of Agriculture estimates, about 1.7 billion metric tons (1.9 billion tons) of topsoil were lost annually from U.S. farmland from 1992 to 1997—840 million tons from wind erosion and 1.06 billion tons from water erosion. Although soil erosion is down from earlier years, the average rate of erosion on U.S. farmland is approximately seven times greater than soil formation, a situation that is clearly unsustainable.

Worldwide, about 25 billion tons of soil is eroded from farmland each year. To help put this into perspective, at this rate, in a decade total soil losses would equal 250 billion tons. That is equivalent to half the topsoil on U.S. farmland.

Globally, annual erosion rates are 18–100 times greater than rates at which soil is reformed. (The average renewal time is 500 years, but it ranges from 200 to 1000 years.) The annual loss of topsoil has caused farmers to retire millions of acres of once-productive farmland and, in many cases, to cut down forests or plow up grassland to replace what has been lost. Approximately 25% of the tropical rain forests cut down each year are leveled to replace farmland destroyed by human activities.

Making matters worse, millions of acres of farmland are lost to urban and suburban sprawl, highway construction, and other human activities (**FIGURE 24-11**). In the United States, at least 3500 acres of rural land—ac-

FIGURE 24-10 Soil Erosion Millions of acres of farmland are destroyed each year because of poor land management practices that lead to severe soil erosion.

FIGURE 24-11 Farmland Conversion Cities are often surrounded by excellent farmland soils that drain well and are flat and highly productive. Many of the features that make soils suitable for farmland also make them suitable for building. This scene, unfortunately, is all too common in expanding urban areas.

well. Worldwide, an area the size of Ohio becomes desert each year, principally because of overgrazing by livestock and poor land management practices.

These figures paint a rather grim picture for the long-term future of food production here and abroad, especially when viewed in light of increasing populations. But this trend need not be our destiny. The loss of topsoil can be stopped, and soils can be replenished. However, worldwide conservation efforts are needed as are population growth measures, which help to reduce the conversion of farmland to other uses such as housing. Additional solutions shown in **TABLE 24-3** (page 551) could alleviate world hunger and could also reduce the loss of productive farmland and rangeland. For these actions to be effective, society must begin work soon.

Many Areas of the World Are Facing Water Shortages or Will Soon Face Them as Population and Demand Increase

FIGURE 24-12 is a map of areas in the United States that will face a water shortage in the near future. Regional water shortages generally result because too many people are drawing on limited water supplies. Long-term

tual or potential farmland, pasture, and rangeland—are lost every day. That's equivalent to 1.25 million acres a year, or a strip 0.3 mile wide extending from New York City to San Francisco. Overgrazing and poor land management are destroying millions of acres of farmland as

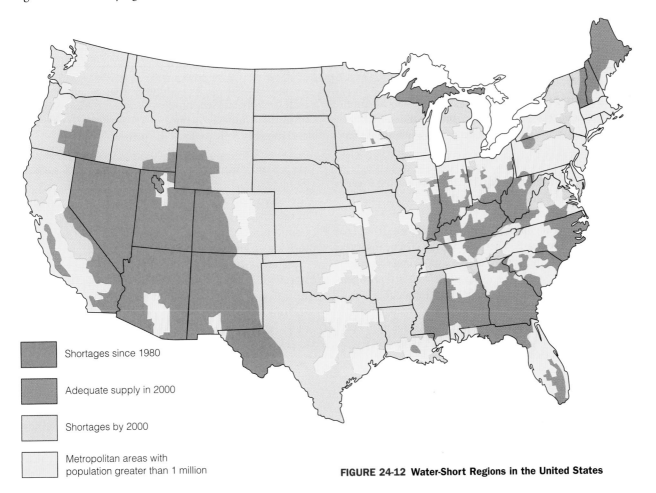

Shortages since 1980

Adequate supply in 2000

Shortages by 2000

Metropolitan areas with population greater than 1 million

FIGURE 24-12 Water-Short Regions in the United States

FIGURE 24-13 The Ogallala Aquifer The water of the Ogallala is replenished very slowly and is currently being withdrawn much faster than it can be replaced. Farmers' wells are running dry, and eventually many irrigated farms will go out of business.

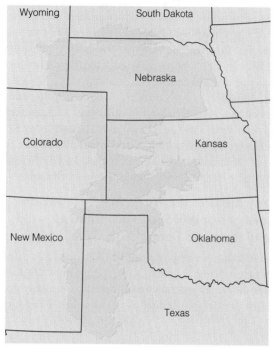

prospects here and abroad appear bleak as agricultural, industrial, and residential water use climbs.

FIGURE 24-13 shows the location of an enormous **aquifer**, a porous underground zone saturated with water. Known as the **Ogallala aquifer**, this zone supplies irrigation and drinking water for farms in Nebraska, Kansas, Colorado, Oklahoma, and Texas. Unfortunately, severe **groundwater overdraft**, withdrawals that exceed natural replenishment, may put an end to irrigated farming in these states.

Reducing the mining of groundwater is essential to meeting future needs. That will require strict conservation efforts. In the agricultural sector, lining irrigation ditches with concrete or using pipes rather than open ditches to transport water to fields can dramatically reduce losses due to evaporation. More efficient sprinklers, computerized systems that monitor soil moisture so that farmers know exactly how much irrigation water is required, and other measures can also help.

Many Essential Minerals Will Be Depleted in the Next Four Decades

Metals such as steel and aluminum are produced from the Earth's mineral deposits. More than 100 minerals, worth billions of dollars to the global economy, are traded on the world market each year. Several dozen of

these minerals are so important to modern society that if they were suddenly no longer available or were unavailable at a reasonable price, the U.S. economy, like those of other industrialized countries, would come to a standstill.

At least 18 economically important minerals will fall into short supply in the next 30 years, even if countries expand their recycling programs. Silver, mercury, lead, sulfur, tin, tungsten, and zinc are among this group. Even if new discoveries and new technologies make it possible to extract five times the currently known reserves, this group will be 80% depleted by or before 2040.

Oil Supplies Are Limited, and Most Students Alive Today Will See the End of Oil in Their Lifetimes

Oil is the lifeblood of modern society. In the United States, for example, oil supplies approximately 40% of our annual energy demand. But the supply of oil is finite. No one knows how much oil is left in Earth's crust, but this we do know: Oil reserves could be depleted within the next 40 to 100 years, depending on demand. If demand continues to increase as it has, oil supplies could be gone by 2038. Many analysts believe that world oil supply will peak between 2005 and 2010, after which demand will outstrip supply. Clearly, time is running out for oil. You will probably see the end of oil within your lifetime. So what do we do?

The first step in meeting future demand is to make current energy use much more efficient. Efficiency will no doubt occur as fuel supplies decrease and citizens shift to more efficient modes of transportation. Waiting until that time, say many experts, wastes precious fuel and unnecessarily pollutes the planet.

Enormous supplies of energy exist today—in our waste. The efficient use of oil and oil products, such as gasoline, diesel fuel, and home heating oil, can help us stretch current oil supplies considerably while actually improving the economy. In fact, many of the leading economic powers, such as Japan and West Germany, are thriving in large part because they are so energy-efficient.

Energy-efficient investments such as storm doors, storm windows, and added insulation coupled with measures to cut air inflow (infiltration) are often inexpensive and can reduce home energy consumption by 30%–50%. More efficient cars could cut demand enormously. Even higher mileage is possible. The Japanese, for example, have a car that gets 98 miles per gallon on the highway and seats four people! Even newer models are being developed. One newcomer is the hybrid car. It has a small gasoline engine and an electric motor. When driving at slow speeds, the electric motor provides power. When additional power is needed, the gasoline engine kicks in. Unlike true electric cars, the batteries of a hybrid vehicle do not require the owner to plug the car into an electrical outlet each night for charging. Electricity is generated by the gas engine and by the wheels when the car is slowing down. With space age materials and aerodynamic design, some people think that hybrid vehicles could get over 150 miles per gallon. Current models fall well short of this goal. Toyota's four-seater Prius, which was released in 1998 in Japan and in 2000 in the United States, gets about 53 miles per gallon in city driving. Honda's two-seater, the Insight, gets close to 70 miles per gallon.

Another important step in increasing energy efficiency is mass transit—buses and trains to transport commuters to and from work. Mass transit is four times more efficient than the automobile.

Energy efficiency is the cheapest and most cost-effective means of meeting future demand. Amory Lovins, a world-renowned energy expert, calculates that Americans could reduce oil demand by 80% without changing life-styles by using energy-efficient technologies currently on the market. Lovins's calculations also show that U.S. electrical demand could be cut by 75% by using energy-efficient light bulbs, motors, and other technologies that are currently available (**FIGURE 24-14**). These measures could save us hundreds of billions of dollars a year.

Alternative fuels can also help meet future demand. Bear in mind that the immediate need is for an alternative source of energy to replace oil, which is used chiefly in transportation and home heating. One example is ethanol. Produced from corn, wheat, and other crops, ethanol can power automobiles and trucks. Grown on special fuel farms, ethanol could virtually replace gasoline, but a shift to ethanol in the United States would not be without its costs. One of those might be a reduction in food output. Brazil is a leader in ethanol use: 98% of the new cars sold in Brazil are equipped to use it.

Another potentially important fuel is hydrogen. Made from water, hydrogen is the ultimate in renewable fuels. It burns cleanly and is available from an abundant resource. Unfortunately, hydrogen is difficult to store.

Renewable energy could provide enormous amounts of fuel in the years to come. Unknown to many, the renewable energy supply is enormous and, in some cases, can be tapped quickly and inexpensively. According to one estimate, nonrenewable energy reserves (coal, oil, natural gas, and so on) would provide the equivalent of 8.8 trillion barrels of oil. Renewable energy could provide 10 times that amount of energy every year!

Pollution: Fouling Our Nest

Like death and taxes, waste is an inescapable fact of life. All organisms produce it. Humans, however, are by far

FIGURE 24-14 Energy-Efficient Many new light bulbs use only 25% of the energy a standard light bulb requires. Although they cost more, they last as long as 10 standard bulbs and save $20–$40 in electricity over their lifetime.

the most prolific generators of waste on the planet. Today, waste from human society is overwhelming many nutrient cycles, poisoning other species (and ourselves), and filling up landfills. This section recaps four of the most serious waste problems.

Global Warming Results from the Release of Carbon Dioxide and Other Greenhouse Gases

Carbon dioxide is produced during cellular respiration and the combustion of all organic materials—most importantly, fossil fuels. In normal concentrations in the atmosphere, carbon dioxide has a warming effect on the planet. Acting much like the glass in a greenhouse, it traps heat escaping from the Earth and radiates it back to the surface. Carbon dioxide is, therefore, also known as a **greenhouse gas.** A little bit of carbon dioxide is essential to life on Earth. In fact, without carbon dioxide in the atmosphere, the planet would be about 55°F (30°C) cooler than it is. Too much, however, may lead to overheating.

Over the past 100 years, global carbon dioxide levels have increased about 32.5%, principally as a result of industrialization (powered by the combustion of fossil fuels) and deforestation. Today, atmospheric carbon dioxide levels continue to rise at a rate of about 0.5% per year (**FIGURE 24-15A**).

Several other pollutants also contribute to global warming. Methane, chlorofluorocarbons, nitrous oxide, and even water vapor all radiate heat back to the Earth, causing the atmosphere to heat up. Methane is released from livestock and the manure they produce; humankind's nearly 1 billion cattle annually release about 73 million metric tons of this gas (providing another good reason to reduce or eliminate one's consumption of beef). Methane production has increased 435% in the last century. Incidentally, termites, which thrive in the

FIGURE 24-15 Global Carbon Dioxide and Temperature Trends
(a) Carbon dioxide levels in the atmosphere have risen dramatically since 1958. *(b)* Graph of average global temperature since 1950.

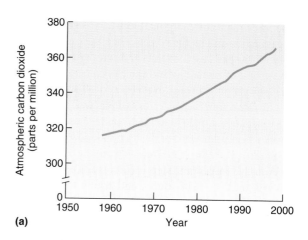

(a)

deforested tropics, also excrete methane. Methane output from all sources is increasing at a rate of about 1% per year and is 20 times more effective at trapping heat than carbon dioxide.

Chlorofluorocarbons, or CFCs, are best known for their effect on the ozone layer and are released from refrigerators, air conditioners, and freezers.[4] One class of CFCs was used to clean circuit boards used in computers and other electronic equipment. In the lower atmosphere, CFCs also trap heat, contributing to the greenhouse effect.

Because of the dramatic increase in the release of greenhouse gases, many atmospheric scientists believe that global temperature is on the rise and may rise dra-

---

[4]CFCs used in spray cans were banned in the United States and several other countries in the late 1970s.

FIGURE 24-16 Changing Rainfall Patterns Possible future changes in climate resulting from the greenhouse effect. This map is based on climatic conditions thought to have existed 4500 to 8000 years ago, when the average temperature was highest. Note that this is a generalized map and may miss regional changes.

(b)

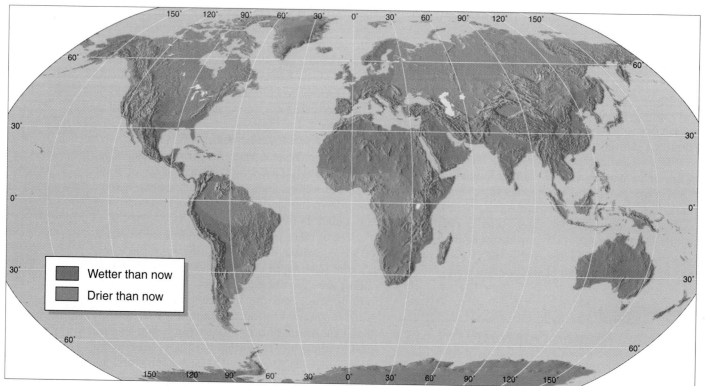

Wetter than now

Drier than now

FIGURE 24-17 Mount Rainier Glaciers This enormous glacier and others like it could melt as the Earth gets warmer, raising the sea level.

FIGURE 24-18 Miami Underwater? A rising sea level due to global warming could flood many coastal cities the world over.

matically in the coming decades, causing an extraordinary shift in climate. **FIGURE 24-15B** shows average global temperature over the past fifty years.

The Impacts of Global Warming Could Be Ecologically Devastating. According to latest projections based on the present rate of increase in greenhouse gases, global temperatures could be 5° to 10°F hotter by 2100. The models suggest that global rainfall patterns will shift dramatically as a result of warming (**FIGURE 24-16**). Computer simulations of U.S. climate suggest that the Midwest and much of the western United States will be drier and hotter than they are today. If that happens, many midwestern farmers will be driven out of business. As rainfall declines in this agriculturally productive region, farming may intensify in the northern states. Overall agricultural productivity in the United States may fall, because northern soils are not as rich as those in the Midwest. Food shortages caused by the decline in U.S. agriculture in the Midwest and rising food prices could affect the economy in profound ways. Computer climate models predict that the southern United States and Pacific Coast may be wetter but hotter.

A rise in global temperature is expected to melt glaciers and the polar ice caps (**FIGURE 24-17**). Warmer temperatures would also expand the volume of the seas. Together, melting ice and expanding oceans would result in an increase in sea level. In the past 50 years, sea level has risen 10–12 centimeters (4–6 inches). By 2100, the computer models suggest that the sea level will rise

50 centimeters (2 feet) because of global warming. What impact would this have?

In the United States, approximately half of the population lives within 50 miles of the ocean, and many large cities such as Miami are located only a few feet above sea level (**FIGURE 24-18**). A rising sea level would flood many low-lying regions. Storms could cause more damage than they do now because high water would be able to move farther inland. Expensive dikes and levees would be needed to protect cities such as Miami and New Orleans. Other coastal cities would have to be rebuilt on higher ground, at a staggering cost.

A rising sea level would be particularly hard on Bangladesh and other Asian countries with extensive lowland rice paddies. Approximately 17% of Bangladesh would be reclaimed by the sea if sea level rose 2–3 feet.

Rising temperatures would also have an impact on many species. In 2000, a report by the National Research Council predicted an increase in average temperature in North America of 3° to 6°C (5° to 10°F) over the next 100 years. In this report, scientists predicted a major shift in climate zones in North America. The authors suggest that the tropical climate of equatorial regions will shift northward into the lower-tier states. Their climate, in turn, will shift to the mid-tier states and the climate of the top-tier states would move into Canada. The effect of such a rapid shift on vegetation and wildlife could be devastating, with many trees simply dying as temperatures climb outside of their range of tolerance.

Some species might adapt or find new habitat; many plants, however, would be wiped out by a relatively rapid increase in temperature, for temperature would probably increase far faster than many species could adapt. As a result, forests would dry out and die off. The incidence of forest fires may increase, further adding to global warming.

Some species may actually thrive amid global warming—for example, organisms that are responsible for infectious diseases. Robert Shope of the Yale University School of Medicine predicts that some diseases now restricted to tropical areas could invade new territory as the planet warms. For example, one form of rabies, now transmitted by vampire bats, could spread northward from Mexico and could result in damage of about $1 billion a year to the Texas cattle industry. Some scientists believe that the recent outbreaks of the deadly Hanta virus, which is transmitted by rodents in the desert Southwest, may be a result of rising global temperature.

Warmer climates are already causing the spread of insects that carry malaria and dengue fever to higher altitudes and higher latitudes. In Africa, studies show that malaria is spreading to higher altitude regions in five countries, which scientists attribute to the warming climate. In Mexico and Costa Rica, dengue fever is spreading into the highlands as well. "The control issue looms largest in the developing world, where resources for prevention and treatment can be scarce," writes Dr. Paul Epstein, Associate director of the Center for Health and the Global Environment at Harvard Medical School in an article in Scientific American. "But the technologically advanced nations, too, can fall victim to surprise attacks—as happened last year (1999) when the West Nile virus broke out for the first time in North America, killing seven New Yorkers. In these days of international commerce and travel, an infectious disorder that appears in one part of the world can quickly become a problem continents away if the disease-causing agent, or pathogen, finds itself in a hospitable environment."

Global warming could cause considerable human suffering. Heat and drought are taking their toll on agriculture worldwide, causing severe economic problems in some areas. In 1999, severe drought plagued many parts of the United States. Heat waves are also responsible for numerous deaths. In 1998, 455 Americans died as a result of sweltering summer heat.

Global warming may also trigger more violent weather, especially hurricanes and tornados that cause billions of dollars worth of damage. A recent study of severe storms in the United States showed that violent downpours are on the rise. Studies also show that the occurrence of tornadoes is on the rise. In fact, 1999 was the fourth "busiest" year for tornadoes in U.S. history with 1225 reported twisters. Worldwide, the incidence of major weather events has also increased. In 1999, there were four times as many major storms and floods as there were in the 1960s and damage was seven times higher. Europe has been plagued by devastating floods in recent years, which many experts think were caused by global warming.

These predictions sound dire—and indeed they are. But a small number of scientists believe that we don't know enough about the atmosphere and the impact of greenhouse gases to know for certain whether the predictions will come true. Global climate is extremely complex and several factors could dampen the warming trend. Other factors could worsen it.

Solving Global Warming Requires Massive Action, and Soon. While scientists and politicians debate global warming, the Earth appears to be getting hotter. In fact, 17 of the hottest years in the past 100 years have occurred from 1980 to 1999. Although warm years are not unusual, having so many record-breaking years in such a short period is highly unlikely. In 1997, these and other statistics spurred the world's nations to agree to measures that will decrease CO_2 emissions.

Sharp reductions in fossil-fuel consumption by energy efficiency, conservation, and the use of alternative sources of fuel will be required. Global reforestation is essential. For each family of four in the United States, 6 acres of fast-growing trees would have to be planted to offset the carbon dioxide the family will produce during its life. Additional strategies are shown in **TABLE 24-4**. We as individuals can also help. On average, each gallon of gasoline you consume in your automobile produces 5 pounds of carbon dioxide. Every hour you watch television results in the production of 0.64 pound of carbon dioxide while your frost-free refrigerator accounts for nearly 13 pounds daily (**TABLE 24-5**). We can play a role in reducing the problem by using energy much more efficiently: using mass transit, recycling, insulating our homes, and a great many other strategies (**TABLE 24-6**).

Large Portions of the World Are Threatened by Acid Deposition

In the Adirondack Mountains of New York, hundreds of lakes are dying. Fishes have vanished as the lakes turn acidic (**FIGURE 24-19**, page 562). A similar phenomenon is occurring in southeastern Canada and in Sweden and Norway, where dying lakes number in the thousands.

The acidification of lakes is a result of acids falling from the skies. They are produced from two atmospheric pollutants, sulfur dioxide and nitrogen dioxide. These pollutants arise chiefly from the combustion of

TABLE 24-4

Measures to Reduce Global Climate Change

Reduce the rate of population growth.

Switch from coal- and oil-fired power plants to natural gas, which produces much less carbon dioxide per unit of electricity.

Implement the technologies that burn coal more efficiently.

Expand cogeneration—processes that trap waste heat and put it to good use.

Boost automobile efficiency.

Expand mass transit.

Develop alternative liquid fuels for the transportation sector.

Improve the efficiency of industry.

Make new and existing homes more energy-efficient through insulation, weather stripping, storm doors, and storm windows.

Build many new homes that use solar energy for space heating.

Reduce global deforestation.

Begin a massive global reforestation effort.

Phase out all CFCs and other CFC-damaging chemicals soon.

Reduce consumption of unnecessary items.

Expand recycling efforts.

TABLE 24-5

Carbon Dioxide Production from Common Activities

Electrical Appliances	Pounds of Carbon Dioxide Added to Atmosphere*
Color television	0.64 per hour
Steam iron	0.85 per hour
Vacuum cleaner	1.70 per hour
Air conditioner, room	4.00 per hour
Toaster oven	12.80 per hour
Ceiling fan	4.00 per day
Refrigerator, frost-free	12.80 per day
Waterbed heater with thermostat	24.00 per day
	12.80 per day
Clothes dryer	10.00 per load
Dishwasher	2.60 per load
Toaster	0.12 per use
Microwave oven	0.25 per 5-minute use
Coffeemaker	0.50 per brew

*At room temperature and sea level, every pound of carbon dioxide occupies 8.75 cubic feet, about half the size of a refrigerator.

Source: Reprinted from the February/March 1990 issue of *National Wildlife.* Copyright © 1990 by the National Wildlife Federation.

TABLE 24-6

Individual Actions That Can Reduce Global Climate Change

Automobile energy savings
Buy energy-efficient vehicles.
Reduce unnecessary driving.
Car-pool, take mass transit, walk, or bike to work.
Combine trips.
Keep your car tuned and your tires inflated to the proper level.
Drive at or below the speed limit.

Home energy savings
Increase your attic insulation to R30 or R38.
Caulk and weather-strip your house.
Add storm windows and insulated curtains.
Install an automatic thermostat.
Turn the thermostat down a few degrees in winter, and wear warmer clothing.
Replace furnace filters when needed.
Lower water heater setting to 120–130°F.
Insulate water heater and pipes, install a water heater insulation blanket, and repair or replace all leaky faucets.
Take shorter showers.
Use cold water as much as possible.
Avoid unnecessary appliances.
Buy energy-efficient appliances.
Use low-energy light bulbs.

Reducing waste and resource consumption
Recycle at home and at work.
Avoid products with excessive packaging.
Reuse shopping bags.
Refuse bags for single items.
Use a diaper service instead of disposable diapers.
Reduce consumption of throwaways.
Donate used items to Goodwill, Disabled American Veterans, the Salvation Army, or other charities.
Buy durable items.
Give environmentally sensitive gifts.

fossil fuels: coal, oil, gasoline, natural gas and jet fuel. In the atmosphere, these gases, or **acid precursors**, combine with water and oxygen to form sulfuric and nitric acids, which are responsible for **acid deposition.** Rain and snow wash acids from the sky. Fog and clouds also carry heavy loads of acids that are deposited on trees. Acid rain, snow, and fog are forms of wet deposition. Some acid precursors are deposited in particulates and on dry surfaces, creating dry deposition. Here they combine with water to form acid.

In the United States and Europe, acid deposition has been worsening for four decades, largely as a result of increased fossil-fuel combustion. The map in **FIGURE 24-20** shows that the region of the United States affected by acid deposition is growing larger and that the level of acidity, measured by pH, is increasing. Today, acid deposition is commonly encountered downwind from virtually all major population centers. It comes from power plants, motorized vehicles, factories, and even our own homes.

Acid deposition changes the pH of lakes and streams, killing fishes and other aquatic organisms. Acids on land dissolve toxic minerals such as aluminum from the soil and wash them into surface waters. Aluminum causes the gills of fishes to clog with mucus, suffocating them. Extensive acidification of lakes and rivers is putting resort owners out of business in the Northeast, upper Midwest, and southern Canada.

FIGURE 24-21 shows areas most susceptible to acid deposition. These regions are generally mountainous and contain soils with little capacity to neutralize acids. Consequently, acids that fall on the land quickly wash to nearby lakes and streams.

Acids also damage crops and trees, directly and indirectly. Direct damage results when acids fall on growing buds or leaves. Indirect damage occurs when acids alter soil chemistry, inhibiting the soil bacteria necessary for nutrient recycling. Acids also leach important minerals from the soil, resulting in slower plant growth.

FIGURE 24-19 Victims of Modern Society These fish were killed by acids from acid deposition.

Some scientists believe that massive forest diebacks occurring throughout the world may be the result of acidic rainfall and fog that often blankets forests (**FIGURE 24-22**). Finally, acid deposition also damages buildings, statues, and other structures. The estimated cost in the United States is about $5 billion per year.

Reducing the deposition of acids will require a dramatic reduction in the release of sulfur dioxide and nitrogen dioxide from power plants, factories, and automobiles. One way of reducing sulfur dioxide is the smokestack scrubber, a device that traps sulfur dioxide gas escaping from power plants, removing up to 95% of this pollutant. Installing and operating a scrubber is rather expensive, and some utilities have objected to this strategy. Using low-sulfur coal can also help, but eastern coal producers find this strategy objectionable because their coal is especially high in sulfur. So far, most utili-

FIGURE 24-20 Acid Precipitation: A Growing Problem As shown here, acid precipitation in the eastern United States has increased between 1955 and 1999. Note the worsening of acid rain and the wider area experiencing it.

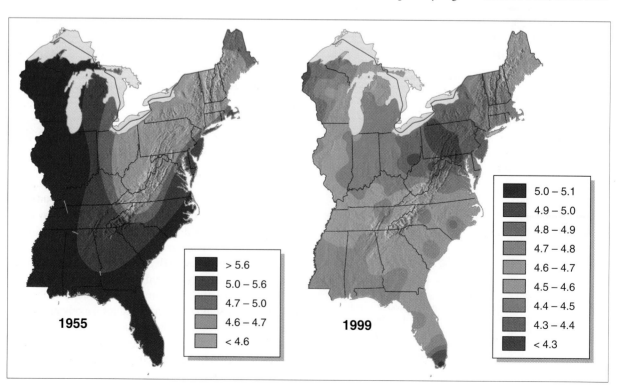

1955

■	> 5.6
■	5.0 – 5.6
■	4.7 – 5.0
■	4.6 – 4.7
■	< 4.6

1999

■	5.0 – 5.1
■	4.9 – 5.0
■	4.8 – 4.9
■	4.7 – 4.8
■	4.6 – 4.7
■	4.5 – 4.6
■	4.4 – 4.5
■	4.3 – 4.4
■	< 4.3

FIGURE 24-21 Sensitive Areas This map of North America shows areas experiencing acid deposition and the most geologically vulnerable regions.

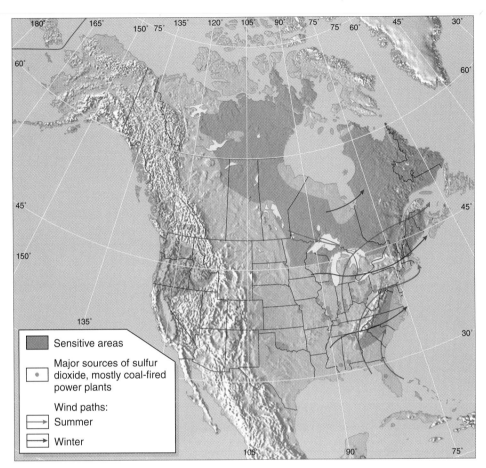

ties have chosen the low-sulfur coal strategy, because it is cheaper.

A far better strategy is energy efficiency. By using less fossil-fuel energy, we cut the combustion of polluting fuels. This action reduces both sulfur dioxide and nitrogen dioxide release and also reduces carbon dioxide, a major contributor to global warming. Energy efficiency therefore has multiple environmental benefits. Add the economic benefits, and it becomes an even more attractive strategy for environmental protection. Renewable energy is an even more important strategy for reducing acid deposition. Solar and wind energy, for example, meet our needs, but release no acid precursors.

The Ozone Layer is Endangered by Human Pollutants

Encircling the Earth, 20–30 miles above its surface, is a region of the atmosphere, the **ozone layer**, containing a slightly elevated level of ozone gas. The ozone layer shields the Earth from harmful ultraviolet radiation from the Sun. Early in the evolution of life, in fact, the formation of the ozone layer probably "allowed" the colonization of land by plants and animals.

Today, however, the ozone layer is being destroyed by chemicals released into the atmosphere by modern society. The most potent destroyer of ozone is a class of chemicals known as the chlorofluorocarbons (CFCs).[5] Once used as spray can propellants, refrigerants, blowing agents for plastic foam, and cleansing agents, CFCs are highly stable molecules. Scientists, in fact, selected them for use in spray cans in large part because of their lack of chemical reactivity. In the early 1970s, however, a U.S. scientist discovered that CFCs were broken down by sunlight. Another scientist showed that CFCs released from human activities gradually drift into the upper atmosphere. Here, the scientists hypothesized, the breakdown products react with and destroy ozone molecules.

[5] Nitric oxide from high-flying jet airplanes such as the supersonic transport can also destroy the ozone layer.

Estimates of ozone depletion came and went over the years, but scientists were hard pressed to detect any measurable decline, in large part because ozone levels fluctuate naturally from year to year. In 1988, however, a panel of atmospheric scientists reviewing 20 years of satellite data on ozone levels concluded that the ozone layer is indeed on the decline. What they found was that satellite measurements of ozone automatically logged into their computer had shown a consistent decline. It hadn't shown up because the computer was programmed to delete low levels on the belief that such readings represented instrument errors. When scientists reexamined the data, they found that over North America ozone levels had fallen 1.7%–3% (**FIGURE 24-23**). Much larger declines were evident at the poles. In fact, scientists found that each year a giant hole in the ozone layer about the size of the United States formed over Antarctica. Ozone levels in the hole declined by as much as 50%. In 1992, the ozone hole reached a record high—almost three times the size of the United States. Studies strongly suggested that the main reason for the decline in the ozone layer was the accumulation of chlorofluorocarbons.

What impacts could ozone depletion have? Like many natural components of our environment, ultraviolet light is beneficial. In small amounts, ultraviolet radiation tans light skin and stimulates vitamin D production in the skin. However, excess ultraviolet exposure can cause problems. In humans, it can cause serious skin burns, cataracts (clouding of the eye's lens), skin cancer, and premature aging. Increased exposure to ultraviolet light may also suppress the human immune system, making us more susceptible to infectious diseases.

EPA researchers estimate that a 1% depletion of the ozone layer would lead to a 0.7 to 2% increase in ultraviolet light striking the Earth. This, in turn, would lead to an increase in skin cancer of about 4%. Over the next five decades, the EPA estimates that ozone depletion will result in approximately 200,000 cases of skin cancer in the United States.

In November 1991, a panel of scientists convened by the United Nations released a report on the predicted effects of global ozone depletion. They estimated that a 10% decrease in stratospheric ozone concentrations will cause 300,000 additional cases of skin cancer and an additional 1.6 million cases of cataracts (loss of opacity) per year worldwide.

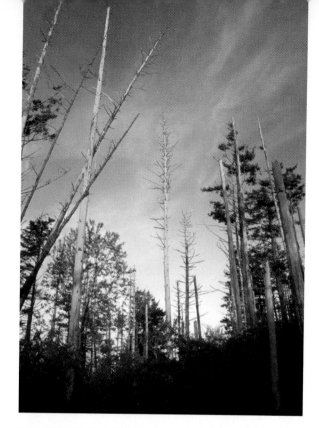

FIGURE 24-22 Forest Die-off Ghostly remains of trees killed by acid deposition in the Pisgah National Forest, North Carolina.

Studies of skin cancer show that light-skinned people are much more sensitive to ultraviolet radiation than more heavily pigmented individuals. In addition, studies show that some chemicals, which are commonly found in drugs, soaps, cosmetics, and detergents, may sensitize the skin to ultraviolet radiation. Thus, exposure to sunlight may increase the incidence of skin cancers among light-skinned people and users of many commercial products.

Land- and water-dwelling plants could also suffer from increasing ultraviolet radiation. Intense ultraviolet radiation is usually lethal to plants; smaller, nonfatal doses damage leaves, inhibit photosynthesis, cause mutations, or stunt growth. Declining ozone and increasing ultraviolet radiation could also cause dramatic declines in commercial crops such as corn, rice, and wheat, costing billions of dollars a year. It may also affect certain commercially valuable tree species such as the loblolly pine.

In a hearing before the U.S. Senate in November 1991, Susan Weiler, head of the American Society of Limnology and Oceanography, testified that studies in Antarctica by other scientists have shown that phytoplankton (algae and other free-floating photosynthetic organisms) populations decrease about 6% to 12% when stratospheric ozone concentrations over the region drop by 40%. Because phytoplankton form the base of the aquatic food chain, damage to them could cause widespread ecological problems. One scientist thinks that ozone depletion and subsequent effects on the food chain may be the reason why two species of penguin are declining in Antarctica.

Finally, ultraviolet light is harmful to many products. Paints, plastics, and other materials deteriorate when ex-

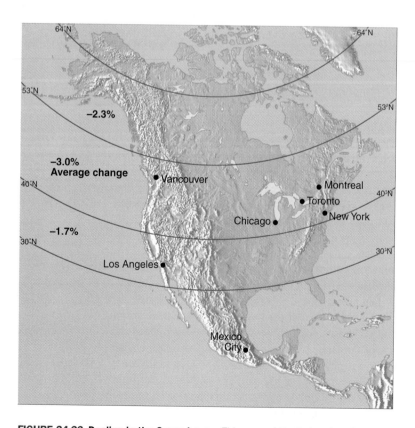

FIGURE 24-23 Decline in the Ozone Layer This map of North America shows the ozone depletion at different latitudes between 1969 and 1988.

posed to ultraviolet light. Losses from further decreases in the ozone layer could cost society enormous amounts of money.

In a show of solidarity on September 1988, 23 nations met in Montreal to sign an agreement to cut back on the production of many ozone-destroying chemicals. By 1999, the treaty was to achieve a 50% reduction in CFC manufacture and release. Some critics objected, saying that a 50% cut, while important, would still result in a 10% decline in the ozone layer. Clearly, greater reductions were needed. Because of these concerns and the cooperation of the CFC industry, the Montreal treaty was revised. The new plan signed in London in 1990 called for a complete phase-out of many CFCs by 1999. After recent findings suggesting an even greater loss than previously suspected, a new treaty was signed in 1992. It called for a faster phase-out of ozone-depleting chemicals and included more chemicals than previous agreements. In 1997, CFC production had been nearly eliminated.

Health, Homeostasis, and the Environment

Building a Sustainable Future

The trends and problems discussed in the previous sections could spawn a crisis of epic proportions. What many people forget when they deal with such issues is that these problems could combine to produce impacts far greater than anticipated. That is, they produce a synergistic effect. For example, soil erosion, global warming, farmland conversion, acid deposition, ozone depletion, and population growth together could produce incredible food shortages.

Solving these problems will require tougher laws and regulations, reductions in population growth, more efficient technologies, and changes in human behavior. Many people, according to opinion polls, believe that broader societal changes are required. One suggestion is that we build a **sustainable society**, one that lives within the carrying capacity of the environment. Living within the limits of nature means achieving a population size and a way of life that do not exceed the planet's ability to supply food and other resources and to handle wastes. It means promoting human societies that manage their affairs in ways that protect the Earth's homeostatic mechanisms.

Building a sustainable society will require a shift to the patterns seen in nature. It will require that we become more efficient in our use of resources; recycle to the maximum extent possible; shift to renewable resources, especially energy; restore ecosystem damage; and stabilize, if not reduce, world population.

FIGURE 24-24 Beyond Petroleum British Petroleum-Amoco, the world's largest oil company, is changing to renewable fuels. In this BP-Amoco gas station, the glass canopy not only lets light through, it produces electricity when struck by sunlight thanks to a thin film of material like that used to make calculators and watches. Solar electricity operates lights and pumps.

Building a sustainable society will also depend on a profound change in attitudes. The prevalent frontier notions of unlimited resources and human dominance over nature, say proponents, must be replaced with a new ethic, a **sustainable-Earth ethic**. This new ethic is based on three tenets: (1) the world has a limited supply of resources, which must be shared with all living things; (2) humans are a part of nature and subject to its rules; and (3) nature is not something to conquer but, rather, a force with which we must learn to cooperate. New attitudes will not come easily, but they are essential as we attempt to strike a balance with nature.

Building a sustainable society will require a lifetime of commitment on the part of businesses, governments, and individuals. Given the course of modern society, it means taking a 180-degree turn. By comparison, the moon landing will seem like a weekend fix-it project.

Some changes required to create an enduring human presence may come as a result of legislative actions—new laws and regulations—that force us to rely more heavily on conservation, recycling, and renewable resources and to restore damaged ecosystems and reach a stable, sustainable population size.

Technological innovations will also help us become a sustainable society. For example, a new line of compact fluorescent light bulbs is now available. These bulbs fit into a regular light socket and use one-fourth as much energy as a regular incandescent bulb (see **FIGURE 24-14**). Photovoltaics, thin silicon wafers that produce electricity from sunlight, could also help us make the transition to solar energy. That's how I power my home in Colorado. Water-sensing computers can help farmers prevent overwatering. Improvements in automobile efficiency can help us cut back on fossil-fuel consumption and clean up the air. But new technologies are not the only, or even the most important, answer. Many existing technologies simply need to be installed. Insulation, weather stripping, flow restrictors for shower heads and faucets, and efficient appliances already on the market can make tremendous inroads into waste.

Many proponents also believe that we will eventually need to reduce consumption and alter our lifestyles. Taking shorter showers, shaving without the water running, turning off lights, and hundreds of other small actions on the part of individuals, when combined with similar actions by millions of other people, can result in significant cuts in resource demand.

The days of profligate resource use are quickly coming to an end. Ending the waste and pollution—and soon—is crucial if we are to protect the environment and ourselves. The balance of nature is, after all, the balance that sustains us. We risk upsetting it at our own peril. Protecting the planet is the ultimate form of health-care.

Summary

1. The economy of nature and the human economy are at odds. Today, that "conflict" manifests itself in a global environmental crisis characterized by overpopulation, resource depletion, and pollution.

Overshooting the Earth's Carrying Capacity

2. Although environmental problems vary from one nation to another, they are all the result of human populations exceeding the carrying capacity of the environment.

3. *Carrying capacity* is the number of organisms an ecosystem can support indefinitely. It is determined by food and resource supplies and by the capacity of the environment to assimilate or destroy waste products of organisms.

Overpopulation: Problems and Solutions

4. *Overpopulation* occurs anytime a population overshoots its carrying capacity. It is manifest in shortages of food, lack of other resources, or excessive pollution—sometimes all three.

5. The world population is nearly 6.2 billion and is growing at a rate of 1.4% per year, a doubling time of 47 years.

6. The most rapid growth in human population is occurring in the developing world in parts of Africa, Asia, and Latin America. Resource depletion and food shortages are the most common problems in these regions.

7. Many experts believe that the industrialized countries are also overpopulated. Judging from the quality of our air, water, and soils, we are clearly exceeding the Earth's carrying capacity.

8. Because of our excessive resource demand, in fact, an average American has 20–40 times as much impact on the environment as a resident of a developing country.

9. The human population is growing exponentially. *Exponential growth* occurs anytime a value, such as population size, grows by a fixed percentage with the "interest" (increase) being applied to the base amount.

10. Exponential growth of population, resource demand, and pollution are at the heart of all environmental problems.

11. The human population problem can be summed up in six words: too many people, reproducing too rapidly. The size of our population and its rapid rate of growth result in resource shortages, excessive pollution, and poverty.

12. A decline in *total fertility rate*, the number of children a woman will have over her lifetime, to *replacement-level fertility*, the rate at which parents replace themselves, is required to reduce the rate of population growth.

Resource Depletion: Eroding the Prospects of All Organisms

13. The human population requires a variety of renewable and nonrenewable resources for survival, and many of these resources are being depleted.

14. Worldwide, forests are being cut faster than they can regenerate. Forests are important sources of wood and wood products, but they also provide wildlife habitat, protect watersheds, regenerate oxygen, and remove pollutants such as carbon dioxide.

15. To prevent the destruction of the world's forests, tree planting, paper recycling, and other strategies are needed.

16. Worldwide, soils are being eroded from rangeland and farmland at an unsustainable rate, and millions of acres of farmland are being destroyed by human encroachment. The destruction of productive soils threatens the long-term prospects for food production. Soil conservation and population control measures can help ensure an adequate supply of soil, but serious efforts must begin soon.

17. Because of regional overpopulation, many areas suffer water shortages. The rise in population and the rise in demand are likely to cause further shortages over the coming decades. Reducing the growth of the human population and strict water conservation are needed.

18. At least 18 economically important metals could fall into short supply in the next 20 years. The more efficient use of metals, recycling, and a reduction in demand are needed to help offset inevitable shortages.

19. Oil supplies, like mineral supplies, are also finite. Given the most optimistic projections of oil supplies, the world will run out of oil by 2038.

20. By reducing population growth, using oil much more efficiently, and seeking clean, renewable alternative fuels, modern society can make a smooth transition to a sustainable energy supply.

Pollution: Fouling Our Nest

21. All organisms produce waste, but humans are by far the most prolific generators of waste on the planet. Today, our waste is overwhelming nutrient cycles, poisoning other species (and ourselves), and destroying the planet's homeostatic mechanisms.

22. One of the most serious threats from pollution comes from carbon dioxide. Global atmospheric concentrations of carbon dioxide have increased 25% in the past century, in large part due to the combustion of fossil fuels and deforestation.

23. Carbon dioxide is a *greenhouse gas*, trapping heat in the Earth's atmosphere. A little carbon dioxide is beneficial, but too much will increase the planet's surface temperature, altering its climate, shifting rainfall patterns and agricultural zones, flooding low-lying regions, and destroying many species that cannot adapt to the sudden change in temperature.

24. Chlorofluorocarbons and methane are also greenhouse gases that are on the increase.

25. Many scientists believe that global warming has begun. To slow it down or stop it, they recommend massive reforestation projects and dramatic improvements in the efficiency of fossil-fuel combustion. Alternative fuels and reductions in population growth can also help.

26. Sulfur dioxide and nitrogen dioxide are two gaseous pollutants released from power plants, factories, automobiles, and other sources. In the atmosphere, they are converted to sulfuric and nitric acid, respectively.

27. Acids fall from the sky in wet and dry deposition. Acids alter the pH of lakes and streams, killing fish and other organisms. They also leach toxic metals from soils that kill fishes. They destroy trees and crops and deface buildings, costing society billions of dollars a year.

28. Pollution-control devices called *scrubbers*, which are now in use on some power plants, can remove sulfur dioxide from smokestack gases. Stopping acid rain requires a multifaceted approach, but conservation, use of cleaner coal, and pollution control devices are the three prominent strategies.

29. The ozone layer encircles the Earth, trapping ultraviolet light. It is being destroyed by chlorofluorocarbons, or CFCs, and other pollutants.

30. Fears over the decline in ozone led to several international agreements to reduce CFC production by 100% at the end of the twentieth century

Health, Homeostasis, and the Environment: Building a Sustainable Future

31. Solving our problems will not only require tougher laws and tighter regulations, but also a profound change in the way we live and conduct business.

32. A sustainable society is built on five operating principles: conservation, recycling, renewable resources, restoration, and population control.

33. A sustainable society is based on respect for nature and a willingness to cooperate with natural processes.

Critical Thinking

Thinking Critically— Analysis

This Analysis corresponds to the Thinking Critically scenario that was presented at the beginning of this chapter.

Critical thinking rules encourage us to question sources of information and their conclusions. In this example, we find that the author of this article is grossly in error when he claims that the scientific community is divided on the issue. About 99% of the nation's 700 atmospheric scientists believe that global warming is a reality; only a handful embrace the opposite view. Critics say they're on the payroll of oil companies, too. The evidence the author introduces to support his assertion—a quote from each side of the issue—is terribly misleading.

This type of reporting is quite common in newspapers, television, and magazines. Although it is intended to give a balanced view of issues, in reality it provides an extremely unbalanced view.

What would have been a more accurate conclusion? Perhaps that not all scientists agree that global warming is occurring, but that the vast majority do. It's important to note that even though the majority of the world's atmospheric scientists agree that global warming is happening, this doesn't mean they're right.

Digging a little deeper, finding out more, often throws conclusions into question.

Test of Concepts

1. In what ways are the economy of nature and the human economy working in opposite directions? In your estimation, is this a serious problem, and, if so, how can it be reduced or eliminated?

2. Human populations in both the industrialized and nonindustrialized countries are overshooting the Earth's carrying capacity. Do you agree or disagree with this statement? Be sure to describe what is meant by overshooting the carrying capacity.

3. The global human population is growing at a rate of 1.8% per year, so there's nothing to worry about. Do you agree or disagree with this statement? Support your position.

4. Why is overpopulation as much a problem in the United States as it is in Bangladesh?

5. The U.S. population fell below replacement-level fertility in 1972, yet it continues to increase. Why?

6. Describe key trends in the use of forests, soils, water, minerals, and oil suggesting that humanity is on an unsustainable course. List and discuss solutions to each of the problems.

7. Given trends in natural resource use, many experts believe that global population growth must stop. Do you agree or disagree? Why? Is your position supported by scientific fact or based more on a general feeling?

8. Describe the cause and impacts of each of the following: global warming, acid deposition, stratospheric ozone depletion, and hazardous wastes.

9. Make a list of solutions for each of the problems you identified in Question 8. How could conservation (efficiency), recycling, renewable resources, and population control factor into the solutions?

10. Explain what is meant by the following statement: A sustainable society is based on a design from nature.

11. Outline the operational and ethical principles of a sustainable society. Using your critical thinking skills, determine how they differ from the principles of modern society.

www.jbpub.com/humanbiology

Connect to this book's web site: www.jbpub.com/humanbiology
The site features eLearning, an online review area that provides quizzes, chapter outlines, and other tools to help you study for your class. You can also follow useful links for in-depth information, research the differing views in the Point/Counterpoints, or keep up on the latest environmental and health news.

Appendix A

Periodic Table of Elements

Lanthanides (rare earth metals)

| 58 Ce 140.1 | 59 Pr 140.9 | 60 Nd 144.2 | 61 Pm (145) | 62 Sm 150.4 | 63 Eu 152.0 | 64 Gd 157.3 | 65 Tb 158.9 | 66 Dy 162.5 | 67 Ho 164.9 | 68 Er 167.3 | 69 Tm 168.9 | 70 Yb 173.0 | 71 Lu 175.0 |

Actinides

| 90 Th 232.0 | 91 Pa (231) | 92 U 238.0 | 93 Np (244) | 94 Pu (242) | 95 Am (243) | 96 Cm (247) | 97 Bk (247) | 98 Cf (251) | 99 Es (252) | 100 Fm (257) | 101 Md (258) | 102 No (259) | 103 Lr (260) |

KEY

16 — Atomic number
S — Symbol of element
32.06 — Atomic mass

Metals

Nonmetals

Metalloids

Noble Gases

Appendix B

The Metric System

Most Common English Units and the Corresponding Metric Units

Measure	English Unit	Metric Unit
Weight	tons	metric tons
	pounds	kilograms
	ounces	grams
Length	miles	kilometers
	yards	meters
	inches	centimeters
Square Measure	acres	hectares
	square miles	square kilometers
Volume	quarts and gallons	liters
	fluid ounces	milliliters

Converting English Units to Metric Units

Measure	English Unit	Metric Unit
Weight	1 ton (2000 pounds)	0.9 metric tons
	1 pound	0.454 kilograms
	1 ounce	28.35 grams
Length	*1 mile	1.6 kilometers
	1 yard	0.9 meters
	*1 inch	2.54 centimeters
Square Measure	1 acre	0.4 hectares
	1 square mile	2.59 square kilometers
Volume	1 quart	0.95 liters
	*1 gallon	3.78 liters
	1 fluid ounce	29.58 milliliters

*Most useful conversions to know.

Converting Metric Units to English Units

Measure	Metric Unit	English Unit
Weight	*1 metric ton	2204 pounds
	1 metric ton	1.1 tons
	*1 kilogram	2.2 pounds
	1 gram	28.35 ounces
Length	*1 kilometer	0.6 miles
	1 meter	1.1 yards
	1 centimeter	0.39 inches
Square Measure	*1 hectare	2.47 acres
	1 square kilometer	0.386 square miles
Volume	1 liter	1.057 quarts
	1 liter	0.26 gallons
	1 milliliter	0.0338 fluid ounces

*Most useful conversions to know.

Glossary

Abiotic factors Physical and chemical components of an organism's environment.

Abortion Natural or induced expulsion of the embryo or fetus from the uterus.

Abstinence Refraining from sexual intercourse.

Accommodation Change in the shape of the lens caused by contraction or relaxation of the smooth muscle of the ciliary body. Through accommodation, the lens adjusts the degree to which incoming light rays are bent, permitting objects to be focused on the retina.

Acetylcholine Neurotransmitter substance in the central and peripheral nervous systems of humans.

Acetylcholinesterase Enzyme that destroys the neurotransmitter acetylcholine in the synaptic cleft.

Achondroplasia Genetic disease that results from an autosomal dominant gene. Individuals with the disease have short legs and arms, but a relatively normal body size.

Acid Any chemical substance that adds hydrogen ions to a solution, such as sulfuric acid.

Acid deposition Deposition of sulfuric and nitric acids in the atmosphere onto the Earth's surface. Acid deposition damages buildings, lakes, streams, crops, and forests. Acids come from sulfur dioxide and nitrogen dioxide produced during the combustion of fossil fuels.

Acid precipitation Refers to the deposition of acid in rain and snow.

Acid precursors Sulfur dioxide and nitrogen dioxide gases that combine with water and oxygen to form sulfuric and nitric acids in the atmosphere.

Acne A skin condition in males and females caused by the build-up of sebum in sebaceous glands, resulting in the formation of pimples.

Acne pimple A protrusion on the skin caused by the build-up of sebum in sebaceous glands. May become infected by bacteria.

Acromegaly A condition in adults caused by the release of excess growth hormone; causes hands and feet to grow and the bones of the face to become enlarged.

Acrosome Enzyme-filled cap over the head of a sperm. Helps the sperm dissolve its way through the corona radiata and zona pellucida of the ovum.

Actin microfilaments Contractile filaments made of protein and found in cells as part of the cytoskeleton. Especially abundant in the microfilamentous network beneath the plasma membrane and in muscle cells.

Action potential Recording of electrical change in membrane potential when a neuron is stimulated.

Activation energy The energy needed to force the electron clouds of reactants together before the formation of products; also, the energy needed to break internal chemical bonds.

Active immunity Immune resistance gained when an antigen is introduced into the body either naturally or through vaccination.

Active site The region of an enzyme molecule that binds substrates and performs the catalytic function of the enzyme.

Active transport Movement of molecules across membranes using protein molecules and energy supplied by ATP. Moves molecules and ions from regions of low to high concentration.

Adaptation Genetically based characteristic that increases an organism's chances of passing on its genes. This term is also used to describe a phenomenon in the nervous system in which pain, temperature, and pressure receptors cease generating impulses even though the stimulus remains.

Adaptive radiation Process in which one species gives rise to many others that occupy different environments. Also known as *divergent evolution.*

Adenine One of the purine bases found in nucleotides such as ATP.

Adenosine diphosphate (ADP) Precursor to ATP; consists of adenine, ribose, and two phosphates; *see also* Adenosine triphosphate.

Adenosine triphosphate (ATP) A molecule composed of ribose sugar, adenine, and three phosphate groups. The last two phosphate groups are attached by "high-energy bonds" that require considerable energy to form but release that energy again when broken. ATP serves as the major energy carrier in cells.

Adenylate cyclase Enzyme bound to the inner surface of the plasma membrane. Linked to plasma membrane hormone receptors. Responsible for the conversion of ATP to cyclic AMP (a second messenger).

Adipose tissue Type of loose connective tissue containing numerous fat cells. Important storage area for lipids.

Adolescence Period of human life from puberty until adulthood. Characterized by sexual maturity.

Adrenal cortex Outer portion of the adrenal gland. Produces a variety of steroid hormones, including cortisol and aldosterone.

Adrenal gland Endocrine gland located on top of the kidney. Consists of two parts: adrenal cortex and medulla, each with separate functions.

Adrenal medulla Inner portion of the adrenal glands. Produces epinephrine (adrenalin) and norepinephrine (noradrenalin).

Adrenalin (epinephrine) Hormone secreted under stress. Contributes to the fight-or-flight response by increasing heart rate, shunting blood to muscles, increasing blood glucose levels, and other functions.

Adrenocorticotropic hormone (ACTH) Polypeptide hormone produced by the anterior pituitary. Stimulates the cells of the adrenal cortex, causing them to synthesize and release their hormones, especially glucocorticoids.

Aerobic exercise Exercise, such as swimming, that does not deplete muscle oxygen. Excellent for strengthening the heart and for losing weight.

Age-structure diagram (population histogram) Graphical representation of the number or percentage of males and females in various age groups in a population.

Agglutination Clumping of antigens that occurs when antibodies bind to several antigens.

Aging Inevitable and progressive deterioration of the body's function, especially its homeostatic mechanisms.

AIDS Acquired immune deficiency syndrome. Fatal disease caused by the HIV virus, which attacks T helper cells, greatly reducing the body's ability to fight infection.

Albinism Genetic disease resulting in a lack of pigment in the eyes or the eyes, skin, and hair. An autosomal recessive trait.

Aldosterone Steroid released by the adrenal cortex in response to a decrease in blood pressure, blood volume, and osmotic concentration. Acts principally on the kidney.

Alga (algae, plural) Heterogeneous group of aquatic plants consisting of three major groups: green, red, and brown. Important producer essential to aquatic food chains.

Alleles Alternative form of a gene.

Allergen Antigen that stimulates an allergic response.

Allergy Extreme overreaction to some antigens, such as pollen or foods. Characterized by sneezing, mucous production, and itchy eyes.

Allopatric speciation The formation of a new species when an existing species becomes geographically separated.

Allosteric inhibition Enzyme regulation in which an inhibitor molecule binds to an enzyme at a site away from the active site, changing the shape or charge of the active site so that it can no longer bind to substrate molecules.

Allosteric site Region of an enzyme where products of metabolic pathways bind, changing the shape of the active site. In some enzymes, this prevents substrates from binding to the active site; in others, it allows them to bind. Thus, allosteric sites can either turn on or turn off enzymes.

Alpine tundra A relatively cold, treeless region similar to the Arctic tundra but found on the tops of mountains.

Altitudinal biomes Regions of a mountain, each characterized by a distinct group of plants and animals. Results from the varying climatic conditions at different altitudes.

Alveolar macrophage Also known as a *dust cell*. A mobile cell that travels through the lungs phagocytizing particulates such as dust, soot, and carbon particles inhaled from tobacco smoke.

Alveoli Tiny, thin-walled sacs in the lung where oxygen and carbon dioxide are exchanged between the blood and the air.

Alzheimer's disease A neurological disorder occuring in older adults. Characterized initially by irritability and lack of initiative, followed by gradual loss of memory.

Ameboid motion Cellular locomotion common in single-celled organisms and some cells in the human body. The cells send out slender cytoplasmic projections that attach to the substrate "ahead" of the cell. The cytoplasm flows into the projections, or pseudopodia, advancing the organism.

Amniocentesis Procedure whereby physicians extract cells and fluid from the amnion surrounding the fetus. The cells are examined for genetic defects, and the fluid is studied biochemically.

Amnion Layer of cells that separates from the inner cell mass of the embryo and eventually forms a complete sac around the fetus.

Amniotic cavity A fluid-filled cavity that forms early in embryonic development and remains throughout, providing protection for the developing embryo and fetus.

Amniotic fluid Liquid in the amniotic cavity surrounding the embryo and fetus during development. Helps protect the fetus.

Ampulla Enlarged area of each semicircular canal that houses receptor cells for movement.

Amylase Enzyme in saliva that helps break down starch molecules.

Anabolic reaction A reaction in which substances are formed; for example, the synthesis of glucose during photosynthesis is an anabolic reaction.

Anabolic steroids Synthetic androgen hormones that promote muscle development.

Analogous structures Anatomical structures that function similarly but differ in structure; for example, the wing of a bird and the wing of an insect.

Anaphase Phase of mitosis during which the chromatids of each chromosome begin to uncouple and are pulled in opposite directions with the aid of the mitotic apparatus.

Anaphylactic shock A condition caused by a massive release of histamine and other chemicals, which causes extensive dilation of blood vessels in the skin and other tissues and a drop in blood pressure, shutting down the circulatory system. Histamine released by mast cells also causes severe constriction of the bronchioles, making breathing difficult. Can result in death if not treated quickly.

Androgen A general term for any male sex hormone such as testosterone produced by the testes or adrenal cortex or synthesized in the laboratory.

Androgen-binding protein (ABP) Cytoplasmic receptor protein that binds to and concentrates testosterone within the Sertoli cell of the seminiferous tubule. Production of ABP is stimulated by FSH.

Anemia Condition characterized by an insufficient number of red blood cells in the blood or insufficient hemoglobin. Often caused by insufficient iron intake.

Anesthetic A substance used by doctors to deaden an area of the body (as in a local anesthetic) or to put a patient to sleep (general anesthetic). They operate by either blocking synaptic transmission or altering the function of the nerve cell membranes.

Aneuploidy Describes a genetic condition in which there is an abnormal number of chromosomes.

Aneurysm Ballooning of the arterial wall caused by a degeneration of the tunica media.

Angina A pain felt in the chest and left arm during heart attacks when blood flow to the heart muscle is reduced due to an occlusion of one or more of the coronary arteries.

Angiogenesis The formation of new blood vessels in tissues and malignant tumors.

Anoxia Lack of oxygen.

Antagonistic Refers to hormones or muscles that exert opposite effects.

Anterior pituitary Major portion of the pituitary gland, which is controlled by hypothalamic hormones. Produces seven protein and polypeptide hormones.

Anthropoids Monkeys, the great apes, and humans.

Antibodies Proteins produced by immune system cells that destroy or inactivate antigens, including pollen, bacteria, yeast, and viruses.

Anticodon Sequence of three bases found on the transfer RNA molecule. Aligns with the codon on messenger RNA and helps control the sequence of amino acids inserted into the growing protein.

Anticodon loop Part of the transfer RNA molecule that bears three bases that bind to the three bases of the codon on messenger RNA.

Antidiuretic hormone (ADH) Hormone released by the posterior pituitary. Increases the permeability of the distal convoluted tubule and collecting tubules, increasing water reabsorption.

Antigens Any substance that is detected as foreign by an organism and elicits an immune response. Most antigens are proteins and large molecular weight carbohydrates.

Antihistamine A drug given to people with allergies to reduce the secretion of histamine, which is responsible for many of the annoying symptoms of this condition.

Antioxidant A chemical substance that reacts with and eliminates oxidants from the body. Many plants contain naturally occurring antioxidants.

Antral follicle A large fluid-filled structure found in the ovarian cortex of sexually mature females that houses the developing egg (oocyte). When it bursts, it releases the oocyte into the oviduct. Also known as a *tertiary follicle.*

Anvil (incus) One of three bones of the middle ear that helps transmit sound waves to the receptor for sound in the inner ear.

Aorta Largest artery in the body; carries the oxygenated blood away from the heart and delivers it to the rest of the body through many branches.

Appendicitis Infection of the appendix.

Appendicular skeleton Bones of the arms, legs, shoulders, and pelvis. Contrast with axial skeleton.

Appendix A vestigial (nonfunctional) wormlike organ at the junction of the large and small intestine. May become infected, and if it is not removed, it may burst.

Aquatic life zones Ecologically distinct regions in fresh water and salt water.

Aqueous humor Liquid in the anterior and posterior chambers of the eye.

Aquifer Porous underground zone containing water.

Arctic tundra Massive biome north of taiga characterized by low precipitation and cold temperatures.

Arteries Vessels that transport blood away from the heart.

Arteriole Smallest of all arteries; usually drains into capillaries.

Arthropods Phylum of invertebrate animals with jointed appendages and chitinous exoskeletons such as insects, arachnids (spiders), and crustaceans. Many arthropods inhabit freshwater and marine ecosystems, but the vast majority live on land.

Arthroscope Device used to examine internal injuries, such as in joints.

Asbestos A naturally occuring mineral fiber with many useful applications. Unfortunately, when inhaled, it causes severe problems in the lungs, including asbestosis and two types of cancer.

Asbestosis Build-up of scar tissue in the lungs caused by inhalation of asbestos fibers.

Asexual reproduction Reproductive strategy common in single-celled organisms, such as the amoeba. Reproduction occurs by cell division.

Association cortex Area of the brain where integration occurs.

Association neurons Nerve cells that receive input from many sensory neurons and help process them, ultimately carrying impulses to nearby multipolar neurons.

Aster Array of microtubules found in the cell in association with the spindle fibers during cell division.

Atherosclerosis A disease characterized by the build-up of plaque in the linings of the arteries. Can block blood flow to vital organs.

Atherosclerotic plaque A cholesterol-rich deposit in the lining of arteries that can block blood flow.

Asthma Respiratory disease resulting from an allergic response. Allergens cause histamine to be released in the lungs. Histamine causes the air-carrying ducts (bronchioles) to constrict, cutting down airflow and making breathing difficult.

Astigmatism Unequal curvature of the cornea (sometimes the lens) that distorts vision.

Atom Smallest particles of matter that can be achieved by ordinary chemical means, consisting of protons, neutrons, and electrons.

Atomic mass unit Unit used to measure atomic weight. One atomic mass unit is 1/12 the weight of a carbon atom.

Atomic number The number assigned to each atom which corresponds to the number of protons in the nucleus of an atom.

Atomic weight Average mass of the atoms of a given element, measured in atomic mass units.

ATP *See* adenosine triphosphate.

Atrioventricular bundle Tract of modified cardiac muscle fibers that conduct the pacemaker's impulse into the ventricular muscle tissue.

Atrioventricular node (AV node) Knot of tissue located in the right ventricle. Picks up the electrical signal arriving from the atria and transmits it down the atrioventricular bundle.

Atrioventricular valves Valves between the atria and ventricles.

Auditory (eustachian) tube Collapsible tube that joins the nasopharynx and middle ear cavities and helps equalize pressure in the middle ear.

Auricle (or pinna) Skin-covered cartilage portion of the outer ear.

Autocrines Chemical substances produced by cells, which affect the function of the cells producing them.

Autoimmune reaction Immune response directed at one's own cells.

Autonomic nervous system That part of the nervous system not under voluntary control.

Autosomal dominant trait Trait that is carried on the autosomes and is expressed in heterozygotes and homozygote dominants.

Autosomal recessive trait Trait that is carried on the autosomes and is expressed only when both recessive genes are present.

Autosomes All human chromosomes except the sex chromosomes.

Autotrophs Organisms such as plants and algae that, unlike animals, are able to synthesize their own food.

Axial skeleton The skull, vertebral column, and rib cage. Contrast with appendicular skeleton.

Axon Long, unbranched process attached to the nerve cell body of a neuron. Transports bioelectric impulses away from the cell body.

B cell *See* B lymphocyte.

B lymphocyte A lymphocyte that is converted into a plasma cell which produces antibodies to ward off infections.

Bacteria Widely distributed group of microscopic prokaryotic organisms that serve many useful functions, although some species can cause illnesses that are sometimes severe.

Bacterial toxin Any one of several toxic chemicals produced by disease-causing bacteria.

Balanced diet A diet containing all of the nutrients in proper amounts for good health.

Ball-and-socket joint A joint in which the articular surface of one bone is shaped like a ball; the other is a cavity in which the gall fits. Example: hip joint.

Balloon angioplasty The expansion of a clogged artery of the heart carried out by a physician using a device that is snaked through the blood vessels of the heart. Once the clogged section is located, the balloon is expanded to open the artery. A small metal device called a *stent* is usually inserted in the vessel to keep it open.

Basal body Organelle located at the base of the cilium and flagellum. Consists of nine sets of microtubules arranged in a circle. Each "set" contains three microtubules.

Basilar membrane Membrane that supports the organ of Corti in the cochlea.

Batesian mimicry Strategy in which one species evolves a warning coloration similar to a species with active defense mechanisms such that the imitating species benefits from the outward similarity.

Behavior An individual's response to environmental stimuli such as other individuals of the same species, members of other species, or some aspect of the physical environment.

Benign tumor Abnormal cellular proliferation. Unlike a malignant tumor, the cells in a benign tumor stop growing after a while, and the tumor remains localized.

Beta cells Insulin-producing cells of the islets of Langerhans in the pancreas.

Bicuspid valve The valve between the right atrium and right ventricles of the heart.

Bile Fluid produced by the liver and stored and concentrated in the gallbladder.

Bile salts Steroids produced by the liver, stored in the gallbladder, and released into the small intestine, where they emulsify fats, a step necessary for enzyme digestion.

Binary fission Bacterial cellular division.

Bioelectric impulse Nerve impulse resulting from the influx of sodium ions along the plasma membrane of a neuron.

Biogeochemical cycle Same as a nutrient cycle.

Biological community An multispecies assemblage of organisms occupying the same region.

Biomass The dry weight of living material in an ecosystem.

Biomass pyramid Diagram of the amount of biomass at each trophic level in an ecosystem or, more commonly, a food chain.

Biome Terrestrial region characterized by a distinct climate and a characteristic plant and animal community.

Biorhythms (biological cycles) Naturally fluctuating physiological process.

Biosphere Region on Earth that supports life. Exists at the junction of the atmosphere, lithosphere, and hydrosphere.

Biotic factor Biological components of ecosystems.

Bipedal Refers to the ability to walk on two legs.

Birth control Any method or device that prevents conception and birth.

Birth control pill Pill generally taken to inhibit ovulation. The most commonly used pills contain both synthetic estrogen and progesterone.

Birth defects Physical or physiological defects in newborns. Caused by a variety of biological, chemical, and physical factors.

Blastocyst The early embryo formed from the morula. Contains an inner fluid-filled cavity. Consists of the inner cell mass and the trophoblast.

Blind spot That portion of the retina at which the neurons converge to form the optic nerve. Because no photo receptors are present at this site, it is insensitive to light.

Blood Specialized form of connective tissue. Consists of white blood cells, platelets, red blood cells, and plasma.

Blood clot Mass of fibrin containing platelets, red blood cells, and other cells. Forms in walls of damaged blood vessels, halting the efflux of blood.

Blood pressure The force that propels blood through the arteries of the body. Generated by the pumping of the heart and the ballonlike contraction of musular and elastic arteries.

B-lymphocytes Type of lymphocyte that transforms into a plasma cell when exposed to antigens.

Bone (organ) Structure composed of bone tissue. Provides internal support, protects organs, and helps maintain blood calcium levels.

Bone (tissue) Tissue consisting of a calcified extracellular material with numerous cells (osteocytes) embedded in it.

Boreal forest Same as Northern Coniferous biome.

Bowman's capsule Cup-shaped end of the nephron that participates in glomerular filtration.

Bowman's space Cavity between the inner and outer layer of Bowman's capsule.

Bradley method Technique used by women during childbirth. Teaches relaxation during uterine contractions to reduce pain and the need for pain-killing drugs. No special breathing is required. Contrast with the Lamaze technique.

Brain stem Part of the brain that consists of the medulla and pons. Houses structures such as the breathing control center and reticular activating systems that control many basic body functions.

Braxton-Hicks contractions Contractions that begin a month or two before childbirth. Also known as *false labor.*

Breast Female external genitalia. Produces milk to nourish infants.

Breathing center Aggregation of nerve cells in the brain stem that controls breathing.

Breech birth Delivery of a baby feet first.

Bronchi Ducts that convey air from the trachea to the bronchioles and alveoli.

Bronchioles Smallest ducts in the lungs. Their walls are largely made of smooth muscle that contracts and relaxes, regulating the flow of air into the lungs.

Bronchitis Infection or persistent irritation of the bronchi characterized by cough.

Budding A type of asexual reproduction in which new organisms form from evaginations or buds that develop in adult form.

Buffer A chemical substance that helps resist changes in acidity.

Bulimia Eating disorder characterized by recurrent binge eating followed by vomiting.

Caeserian section A surgical technique used to deliver a baby involving an incision in the lower abdomen and uterus. Used when birth is prolonged or complications arise (e.g., the umbilical cord wraps around the baby's neck)

Calcitonin (thyrocalcitonin) Polypeptide hormone produced by the thyroid gland that inhibits osteoclasts and stimulates osteoblasts to produce bone, thus lowering blood calcium levels.

Callus A bridge between ends of a broken bone. Made of collagen.

Canaliculi Tiny canals in compact bone that provide a route for nutrients and wastes to flow to and from the osteocytes.

Cancer Any of dozens of diseases, all characterized by the uncontrollable replication of various body cells.

Capillaries Tiny vessels in body tissues whose walls are composed of a flattened layer of cells that allow water and other molecules to flow freely into and out of the tissue fluid.

Capillary bed Branching network of capillaries supplied by arterioles and drained by venules.

Capsid Protein coat of a virus.

Capsomere Globular proteins that make up the capsid of viruses.

Carbohydrate Organic compound consisting of carbon, hydrogen, and oxygen. A structural component of plant cells, it is used principally as a source of energy in animal cells.

Carbon cycle Nutrient cycle responsible for the recycling of carbon dioxide.

Carbon monoxide A clear, odorless gase given off during the incomplete combustion of fossil fuels and other forms of organic matter. Binds with hemoglobin in the blood, reducing the ability of RBCs to carry oxygen.

Carbonic anhydrase Enzyme found in red blood cells that catalyzes the conversion of carbon dioxide to carbonic acid.

Carcinogens A general term used to describe any chemical, biological, or physical agent that is involved in the conversion of normal body cells to malignant ones. Includes promoters and co-carcinogens.

Cardiac muscle Type of muscle found in the walls of the heart; it is striated and involuntary.

Cardiac output The amount of blood that is pumped by the heart in a given period. Related to heart rate and stroke volume, the amount of blood pumped with each contraction of the heart.

Cardiopulmonary resuscitation Also known as CPR. A technique used to revive people whose hearts have stopped beating that involves application of pressure on the breast bone over the heart. During this procedure air must be forced into the lungs either orally or using a special bag-like device.

Carnivores Meat eaters; organisms that feed on other animals.

Carotid artery Large, muscular artery that supplies the brain.

Carrier proteins Class of proteins that transport smaller molecules and ions across the plasma membrane of the cell. Are involved in facilitated diffusion.

Carriers Individuals who carry a gene for a particular trait that can be passed on to their children, but who do not express the trait.

Carrion Dead remains of animals consumed by scavengers.

Carrying capacity The number of organisms an ecosystem can support on a sustainable basis.

Cartilage Type of specialized connective tissue. Found in joints on the articular surfaces of bones and other locations such as the ears and nose.

Catabolic reaction A reaction in which molecules are broken down; for example, the breakdown of glucose is a catabolic reaction.

Catalyst Class of compounds that speed up chemical reactions. Although they take an active role in the process, they are left unchanged by the reaction. Thus, they can be used over and over again. Catalysts lower the activation energy of a reaction. *See also* Enzyme.

Cataracts Disease of the eye resulting in cloudy spots on the lens (and sometimes the cornea) that cause cloudy vision.

Cauda equina Term used to describe the many spinal nerves that emanate from the terminal end of the spinal cord.

Cavity A small to large depression in the enamel of teeth produced by acids released from bacteria trapped by plaque on the teeth.

Cecum The pouchlike structure at the junction of the small and large intestine. The appendix is attached to the cecum.

Cell body Part of the nerve cell that contains the nucleus and other cellular organelles; the center of chemical synthesis.

Cell culture Glass bottle or shallow dish containing nutrient medium and designed to permit cells to grow in the laboratory under controlled conditions.

Cell cycle Repeating series of events in the lives of many cells. Consists of two principal parts: interphase and cellular division.

Cell division Process by which the nucleus and the cytoplasm of a cell are split, creating two daughter cells. Consists of mitosis and cytokinesis.

Cell wall A thick, fairly rigid layer surrounding bacterial cells.

Cellular respiration The complete breakdown of glucose in the cell, producing carbon dioxide and water. Composed of four separate but interconnected parts: glycolysis, the intermediate reaction, the citric acid cycle, and the electron transport system.

Cellulose A water-insoluble fiber made of many molecules of glucose and found in many plants.

Central nervous system The brain and spinal cord.

Centriole Organelle consisting of a ring of microtubules, arranged in nine sets of three. Structurally identical to basal bodies, but associated with the spindle apparatus. Gives rise to the basal body in ciliated cells.

Centromere The region of the chromosome to which the spindle fibers attach. Participates in chromosome movement during mitosis and meiosis.

Cerebellum Structure of the brain that lies above the pons and medulla. It has many important functions including synergy.

Cerebral cortex Outer layer of each cerebral hemisphere, consisting of many multipolar neurons and nerve cell fibers.

Cerebral hemisphere Convoluted mass of nervous tissue located above the deeper structures, such as the hypothalamus and limbic system. Home of consciousness, memory, and sensory perception; originates much conscious motor activity.

Cerebral palsy A neurological disorder usually caused by an interruption of blood flow to the brain at birth. Mild cases result in slight rigidity of muscles (called *spasticity*). More severe cases result in serious problems controlling muscles of speech and skeletal muscles involved in movement.

Cerebrospinal fluid (CSF) A watery fluid found in the ventricles of the brain, in the meninges of the brain and spinal cord.

Cerebrum The largest portion of the brain consisting of two cerebral hemispheres.

Cervical cap Birth control device consisting of a small cup that fits over the tip of the cervix.

Cervix Lowermost portion of the uterus; it protrudes into the vagina.

Cesarean section Delivery of a baby via an incision through the abdominal and uterine walls.

Chemical equilibrium The point at which the "forward" reaction from reactants to products proceeds at the same rate as the "backward" reaction from products to reactants, so that there is no net change in chemical composition.

Chemical evolution Formation of organic molecules from inorganic molecules early in the history of the Earth.

Chemiosmosis Production of ATP in the chloroplast's and the mitochondrion's electron transport systems. H^+ flowing through pores in ATPase molecules drives the endergonic synthesis of ATP.

Chemoreceptor Any sensory receptor that detects levels of ions and chemicals in the blood or cerebrospinal fluid.

Chemosynthetic organisms Autotrophic cells that lack chlorophyll and acquire electrons from inorganic molecules.

Chemotherapy Refers to the treatment of cancers using cancer-killing drugs administered alone or in conjunction with radiation or surgery.

Chlamydia Bacterium that causes nonspecific urethritis, a type of sexually transmitted disease.

Chlorofluorocarbons (CFCs) Chemical substances once used as spray can propellants and refrigerants. These substances drift to the upper stratosphere and dissociate. Chlorine released by CFCs reacts with ozone, thus eroding the ozone layer.

Chlorophyll A green pigment that acts as the primary light-trapping molecule for photosynthesis.

Cholecystokinin (CCK) Hormone produced by cells of the lining of the duodenum when chyme is present. Causes the gallbladder to contract, releasing bile.

Chordae tendineae Tendinous cords that anchor the atrioventricular valves to the inner walls of the ventricles.

Chorionic villus biopsy Medical procedure to detect genetic defects; involves removing a small portion of the villi and then examining it for chromosomal abnormalities.

Choroid Middle layer of the eye that absorbs stray light and supplies nutrients to the eye.

Chromatid Strand of the chromosome consisting of DNA and protein.

Chromatin Long, threadlike fibers containing DNA and protein in the nucleus.

Chromosome A strand of DNA and protein found in the nucleus of cells that houses the genetic information.

Chromosome-to-pole fibers Microtubules of the spindle that extend from the centriole to the chromosome where they attach. They play a crucial role in separating the double-stranded chromosomes during mitosis.

Chronic bronchitis Persistent irritation of the bronchi, which causes mucous build-up, coughing, and difficulty breathing.

Chylomicrons Small globules of fat found in cells lining the small intestine.

Chyme Liquified food in the stomach.

Ciliary body Portion of the middle layer of the eye that is located near the lens. Contains smooth muscle that constricts, thus helping control the shape of the lens and permitting the eye to focus.

Cilia Tiny motile surface projections from certain cells of the body like those lining the respiratory tract. Cilia aid in the movement of mucus or fluids along the surface of the cells.

Circadian rhythm Biorhythm that occurs on a daily cycle.

Circulatory system Organ system consisting of the heart, blood vessels, and blood.

Circumcision Operation to remove the foreskin of the penis. Generally performed on newborns.

Cisterna Channels of the endoplasmic reticulum and Golgi.

Citric acid Six-carbon compound produced in the first reaction of the citric acid or Krebs cycle. Formed when oxaloacetate reacts with acetyl Coenzyme A.

Citric acid cycle A cyclic series of reactions in which the pyruvates produced by glycolysis are broken down to CO_2, accompanied by the formation of ATP and electron carriers. Occurs in the matrix of mitochondria.

Class Subgroup of a phylum.

Clitoris Small knot of tissue located where the labia minora meet. Consists of erectile tissue.

Clone Refers to an organism produced from cells of another.

Cloning Technique of genetic engineering whereby many copies of a gene are produced. Also refers to a technique in which the nucleus of an organism is transferred to an enucleated egg, then allowed to develop, producing an organism identical to the one whose nucleus was used. Clones can be produced by cells taken from embryos, too.

Closed system System that receives no materials from the outside.

Coacervates Microscopic globules that selectively incorporate molecules from their environment. Coacervates existing on Earth over 3 billion years ago may have given rise to the earliest cells.

Co-carcingoen A chemical, biological, or physical agent that causes a mutation in one of the many genes of a cell involved in replication. This step is the first step in the production of a malignant tumor.

Cochlea Sensory organ of the inner ear that houses the receptor for hearing.

Cochlear implant A small device that picks up sound, then transmits it to electrodes that are imbedded in the vestibulocochlear nerve. It enables deaf people to hear.

Codominant gene Refers to two equally expressed alleles.

Codon Three adjacent bases in the messenger RNA that code for a single amino acid.

Coelom Body cavity (a space between the body wall and internal organs) lined by mesoderm.

Coevolution Process in which two or more species act as selective forces on each other, resulting in anatomical, behavioral, and functional changes in each other.

Coitus interruptus A fairly ineffective form of birth control involving the withdrawl of the penis from the vagina right before ejaculation.

Collagen A protein found in the body in connective tissue, cartilage, and bone.

Collecting tubules Tubules in the kidney into which nephrons drain. They converge and drain into the renal pelvis.

Colon Another name for the large intestine.

Color blindness Condition that occurs in individuals who have a deficiency of certain cones. The most common form involves difficulty in distinguishing between red and green.

Colostrum Protein-rich product of the breast, produced for two to three days immediately after delivery and prior to milk production.

Community All of the plants, animals, and microorganisms in an ecosystem.

Compact bone Dense bony tissue in the outer portion of all bones.

Competition Struggle by two or more individuals for the same limited resource.

Competitive exclusion principle A natural law stating no two organisms can occupy the exact same niche.

Complement system Group of blood proteins that circulate in the blood in an inactive state until the body is invaded by bacteria; then they help destroy the bacteria.

Complementary base pairing Unalterable coupling of the purine adenine to the pyrimidine thymine, and the purine guanine to the pyrimidine cytosine. Responsible for the accurate transmission of genetic information from parent to offspring.

Complementary strand A strand of DNA produced on a template formed when the double-stranded DNA molecule unwinds.

Complete protein A protein that contains all of the amino acids one needs for a healthy life-style. Contast with incomplete protein.

Compound A chemical substance that consists of two or more atoms.

Condom Birth control device, consisting of a thin latex rubber sheath or other material that is rolled onto the erect penis. Prevents sperm from entering the vagina and helps prevent the spread of sexually transmitted diseases.

Conduction deafness Loss of hearing that occurs when the conduction of sound waves to the inner ear is impaired. May be caused by ruptured eardrum or damage to ossicles.

Cone Type of photoreceptor that operates in bright light; is responsible for color vision.

Connective tissue One of the primary tissues. It contains cells and varying amounts of extracellular material and holds cells together, forming tissues and organs.

Connective tissue proper Name referring to loose and dense connective tissue; supports and joins various body structures.

Constipation Blockage of the large intestine by dry fecal matter.

Consumers Organisms that eat plants and algae (producers) and other consumers.

Contact inhibition Cessation of growth that results when two or more cells contact each other. A feature of normal cells but absent in cancer cells.

Continental shelf Gradually sloping ocean bottom next to continents.

Contraception Practice of birth control using preventive means such as condoms, diaphragms, or birth control pills.

Contraceptive Any measure that helps prevent fertilization and pregnancy.

Contractile vacuole Vacuole in amoeboid protists that collects excess water from the cytoplasm and, when full, contracts, voiding the water through a temporary opening in the plasma membrane.

Control group A group of subjects (plants, animals, etc.) that is used in an experiment; this group is identical to the experimental group in all regards except that it does not receive the experimental treatment.

Convergence Inward turning of the eyes to focus on a nearby object.

Conversion The first step in the production of cancer. Usually involves a mutation caused by a chemical, physical, or biological agent in one of the many genes of the cell that control the replication of cells.

Coral reef Biologically rich life zones, found in relatively warm and shallow waters in the tropics or nearby regions consisting of calcium carbonate or limestone produced by calcarous red and green algae and by colonies of organisms called stony corals.

Corepressor Molecule that binds to a repressor protein, allowing it to bind to the operator site, which, in turn, shuts down the structural genes by blocking RNA polymerase.

Cornea Clear part of the wall of the eye continuous with the sclera; allows light into the interior of the eye.

Coronary bypass surgery Surgical technique used to reestablish blood flow to the heart muscle by grafting a vein to shunt blood around a clogged coronary artery.

Corpus luteum (CL) Structure formed from the ovulated follicle in the ovary; produces estrogen and progesterone.

Cortical granules Secretory vesicles lying beneath the plasma membrane of the oocyte that are released when a sperm cell contacts the oocyte membrane. They block additional sperm from fertilizing the ovum.

Cortisol Glucocorticoid hormone that increases blood glucose by stimulating gluconeogenesis. Also stimulates protein breakdown in muscle and bone.

Coupled reactions A pair of reactions, one exergonic and one endergonic, that are linked so that the energy produced by the exergonic reaction provides the energy to drive the endergonic reaction.

Cowper's gland Smallest of the sex accessory glands; empties into the urethra.

Cranial nerves Nerves arising from the brain and brain stem.

Creatine phosphate High-energy molecule in skeletal muscle.

Creationist A term used to describe an individual who subscribes to the view that God created the Earth and living things. Generally opposed to the idea of evolution.

Cristae Folds formed by the inner membrane of the mitochondrion.

Critical thinking Process in which one seeks to determine the validity of conclusions based on sound reasoning. This often requires one to examine hidden bias, the appropriateness of experimental design, and other factors.

Cro-Magnons Earliest known members of *Homo sapiens sapiens*.

Crossing over Exchange of chromatin by homologous chromosomes during prophase I of meiosis. Increases genetic variation in gametes and offspring.

Crystallin Protein inside the lens that may denature, causing cataracts.

Culture The ideas, customs, skills, and arts of a given people at a given time that can change or evolve over time.

Cushing's disease Disease that results from pharmacologic doses of cortisone usually administered for rheumatoid arthritis or allergies.

Cyanobacteria The most abundant of the photosynthetic bacteria; once called blue-green algae.

Cyclic AMP Nucleotide derived from ATP. Its synthesis is stimulated when protein and polypeptide hormones bind to the plasma membrane of cells. In the cytoplasm, it activates protein kinase, which, in turn, activates other enzymes.

Cyclosporin One of numerous drugs used to suppress graft rejection.

Cystic fibrosis Autosomal recessive disease that leads to problems in sweat glands, mucous glands, and the pancreas. Pancreas may become blocked, thus reducing the flow of digestive enzymes to the small intestine. Mucus build-up in the lungs makes breathing difficult.

Cytokinesis Cytoplasmic division brought about by the contraction of a microfilamentous network lying beneath the plasma membrane at the midline. Usually begins when the cell is in late anaphase or early telophase.

Cytoplasm Material occupying the cytoplasmic compartment of a cell. Consists of a semifluid substance, the cytosol, containing many dissolved substances, and formed elements, the organelles.

Cytosine A nitrogen-containing base known as a pyrimidine and found in RNA and DNA.

Cytoskeleton A network of protein tubules in the cytoplasmic compartment of a cell. Attaches to many organelles and enzyme molecules and thus helps organize cellular activities, increasing efficiency.

Cytotoxic T cells Type of T cell (T-lymphocyte) that attacks and kills virus-infected cells, parasites, fungi, and tumor cells.

Darwin, Charles An eighteenth century British naturalist who with Alfred Russell Wallace, another scientist working independently, proposed the theory of natual selection.

Daughter cells Cells produced during cell division.

Decibel Unit used to measure the intensity of sound.

Deciduous Term referring to trees that shed their leaves during the fall.

Decomposer Any organism involved in the decomposition of organic matter. Includes many species of bacteria and fungi.

Decomposer food chain Series of organisms that feed on organic wastes and the dead remains of other organisms.

Defecation reflex An automatic response that causes feces to be voided in babies. The reflex is present in adults but is overridden by conscious control.

Defibrillation Procedure to stop fibrillation (erratic electrical activity) of the heart.

Deletion Loss of a piece of a chromosome.

Demographer Scientist who studies populations.

Dendrite Short, highly branched fiber that carries impulses to the nerve cell body.

Dense connective tissue Type of connective tissue that consists primarily of densely packed fibers, such as those found in ligaments and tendons.

Deoxyribonuclease Pancreatic enzyme that breaks RNA and DNA into shorter chains.

Deoxyribonucleic Acid *See* DNA.

Demineralized bone matter A collagen-rich material produced by dissolving away the minerals found in bone. Used to repair bones.

Depolarization Refers to a change in the potential difference, measured in millivolts, occurring across the plasma membrane when muscle cells and nerve cells are stimulated.

Depth perception Ability to judge the relative position of objects in our visual field. Also known as *stereoscopic vision.*

Dermis Layer of dense irregular connective tissue that binds the epidermis to underlying structures.

Desert Biome characterized by low rainfall and a hot climate. Contains organisms well adapted to these conditions.

Detrivores Organisms that feed on animal waste or the remains of plants and animals.

Development and progression The second stage in the formation of malignant cells during which converted cells are fully released by a promoter from constraints that keep it from dividing uncontrollably.

Diabetes insipidus Condition caused by lack of the pituitary hormone ADH. Main symptoms are polydipsia (excessive drinking) and polyuria (excessive urination).

Diabetes mellitus Insulin disorder either resulting from insufficient insulin production or decreased sensitivity of target cells to insulin. Results in elevated blood glucose levels unless treated.

Dialysis Procedure used to treat patients whose kidneys have failed. Blood is removed from the body and pumped through an artificial filter that removes impurities.

Diaphragm (birth control) Birth control device consisting of a rubber cup that fits over the end of the cervix. Used in conjunction with spermicidal jelly or cream.

Diaphragm (muscle) Dome-shaped muscle that separates the abdominal and thoracic cavities.

Diaphysis Shaft of the long bones. Consists of an outer layer of compact bone and an inner marrow cavity.

Diastolic pressure The pressure at the moment the heart relaxes. The lower of the two blood pressure readings.

Differentiation Structural and functional divergence from the common cell line. Occurs during embryonic development.

Diffusion The movement of molecules or ions from a region of high concentration to a region of low concentration.

Dihybrid cross Procedure where one plant is bred with another to study two traits.

Dilation stage The first stage during birth. Characterized by the dilation of the cervix due to the pressure placed upon it by the baby.

Diploid A term used to describe a cell that has the full number of chromosomes. In humans, it would refer to all cells that contain 46 chromosomes—half from the mother and half from the father. Contrast with haploid.

Diplopia Double vision. May occur when the eyes fail to move synchronously.

Disaccharide A carbohydrate like sucrose consisting of two monosaccharides.

Dislocation Refers to an injury of a joint in which one of the bones is dislodged from its normal position.

Distal convoluted tubule Section of the nephron that connects the loop of Henle to the collecting tubule. Site of tubular reabsorption.

Diuretic Any substance that increases the excretion of water by the kidneys; for example, caffeine.

Divergent evolution Process in which organisms evolve in different directions due to exposure to different environmental influences. Synonymous with adaptive radiation.

Diverticulitis Expansion of the large intestine due to obstruction.

DNA The genetic material of all living organisms. Consists of two polynucleotide strands (consisting of many nucleotides) that form a double helix. In the nucleus of cells, DNA is associated with protein to form chromosomes.

DNA fingerprinting Use of DNA taken from the scene of a crime to determine culpable parties.

DNA ligase An enzyme used in genetic engineering to attach a piece of inserted DNA into a vacant segment of another.

DNA polymerase Enzyme that helps align the nucleotides and join the phosphates and sugar molecules in a newly forming DNA strand.

DNA probe Small fragments of single-stranded DNA produced by DNA synthesizers. Used to determine the sequence of bases in DNA during criminalistic inquiries and in mapping chromosomes.

DNA-reactive carcinogens Chemical, biological, or physical agents that react with genes to stimulate the production of a cancer.

Dominant Adjective used in genetics to refer to an allele that is always expressed in heterozygotes. Designated by a capital letter.

Dorsal root (of a spinal nerve) Inlet for sensory nerve fibers to the spinal cord.

Double helix Describes the helical structure formed by two polynucleotide chains making up the DNA molecule.

Doubling time Time it takes a population to double.

Down syndrome Genetic disorder caused by an additional chromosome 21 that results in distinctive facial characteristics and mental retardation. Also known as *Trisomy 21*.

Dry deposition Refers to the deposition of acid precursors such as sulfur dioxide or sulfate particulates independently of precipitation such as rain or snow.

Dryopithecus Genus of apelike creatures that is thought to have given rise to the gibbons, gorillas, orangutans, and chimpanzees.

Duodenum First portion of the small intestine; site where most food digestion and absorption takes place.

Dust cell Also known as an *alveolar macrophage*. Cell found in and around the alveoli; phagocytizes particulate matter that has entered the lung.

Dynamic balance Balance maintained while an individual is moving.

Eardrum Also known as the *tympanic membrane.*

E. coli Common bacterium that lives in the large intestine of humans and other mammals. Digests leftover glucose and other materials from food. Used in much genetic research.

ECG *See* electrocardiogram.

Ecological niche An organism's habitat and all of the relationships that exist between that organism and its environment.

Ecological system (ecosystem) System consisting of organisms and their environment and all of the interactions that exist between these components.

Ecology Study of living organisms and the web of relationships that binds them together in the economy of nature. The study of ecosystems.

Ecosystem *See* eological system.

Ecosystem balance Dynamic equilibrium in ecosystems. Maintained by the interplay of growth and reduction factors.

Ectoderm One of the three types of cells that emerges in human embryonic development. Gives rise to the skin and associated structures, including the eyes.

Ectopic pregnancy A pregnancy occurring outside the body of the uterus often in the oviducts (called a *tubal pregnancy*). Fetus or embryo must usually be removed to protect the mother's life.

Edema Swelling resulting from the build-up of fluid in the tissues.

Effector General term for any organ or gland that is controlled by the nervous system.

Ejaculate The product of ejaculation in males; a fluid containing sperm and secretions of the sex accessory glands. Also known as *semen.*

Ejaculation Ejection of semen from the male reproductive tract.

EKG *See* electrocardiogram.

Elastic arteries Arteries that contain numerous elastic fibers interspersed among the smooth muscle cells of the tunica media.

Elastic cartilage Type of cartilage containing many elastic fibers found in regions where support and flexibility are required.

Electrocardiogram A graph showing the electrical activity of the heart as it pumps blood throughout the body. Also known as an *EKG* or *ECG.*

Electroencephalogram (EEG) A recording of the electrical activity of the brain used to diagnose neurological disorders.

Electron Highly energetic particle carrying a negative charge that orbits the nucleus of an atom.

Electron carrier A molecule that can reversibly gain and lose electrons. Electron carriers generally accept high-energy electrons produced during an exergonic reaction and donate the electrons to acceptor molecules that use the energy to drive endergonic reactions.

Electron cloud A region surrounding the nucleus of an atom where electrons orbit.

Electron microscope A microscope that uses a beam of electrons cast on a thin slice of tissue that allows researchers to examine the detailed structure of cells. There are two types, scanning electron microscopes, which produce a detailed topographical view, and transmission electron microscopes, which allow researchers to see the internal structures of cells and organs.

Electron transport system Series of protein molecules in the inner membrane of the mitochondrion that pass electrons from the citric acid cycle from one to another, eventually donating them to oxygen. The electrons come from the citric acid cycle. During their journey along this chain of proteins, the electrons lose energy, which is used to make ATP. *See also* Chemiosmosis.

Elements Purest form of matter; substances that cannot be separated into different substances by chemical means.

Emphysema Progressive, debilitating disease that destroys the tiny air sacs in the lung (alveoli), caused by smoking and air pollution.

Enamel The extremely hard, white outer layer on teeth.

Endergonic reaction A chemical reaction that requires an input of energy to proceed.

Endochondral ossification The formation of bone from a hyaline cartilage template in the fetus.

Endocrine glands Glands of internal secretion that produce hormones secreted into the bloodstream.

Endocrine system Numerous, small, hormone-producing glands scattered throughout the body.

Endocytosis Process by which cells engulf solid particles, bacteria, viruses, and even other cells.

Endoderm One of the three types of cells that emerges during embryonic development. Gives rise to the intestinal tract and associated glands.

Endolymph Fluid inside the semicircular canals that deflects the cupula, signaling rotational movement of the head and body.

Endometrium Uterine endothelium or lining.

Endoplasmic reticulum Branched network of channels found throughout the cytoplasm of many cells. Formed from flattened sheets of membrane derived from the nuclear membrane. *See* rough and smooth endoplasmic reticulum for functions.

Endosymbiotic evolution Theory that accounts for the development of the first eukaryotes. Says that free-living bacteria-like organisms were engulfed by other cells and became internal symbionts. Internal symbionts later became the organelles of eukaryotes.

Endothelium Single-celled lining of blood vessels.

End-product inhibition The inhibition of an enzyme by a product of the chemical reaction it catalyzes or by the product of a series of chemical reactions of which the enzyme is a part; may result from binding of the end product to the allosteric site or active site of the enzyme.

Energy The capacity to do work.

Energy carrier A molecule that stores energy in "high-energy" chemical bonds and releases the energy again to drive coupled endergonic reactions. ATP is the most common energy carrier in cells; NAD and FAD are others.

Energy pyramid Diagram of the amount of energy at various trophic levels in a food chain or ecosystem.

Enhancement An increase of gene activity caused by an enhancer.

Enhancer Segment of DNA that increases the activity of nearby genes several hundred times.

Envelope Protective membrane of some viruses; lies outside the capsid.

Environmental resistance Refers to the biotic and abiotic factors in an environment that reduce the size of populations.

Enzyme A protein catalyst that speeds up the rate of specific biochemical reactions.

Epidemiology The study of diseases in populations using statistical methods to find links between causes and diseases.

Epidermis Outermost layer of the skin that protects underlying tissues from drying out and from bacteria and viruses.

Epididymal duct Duct within the epididymis; site where sperm are stored until ejaculation.

Epididymis Storage site of sperm. Located on the testis, it consists of a long, tortuous duct, the epididymal duct.

Epidural anaesthesia A procedure in which a pain-killing drug is injected into the fluid surrounding the spinal cord. Given to a women prior to the birth of a child.

Epigenetic carcinogen Any agent that causes a cancer to form through ways that do not involve mutations of the growth-control genes of the cell.

Epiglottis Flap of tissue that closes off the trachea during swallowing.

Epilepsy A neurological disorder characterized by seizures (rapid firing of many neurons in the brain) often accompanied by involuntary spasms of skeletal muscles and alterations in behavior.

Epilimnion The warm-water layer of a lake located along the surface.

Epiphyseal plate Band of cartilage cells between the shaft of the bone and the epiphysis. Allows for bone growth.

Epiphysis Expanded end of the long bones.

Episiotomy Surgical incision that runs from the vaginal opening toward the rectum. Enlarges the vaginal opening, easing childbirth.

Epithelium One of the primary tissues. Forms linings and external coatings of organs.

Erectile tissue Spongy tissue of the penis that fills with blood during sexual excitement, making the penis turgid.

Erythropoietin Hormone produced by the kidney when oxygen levels decline. Stimulates red blood cell production in the bone marrow. Also known as *EPO*.

Esophagus Muscular tube that transports food to the stomach.

Essential amino acid One of eight amino acids that must be provided in the human diet.

Estuarine zone Estuary and coastal wetland. One of the richest coastal life zones.

Euchromatin Metabolically active chromatin.

Euglenoids Protists with characteristics of both plants and animals. They get their name from the best-known of their kind, Euglena.

Eukaryote Any cell containing a distinct nucleus and organelles. They are found in single-celled organisms of the kingdom Protista and all multicellular organisms of the kingdoms Plantae, Animalia, and Fungi.

Euthanasia Refers to active (withholding life-saving treatment) and passive (lethal injection) means to bring about a person's death.

Evolution Process that leads to structural, functional, and behavioral changes in species, making them better able to survive in their environment; also leads to the formation of new species. Results from natural genetic variation and environmental conditions that select for organisms best suited to their environment.

Evolutionary tree A graphical representation of evolution showing relationships between various organisms.

Excretion The release of materials from glands via ducts or from the body as in the excretion of feces.

Excretory organs Any of several organs like the kidney and intestinal tract that help rid waste from the body.

Exergonic reaction A chemical reaction that releases energy.

Exhalation Expulsion of air from the lungs.

Exocrine gland Gland of external secretion; empties its contents into ducts.

Exocytosis Process by which cells release materials stored in secretory vesicles. The reverse of endocytosis.

Exon Expressed segment of DNA.

Exophthalmos Bulging eyes caused by swelling of surrounding tissues in patients with hyperthyroidism.

Experiment Test performed to support or refute an hypothesis.

Expiration Same as exhalation.

Exponential growth Type of growth that occurs when a value grows by a fixed percentage and the increase is applied to the base amount.

Expulsion stage The phase in which the baby is expelled from the uterus through the vagina into the world.

Extension Movement of a body part (limbs, fingers, and toes) that opens a joint.

External auditory canal Channel that directs sound waves to the eardrum.

External genitalia External portion of the female reproductive system consisting of the clitoris, labia minora, and labia majora.

External sphincter of the bladder Voluntary muscular valve that controls urine release under conscious control. Formed by a flat band of muscle that forms the floor of the pelvic cavity.

Extracellular fluid Same as interstitial fluid.

Extrinsic eye muscles Six muscles located outside the eye that are responsible for eye movement.

Facilitated diffusion Process in which carrier proteins shuttle molecules across plasma membranes. The molecules move in response to concentration gradients.

FAD *See* flavine adenine dinucleotide.

Fallopian tube *See* oviduct.

False labor Muscular contractions of the uterus that occur in the weeks before birth. Also known as *Braxton-Hicks contractions.*

Fast-twitch fibers A type of muscle cell that permits rapid muscular contraction. Found in muscles that are involved in rapid movements.

Fat cell A cell that's specialized to store fat. In these cells, the cytoplasm becomes filled with fat, which forces the cytoplasm and nucleus to the outer portion of the cell.

Fatty acid A long-chain organic molecule found in triglycerides. It can be broken down to produce energy.

Feces Semisolid material containing undigested food, bacteria, ions, and water; produced in the large intestine.

Feedback mechanism A mechanism in which the product of one process regulates the rate of another process, either turning it on or shutting it off.

Fermentation Process occurring in eukaryotic cells in the absence of oxygen, during which pyruvic acid is converted to lactic acid or ethyl alcohol. Also occurs in those prokaryotes that live in oxygen-free environments.

Fertilization Union of sperm and ovum.

Fetal alcohol syndrome A condition in children caused by their mothers' ingestion of alcohol during pregnancy. Usually results in multiple birth defects.

Fiber (dietary) Any of the indigestible polysaccharides in fruits, vegetables, and grains.

Fibrillation Cardiac muscle spasms occurring during heart attacks due to a loss of synchronized electrical signals.

Fibrin A form of protein found in blood clots. Its filaments form a meshwork that captures red blood cells and platelets forming a clot that stops the leakage of blood out of vessels.

Fibrinogen An protein found in the blood that is converted to fibrin when activated. Fibrin forms fibers that become part of a blood clot.

Fibroblast Connective tissue cell, found in loose and dense connective tissues that produces collagen, elastic fibers, and a gelatinous extracellular material; responsible for repairing damage created by cuts or tears to connective tissue.

Fibrocartilage Type of cartilage whose extracellular matrix consists of numerous bundles of collagen fibers. Principally found in the intervertebral disks.

Fight-or-flight response An automatic response of an organism to danger that enables it to flee or stand and fight; it is activated by the autonomic nervous system and results in an increase in heart rate and breathing and an increase in blood flow to the muscles.

First law of thermodynamics Law stating that energy can be converted from one form to another but is never created or destroyed.

First polar body Cast-off nuclear material produced during the first meiotic division during oogenesis.

Fitness A term used to describe an organism's potential to survive and reproduce; influenced by many factors such as strength, ability to capture prey, or, in the case of prey, to avoid being captured by predators.

Flagellum Long, whiplike extension of the plasma membrane of certain protozoans and sperm cells in humans. Used for motility.

Flavine adenine dinucleotide (FAD) A molecule that carries high-energy electrons from one chemical reaction to another; found in the citric acid cycle.

Flavonoid One of dozens of naturally occuring antioxidants in plant-derived foods.

Flexion Movement of a limb, finger, or toe that involves closing a joint.

Fluid mosaic model of the plasma membrane A model of the structure of the plasma membrane based on scientific observations. It consists of a bilayer of phospholipids with proteins embedded in the membrane and on its inner and outer surfaces.

Foam cell A cell in the lining of arteries that is filled with cholesterol.

Follicle (ovary) Structure found in the ovary. Each follicle contains an oocyte and one or more layers of follicle cells that are derived from the loose connective tissue of the ovary surrounding the follicle.

Follicle (thyroid) Structure found in the thyroid gland. Consists of an outer layer of cuboidal cells surrounding thyroglobulin, a proteinaceous material from which thyroxine is formed.

Follicle-stimulating hormone (FSH) Gonadotropic hormone from the anterior pituitary that promotes gamete formation in both men and women.

Food chain Series of organisms in an ecosystem in which each organism feeds on the organism preceding it.

Food pyramid A schematic developed by the U.S. Department of Agriculture that shows the proper amounts of various food types needed for a healthy diet.

Food vacuole Membrane-bound vacuole in a cell containing material engulfed by the cell.

Food web All of the connected food chains in an ecosystem.

Foreskin Sheath of skin that covers the glans penis. Also known as the *prepuce.*

Formed elements A term that refers to cells or cell fragments found in the blood, including white blood cells, red blood cells, and platelets.

Fossil Remains or imprints of organisms that lived on Earth many years ago, usually embedded in rocks or sediment.

Founder effect A term evolutionary biologists use to describe the formation of a new population from a very small, genetically homogenous stock.

Fovea centralis Tiny spot in the center of the macula of the eye that contains only cones. Objects are focused onto the fovea for sharp vision.

Free radical A highly reactive chemical in the body containing an unpaired electron. Formed naturally and by radiation. Can react with other naturally occurring biochemicals, causing damage to tissue, even cancer.

Functional food A food that provides benefit (for example, it contains antioxidants) beyond its direct nutrient value.

Fusion Joining of two atoms, which releases large amounts of energy. Occurs in the sun.

Gallbladder Sac on the underside of the liver that stores and concentrates bile.

Gall stone A hard deposit formed in the gallbladder.

Gastric glands Tiny glands in the wall of the stomach that produce hydrochloric acid.

Gastic juice A name given to the watery secretions of the gastric glands of the stomach.

Gastrin Stomach hormone that stimulates HCl production and release by the gastric glands.

Gastroesophageal sphincter Ring of muscle located in the lower esophagus that opens when food arrives, allowing food to pass into the stomach, and then closes to keep food and stomach acid from percolating upward.

Gene Segment of the DNA that controls cell structure and function.

Gene flow Introduction of new genes into a population when new individuals join the population.

Gene pool All the genes of all of the members of a population or species.

Gene therapy The use of artificially produced genes to treat, even cure, diseases.

Genera Plural of *genus.*

General senses Refers to pain, light touch, and pressure. Contrast with special senses.

Genetic drift A term used to describe a phenomenon in which the frequency of genes in a population changes due to some chance happening, for example, a natural event that wipes out many members of a population.

Genetic engineering The artificial manipulation of genes in which certain genes from one organism are removed and transferred to another organism of the same or a different species. This permits scientists to transfer important genes to improve species, for example, to increase resistance to disease.

Genetic resistance A term that describes a naturally occurring resistance to organisms, for example, insects or bacteria to pesticides or antibiotics, respectively.

Genital herpes A sexually transmitted disease caused by a virus. Infection with the virus causes small, painful lesions on the skin of the external genitalia of men and women and on the skin on their thighs.

Genital warts A sexually transmitted disease caused by the human papillomavirus (HPV). Results in benign growths on external genitalia and around the anuses of men and women. Warts also grow inside the vagina of women. Generally occurs in individuals whose immune systems are suppressed.

Genome All of the genes of an organism.

Genotype Genetic makeup of an organism.

Genus Subgroup of a family of organisms.

Geographic isolation Physical separation of a population by some barrier. Sometimes results in reproductive isolation and the formation of new species.

Germ cell Refers to the sperm or ovum (egg) and the cells from which they are derived; germ cells contain half the chromosomes of somatic cells.

Germinal epithelium Germ cells in the wall of the seminiferous tubule that give rise to sperm.

Gestation The period of pregnancy.

Giantism An endocrine disorder caused by excess growth hormone early in life which results in excessive growth of long bones. Individuals end up much taller than normal adults.

Gingivitis An inflammation of the gums caused by the build-up of bacteria trapped by plaque.

Glans penis Slightly enlarged tip of the penis.

Glaucoma Disease of the eye caused by pressure resulting from a build-up of aqueous humor in the anterior chamber.

Global warming Warming of the Earth's atmosphere and oceans due to the accumulation of heat trapping gases, mostly from human sources, in the atmosphere.

Glomerular filtration Movement of materials out of the glomeruli into Bowman's capsule in the kidney.

Glomerulus Tuft of capillaries that make up part of the nephron; site of glomerular filtration.

Glucagon Hormone released by the pancreas that stimulates the breakdown of glycogen in the liver and the release of glucose molecules, thus increasing blood levels of glucose.

Glucocorticoids Group of steroid hormones produced by the adrenal cortex that stimulate gluconeogenesis.

Gluconeogenesis Synthesis of glucose from fatty acids and amino acids. Takes place in the liver where amino acids and fatty acids are stored.

Glucose A simple sugar that is used to produce energy and is combined to form large polymers such as cellulose, starch, and glycogen.

Glycogen A polysaccharide found in animals cells, especially in the muscle and liver where it serves as means of storing glucose.

Glycogenolysis Breakdown of glycogen, releasing glucose.

Glycolysis Metabolic pathway in the cytoplasm of the cell, during which glucose is split in half, forming two molecules of pyruvic acid. The energy released during the reaction is used to generate two molecules of ATP.

Glycoproteins Proteins that have carbohydrate attached to them.

Goiter Condition in which the thyroid gland enlarges due to lack of dietary iodide.

Golgi complex Organelle consisting of a series of flattened membranes that form channels. It sorts and chemically modifies molecules and repackages its proteins into secretory vesicles.

Golgi tendon organs Special receptors found in tendons that respond to stretch. Also known as *neurotendinous organs*.

Gonadotropin General term for FSH and LH, which are produced by the anterior pituitary and target male and female gonads.

Gonadotropin-releasing hormone or GnRH Hormone produced by the hypothalamus that controls the release of FSH (ICSH in males) and LH.

Gonorrhea Sexually transmitted disease caused by a bacterium.

Gout A disorder caused by the build-up of uric acid crystals in the blood and joints. Can be very painful.

Grassland One of the Earth's major biomes. Receives intermediate level of precipitation, enough to support grasses but not trees. Highly valued by humans for agricultural uses.

Gray matter Gray, outermost region of the cerebral cortex.

Grazer Herbivorous organism.

Grazer food chain Food chain beginning with plants and grazers (herbivores).

Greenhouse effect A warming of the Earth caused by the entrapment of heat by carbon dioxide and other greenhouse gases. So named because of its approximate similarity to the heat-trapping effect of glass in a greenhouse. *See* global warming.

Greenhouse gas Gas, such as carbon dioxide and chlorofluorocarbons, that traps heat escaping from the Earth and radiates it back to the surface.

Groundwater Water found in the Earth's crust in porous subsoils and porous rock, beneath the Earth's surface.

Groundwater overdraft The removal of groundwater from an aquifer faster than it can be replaced or recharged.

Growth factor Any biotic or abiotic factor that causes a population to grow.

Growth hormone A protein hormone produced by the anterior pituitary that stimulates cellular growth in the body, causing cellular hypertrophy and hyperplasia. Its major targets are bone and muscle.

Growth rate (of a population) Determined by subtracting the death rate from the birth rate.

Guanine A nitrogen-containing base known as a purine found in RNA and DNA.

Habitat Place in which an organism lives.

Habituation Condition where sensory receptors stop generating impulses, even though a stimulus is still present.

Hammer (malleus) One of three bones of the middle ear. Abuts the tympanic membrane and helps transmit sound from the eardrum to the inner ear.

Haploid A term used to describe a cell with half the number of chromosomes of a somatic or diploid cell. The only haploid cells in the body are the germ cells.

Heart The muscular organ in the chest cavity that pumps blood through the pulmonary and systemic circulatory circuits of the circulatory system.

Heart murmur A sloshing sound made when the valves of the heart fail to close completely.

Helper T cell Type of T-lymphocyte that stimulates the proliferation of T and B cells when antigen is present. Also called *T4 cell.*

Hematocrit A measure of the volume of blood occupied by red blood cells.

Heme group Subunit of the hemoglobin molecule. Consists of a porphyrin ring and a central iron ion to which oxygen binds.

Hemoglobin Protein molecules inside red blood cells; binds to oxygen.

Hemolyze Refers to the bursting of red blood cells when they are immersed in a hypotonic solution or during a transfusion reaction (that is, when the wrong type of blood is given to a patient).

Hemophilia Disease caused by a gene defect occurring on the Y chromosome. Results in the absence of certain blood-clotting factors.

Hemorrhoids A condition characterized by a swelling of the internal hemorrhoidal veins around the anus. Results in an itchy sensation and can cause considerable pain.

Herbicide Any chemical applied to crops to control weeds.

Herbivore Any organism that feeds directly on plants. Also known as a *grazer.*

Herniated disk An intervertebral disk whose center portion has pushed out, causing the disk to bulge. It may press on a nerve or the spinal cord, causing pain.

Herpes One of the most common sexually transmitted diseases; caused by a virus.

Heterochromatin Inactive chromatin that is slightly coiled or compacted in the interphase nucleus.

Heteroculture A term used to describe farm fields deliberately planted in several species to naturally control pests.

Heterotrophic fermenter Evolutionarily probably one of the first cells. Absorbed glucose from the environment and broke it down by anaerobic glycolysis.

Heterotrophs Organisms such as animals that, unlike plants, are unable to synthesize their own food. Consume plants and other organisms.

Heterozygous Adjective describing a genetic condition in which an individual contains one dominant and one recessive gene in a gene pair.

Heterozygous dominant Refers to a situation in which an individual has one dominant and another recessive gene for a particular trait. Because of the presence of one dominant allele, that gene is expressed and the organism is indistinguishable from a homozygous individual for that trait.

High-density lipoproteins (HDLs) Complexes of lipid and protein that transport cholesterol to the liver for destruction.

Hinge joint A type of joint that opens and closes like a hinge, not permitting any other kind of movement.

Histamine Potent vasodilator released by certain cells in the body during allergic reactions.

Histone Globular protein thought to play a role in regulating the genes.

Homeostasis A condition of dynamic equilibrium within any biological or social system. Achieved through a variety of automatic mechanisms that compensate for internal and external changes.

Hominid First humanlike creatures.

Hominoids Group consisting of the great apes, the lesser apes, and humans, which diverged from the Old World monkeys over 20 million years ago.

Homo sapiens neanderthalensis The Neanderthals. Subspecies of *Homo sapiens.*

Homo sapiens sapiens Species of modern humans that emerged about 400,000 years ago.

Homologous chromosomes Two chromosomes in a somatic (dipoid) cell that contain the same genes. One member of a homologous pair is derived from the mother and the other is derived from the father.

Homologous structures Structures thought to have arisen from a common origin.

Homozygous Adjective describing a genetic condition marked by the presence of two identical alleles for a given gene.

Homozygous dominant Refers to an organism that has two alleles for a given trait.

Hormone Chemical substance produced in one part of the body that travels to another, typically through the bloodstream, where it elicits a response.

Human chorionic gonadotropin (HCG) Hormone produced by the embryo that stimulates the corpus luteum in the mother's body to produce estrogen.

Human chorionic somatomammotropin A hormone produced by the placenta that stimulates milk production by the breasts. Released near the end of pregnancy.

Human papillomavirus (HPV) A fairly common virus spread by sexual contact. In people with suppressed immune systems, HPV causes the formation of benign growths on the skin on and around the external genitalia.

Humoral immunity Immune reaction that protects the body primarily against viruses and bacteria in the body fluids via antibodies produced by plasma cells.

Hyaline cartilage One of the three main types of cartilage. It is found on the articular surfaces of bone, where it reduces friction, and in other places. The skeleton of humans starts out as hyaline cartilage which is converted into bone.

Hydrocephalus Accumulation of fluid inside the cavities of the brain. Typically found in newborns. Can cause severe damage to the brain if not corrected immediately.

Hydrogen bond A weak electrostatic attraction between two atoms on different molecules, usually involving hydrogen and either nitrogen or oxygen. Responsible for many of the unique characteristics of water.

Hydrolysis The breakdown of a molecule involving water.

Hyperglycemia High blood glucose levels.

Hyperopia (farsightedness) Condition that occurs when the eyeball is too short or the lens is too weak, resulting in poor focus on nearby objects.

Hypersecretion Refers to increased rate of hormonal secretion by an endocrine gland.

Hypersensitivity A dramatic immune response to small quantities of an antigen created by earlier exposure to the substance.

Hypertension High blood pressure.

Hyperthyroidism An endocrine disorder caused by excessive secretion of thyroid hormones. Results in elevated metabolism, excessive sweating (due to overheating), weight loss, increased heart rate, insomnia, and increased mental activity, resulting in nervousness and anxiety.

Hypertonic Adjective describing a solution with a higher solute concentration than the cell's cytoplasm, causing the cell to shrivel.

Hypolimnion The coldest water of a lake, which lies below the thermocline.

Hyposecretion A lower rate of secretion by an endocrine gland.

Hypothalamus Structure in the brain located beneath the thalamus. It consists of many aggregations of nerve cells and controls a variety of autonomic functions aimed at maintaining homeostasis.

Hypothesis Tentative and testable explanation for a phenomenon or observation.

Hypothyroidism A condition characterized by a reduction in thyroid hormone secretion which results in a decrease in the metabolic rate, a feeling of being cold much of the time, fatigue, decreased heart rate, and decreased mental activity.

Hypotonic Adjective describing a solution with a solute concentration lower than the cell's cytoplasm, resulting in a swelling of the cell.

I gene Gene that controls blood type through the synthesis of glycoproteins that end up on the plasma membrane of the red blood cell.

Immune system Diffuse system consisting of trillions of cells that circulate in the blood and lymph and take up residence in the lymphoid organs, such as the spleen, thymus, lymph nodes, and tonsils, as well as other body tissues. Helps protect the body against foreign cells, such as bacteria and viruses, and protects against cancer cells.

Immunity Term referring to the resistance of the body to infectious disease.

Immunocompetence Process in which lymphocytes mature and become capable of responding to specific antigens.

Immunoglobulins Antibodies.

Implantation Process in which the blastocyst embeds in the uterine lining.

Impotence Inability of a male to achieve an erection.

Imprinting Attachment of young animals such as birds to their mothers or artificial substitutes during a critical period early in life.

Incomplete dominance Occurs when an allele exerts only partial dominance over another allele, resulting in an intermediate trait. Also known as *partial dominance.*

Incomplete protein A protein source that does not provide all of the amino acids you need to be healthy. That is, it is missing one or more essential amino acids.

Incontinence Inability to control urination.

Induced abortion Deliberate expulsion of a fetus or embryo.

Inducer Chemical substance that activates inducible genes.

Inducible operon An operon that is in an off state until switched on by an inducer substance.

Infarct A region of the body, usually part the brain or heart muscle, that is cut off from blood by a clogged artery.

Industrial Revolution A period in history marked by the emergence of machine production powered by fossil fuels, replacing manufacturing by hand.

Infectious mononucleosis White blood cell disorder caused by a virus. Characterized by a rapid increase in the number of monocytes and lymphocytes in the blood.

Inferior vena cava Large vein that empties deoxygenated blood from the body below the heart into the right atrium of the heart.

Infertility Inability to conceive; can be due to problems in either the male or the female or both partners.

Inflammatory response Response to tissue damage including an increase in blood flow, the release of chemical attractants, which draw monocytes to the scene, and an increase in the flow of plasma into a wound.

Inguinal canal Two small openings in the lower anterior wall of the abdomen of men that permit the vas deferentia to enter the pelvic cavity. This area, if weakened, may be the site of inguinal hernias.

Inguinal hernia A protrusion of the intestines through the inguinal canal in men.

Inhalation Process of air being drawn into the lungs.

Inhibin Hormone produced by the seminiferous tubules that inhibits the production of FSH by the anterior pituitary.

Inhibiting hormone Hormone from the hypothalamus that inhibits the release of hormones from the anterior pituitary.

Initiator codon Codon found on a messenger RNA strand that marks where protein synthesis begins.

Inner cell mass Cells of the blastocyst that become the embryo and amnion.

Inorganic molecule Any molecule that is not organic. Usually smaller molecules such as water. Many inorganic molecules consist of atoms joined by ionic bonds.

Inspiration Same as inhalation.

Insulin Hormone that stimulates the uptake of glucose by body cells, especially muscle and liver cells. Stimulates the synthesis of glycogen in liver and muscle cells.

Insulin-dependent diabetes Type of diabetes that can only be treated with injections of insulin. May be caused by an autoimmune reaction. Also known as *early-onset diabetes.*

Insulin-independent diabetes Type of diabetes that often occurs in obese people. In most patients, it can be controlled by diet. Also known as *late-onset diabetes.*

Insulin shock A condition in diabetics resulting from the administration of excess insulin; results in hypoglycemia, tremor, fatigue, sleepiness, and the inability to concentrate. In severe cases, unconsciousness and death may occur.

Integral protein Large protein molecules in the lipid bilayer of the plasma membrane.

Integration Process of making sense of various nervous inputs so that a meaningful response can be achieved.

Intercostal muscles Short, powerful muscles that lie between the ribs. Involved in inspiration and active exhalation.

Interferon Protein released from cells infected by viruses that stops the replication of viruses in other cells.

Interleukin 1 Substance released by macrophages. Enhances the proliferation and differentiation of B cells into plasma cells.

Interleukin 2 Chemical released by helper cells that increases the activity of cytotoxic T as well as that of suppressor T and other helper T cells.

Internal sphincter (of the bladder) Involuntary muscular valve that relaxes reflexively, releasing urine. Formed by a smooth muscle in the neck of the bladder at the junction of the bladder and the urethra.

Interphase Period of cellular activity occurring between cell divisions. Synthesis and growth occur in preparation for cell division.

Interstitial cells Testosterone-producing cells located in the loose connective tissue between the seminiferous tubules of the testes.

Interstitial cell stimulating hormone (ICSH) Luteinizing hormone in males. Stimulates testosterone secretion.

Interstitial fluid Fluid surrounding cells in body tissues. Provides a path through which nutrients, gases, and wastes can travel between the capillary and the cells. Also called *extracellular fluid.*

Intervertebral disks Shock-absorbing material between the bones of the spine.

Intrauterine device (IUD) Birth control device that consists of a small plastic or metal object with a string attached that is inserted into the uterus through the cervix to prevent implantation.

Intron Segment of DNA that is not expressed. Lies between exons (expressed segments).

Invertebrates Animals without a spinal column such as insects.

In vitro A term referring to any procedure carried out in a test tube or petri dish, such as *in vitro* fertilization.

Ion Atom that has gained or lost one or more electrons. May be either positively or negatively charged.

Ionic bond Weak bond that forms between oppositely charged ions.

Iris Colored segment of the middle layer of the eye visible through the cornea.

Irritability Ability to perceive and respond to stimuli.

Islets of Langerhans Group of endocrine cells found in the pancreas that produce insulin and glucagon.

Isotonic Having the same solute concentration as a cell or body fluid.

Isotope Alternative form of an atom; differs from other atoms in the number of neutrons found in the nucleus.

Joint A juncture of two bones. Some joints permit a great deal of movement; others permit none.

Joint capsule Connective tissue that connects to the opposing bones of a joint and forms the synovial cavity. The inner layer of the joint capsule produces synovial fluid.

Kaposi's sarcoma A rare form of skin cancer that develops in people infected with HIV. May also affect internal organs.

Karyotype The term used to describe a photographic display of the chromosomes of a cell. Used to diagnose some genetic disorders.

Keratin A body protein found in hair, nails, and skin cells.

Kidney Organ that rids the body of wastes and plays a key role in regulating the chemical constancy of blood.

Kingdom A large grouping of organisms; scientists typically recognize five major kingdoms: Monera, Protista, Animalia, Plantae, and Fungi.

Klinefelter syndrome Genetic disorder that results from an XXY genotype.

Krebs cycle *See* citric acid cycle.

Labia majora Outer folds of skin of the external genitalia in women.

Labia minora Inner folds of the external genitalia in women.

Labor The process or period of childbirth.

Lactation Milk production in the breasts. Stimulated by prolactin and HCS.

Lacteal A small lymphatic vessel in the villi of the small intestine.

Lamaze technique A technique women use to lessen the pain of childbirth. Uses breathing techniques to reduce pressure from the diaphragm on the baby.

Laparoscope Instrument used to examine internal organs through small openings made in the skin and underlying muscle.

Laryngitis Inflammation of the lining of the larynx, resulting in hoarseness. Caused by bacterial and viral infection and also excessive use of the voice.

Larynx Rigid but hollow cartilaginous structure that houses the vocal cords and participates in swallowing.

Latent period The period between exposure to a cancer-causing agent and the emergence of a malignant tumor.

Learning Process in which stored information can lead to changes in innate behavior.

Lens Transparent structure that lies behind the iris and in front of the vitreous humor. Focuses light on the retina.

Leukemia Cancer of white blood cells.

Leukocyte A general term for white blood cells such as lymphocytes, monocytes, and neutrophils.

Leukocytosis An increase in the concentration of white blood cells, which often occurs during a bacterial or viral infection.

Life expectancy Average length of time a person will live.

Ligament Connective tissue structure that runs from bone to bone, located alongside and sometimes inside the joint. Offers support for joints.

Light microscope A device that uses light and a series of lenses to magnify structures.

Limbic system Array of structures in the brain that work in concert with centers of the hypothalamus. Site of instincts and emotions.

Limiting factor One factor that is most important in regulating growth in an ecosystem.

Linked trait Refers to traits that are inherited together because the genes responsible for them are on the same chromosome.

Lipase Enzyme that removes some of the fatty acids from the glycerol molecule, forming a monoglyceride. Produced by the salivary glands and the pancreas.

Lipid Commonly known as fats. Water-insoluble organic molecules that provide energy to body cells, help insulate the body from heat loss, and serve as precursors in the synthesis of certain hormones. A principal component of the plasma membrane.

Liposuction Surgical technique used to remove subcutaneous fat.

Liver Organ located in the abdominal cavity that performs many functions essential to homeostasis. It stores glucose and fats, synthesizes some key blood proteins, stores iron and certain vitamins, detoxifies certain chemicals, and plays an important role in digestion by producing bile.

Long bones Bones of the skeleton that form parts of the extremities.

Loose connective tissue Type of connective tissue that serves primarily as a packing material. Contains many cells among a loose network of collagen and elastic fibers. Often contains cells that help protect the body from foreign organisms.

Low-density lipoproteins (LDLs) Complexes of protein and lipid that transport cholesterol, depositing it in body tissues.

Lungs Two large saclike organs in the thoracic cavity where the blood and air exchange carbon dioxide and oxygen.

Luteinizing hormone (LH) Hormone produced by the anterior pituitary that stimulates gonadal hormone production. In men, LH stimulates the production of testosterone, the male sex steroid. In women, LH stimulates estrogen secretion.

Lymph Fluid contained in the lymphatic vessels. Similar to tissue fluid, but also contains white blood cells and may contain large amounts of fat.

Lymph capillary Tiny vessel that transports excess tissue fluid to larger vessels that eventually return the fluid to the bloodstream.

Lymph node Small nodular organ interspersed along the course of the lymphatic vessels. Serves as a filter for lymph.

Lymphatic system Network of vessels that drains extracellular fluid from body tissues and returns it to the circulatory system.

Lymphocyte Type of white blood cell. *See also* B-lymphocyte and T-lymphocyte.

Lymphoid organs Organs, such as the spleen and thymus, that belong to the lymphatic system.

Lymphokine Chemical released by suppressor T cells that inhibits the division of B and T cells.

Lysosome Membrane-bound organelle that contains enzymes. Responsible for the breakdown of material that enters the cell by endocytosis. Also destroys aged or malfunctioning cellular organelles.

Lysozyme Enzyme produced in saliva that dissolves the cell walls of bacteria, killing them.

Macronutrients Nutrients required in relatively large amounts by organisms. Includes water, proteins, carbohydrates, and lipids.

Macrophage Phagocytic cell derived from monocytes that resides in loose connective tissues and helps guard tissues against bacterial and viral invasion.

Macula lutea Region of the retina located lateral to the optic disc where cones are most abundant.

Maculae Receptor organs in the saccule and utricle that play a role in position sense.

Malignant tumor Structure resulting from uncontrollable cellular growth. Cells often spread to other parts of the body.

Mammals Class of vertebrates with a single jaw bone, specialized teeth, hair, mammary glands, a four-chambered heart, and an advanced brain. Reproduction is the most complex of animals.

Marfan's syndrome Autosomal dominant genetic disorder that affects the skeletal system, the eye, and the cardiovascular system.

Marrow cavity Cavity inside a bone containing either red or yellow marrow.

Mast cell Cell found in many tissues, especially in the connective tissue surrounding blood vessels. Contains large granules containing histamine.

Matrix Extracellular material found in cartilage. Also the material in the inner compartment of the mitochondrion.

Matter Anything that has mass and occupies space.

Mechnoreceptor A sensory receptor that is activated by mechanical stimulation such as touch or pressure.

Medulla Term referring to the central portion of some organs; for example, the adrenal medulla.

Megakaryocyte Large cell found in bone marrow that produces platelets.

Meiosis Type of cell division that occurs in the gonads during the formation of gametes. Requires two cellular divisions (meiosis I and meiosis II). In humans, it reduces the chromosome number from 46 to 23.

Meiosis I First meiotic division.

Meiosis II Second meiotic division.

Meissner's corpuscle Encapsulated sensory receptor thought to respond to light touch.

Melanin A dark brown pigment found in skin, hair, and the eye.

Membranous epithelium Refers to any sheet of epithelium that forms a continuous lining on organs.

Membrane potential Same as resting potential.

Memory cells T or B cells produced after antigen exposure. They form a reserve force that responds rapidly to antigen during subsequent exposure.

Meninges The connective tissue covering of the brain and spinal cord. Consists of three parts, the dura mater, the arachnoid, and the pia mater.

Meningitis Infection of the connective tissue layers surrounding the brain, the meninges. Can be lethal if not treated.

Menopause End of the reproductive function (ovulation) in women. Usually occurs between the ages of 45 and 55.

Menstrual cycle Recurring series of events in the reproductive functions of women. Characterized by dramatic changes in ovarian and pituitary hormone levels and changes in the uterine lining that prepare the uterus for implantation.

Menstruation Process in which the endometrium is sloughed off, resulting in bleeding. Occurs approximately once every month.

Merkel disk Light touch receptor. Consists of dendrites that end on cells in the epidermis.

Mesoderm One of the three types of cells that emerge in human embryonic development. Lies in the middle of the forming embryo. Gives rise to muscle, bone, and cartilage.

Mesosome A structure found in bacterial cells. Consists of an infolding of the plasma membrane that encompasses the DNA, forming a pseudonucleus.

Messenger RNA (mRNA) Type of RNA that carries genetic information needed to synthesize proteins to the cytoplasm of a cell.

Metabolic pathway Series of linked chemical reactions in which the product of one reaction becomes the reactant in another.

Metabolic water Water produced during cellular respiration by the addition of protons (hydrogen ions) and electrons to oxygen. Occurs in the electron transport system.

Metabolism The chemical reactions of the body, including all catabolic and anabolic reactions.

Metaphase Stage of cellular division in which chromosomes line up in the center of the cell.

Metarterioles Arterioles that serve as circulatory short cuts, connecting arterioles with venules in a capillary bed. Also known as *thoroughfare channels*.

Metastasis Spread of cancerous cells throughout the body, through the lymph vessels and circulatory system or directly through tissue fluid.

Microfilament Solid fiber consisting of contractile proteins that is found in cells in a dense network under the plasma membrane. Forms part of the cytoskeleton.

Micronutrients Nutrients required in small quantities. They include two broad groups: vitamins and minerals.

Microscope A device used to obtain a magnified view of structures, which, in some cases, may be invisible to the unaided eye. Two main types of microscopes are the light microscope and the electron microscope.

Microspheres Small globules consisting of protein that may have been precursors of the first cells. Also known as *proteinoids*.

Microtubules Hollow protein tubules in the cytoplasm of cells that form part of the cytoskeleton. Also form spindles.

Microvilli Tiny projections of the plasma membranes of certain epithelial cells that increase the surface area for absorption.

Middle ear Portion of the ear located within a bony cavity in the temporal bone of the skull. Houses the ossicles.

Milk letdown The expulsion of milk from the mammary glands in a woman caused by the hormone oxytocin whose release is stimulated by suckling.

Mineral Any of dozens of inorganic substances required for good health such as calcium and iron. Major minerals are needed in large quantities. Trace minerals are required in tiny amounts.

Mineralocorticoids Group of steroid hormones produced by the adrenal cortex. Involved in electrolyte or mineral salt balance.

Mitochondrion Membrane-bound organelle where the bulk of cellular energy production occurs in eukaryotic cells. Houses the citric acid cycle and electron transport system.

Mitosis Term referring specifically to the division of a cell's nucleus. Consists of four stages: prophase, metaphase, anaphase, and telophase.

Mitotic spindle Array of microtubules constructed in the cytoplasm during prophase. Microtubules of the mitotic spindle connect to the chromosomes and help draw them apart during mitosis.

Molecular genetics The study of RNA, DNA, and genes at the molecular level.

Molecule A stucture formed by two or more atoms.

Monerans Organisms belonging to the Kingdom Monera, which consists of prokaryotic organisms, the bacteria.

Monocyte White blood cell that phagocytizes bacteria and viruses in body tissues.

Monoculture A term used to refer to farm fields planted in a single crop. Highly susceptible to insect pests and diseases.

Monohybrid cross Procedure in which one plant is bred with another to study the inheritance of a single trait.

Monosaccharide A simple sugar such as glucose or ribose. Often combines to form large polymers such as starch and glycogen.

Monosomy A term used to denote a genetic condition caused by a missing chromosome.

Morning sickness Nausea that often occurs in the first two to three months of pregnancy.

Morula Solid ball of cells produced from the zygote by numerous cellular divisions.

Motor neuron or nerve A nerve cell that innervates muscles.

Motor cortex That portion of the cerebral cortex that controls voluntary muscles.

Motor unit Muscle fibers supplied by a single axon and its branches.

Mucous cell A cell in the lining of many parts of the respiratory tract that produces mucus.

Mucus Thick, slimy material produced by the lining of the respiratory tract and parts of the digestive tract. Moistens and protects them.

Mullerian mimicry Phenomenon of several species, each with toxic characteristics, evolving similar color patterns.

Multiple alleles Refers to a genetic trait that is controlled by two or more genes.

Multiple chemical sensitivity (MCS) A condition characterized by mild to life-threatening reaction to chemicals in the environment. The most common symptoms are tension, memory loss, fatigue, sleepiness, headaches, confusion, and depression. Many victims of MCS experience gastrointestinal problems such as nausea, indigestion, and cramps. Some exhibit respiratory symptoms as well, including frequent colds, bronchitis, and shortness of breath. Skin rashes are not uncommon. Many people report allergylike symptoms such as nasal stuffiness and sinus infections.

Multiple sclerosis A neurological disorder caused by damage to myelin sheath of neurons, which results in nerve cell death that leads to numbness, slurred speech, and paralysis. Thought to be an autoimmune disease, multiple sclerosis can affect any part of the CNS.

Multipolar neuron Motor neuron found in the central nervous system. Contains a prominent, multiangular cell body and several dendrites.

Muscle A highly differentiated cell that is capable of contraction upon stimulation. The body contains three types: smooth muscle, cardiac muscle, and skeletal muscle.

Muscle fiber Long, unbranched, multinucleated cell found in skeletal muscle.

Muscle spindles Stretch receptors found in skeletal muscle. Also known as *neuromuscular spindles.*

Muscle tone Inherent firmness of muscle, resulting from contraction of muscle fibers during periods of inactivity.

Muscular artery Any one of the main branches of the aorta. Tunica media consists primarily of smooth muscle cells.

Mutation Technically, a change in the DNA caused by chemical and physical agents. Also refers to a wide range of chromosomal defects.

Myelin sheath Layer of fatty material coating the axons of many neurons in the central and peripheral nervous systems.

Myocardial infarction A type of heart attack caused by blockage of one or more of the coronary arteries; usually a result of the build-up of atherosclerotic plaque.

Myofibril Bundle of contractile myofilaments in skeletal muscle cells.

Myoglobin Cytoplasmic protein in muscle cells that binds to oxygen.

Myometrium Smooth muscle in the wall of the uterus that aids in the expulsion of the fetus at birth.

Myopia (nearsightedness) Visual condition that results when the eyeball is slightly elongated or the lens is too strong. In the uncorrected eye, light rays from distant images come into focus in front of the retina.

Myosin Protein filament found in many cells in the microfilamentous network. Also found in muscle cells.

NAD *See* nicotine adenine dinucleotide.

Naked nerve ending Unmodified dendritic ending of the sensory neurons. Responsible for at least three sensations: pain, temperature, and light touch.

Natural childbirth Childbirth without the use of drugs.

Natural selection Evolutionary process in which environmental abiotic and biotic factors "weed" out the less fit—those organisms not as well adapted to the environment as their counterparts.

Nearsightedness *See* myopia.

Necrosis The death of tissues usually due to a loss of their blood supply.

Negative feedback loop In biology, a process in which the end product (e.g., hormone) feeds back on the system, causing it to shut down.

Nephron Filtering unit in the kidney. Consists of a glomerulus and renal tubule.

Nerve Bundle of nerve fibers. May consist of axons, dendrites, or both. Carries information to and from the central nervous system.

Nerve deafness Loss of hearing resulting from nerve or brain damage.

Nervous tissue One of the primary tissues. Found in the nervous system and consists of two types of cells: conducting cells (neurons) and supportive cells.

Neural groove Ectodermal groove that forms early in embryonic development and runs the length of the embryo, later forming the neural tube.

Neural tube Tube of ectoderm that arises from the neural groove and will become the spinal cord.

Neuroendocrine reflex A reflex involving the endocrine and nervous systems.

Neuron Highly specialized cell that generates and transmits bioelectric impulses from one part of the body to another.

Neurosecretory neurons Specialized nerve cells of the hypothalamus and posterior pituitary that produce and secrete hormones.

Neurotransmitter Chemical substance released from the terminal ends (terminal boutons) of axons when a bioelectric impulse arrives. May stimulate or inhibit the next neuron.

Neutraceutical A term used to describe foods that provide a healing benefit in addition to a nutritional benefit.

Neutron Uncharged particle in the nucleus of the atom.

Neutrophil Type of white blood cell that phagocytizes bacteria and cellular debris.

NGU *See* nonspecific gonococcal urethritis.

Niche *See* ecological niche.

Nicotinamide adenine dinucleotide (NAD) Electron acceptor molecule that shuttles energetic electrons from glycolysis, the transition reaction, and the citric acid cycle to the electron transport system.

Nipple An elevated portion of the breast in which the ducts from the breast converge.

Nitrogen fixation Process in which bacteria and a few other organisms convert atmospheric nitrogen to nitrate or ammonia, forms usable by plants.

Nocireceptor A receptor for pain stimulated by pinching, tearing, or burning.

Node of Ranvier Small gap in the myelin sheath of an axon; located between segments formed by Schwann cells. Responsible for saltatory conduction.

Nondisjunction Failure of a chromosome pair or chromatids of a double-stranded chromosome to separate during mitosis or meiosis.

Nonpoint source (of pollution) A source that does not release pollutants via an easily identifiable route. *See also* Point source.

Nonrenewable resources Refers to natural resources such as coal, copper, and oil that are finite and cannot be renewed by natural processes.

Nonspecific gonococcal urethritis (NGU) A very common sexually transmitted disease caused by one of several bacteria, often chlamydia.

Nonspecific urethritis (NSU) One of the most common sexually transmitted diseases. Caused by several different bacteria.

Noradrenaline (norepinephrine) Hormone produced by adrenal medulla and secreted under stress. Contributes to the fight-or-flight response.

Northern coniferous forest biome Same as boreal forest. A large northern biome dominated by evergreen trees. Lies between the tundra to the north and warmer biomes to the south.

Nuclear envelope Double membrane delimiting the nucleus.

Nuclear pores Minute openings in the nuclear envelope that allow materials to pass to and from the nucleus.

Nucleic acid A general term for the two polynucleotides DNA and RNA.

Nucleoli Temporary structures in the nuclei of cells during interphase. Regions of the DNA that are active in the production of RNA.

Nucleoplasm General term referring to the material inside the nucleus of a cell.

Nucleotide Chemical building blocks of DNA and RNA. Consists of a purine or pyrimidine base, a sugar, and phosphate group.

Nucleus (atom) Dense, center region of the atom that contains neutrons and protons.

Nucleus (cell) Cellular organelle that contains the genetic information that controls the structure and function of the cell.

Nutrient cycle Circular flow of nutrients from the environment through the various food chains back into the environment.

Olfactory cilia The six to eight hairlike projections found on each of the estimated 50 million olfactory receptor cells (modified neurons) in the olfactory membrane. The olfactory hairs contain protein receptors for molecules in the atmosphere. When a molecule binds to the receptor it activates the neuron causing an impulse to be sent to the olfactory cortex.

Olfactory membrane Receptor for smell; found in the roof of the nasal cavity.

Olfactory nerve Nerve that transmits impulses from the olfactory membrane to the brain.

Omnivores Organisms that feed on both plants and animals.

Oncotoxin A chemical or any other agent (for example, radiation) that kills cancer cells.

Oocyte A cell found in the ovaries of sexually mature women formed from oogonia. Develops into an ovum if fertilization occurs.

Oogenesis Production of ova.

Oogonium Germ cell in ovary that contains 46 double-stranded chromosomes. Forms primary oocytes.

Operator site Region of the DNA molecule adjacent to the structural genes that acts as a switch to turn the operon on or off.

Operon Functional unit of the DNA of bacteria. Consists of structural and regulatory genes. Produces mRNA responsible for the production of enzymes and other proteins required by cells.

Optic disk Site in the retina where the optic nerve exits. Also known as the *blind spot*.

Optic nerve Nerve that carries impulses from the retina to the brain.

Optimum range Refers to the range of conditions that are optimum for the survival and reproduction of a species.

Orbit The bony socket in the skull in which the eye is located.

Order Taxonomic term that refers to a subgroup of a class.

Organ Discrete structure that carries out specialized functions.

Organelle Refers to any of the membrane- and nonmembrane-bound structures found inside cells that carry out specific functions. Includes structures such as the mitochondria, endoplasmic reticulum, ribosomes, the Golgi Complex, and nucleus.

Organ of Corti Receptor for sound; located in the inner ear within the cochlea.

Organ system Group of organs that participate in a common function.

Organic molecule or compond A chemical made primarily of carbon and hydrogen atoms. Proteins, amino acids, fatty acids, and other biochemicals are all organic compounds.

Organogenesis Organ formation during embryonic development.

Original strand Refers to the template on which a new strand of DNA is made.

Osmosis Diffusion of water across a selectively permeable membrane.

Osmotic pressure Force that drives water across a selectively permeable membrane. Created by differences in solute concentrations.

Ossicles Three small bones inside the middle ear that transmit vibrations created by sound waves to the organ of Corti.

Osteoarthritis Degenerative joint disease caused by wear and tear that impairs movement of joints.

Osteoblast Bone-forming cell; secretes collagen.

Osteoclast Cell that digests the extracellular material of bone. Stimulated by the parathyroid hormone.

Osteocyte Bone cell derived from osteoblasts that has been surrounded by calcified extracellular material.

Osteoporosis Degenerative disease resulting in the deterioration of bone. Due to inactivity in men and women and loss of the ovarian hormone estrogen in postmenopausal women.

Outer ear External portion of the ear.

Oval window Membrane-covered opening in the cochlea where vibrations are transmitted from the stirrup to the fluid within the cochlea.

Ovary Female gonad. Produces ova (eggs) and steroid hormones, estrogen and progesterone.

Overnutrition A condition characterized by an excess intake of food resulting in the accumulation of body fat.

Overpopulation Condition in which a species has exceeded the carrying capacity of the environment.

Oviduct Two hollow, muscular tubes that are part of the uterus. Connected to the upper part of the uterus. The site of fertilization. Also known as a *uterine tube* or *Fallopian tube*.

Ovulation Release of the oocyte from ovary. Stimulated by hormones from the anterior pituitary.

Ovum (ova, plural) Germ cell containing 23 single-stranded chromosomes. Produced during the second meiotic division. Commonly referred to as an *egg*.

Oxaloacetate Four-carbon compound of the citric acid cycle. It is involved in the very first reaction of the cycle and is regenerated during the cycle.

Oxidation The loss of hydrogens or electrons from a substance.

Oxygen debt Depletion of oxygen during muscle contraction.

Oxytocin Hormone from the posterior pituitary hormone. Stimulates contraction of the smooth muscle of the uterus and smooth-muscle-like cells surrounding the glandular units of the breast.

Ozone (O_3) Molecule produced in the stratosphere (upper layer of the atmosphere) from molecular oxygen. Helps screen out incoming ultraviolet light. *See also* Ozone layer.

Ozone layer Region of the atmosphere located approximately 12 to 16 miles above the Earth's surface where ozone molecules are produced. Helps protect the Earth from ultraviolet light.

Pacinian corpuscle Large encapsulated nerve ending that is located in the deeper layers of the skin and near body organs. Responds to pressure.

Pancreas Organ found in the abdominal cavity under the stomach, nestled in a loop formed by the first portion of the small intestine. Produces enzymes needed to digest foodstuffs in the small intestine and hormones that regulate blood glucose levels.

Pap smear Procedure in which cells are retrieved from the cervical canal to be examined for the presence of cancer.

Papillae Small protrusions on the upper surface of the tongue. Some papillae contain taste buds.

Pap smear A technique to detect cervical cancer in women. The physician first swabs the interior of the cervix of women. Cells obtained from the swab are spread on a microscope slide, stained, and observed.

Paracrines Chemicals released by cells that elicit a response in nearby regions.

Parasitism Process in which an individual feeds on (usually without killing) another larger individual—the host.

Parasympathetic division (of the autonomic nervous system) Portion of the autonomic nervous system responsible for a variety of involuntary functions.

Parathormone Same as parathyroid hormone.

Parathyroid glands Endocrine glands located on the posterior surface of the thyroid gland in the neck. Produce parathyroid hormone.

Parathyroid hormone (PTH) Hormone that helps regulate blood calcium levels. Stimulates osteoclasts to digest bone, thus raising blood calcium levels. Also known as *parathormone.*

Parkinson's disease A neurological disorder that causes tremors of the hands, arms, and head. Caused by a progressive detioration of certain brain centers, those that control movement, especially semiautomatic movements.

Passive immunity Temporary protection from antigen (bacteria and others) produced by the injection of immunoglobulins.

Pattern baldness Refers to partial baldness occurring in men and, much less commonly, in women. Hair loss results in a rim of hair on the sides and back of the head. Caused by a sex-influenced gene.

Pedigree A display that allows one to see how members of a family are related to one another.

Penis Male organ of copulation.

Pepsin Enzyme released by the gastric glands of the stomach. Breaks down proteins into large peptide fragments.

Pepsinogen Inactive form of pepsin.

Peptide A short-chained polymer of amino acids too short to be classified as a true protein.

Perforin Chemical released by cytotoxic cells that destroys bacteria. Binds to plasma membrane of target cells, forming pores that make the target cells leak and die.

Perichondrium Connective tissue layer surrounding most types of cartilage. Contains blood vessels that supply nutrients to cartilage cells.

Periodic table of elements Table that lists elements by ascending atomic number. Also lists other vital statistics of each element.

Periosteum The thin, connective tissue external lining of bones; contains numerous pain fibers.

Peripheral nervous system Portion of the nervous system consisting of the cranial and spinal nerves and receptors.

Periplegia Paralysis of the lower limbs caused by spinal cord injury.

Peristalsis Involuntary contractions of the smooth muscles in the wall of the esophagus, stomach, and intestines, which propel food along the digestive tract.

Periotoneum The lining of the abdominal cavity and the major organs in the abdomen.

Peritubular capillaries Capillaries that surround nephrons. They pick up water, nutrients, and ions from the renal tubule, thus helping maintain the osmotic concentration of the blood.

Permafrost Permanently frozen subsoil in the Arctic tundra.

Permanent threshold shift Permanent hearing loss caused by repeated exposure to noise.

pH A measure of acidity. The pH scale ranges from zero to 14. Substances with a pH of 7 are said to be neutral, that is, neither acidic nor basic. Substances with a pH of less than 7 are acidic and greater than 7 are basic.

Phagocytosis A type of endocytosis in which cells engulf solid materials. Compare to pinocytosis.

Pharynx Chamber that connects the oral cavity with the esophagus.

Phenotype Outward appearance of an organism.

Phenotypic variation Variation in the external appearance of organisms in a population due to genetic differences.

Phonation Production of sound.

Phosphofructokinase Enzyme in the glycolytic pathway that catalyzes the conversion of glucose-6-phosphate to fructose-6-phosphate; regulated by ATP and citric acid.

Phosphoglyceraldehyde A three-carbon monosaccharide produced during glycolysis by the splitting of the glucose molecules.

Photoreceptors Modified nerve cells that respond to light. Located in the retina of humans and other animals.

Photosynthesis The series of chemical reactions in which the energy of light is used to synthesize high-energy organic molecules, usually carbohydrates, from low-energy inorganic molecules, usually carbon dioxide and water.

Phylum (phyla, plural) Major grouping of organisms. Animal kingdom contains about two dozen primary phyla, nearly all of which are represented today.

Phytochemical A chemical found in plants. The term is used specifically to refer to the beneficial substances in plants that protect against mutations and cancer or have other beneficial effects.

Phytoplankton Microscopic, free-floating organisms, principally algae, which capture sunlight energy, using it to produce carbohydrates from carbon dioxide dissolved in the water.

Pineal gland Small gland located in the brain that secretes a hormone thought to help control the biological clock.

Pinocytosis A type of endocytosis in which cells engulf liquids.

Pituitary gland Small pea-sized gland located beneath the brain in the sella turcica. It produces numerous hormones and consists of two main subdivisions: anterior and posterior pituitary.

Placenta A structure embedded in the wall of the uterus in pregnant women. Produced by embryonic and maternal tissue, the placenta helps rid the embryo and fetus of wastes and provides nutrients and oxygen. Also produces important hormones such as HCG and HCS.

Placental stage The final stage of birth marked by the delivery (expulsion) of the placenta.

Plasma Extracellular fluid of blood. Comprises about 55% of the volume of blood.

Plasma cell Cell produced from B-lymphocytes (B cells); synthesizes and releases antibodies.

Plasma membrane Outer layer of the cell. Consists of lipid and protein and controls the movement of materials into and out of the cell.

Plasmids Small circular strands of DNA found in bacterial cytoplasm separate from the main DNA.

Plasmin Enzyme in the blood that helps dissolve blood clots.

Plasminogen Inactive form of plasmin.

Platelet Cell fragment produced from megakaryocytes in the red bone marrow. Plays a key role in blood clotting.

PMS *See* premenstrual syndrome.

Point source (of pollution) A discrete, easily identifiable source, usually releasing pollutants directly into waterways via pipes.

Polar body Discarded nuclear material produced during meiosis I and meiosis II of oogenesis. The polar body is small structure lying against the plasma membrane of secondary oocytes and ova.

Polar covalent bond A covalent bond formed by two atoms with slightly different electron affinities, resulting in the production of a small charge difference between the atoms.

Polar fibers Type of microtubule found in the spindle. Extend from one centriole to the center of the cell.

Polygenic inheritance A term used to describe the inheritance of traits determined by two or more alleles, i.e., multiple alleles.

Polymer A general term used to describe a molecule such as DNA and protein that consists of many smaller molecules covalently linked together.

Polymerase chain reaction A way of producing numerous identical copies of a strand of DNA.

Polyploidy Term referring to a genetic disorder caused by an abnormal number of chromosomes. Includes tetraploidy and triploidy.

Polyribosome Also known as *polysome*. Organelle formed by several ribosomes attached to a single messenger RNA. Synthesizes proteins used inside the cell.

Polysaccharide A carbohydrate molecule such as glycogen and starch which is made of many smaller molecules (monosaccharides).

Population Group of like organisms occupying a specific region.

Population histogram (profile) A graph showing the age and sex distribution of a population. Gives a view of the future growth potential of any given population.

Porphyrin ring Part of the chlorophyll molecule that absorbs sunlight.

Portal system Arrangement of blood vessels in which a capillary bed drains to a vein, which drains to another capillary bed.

Positive feedback loop or mechanism A rare biological process in which the product of a process causes it to speed up.

Posterior chamber Posterior portion of the anterior cavity of the eye.

Posterior pituitary Neuroendocrine gland that consists of neural tissue and releases two hormones: oxytocin and antidiuretic hormone.

Premature birth Birth of a baby before 37 weeks of gestation.

Premenstrual syndrome (PMS) A fairly common condition occurring in women right before menstruation. Many women suffer from irritability, depression, fatigue, headaches, bloating, tension, joint pain, and swelling and tenderness of the breasts.

Premotor area Region of the brain in front of the primary motor area. Controls muscle contraction and other less voluntary actions (playing a musical instrument).

Presbyopia Visual impairment caused by aging. Lens becomes stiffer, making it more difficult to focus on nearby objects.

Primary follicle Structure in the ovary consisting of a primary oocyte and a complete single layer of cuboidal follicle cells.

Primary motor area Ridge of tissue in front of a central groove (the central sulcus). Controls voluntary motor activity.

Primary oocyte Germ cell produced from oogonium in the ovary. Undergoes the first meiotic division.

Primary response Immune response elicited when an antigen first enters the body.

Primary sensory area Region of the brain located just behind the central sulcus. The point of destination for many sensory impulses traveling from the body into the spinal cord and up to the brain.

Primary spermatocyte Cell produced from spermatogonium in the seminiferous tubule. Will undergo first meiotic division.

Primary succession Process of sequential change in which one community is replaced by another. Occurs where no biotic community has existed before.

Primary tissue One of the major tissue types, including epithelial, connective, muscle, and nervous tissue.

Primary tumor Cancerous growth that gives rise to cells that spread to other regions of the body.

Primates An order of the kingdom Animalia. Includes prosimians (premonkeys), monkeys, apes, and humans.

Primordial follicle Structure in the ovary that consists of a primary oocyte surrounded by a layer of flattened follicle cells. Gives rise to the primary follicle.

Primordial germ cells Cells that originate in the wall of the yolk sac and eventually become either spermatogonia or oogonia.

Principle of independent assortment Mendel's second law. Hereditary factors are segregated independently during gamete formation. Occurs only when genes are on different chromosomes.

Principle of segregation One of Mendel's discoveries stating that paired hereditary factors of the mother and father must separate during gamete formation so that each gamete contributes one and only one hereditary factor to the zygote.

Producers Generally refers to organisms that can synthesize their own foodstuffs. Major producers are the algae and plants that absorb sunlight and use its energy to synthesize organic foodstuffs from water and carbon dioxide.

Prokaryote A cell that has no nucleus and no organelles such as a bacterium. All prokaryotes are members of the Kingdom Monera.

Prolactin Protein hormone secreted by the posterior pituitary. In humans, it is responsible for milk production by the glandular units of the breast. Its release is stimulated by suckling.

Promoter (in cancer) A chemical, physical, or biological agent that stimulates the second stage of cancer formation (development and progression).

Promoter (in gene control) Region of the operon between the regulator gene and operator site. Binds to RNA polymerase.

Pronucleus Name of the ovum and sperm cell nuclei shortly after fertilization occurs. Each contains 23 chromosomes.

Prophase First phase of mitosis during which chromosomes condense, the nuclear membrane disappears, and the spindle forms.

Proprioception Sense of body and limb position.

Prosimians The primates that preceeded monkeys including lemurs, tarsiers, and tree shrews.

Prostaglandins Group of chemical substances that have a variety of functions. Act on nearby cells.

Prostate gland Sex accessory gland that is located near the neck of the bladder and empties into the urethra. Produces fluid that is added to the sperm during ejaculation.

Prosthesis An artificial body part such as a limb or joint used to replace a nonfunctional, lost, or damaged part.

Protease inhibitor A drug used to treat individuals who have been infected with HIV. Blocks protease, an enzyme vital to viral replication.

Protein A polymer consisting of many amino acids.

Proteinoids Spherical structures composed of small amino acid chains formed when amino acids are heated in air. May have been an early precursor of the first cells.

Prothrombin An inactive form of thrombin, a chemical in the blood that is required to convert fibrinogen into fibrin during clot formation.

Protista A major grouping (kingdom) or organisms.

Protistan Any organism belonging to the Kingdom protista. Includes all free-living single-celled eukaryotic organisms such as ameba and paramecia.

Protists Unicellular eukaryotic organisms such as protozoans and amoebae. Some are autotrophic and some are heterotrophic.

Protocell A term used to describe structures (formed abiotically) that may have given rise to the first cells.

Proton Subatomic particle found in the nucleus of the atom. Each proton carries a positive charge.

Proto-oncogene A gene in a cell that is involved in the regulation of the cell cycle, specifically cellular replication. When mutated, these genes can result in uncontrolled cellular divisions characteristic of cancer.

Pseudopodia Small protoplasmic projections of single-celled organisms and mobile cells in the body that are vital to ameboid movement. These projections extend forward, then attach to a solid surface. Cytoplasm flows into the pseudopodia causing the cell to move forward.

Puberty Period of sexual maturation in humans.

Pudendal block An injection of nerve-deadening substance in the region around the vaginal opening to block pain caused by an episiotomy.

Pulmonary circuit (or circulation) Short circulatory loop that supplies blood to the lungs and transports it back to the heart.

Pulmonary veins Veins that carry oxygenated blood from the lungs to the left atrium.

Punctuated equilibrium Hypothesis explaining how evolutionary change occurs. States that long periods of relatively little change are broken up by briefer periods of relatively rapid evolution.

Punnett square A tool to determine the frequency of different genotypes resulting from any given mating in which the parental genotypes are known.

Pupil Central opening in the iris that allows light to penetrate deeper into the eye.

Purine Type of nitrogenous base found in DNA nucleotides. Consists of two fused rings.

Purkinje fiber Modified cardiac muscle fiber that conducts bioelectric impulses to individual heart muscle cells.

Pus Liquid emanating from a wound. Contains plasma, many dead neutrophils, dead cells, and bacteria.

Pyloric sphincter Ring of smooth muscle cells in the lower portion of the stomach where it joins the duodenum. Serves as a gate valve. Opens periodically after a meal, releasing spurts of chyme (liquified, partially digested food) into the small intestine.

Pyramid of numbers Diagram of the number of organisms at various trophic levels in a food chain or ecosystem.

Pyrimidine One of two types of nitrogen base found in DNA nucleotides. Consists of one ring.

Pyrogen Chemical released primarily from macrophages that have been exposed to bacteria and other foreign substances. Responsible for fever.

Quadraplegia Paralysis of skeletal muscles of the body from the neck down caused by spinal cord injury in the neck region.

Race Refers to a subgroup or a phenotypically distinct subpopulation.

Radial keratotomy Procedure to correct nearsightedness. Numerous, small superficial incisions are made in the cornea, flattening it and reducing its refractive power.

Radiation Tiny bursts of energy or particles emitted from the nucleus of some unstable atoms. Results from excess neutrons in the nuclei of some atoms.

Radionuclide Radioactive isotope of an atom.

Ramapithecines One of two primates that may have been the progenitor of apes and humans. Similar to the dryopithecines in many respects.

Range of tolerance Range of conditions in which an organism is adapted.

Receptor Any structure that responds to internal or external changes. Three types of receptors are found in the body: encapsulated, nonencapsulated (naked nerve endings), and specialized (e.g., the retina and semicircular canals).

Recessive Term describing an allele of a gene that is expressed when the dominant factor is missing.

Recombinant DNA technology Procedure in which scientists take segments of DNA from an organism and combine them with DNA from other organisms of the same or different species. Also more commonly known as *genetic engineering.*

Recombination Process of crossing over during meiosis, resulting in new genetic combinations.

Recruitment The engagement of additional muscle fibers during muscle contraction.

Rectum The last portion of the large intestine where feces are stored prior to defecation.

Red blood cells (RBCs) Enucleated cells in blood that transport oxygen in the bloodstream.

Red bone marrow Tissue found in the marrow cavity of bones. Site of blood cell and platelet production.

Reduction The addition of hydrogens or electrons to a molecule.

Reduction factor Any of the factors that cause populations to decline.

Referred pain Pain felt in one part of the body due to painful stimuli in another. For example, heart pain felt along the left arm.

Reflex Automatic response to a stimulus. Mediated by the nervous system.

Refraction Bending of light as it passes from one medium to another of different density.

Regulator gene Gene that codes for the synthesis of repressor protein in an operon.

Relaxin Hormone produced by the corpus luteum and the placenta. It is released near the end of pregnancy and softens the cervix and the fibrocartilage uniting the pubic bones, thus facilitating birth.

Releasing hormone Any of a group of hypothalamic hormones that stimulates the release of other hormones by the anterior pituitary.

Renal dialysis *See* dialysis.

Renal failure Shut-down of the kidney caused by the presence of toxic chemicals in the blood, immune reactions to certain antibiotics, severe kidney infections, and massive loss of blood. Renal failure may occur suddenly, over a period of a few hours or a few days.

Renal pelvis Hollow chamber inside the kidney. Receives urine from the collecting tubules and empties into the ureter.

Renal tubule That portion of the nephron where urine is produced.

Renewable resources Resources that replenish themselves via natural biological and geological processes, such as wind, hydropower, trees, fish, and wildlife.

Renin An enzyme produced by the kidney that cleaves a segment off a plasma protein called angiotensin, producing angiotensin I. It is then activated to form angiotensin II, which stimulates aldosterone secretion.

Replacement-level fertility Number of children that will replace a couple when they die.

Repolarization The return of a depolarized membrane in a nerve or muscle to its resting state.

Repressible operon Operon whose genes remain active unless turned off. Found in bacteria and may be present in eukaryotes as well.

Repressor protein Protein produced by a regulator gene. Binds to a region of the DNA molecule (the operator site) adjacent to the structural genes. Blocks RNA polymerase from transcribing structural genes.

Reproductive isolation Condition in which two groups of similar organisms derived from the same parent stock lose the ability to interbreed. Often due to geographic isolation.

Reptiles Class of vertebrates in which fertilization occurs internally. Includes snakes, lizards, and turtles.

Respiratory distress syndrome (RDS) A potentially life-threatening condition caused by a lack of surfactant in the lungs in premature babies.

Resting potential Minute voltage differential across the membrane of neurons. Also known as the *membrane potential.*

Restriction endonuclease Enzyme used in recombinant DNA technology. Cuts off segments of the DNA molecule for cloning and splicing.

Reticular activating system (RAS) Region of the medulla that receives nerve impulses from neurons transmitting information to and from the brain. Impulses are transmitted to the cortex, alerting it.

Retina Innermost, light-sensitive layer of the eye. Consists of an outer pigmented layer and an inner layer of nerve cells and photoreceptors (rods and cones).

Retrovirus Special type of RNA virus that carries an enzyme enabling it to produce complementary strands of DNA on the RNA template.

Reverse transcriptase Enzyme that allows the production of DNA from strands of viral RNA.

Reverse transcription The production of RNA from a DNA template. Occurs in cells infected by RNA viruses and permits viral replication as the DNA templates then serve as templates to make more viral RNA.

Rh factor An antigen on cells that can cause transfusion reactions if blood types are not well matched. People whose cells contain the Rh antigen, or Rh factor, are said to be Rh-positive. Those without it are Rh-negative.

Rheumatoid arthritis Type of arthritis in which the synovial membrane of the joint becomes inflamed and thickens. Results in pain and stiffness in joints. Thought to be an autoimmune disease.

Rhythm method Birth control method in which a couple abstains from sexual intercourse around the time of ovulation. Also known as the *natural method.*

Ribosomal RNA (rRNA) RNA produced at the nucleolus. Combines with protein to form the ribosome.

Ribosome Cellular organelle consisting of two subunits, each made of protein and ribosomal RNA. Plays an important part in protein synthesis.

Risk factor Factors such as smoking that increase the likelihood that someone will contract a disease.

RNA A nucleic acid consisting of numerous nucleotides. Three types are found in the body, ribosomal RNA, messenger RNA, and transfer RNA.

RNA polymerase Enzyme that helps align and join the nucleotides in a replicating RNA molecule.

Rod Type of photoreceptor in the eye. Provides for vision in dim light.

Root nodule Swelling in the roots of certain plants (legumes) containing nitrogen-fixing bacteria.

Rough endoplasmic reticulum (RER) Ribosome-coated endoplasmic reticulum. Produces lysosomal enzymes and proteins for use outside the cell.

Saccule Membranous sac located inside the vestibule. Contains a receptor for movement and body position.

Saliva A watery secretion produced by the salivary glands. Helps lubricate food for ease of swallowing. Contains a digestive enzyme that helps digest starch.

Salivary gland Any of several exocrine glands situated around the oral cavity. Produces saliva.

Saltatory conduction Conduction of a bioelectric impulse down a myelinated neuron from node to node.

Saprophyte Organism that releases enzymes that digest food materials externally. Smaller food molecules generated in the process are absorbed by the organism. Includes most fungi and nonphotosynthetic bacteria.

Sarcomere Functional unit of the muscle cell. Consists of the myofilaments, actin, and myosin.

Sarcoplasmic reticulum Term given to the smooth endoplasmic reticulum of a skeletal muscle fiber. Stores and releases calcium ions essential for muscle contractions.

Schwann cell Type of neuroglial cell or supportive cell in the nervous system. Responsible for the formation of the myelin sheath.

Science Body of knowledge on the workings of the world and a method of accumulating knowledge. *See also* Scientific method.

Scientific method Deliberate, systematic process of discovery. Begins with observation and measurement. From observations, hypotheses are generated and tested. This leads to more observation and measurement that supports or refutes the original hypothesis.

Sclera Outermost layer of the eye.

Scrotum Skin-covered sac containing the testes.

Sebaceous glands Oil-producing glands of the skin often associated with hair follicles.

Sebum Oil excreted by sebaceous glands onto the surface of the skin.

Second law of thermodynamics Law stating that no energy conversion is ever 100% efficient.

Secondary response Generally, a powerful, swift immune system response occurring the second time an antigen enters the body. Much faster than the primary response.

Secondary sex characteristics Distinguishing features of men and women resulting from the sex steroids. In men, includes facial hair growth and deeper voices. In women, includes breast development and fatty deposits in the hips and other regions.

Secondary succession Process of sequential change in which one community is replaced by another. It occurs where a biotic community previously existed, but was destroyed by natural forces or human actions.

Secondary tumor Cancerous growth formed by cells arising from a primary tumor.

Secretin Hormone produced by the cells of the duodenum. Stimulates the pancreas to release sodium bicarbonate.

Secretory vesicles Membrane-bound vesicles containing protein (hormones or enzymes) produced by the endoplasmic reticulum and packaged by the Golgi complex of some cells. They fuse with the membrane, releasing their contents by exocytosis.

Selective breeding A procedure in which organisms with superior or desirable traits are bred with other similar organisms to produce more of their kind.

Selective permeability Control of what moves across the plasma membrane of a cell.

Semen Fluid containing sperm and secretions of the secondary sex glands.

Semicircular canal Sensory organ of the inner ear. Houses the receptors that detect body position and movement.

Semiessential amino acid An amino acid that can be made in the body in sufficient amounts in adults but not growing children.

Semilunar valve Type of valve lying between the ventricles and the arteries that conduct blood away from the heart.

Seminal vesicles Sex accessory glands that empty into the vas deferens. Produce the largest portion of ejaculate.

Seminiferous tubule Sperm-producing tubule in the testis.

Sensineural deafness Deafness caused by a damage or a defect to the hair cells in the cochlea, the vestibulocochlear nerve, or the auditory cortex.

Sensitization Type of associative learning in which an individual learns to pay heightened attention to stimuli.

Sensory cortex That portion of the cerebral cortex involved in the perception of senses. Receives information from sensory neurons.

Sensory neuron A nerve cell that detects sensations often in conjunction with a specific receptor. It transmits information to the sensory cortex of the brain.

Sertoli cell Cell in the germinal epithelium of the seminiferous tubule. Houses spermatogenic cells as they develop.

Sex accessory gland One of several glands that produce secretions that are added to sperm during ejaculation.

Sex chromosomes X and Y chromosomes that help determine the sex of an individual. They also carry a few other traits.

Sex-influenced traits A term used to describe a trait in which the sex autosomal genes behave differently in the two sexes. In one sex, for example, an allele will be dominant; in the other sex, it will be recessive.

Sex-linked trait Trait produced by a gene carried on a sex chromosome.

Sex steroid Steroid hormones produced principally by the ovaries (in women) and testes (in men). Help regulate secretion of gonadotropins and determine secondary sex characteristics.

Sexually transmitted diseases (venereal diseases) Infections that are transmitted by sexual contact. Commonly referred to as *STDs.*

Sickle-cell anemia Genetic disease common in African Americans that results in abnormal hemoglobin in red blood cells, causing cells to become sickle shaped when exposed to low oxygen levels. Sickling causes cells to block capillaries, restricting blood flow to tissues.

Simple diffusion The movement of molecules or ions down a concentration gradient through pores in the membrane without the aid of a carrier protein.

Simple epithelium A lining of an organ or structure in the body consisting of a single layer of cells.

Sinoatrial node The heart's pacemaker. Located in the wall of the right atrium, it sends timed impulses to the heart muscle, thus synchronizing muscle contractions.

Sinusitis Bacterial and viral infections of the paranasal sinuses.

Skeletal muscle Muscle that is generally attached to the skeleton and causes body parts to move.

Skeleton Internal support of humans and other animals. Consists of bones joined together at joints.

Sliding filament mechanism Sliding of actin filaments toward the center of a sarcomere, causing muscle contraction.

Slow-twitch fibers Muscle fibers that contract slowly, but have high endurance. Found in areas of the body involved in maintaining balance and where rapid movement is not generally needed.

Small intestine A long tubular structure in the abdominal cavity in which food is digested and absorbed into the bloodstream.

Smooth endoplasmic reticulum (SER) Endoplasmic reticulum without ribosomes. Produces phosphoglycerides used to make the plasma membrane. Performs a variety of different functions in different cells.

Smooth muscle Involuntary muscle that lacks striations. Found around circulatory system vessels and in the walls of such organs as the stomach, uterus, and intestines.

Solvent Refers to any liquid capable of dissolving organic and inorganic compounds, such as water and alcohol.

Somatic cell A body cell such as those of bone, muscle, liver, brain, and blood.

Somatic pain Pain emanating from muscle, bones, joints, ligaments, tendons, and the skin, as opposed to visceral pain from internal organs.

Somite Block of mesoderm that gives rise to the vertebrae, muscles of the neck, and trunk.

Special sense Vision, hearing, taste, smell, and balance.

Speciation Formation of new species often as a result of geographic isolation.

Species Group of organisms that is structurally and functionally similar. When members of the group breed, they produce viable, reproductively competent offspring. Also a subgroup of a genus.

Species diversity Refers to the number of different species present in an ecosystem or biome; the higher the diversity, the more species are present.

Specificity The property of an enzyme allowing it to catalyze only one or a few chemical reactions.

Sperm A fully formed male gamete with a tail and a head. Contains 23 single-stranded chromosomes.

Spermatid One of several cells in the progression from spermatogonium to mature sperm. Found in the germinal epithelium of the seminiferous tubule. Produced by the second meiotic division. Contains 23 single-stranded chromosomes.

Spermatocyte (primary and secondary) Two cells in the progression from spermatogonium to mature sperm. Found in the germinal epithelium of the seminiferous tubule. Primary spermatocytes contain 46 double-stranded chromosomes and undergo the first meiotic division to produce secondary spermatocytes.

Spermatogenesis Formation of sperm in the seminiferous tubules.

Spermatogonia Sperm-producing cells in the periphery of the germinal epithelium of the seminiferous tubules.

Spermatozoan Sperm. Male germ cell.

Spinal nerve Nerve that arises from the spinal cord. Involved in motor and sensory functions.

Sponges Phylum of simple, immobile animals that live in colonies, mostly in saltwater. They demonstrate somewhat more complexity than one-celled organisms but less than organisms with distinct tissues.

Spongy bone Type of bony tissue inside most bones. Consists of an irregular network of bone spicules.

Spores (bacterial) Resistant structures produced when environmental conditions become unfavorable. They house the circular chromosome and a tiny amount of cytoplasm and are encased in a thick cell wall.

Starch A polysaccharide found in plants and made of many glucose units.

Stent A tiny metalic cylindrical structure that is inserted into coronary arteries to keep them open after balloon angioplasty.

Stereoscopic vision *See* depth perception.

Sterilization One of several techniques used to render sexually mature males and females infertile, incapable of producing offspring. *See* vasectomy and tubal ligation.

Steroid A type of lipid consisting of four joined ring structures. Examples: cholesterol and testosterone.

Stirrup (stapes) One of three bones of the middle ear that conducts vibrations from the eardrum to the inner ear.

Stoma (plural, *stomata*) Adjustable openings in plant leaves. Most gas exchange between leaves and the air occurs through the stoma.

Stomach A large hollow organ in the abdominal cavity that stores food and begins its breakdown.

Stratified epithelium A multilayered lining of a body surface or organ such as the epidermis of the skin.

Streptococcus A type of bacterium that infects the throat. Antibodies to it also damage the heart valve, making it extremely important to be treated early on.

Streptokinase An enzyme extracted from streptococcal bacteria that is used to dissolve blood clots in heart attack victims soon after they arrive in the emergency room.

Stretch receptor A receptor in tendons, muscles, and lungs that detect stretch. Often involved in spinal cord reflexes.

Stroke Also known as a *cerbrovascular accident*. Caused when blood flow to the brain is blocked due to an occlusion of an artery by an atherosclerotic plaque or a blood clot.

Stroma The semifluid medium of chloroplasts, in which the membranous grana are embedded; the site of the light-independent reactions.

Structural gene Any gene of an operon that codes for the production of enzymes and other proteins.

Subatomic particles Electrons, protons, and neutrons. Particles that can be separated from an atom by physical means.

Substrate Molecule that fits into the active site of an enzyme.

Succession Process of sequential change in which one community is replaced by another until a mature or climax ecosystem is formed. *See also* primary succession and secondary succession.

Sulcus Indented region or groove in the cerebral cortex between ridges.

Suppressor cell Cell of the immune system that shuts down the immune reaction as the antigen begins to disappear.

Surfactant Detergent-like substance produced by the lungs. Dissolves in the thin watery lining of the alveoli; helps reduce surface tension, keeping the alveoli from collapsing.

Suspensory ligament Zonular fibers that connect the lens to the ciliary body.

Sustainable society Society that lives within the carrying capacity of the environment.

Symbiosis Refers to a number of different types of biotic interaction within a community, including mutualism and commensalism.

Sympathetic division Division of the autonomic nervous system that is responsible for many functions, especially those involved in the fight-or-flight response.

Sympatric speciation The formation of a new species without geographic isolation. Common in plants.

Synapse Juncture of two neurons that allows an impulse to travel from one neuron to the next.

Synaptic cleft Gap between an axon and the dendrite or effector (e.g., gland or muscle) it supplies.

Synergist Stabilizing muscles that steady joints, allowing other muscles to act. These muscles help to maintain our posture, permitting us to stand or sit upright.

Synergy Coordination of the workings of antagonistic muscle groups.

Synovial fluid Lubricating liquid inside joint cavities. Produced by the synovial membrane.

Synovial joint Any of the many movable body joints that is filled with synovial fluid.

Synovial membrane Inner layer of the joint capsule.

Syphilis Potentially serious, sexually transmitted disease caused by a bacterium.

Systemic circulation System of blood vessels that transports blood to and from the body and heart, excluding the lungs.

Systolic pressure Peak pressure at the moment the ventricles contract. The higher of the two numbers in a blood pressure reading.

Taiga The northern coniferous forests biome.

Target cell A term used to describe the cell or cells that a hormone affects.

Taste bud Receptor for taste principally found in the surface epithelium and certain papillae of the tongue.

T cell *See* T-lymphocyte.

Telophase Final stage of mitosis in which the nuclear envelope reforms from vesicles and the chromosomes uncoil.

Temperate deciduous forest Biome that in the United States lies east of the Mississippi River and is characterized by broadleafed trees.

Temporary threshold shift Temporary loss of hearing after being exposed to a noisy environment.

Tendons Connective tissue structures that generally attach muscles to bones.

Teratogen Chemical, biological, or physical agent that causes birth defects.

Teratology Study of birth defects.

Terminal boutons Small swellings on the terminal fibers of axons. They lie close to the membranes of the dendrites of other axons or the membranes of the effectors, and transfer bioelectric impulses from one cell to another.

Terminator codon Codon found on each strand of messenger RNA that marks where protein synthesis should end.

Testes Male gonads. They produce sex steroids and sperm.

Testosterone Male sex hormone that stimulates sperm formation and is responsible for secondary sex characteristics, such as facial hair growth and muscle growth.

Tetanus A long sustained muscle contraction, for example, when you are carrying a bag of groceries.

Thalamus A part of the brain that acts as a relay center.

Theory Principles of science—the broader generalizations about the world and its components. Theories are supported by considerable scientific research.

Theory of Endosymbiotic Evolution A theory that explains the formation of eukaryotic cells in which many of the organelles were formed by the incorporation of free-living single-celled organisms in early cells.

Theory of Natural Selection A theory proposed by Charles Darwin to explain how evolution works; it states that the fittest organisms of a population survive and reproduce, thus passing their genes on to future generations. Over time, this results in a shift in the genetic makeup of the population.

Theory of Spontaneous Generation A outdated (and incorrect) theory that says that organisms arise spontaneously from nonliving matter.

Thermocline A layer of water between the epilimnion and hypolimnion; characterized by rapid temperature change.

Thermoreceptor A receptor that detects hot or cold.

Thoracic duct Duct carrying lymph to the circulatory system. Empties into the large veins at the base of the neck.

Thrombin A chemical in the blood that converts fibrinogen into fibrin during clot formation.

Thromboplastin A lipoprotein that acts on an inactive plasma enzyme in the blood known as prothrombin. Thromboplastin causes prothrombin to be converted into its active form, thrombin.

Thrombosis A blood clot that breaks loose and travels in the circulatory system, where it may eventually become lodged in an artery, blocking blood flow to downstream areas.

Thymine A nitrogen-containing base known as a pyrimidine. Found in DNA, not RNA.

Thymus A lymphoid organ found above the heart. Gradually decreases in size as we age. The site at which T cells become immunologically competent.

Thyroglobulin The protein in the interior of the thyroid follicles from which thyroid hormones are made.

Thyroid gland U- or H-shaped gland located in the neck on either side of the trachea just below the larynx. Produces three hormones: thyroxin, triiodothyronine, and calcitonin.

Thyroid-stimulating hormone (TSH) Hormone produced by the pituitary gland. Stimulates production and release of thyroxine and triiodothyronine by the thyroid gland.

Thyroxin Hormone produced by the thyroid gland that accelerates the rate of mitochondrial glucose catabolism in most body cells and also stimulates cellular growth and development.

Tidal volume The air that moves in and out of the lungs during normal breathing.

Tight junction A structure that holds the plasma membrane of cells together in regions of the body like the skin, where it is necessary to prevent the loss of water or the movement of bacteria.

Tissue Component of the body from which organs are made. Consists of cells and extracellular material (fluid, fibers, and so on). See primary tissue.

T-lymphocyte Type of lymphocyte responsible for cell-mediated immunity. Attacks foreign cells, virus-infected cells, and cancer cells directly. Also known as *T cell*.

Total fertility rate (TFR) Number of children a woman is expected to have during her lifetime.

Trachea Duct that leads from the pharynx to the lungs.

Transcription RNA production on a DNA template.

Transfer RNA (tRNA) Small RNA molecules that bind to amino acids in the cytoplasm and deliver them to specific sites on the messenger RNA.

Transformation Conversion of a normal cell to a cancerous one.

Transition reaction Part of cellular respiration in which one carbon is cleaved from pyruvic acid, forming a two-carbon compound, which reacts with Coenzyme A. The resulting chemical enters the citric acid cycle.

Translation Synthesis of protein on a messenger RNA template.

Translocation Process in which a segment of a chromosome breaks off but reattaches to another site on the same chromosome or another one.

Transpiration Process by which water evaporates from leaf surfaces. Creates a tension (reduced pressure) in the xylem that pulls columns of water from the roots to the stems.

Triiodothyronine Hormone produced by the thyroid gland. Nearly identical in function to thyroxin.

Triploidy Genetic disorder in which cells have 69 chromosomes instead of 46.

Trisomy Genetic condition characterized by the presence of one extra chromosome.

Trophic hormones Hormones that stimulate the production and secretion of other hormones. Also known as *tropic hormones*.

Trophic level Feeding level in a food chain.

Trophoblast Outer ring of cells of the blastocyst that form the embryonic portion of the placenta.

Trypsin A proteolytic digestive enzyme produced by pancreas in an inactive form, trypsinogen.

TSH-releasing hormone (TSH-RH) Hormone secreted by the posterior lobe of the pituitary gland. Stimulates thyroxin secretion by the thyroid gland.

T tubules (transverse tubules) Invaginations of the plasma membrane of skeletal muscle fibers that conduct an impulse to the interior of the cell.

Tubal ligation Sterilization procedure in women. Uterine tubes are cut, preventing sperm and ova from uniting.

Tubal pregnancy One type of ectopic pregnancy in which the embryo embeds in the lining of the oviduct or Fallopian tube.

Tubular reabsorption Process in which nutrients are transported out of the nephron into the peritubular capillaries.

Tubular secretion Process in which wastes are transported from the peritubular capillaries into the nephron.

Tumor Mass of cells derived from a single cell that has begun to divide. In malignant tumors, the cells divide uncontrollably and often release clusters of cells or single cells that spread in the blood and lymphatic systems to other parts of the body. Benign tumors grow to a certain size, then stop.

Tumor suppressor genes A gene that is involved in regulation of the cell cycle, suppressing cell division. A mutation in this gene can lead to uncontrolled cellular replication.

Tundra Northernmost biome with long, cold winters and a short growing season.

Turner syndrome Genetic disorder in which an offspring contains 22 pairs of autosomes and a single, unmatched X chromosome. Phenotypically female.

Twitch A muscle contraction followed by relaxation.

Tympanic membrane (eardrum) Membrane between the external auditory canal and middle ear that oscillates when struck by sound waves.

Type I alveolar cell Flattened cell in the lining of the alveoli in the lungs.

Type II alveolar cell Cell found in the lining of the alveoli. Produces surfactant.

Type I diabetes Form of diabetes that occurs mainly in young people and results from an insufficient amount of insulin production and release. Brought on by damage to insulin-producing cells of the pancreas. Also known as *early-onset diabetes*.

Type II diabetes Form of diabetes that occurs chiefly in older individuals (around age of 40) and results from a loss of tissue responsiveness to insulin. Also known as *late-onset diabetes*.

Ulcer A region of the stomach lining eroded by acids and digestive enzymes.

Ultrasound Low-frequency sound waves that are used to break apart kidney stones. They're also used diagnostically to view embryos and intervertebral disks.

Ultraviolet radiation A type of radiation produced by the sun. It is responsible for vitamin D formation in the skin of humans, but excess exposure can lead to cataracts and skin cancer. It is also lethal to plants and other organisms.

Umbilical artery One of two arteries in the umbilical cord that carries blood from the embryo to the placenta.

Umbilical vein Vein in the umbilical cord that carries blood from the placenta to the fetus.

Undernutrition A condition characterize by a lack of nutrients.

Universal donor An individual with Type O blood is so named because Type O blood has neither A nor B antigens and can be transfused into individuals with all four blood types.

Urea A waste product produced during the breakdown of amino acids in cells.

Ureter Hollow, muscular tube that transports urine by peristaltic contractions from the kidney to the urinary bladder.

Urethra Narrow tube that transports urine from the urinary bladder to the outside of the body. In males, it also conducts sperm and semen to the outside.

Uric acid A waste product of the breakdown of nucleic acids in the body. Excreted in the urine.

Urinary bladder Hollow, distensible organ with muscular walls that stores urine. Drained by the urethra.

Urinary incontinence A medical condition created by a loss of control of the urinary bladder so that when urine builds up, it is automatically excreted.

Urine Fluid containing various wastes that is produced in the kidney and excreted out of the urinary bladder.

Urochrome A yellow pigment found that produced by the breakdown of hemoglobin in the liver and excreted in the urine.

Urokinase An enzyme that breaks down blood clots which is given to heart attack victims soon after arriving at the emergency room.

Uterine glands Small glands found in the inner lining of the uterus. Produce secretions that nourish the newly formed zygote and embryo before implantation.

Uterine tubes Same as oviducts or Fallopian tubes.

Uterus (womb) Organ that houses and nourishes the developing embryo and fetus.

Utricle Membranous sac containing a receptor for body position and movement. Located inside the vestibule of the inner ear.

Vaccine Preparation containing dead or weakened bacteria and viruses that, when injected in the body, elicits an immune response. *See also* Active immunity.

Vagina Tubular organ that serves as a receptacle for sperm and provides a route for delivery of the baby at birth.

Vaginal sponge A small sponge device placed over the end of the cervix to prevent fertilization. The sponge is impregnated with spermacidal chemicals.

Vagus nerve Nerve that terminates in the stomach wall and stimulates HCl production by cells in the gastric glands.

Variation Genetically based differences in physical or functional characteristics within a population.

Varicose vein Vein whose wall balloons out because the flow of blood downstream is obstructed.

Vas deferens Duct that carries sperm from the testis to the urethra. Contracts during ejaculation.

Vasectomy Contraceptive procedure in men in which the vas deferens is cut and the free ends sealed to prevent sperm from entering the urethra during ejaculation.

Vasopressin Also known as *antidiuretic hormone* or *ADH*, which in high concentrations increases blood pressure.

Vein Type of blood vessel that carries blood to the heart.

Vena cava One of two large veins that empty into the right atrium of the heart.

Ventral root (of a spinal nerve) The anterior portion of the spinal nerve carrying motor impulses to muscles and glands.

Ventricle (of brain) Any of the several cavities inside the brain containing cerebrospinal fluid.

Ventricle (of heart) The large muscular pumping chambers of the heart. Located below the atria.

Venule Smallest of all veins. Empties into capillary networks.

Vertebra Any of the small bones of the back that form the spinal column.

Vertebral canal The opening in the vertebrae through which the spinal cord passes.

Vertebrates Animals with a spinal column (backbone).

Vestibular apparatus An organ that contains receptors for both movement and body position. Consists of the semicircular canals and vestibule.

Vestigial structure A body part that has no apparent function, such as the appendix.

Visceral pain Pain in the viscera, the internal organs.

Villi Fingerlike projections of the lining of the small intestine that increase the surface area for absorption.

Virus Nonliving entity consisting of a nucleic acid—either DNA or RNA—core surrounded by a protein coat, the capsid. Viruses are cellular parasites, invading cells and taking over their metabolic machinery to reproduce.

Visible light Electromagnetic radiation visible to humans and other animals.

Vitamin Any of a diverse group of organic compounds. Essential to many metabolic reactions.

Vitreous humor Gelatinous material found in the posterior cavity of the eye.

Vocal cords Elastic ligaments inside the larynx that vibrate as air is expelled from the lungs, generating sound.

Watershed A region drained by a river.

Wave summation A piggybacking of muscle fiber contractions that occurs when stimuli arrive before a muscle fiber relaxes.

Wet deposition Deposition of acids in rain, snow, fog, and mist.

White blood cells (WBCs) Cells of the blood formed in the bone marrow. Principally involved in fighting infection.

White matter The portion of the brain and spinal cord that appears white to the naked eye. Consists primarily of white, myelinated nerve fibers.

Withdrawal *See* coitus interruptus.

X-Linked trait A trait that is determined by a gene on the X chromosome.

Yellow marrow Inactive marrow of bones in adults containing fat. Formed from red marrow.

Yolk sac Embryonic pouch formed from endoderm. Site of early formation of red blood cells and germ cells.

Zero population growth (ZPG) Condition in which a population stops growing.

Zona pellucida Band of material surrounding the oocyte.

Zone of intolerance Refers to the biotic and abiotic factors that make survival and reproduction impossible.

Zone of physiological stress Refers to the biotic and abiotic conditions that do not exclude an organism, but are clearly not optimal for survival and reproduction.

Zonular fibers Thin fibers that attach the lens to the ciliary body.

Zygote Cell produced by a sperm and ovum during fertilization. Contains 46 chromosomes.

Index

Note: Page numbers followed by f indicate figures; those followed by t indicate tables.

Photo Credits

■ **Chapter 1**

Chapter opener Vandystadt/Allsport USA; **FIGURE 1-2A**, Marc Epstein/Visuals Unlimited; **FIGURE 1-2B**, Grant Heilman/Grant Heilman Photography; **FIGURE 1-3**, PhotoDisc; **FIGURE 1-4A**, Peter Arnold, Inc.; **FIGURE 1-4B**, Ed Reschke/Peter Arnold, Inc.; **FIGURE 1-5** PNI; **FIGURE 1-6**, Photodisc; **FIGURE 1-7A**, Joe McDonald/Visuals Unlimited; **FIGURE 1-7B**, A.M. Siegelman/Visuals Unlimited; **FIGURE 1-7C**, Cabisco/Visuals Unlimited; **FIGURE 1-8**, Tom Edwards/Visuals Unlimited; Health Note 1-1, **FIGURE 1** Will and Demi McIntyre/Photo Researchers

■ **Chapter 2**

Chapter opener George Musil/Visuals Unlimited; **FIGURE 2-6**, Kim Taylor/Bruce Coleman, Inc.; **FIGURE 2-7**, Walt Anderson/Visuals Unlimited

■ **Chapter 3**

Chapter opener Don W. Fawcett/Visuals Unlimited; **FIGURE 3-1A**, Ralph A. Slepecky/Visuals Unlimited; **FIGURE 3-1B**, K.G. Murty/Visuals Unlimited; **FIGURE 3-2A**, R. Calentine/Visuals Unlimited; **FIGURE 3-2B**, Biodisc/Visuals Unlimited; **FIGURE 3-3A**, W. Ormerod/Visuals Unlimited; **FIGURE 3-3B**, Fred E. Hossler/Visuals Unlimited; **FIGURE 3-5**, M. Schliwa/Visuals Unlimited; **FIGURE 3-18A**, K.G. Murty/Visuals Unlimited; **FIGURE 3-18B**, Don W. Fawcett/Visuals Unlimited; **FIGURE 3-19A**, K.G. Murty/Visuals Unlimited; **FIGURE 3-19B**, L.Lisco/D.W. Fawcett/Visuals Unlimited; **FIGURE 3-20**, from Electron Microscopy, Second Edition by John J. Bozzola and Lonnie D. Russell reprinted with permission from Jones and Bartlett Publishers, Inc.; **FIGURE 3-21B**, Don W. Fawcett/Visuals Unlimited.; **FIGURE 3-21C**, Don W. Fawcett/Visuals Unlimited; **FIGURE 3-22**, RMF/Visuals Unlimited; **FIGURE 3-23**, DonW. Fawcett/Visuals Unlimited; **FIGURE 3-24**, Cabisco/Visuals Unlimited; **FIGURE 3-25**, David M. Philips/Visuals Unlimited; **FIGURE 3-26A**, David M. Phillips/Visuals Unlimited; **FIGURE 3-26B**, David M. Phillips/Visuals Unlimited; **FIGURE 3-27**, Ellen R. Dirksen/Visuals Unlimited; **FIGURE 3-29**, M. Abbey/Visuals Unlimited

■ **Chapter 4**

Chapter opener M. Schliwa/Visuals Unlimited; **FIGURE 4-1**, David M. Phillips/Visuals Unlimited; **FIGURE 4-5A**, Fred Hossler/Visuals Unlimited; **FIGURE 4-5B**, David M. Phillips/Visuals Unlimited; **FIGURE 4-8**, J. Boliver/Custom Medical Stock; **FIGURE 4-9A**, Fred Hossler/Visuals Unlimited; **FIGURE 4-9B**, Cabisco/Visuals Unlimited; **FIGURE 4-11A**, R. Calentine/Visuals Unlimited; **FIGURE 4-11B**, John D. Cunningham/Visuals Unlimited; **FIGURE 4-11C**, R. Kessel/Visuals Unlimited; **FIGURE 4-12A**, John D. Cunningham/Visuals Unlimited; **FIGURE 4-12B**, John D. Cunningham/Visuals Unlimited; **FIGURE 4-12C**, R. Calentine/Visuals Unlimited; **FIGURE 4-13**, John D. Cunningham/Visuals Unlimited

■ **Chapter 5**

Chapter opener Biodisc/Visuals Unlimited; **FIGURE 5-6A**, Cabisco/Visuals Unlimited; **FIGURE 5-6B**, Veronika Burmeister/Visuals Unlimited; **FIGURE 5-8A**, Cabisco/Visuals Unlimited; **FIGURE 5-8B**, William Ober/Visuals Unlimited; **FIGURE 5-9**, AP/Wide World Photos; **FIGURE 5-11**, Tony Cubillas/Visuals Unlimited; **FIGURE 5-15**, John D. Cunningham/Visuals Unlimited; **FIGURE 5-19**, ©Dr. E. Walker/Science Photo Library; **FIGURE 5-21A**, From Edward J. Reith and Michael H. Ross, Atlas of Descriptive Histology, 3/e, 1977 by Harper and Row. Used by permission of J.B. Lippincott Company; **FIGURE 5-21B**, John D. Cunningham/Visuals Unlimited; **FIGURE 5-21C**, John D. Cunningham/Visuals Unlimited; **FIGURE 5-21D**, Michael Webb; **FIGURE 5-21E**, David M. Phillips/Visuals Unlimited

■ **Chapter 6**

Chapter opener Fred Hossler/Visuals Unlimited **FIGURE 6-1**, CNRI/Photo Researchers; **FIGURE 6-4A**, Phillipe Plailly/Photo Researchers; **FIGURE 6-4B**, Science Photo Library/Photo Researchers; **FIGURE 6-6**, Ken Sherman/Medichrome; **FIGURE 6-7**, VAS Comm/Custom Medical Stock Photo; **FIGURE 6-8B**, William Ober/Visuals Unlimited; **FIGURE 6-9**, D.W. Fawcett-Kuwabara/Visuals Unlimited; **FIGURE 6-10**, Cabisco/Visuals Unlimited; **FIGURE 6-13A**, John D. Cunningham/Visuals Unlimited; **FIGURE 6-13B**, John D. Cunningham/Visuals Unlimited; **FIGURE 6-14**, Keith/Custom Medical Stock Photo; **FIGURE 6-18**, Fred Marsik/Visuals Unlimited; Scientific Discoveries 6-1, **FIGURE 1**, Bettmann Archive

■ **Chapter 7**

Chapter opener CNRI/Photo Researchers; **FIGURE 7-2A**, David M. Phillips/Visuals Unlimited; **FIGURE 7-2B**, Stanley Flegler/Visuals Unlimited; **FIGURE 7-3**, Stanley Flegler/Visuals Unlimited; **FIGURE 7-6**, R. Calentine/Visuals Unlimited; **FIGURE 7-7**, G. Prance/Visuals Unlimited; **FIGURE 7-8A**, Science VU/Visuals Unlimited; **FIGURE 7-8B**, Peter K. Ziminski/Visuals Unlimited; **FIGURE 7-9**, John D. Cunningham/Visuals Unlimited; **FIGURE 7-10**, David M. Phillips/Visuals Unlimited; **TABLE 7-2**, John D. Cunningham/Visuals Unlimited

■ Chapter 8

Chapter opener W. Johnson/Visuals Unlimited; **FIGURE 8-1**, Visuals Unlimited/G. Musil; **FIGURE 8-2**, David M. Phillips/Visuals Unlimited; **FIGURE 8-10**, W. Johnson/Visuals Unlimited; **FIGURE 8-12**, Leonard L Rue III/Visuals Unlimited; **FIGURE 8-16A**, Science VU/Visuals Unlimited; **FIGURE 8-16B**, Science VU/Visuals Unlimited; Health Note 8-1, **FIGURE 1**, John D. Cunningham/Visuals Unlimited

■ Chapter 9

Chapter opener CNRI/Photo Researchers; **FIGURE 9-5A**, David M. Phillips/Visuals Unlimited; **FIGURE 9-5B**, David M. Phillips/Visuals Unlimited; **FIGURE 9-5C**, Don Fawcett/Visuals Unlimited; **FIGURE 9-7**, R. Calentine/Visuals Unlimited; **FIGURE 9-8**, Science VU/Visuals Unlimited; **FIGURE 9-9**, Chet Childs/Custom Medical Stock; **FIGURE 9-14A**, SIU/Visuals Unlimited; **FIGURE 9-14B**, SIU/Visuals Unlimited; **FIGURE 9-15**, SIU/Visuals Unlimited; Health Note 9-2, **FIGURE 1A**, American Cancer Society; Health Note 9-2, **FIGURE 1B**, James Stevenson/SPL/Photo Researchers

■ Chapter 10

Chapter opener CNRI/Photo Researchers; **FIGURE 10-1**, SIU/Visuals Unlimited; **FIGURE 10-10A**, NMSB/Custom Medical Stock; **FIGURE 10-10B**, Runk/Schoenberger/Medical Images, Inc.

■ Chapter 11

Chapter opener Cabisco/Visuals Unlimited; **FIGURE 11-4**, David M. Phillips/Visuals Unlimited; **FIGURE 11-6**, C. Raines/Visuals Unlimited; **FIGURE 11-7**, Howard Sochureck/Visuals Unlimited; **FIGURE 11-11A**, Science VU/E.R. Lewis/Visuals Unlimited; **FIGURE 11-11B**, T. Reese, D.W. Fawcett/Visuals Unlimited; **FIGURE 11-24**, SIU/Visuals Unlimited; Health Note 11-1, **FIGURE 1**, TongueDisco/The Image Bank

■ Chapter 12

Chapter opener John D. Cunningham/Visuals Unlimited; **FIGURE 12-3A**, Cabisco/Visuals Unlimited; **FIGURE 12-3B**, Biophoto Associates/Photo Researchers; **FIGURE 12-8**, A.L. Blum/Visuals Unlimited; **FIGURE 12-10**, Bill Beatty/Visuals Unlimited; **FIGURE 12-20**, Beltone Electronics; **FIGURE 12-21**, Science VU/Cochlear Corp./Visuals Unlimited; Health Note 12-1, **FIGURE 1**, © Photodisc

■ Chapter 13

Chapter opener Science Photo Library/Photo Researchers; **FIGURE 13-1**, Jeffrey Howe/Visuals Unlimited; **FIGURE 13-7A**, SIU/Visuals Unlimited; **FIGURE 13-7B**, SIU/Visuals Unlimited; **FIGURE 13-8**, SIU/Visuals Unlimited; **FIGURE 13-9A**, SIU/Visuals Unlimited; **FIGURE 13-9B**, SIU/Visuals Unlimited; **FIGURE 13-10**, Science VU/Visuals Unlimited; **FIGURE 13-13A**, Reprinted with permission from Calcified Tissue Research, 1967; **FIGURE 13-13B**, Reprinted with permission from Calcified Tissue Research, 1967; **FIGURE 13-13C**, Reprinted with permission from Calcified Tissue Research, 1967; **FIGURE 13-13D**, Reprinted with permission from Calcified Tissue Research, 1967; **FIGURE 13-15**, R. Calentine/Visuals Unlimited; **FIGURE 13-18**, John D. Cunningham/Visuals Unlimited; **FIGURE 13-20**, Bruce Bergs/Visuals Unlimited; Health Note 13-1, **FIGURE 1**, Yoav Levy/Phototake

■ Chapter 14

Chapter opener SIU/Visuals Unlimited; **FIGURE 14-7A**, AP/Wide World Photos; **FIGURE 14-7B**, AP/Wide World Photos; **FIGURE 14-8**, Reprinted with permission from American Journal of Medicine, 20 (1956); **FIGURE 14-14A**, R. Calentine/Visuals Unlimited; **FIGURE 14-14B**, David M. Phillips/Visuals Unlimited; **FIGURE 14-15**, Ken Greer/Visuals Unlimited; **FIGURE 14-16**, John D. Cunningham/Visuals Unlimited; **FIGURE 14-20**, Science VU/Visuals Unlimited

■ Chapter 15

Chapter opener M. Schliwa/Visuals Unlimited; **FIGURE 15-1**, Stan W. Elems/Visuals Unlimited; **FIGURE 15-4**, Cabisco/Visuals Unlimited; **FIGURE 15-5**, Custom Medical Stock Photography; **FIGURE 15-6**, Science VU/Visuals Unlimited; **FIGURE 15-7**, SIU/Visuals Unlimited; **FIGURE 15-8A**, Michael Abbey/Visuals Unlimited; **FIGURE 15-8B**, Michael Abbey/Visuals Unlimited; **FIGURE 15-8C**, John D. Cunningham/Visuals Unlimited; **FIGURE 15-8D**, John D. Cunningham/Visuals Unlimited; **FIGURE 15-8E**, John D. Cunningham/Visuals Unlimited; **FIGURE 15-8F**, John D. Cunningham/Visuals Unlimited; **FIGURE 15-11**, David M. Phillips/Visuals Unlimited; Scientific Discovery 15-1, **FIGURE 1**, Cold Spring Harbour Laboratory; Scientific Discovery 15-1, **FIGURE 2**, Science VU/NIHLBL/Visuals Unlimited; Health Note 15-1, **FIGURE 1**, Cabisco/Visuals Unlimited

■ Chapter 16

Chapter opener Biophoto Associates/Photo Researchers; **FIGURE 16-4A**, The Bettmann Archive; **FIGURE 16-4B**, Malcolm Gutter/Visuals Unlimited; **FIGURE 16-9**, Joe McDonald/Visuals Unlimited; **FIGURE 16-10A**, Science VU/Daniel V. Schidlow/Visuals Unlimited; **FIGURE 16-10B**, Science VU/Daniel V. Schidlow/Visuals

Unlimited; **FIGURE 16-11**, Jeffrey Reed/Medichrome; **FIGURE 16-12A**, Bruce Berg/Visuals Unlimited; **FIGURE 16-12B**, Bruce Berg/Visuals Unlimited; **FIGURE 16-13**, Dr. Ira Rosenthal, Department of Pediatrics, University of Illinois at Chicago; **FIGURE 16-16A**, James Alan Brown/Visuals Unlimited; **FIGURE 16-16B**, A.J. Copley/Visuals Unlimited; **FIGURE 16-16C**, M. Long/Visuals Unlimited; **FIGURE 16-16D**, Marek W. Litwin/Visuals Unlimited; **FIGURE 16-16E**, John D. Cunningham/Visuals Unlimited; **FIGURE 16-18**, Cabisco/Visuals Unlimited; **FIGURE 16-20**, Biophoto Associates/Photo Researchers; **FIGURE 16-23A**, Science VU/Valerie Lindgren/Visuals Unlimited; **FIGURE 16-23B**, Bernd Wittich/Visuals Unlimited; **FIGURE 16-26A**, Science VU/Valerie Lindgren/Visuals Unlimited; **FIGURE 16-26B**, Dr. Ira Rosenthal/Department of Pediatrics, University of Illinois at Chicago; **FIGURE 16-27**, S.C.R. Reuman/Visuals Unlimited; Health Note 16-1, **FIGURE 1**, Bill Bachmann/Photo Network/PNI

■ Chapter 17

Chapter opener Science VU/Lawrence Livermore Laboratory/Visuals Unlimited; **FIGURE 17-12**, Ralph A. Slepecky/Visuals Unlimited; **FIGURE 17-16**, Dana Richter/Visuals Unlimited; **FIGURE 17-17**, Courtesy of Thermo Technologies.; Scientific Discoveries 17-1, **FIGURE 1**, AP/Wide World Photos

■ Chapter 18

Chapter opener SIU/Visuals Unlimited; **FIGURE 18-1**, Tom McHugh/Photo Researchers; **FIGURE 18-2**, Ken Lucas/Visuals Unlimited; **FIGURE 18-4**, Huntington Potter and David Pressler/Department of Neurobiology, Harvard Medical School; **FIGURE 18-7**, Science VU/©Jackson Lab/Visuals Unlimited; **FIGURE 18-8**, Keith V. Wood/Science VU/Visuals Unlimited

■ Chapter 19

Chapter opener Visuals Unlimited; **FIGURE 19-3A**, Biophoto Associates/Photo Researchers; **FIGURE 19-3B**, Lester Bergman and Associates; **FIGURE 19-4**, John D. Cunningham/Visuals Unlimited; **FIGURE 19-5**, Fred Hossler/Visuals Unlimited; **FIGURE 19-6**, David M. Phillips/Visuals Unlimited; **FIGURE 19-16**, Carter-Wallace Company; **FIGURE 19-20**, Science-VU-ortho/Visuals Unlimited; **FIGURE 19-21A**, Cabisco/Visuals Unlimited; **FIGURE 19-21B**, Cabisco/Visuals Unlimited; **FIGURE 19-22**, SIU/Visuals Unlimited; **FIGURE 19-23**, SIU/Visuals Unlimited; **FIGURE 19-24**, M. Long/Visuals Unlimited; **FIGURE 19-25**, SIU/Visuals Unlimited; **FIGURE 19-28**, Phototake/PNI; **FIGURE 19-29**, Christopher

Brown/Stock Boston Health Note 19-1, **FIGURE 1** © SIU, Visuals Unlimited; **FIGURE 2** OJ Staats/Custom Medical Stock Photos

■ Chapter 20

Chapter opener Cabisco/Visuals Unlimited; **FIGURE 20-2**, Lennart Nilsson, Behold Man, Little, Brown and Company; **FIGURE 20-11**, SIU/Visuals Unlimited; **FIGURE 20-14**, Ka Botzis; **FIGURE 20-16**, Michael DeMocker/Visuals Unlimited; Health Note 20-1 **FIGURE 1**© SIU/Visuals Unlimited

■ Chapter 21

Chapter opener Kjell Sandved/Visuals Unlimited; **FIGURE 21-3**, Sidney Fox/Science VU/Visuals Unlimited; **FIGURE 21-4**, Science VU-USM/Visuals Unlimited; **FIGURE 21-7**, Rick Wallace/Visuals Unlimited; **FIGURE 21-8**, Ken Lucas/Visuals Unlimited; **FIGURE 21-9**, John D. Cunningham/Visuals Unlimited; **FIGURE 21-10A**, Dale Jackson/Visuals Unlimited; **FIGURE 21-10B**, Daniel D. Chiras; **FIGURE 21-11**, Science VU/Visuals Unlimited; **FIGURE 21-14A**, Nada Pecnick/Visuals Unlimited; **FIGURE 21-14B**, A.J. Copley/Visuals Unlimited; **FIGURE 21-14C**, Dr. P.A. Zahl, Photo Researchers; **FIG-URE 21-16**, John Cancalos/Visuals Unlimited; **FIGURE 21-18 TOP**, Gary Meszaros/Visuals Unlimited; **FIGURE 21-18 BOTTOM**, Arthur Morris/Visuals Unlimited; Health Note 21-1, **FIGURE 1**, Link/Visuals Unlimited

■ Chapter 22

Chapter opener Fred Espenak/NASA/Science Photo Library/Photo Researchers; **FIGURE 22-1**, Milton H. Tierney, Jr./Visuals Unlimited; **FIGURE 22-3A**, Michael Dick/Animals Animals; **FIGURE 22-3B**, Walt Anderson/Visuals Unlimited; **FIGURE 22-4A**, Walt Anderson/Visuals Unlimited; **FIGURE 22-4B**, John D. Cunningham/Visuals Unlimited; **FIGURE 22-5A**, Thomas C. Boyden/Visuals Unlimited; **FIGURE 22-5B**A. Wolfe, Photo Researchers; **FIGURE 22-7**, Charles Rushing/Visuals Unlimited; **FIGURE 22-9**, National Museum of Kenya/VU; **FIGURE 22-10**, Cabisco/Visuals Unlimited; **FIGURE 22-12**, Science VU/Visuals Unlimited; **FIGURE 22-13A**, Henri Sommer/Visuals Unlimited; **FIGURE 22-13B**, Emily Strong/Visuals Unlimited; **FIGURE 22-13C**, Daniel D. Chiras; **FIGURE 22-13D**, Charles Sykes/Visuals Unlimited; **FIGURE 22-13E**, John Cancalosi/Visuals Unlimited; **FIGURE 22-14**, G. Prance/Visuals Unlimited; **FIGURE 22-15**, © Art Wolfe/Tony Stone Images; **FIGURE 22-16**, Clyde H. Smith/Peter Arnold, Inc.

Biological Roots

ONE OF THE MAJOR CHALLENGES of a biology course is mastering new terminology. One of the best ways of learning and remembering technical terms is to first learn their component parts—that is, their roots. But studying common Latin and Greek roots for biological terms before you begin your study can also help. Spend a few minutes early in your course studying these common roots. They will not only help you understand new terms, but also make them easier to remember.

a-, an- [Gk. *an-,* not, without, lacking]: anaerobic, abiotic, anemia

ad- [L. *ad-,* toward, to]: adrenalin

amphi- [Gk. *amphi-,* two, both, both sides of]: amphibian

ana- [Gk. *ana-,* up, up against]: anaphase, anabolic, anatomy

andro- [Gk. *andros,* an old man]: androgen

anti- [Gk. *anti-,* against, opposite, opposed to]: antibiotic, antibody, antigen, antidiuretic hormone

arthro- [Gk. *arthron,* a joint]: arthropod, arthritis

auto- [Gk. *auto-,* self, same]: autoimmune, autotroph

bi-, bin- [L. *bis,* twice; *bini,* two-by-two]: binary fission, binocular vision, bicarbonate

bio- [Gk. *bios,* life]: biology, biomass, biome, biosphere, biotic

blasto-, -blast [Gk. *blastos,* sprout; pertains to embryo]: blastula, trophoblast, osteoblast

broncho- [Gk. *bronchos,* windpipe]: bronchus, bronchi, bronchiole, bronchitis

carb- [L. *carbo,* coal]: carbon, carbohydrate

carcino- [Gk. *karkin,* a crab, cancer]: carcinogen

cardio- [Gk. *kardia,* heart]: cardiac, myocardium, electrocardiogram

cat- [Gk. *kata,* down, downward]: catabolic

chloro- [Gk. *chloros,* green]: chlorophyll, chloroplast, chlorine

chromo- [Gk. *chroma,* color]: chromosome, chromatin

coelo, -coel [Gk. *koilos,* hollow, cavity]: coelom

com-, con-, col-, co- [L. *cum,* with, together]: coenzyme, covalent

cranio- [Gk. *kranios,* L. cranium, skull]: cranial, cranium

cuti- [L. *cutis,* skin]: cutaneous, cuticle

cyto-, cyte [Gk. *kytos,* vessel or container; now, "cell"]: cytoplasm, cytokinesis, erythrocyte, leukocyte

de- [L. *de-,* away, off, removal, separation]: deciduous, decomposer, dehydration

derm-, dermato- [Gk. *derma,* skin]: dermis, epidermis, ectoderm, endoderm, mesoderm

di- [Gk. *dis,* twice, two, double]: disaccharide, dioxide

dia- [Gk. through, passing through, thorough, thoroughly]: diabetes, dialysis, diaphragm

diplo- [Gk. *diploos,* two-fold]: diploid

eco- [Gk. *oikos,* house, home]: ecology, ecosystem, economy

ecto- [Gk. *ektos,* outside]: ectoderm

endo- [Gk. *endon,* within]: endoderm, endometrium

epi- [Gk. *epi,* on, upon, over]: epidermis, epididymis, epiglottis, epithelium

equi- [L. *aequus,* equal]: equilibrium

eu- [Gk. *eus,* good; eu, well, true]: eukaryote

ex, exo-, ec-, e- [Gk., L. out, out of, from, beyond]: emission, ejaculation, excretion, exergonic, exhale, exocytosis, exoskeleton

extra- [L. outside of, beyond]: extracellular, extraembryonic

-fer [L. *ferre,* to bear]: fertile, fertilization, conifer

gam-, gameto- [Gk. *gamos,* marriage; now usually in reference to gametes (sex cells)]: gamete

gastro- [Gk. *gaster,* stomach]: gastric, gastrin, gastrovascular cavity

gen- [Gk. *gen,* born, produced by; Gk. genos, race, kind; L. genus, generare, to beget]: polygenic genotype, geneology, glycogen, pyrogen, heterogenous

gluco-, glyco- [Gk. *glykys,* sweet; now pertaining to sugar]: glucose, glycogen, glycolysis, glycoprotein

hemo-, hemato-, -hemia, -emia [Gk. *haima,* blood]: hematology, hemoglobin, hemophilia

hepato- [Gk. *hepar, hepat-,* liver]: hepatitis, hepatic portal system

hetero- [Gk. *heteros,* other, different]: heterogeneous, heterozygote

histo- [Gk. *histos,* web of a loom, tissue; pertains to biological tissues]: histology, histamine, antihistamine

homo-, homeo- [Gk. *homos,* same; Gk. *homios,* similar]: homeostasis, homogeneous, homologous, homozygote

hydro- [Gk. *hydor,* water; pertains either to water or to hydrogen]: dehydration, carbohydrate